Ultrasonography of the Urinary Tract

THIRD EDITION

Ultrasonography of the Urinary Tract

THIRD EDITION

Edited by

Martin I. Resnick, M.D.

Lester Persky Professor and Chairman
Division of Urology
Case Western Reserve University
Cleveland, Ohio

Matthew D. Rifkin, M.D.

Professor of Radiology and Urology
Director, Division of Magnetic Resonance Imaging
Thomas Jefferson University, Hospital
Philadelphia, Pennsylvania

WILLIAMS & WILKINS
BALTIMORE · HONG KONG · LONDON · MUNICH
SAN FRANCISCO · SYDNEY · TOKYO

Editor: Laurel Craven
Associate Editor: Victoria M. Vaughn
Copy Editor: Thomas Lehr
Designer: JoAnne Janowiak
Illustration Planner: Ray Lowman
Production Coordinator: Barbara J. Felton

Williams & Wilkins
428 East Preston Street
Baltimore, Maryland 21202, USA

Accurate indications, adverse reactions, and dosage schedules for drugs are provided in this book, but it is possible that they may change. The reader is urged to review the package information data of the manufacturers of the medications mentioned.

Printed in the United States of America

First Edition, 1979
Second Edition, 1984

Library of Congress Cataloging-in-Publication Data

Ultrasonography of the urinary tract / edited by Martin I. Resnick,
Matthew D. Rifkin.—3rd ed.
p. cm.
Rev. ed. of: Ultrasound in urology / [edited by] Martin
I. Resnick, Roger C. Sanders. 2nd. © 1984.
Includes bibliographical references and index.
ISBN 0-683-07222-6
1. Genitourinary organs—Ultrasonic imaging. I. Resnick, Martin
I. II. Rifkin, Matthew D. III. Ultrasound in urology.
[DNLM: 1. Urinary Tract—ultrasonography. 2. Urologic Diseases—
diagnosis. WJ 141 U47]
RC874.U36 1991
616.6′07543—dc20
DNLM/DLC
for Library of Congress 91-10350
CIP

91 92 93 94 95
1 2 3 4 5 6 7 8 9 10

Vicki, Andy, and Jeff
—M.I.R.

Susan, Adam, and Jason
—M.D.R.

Preface

Ultrasonography of the Urinary Tract is the third edition of a monograph previously published as *Ultrasound in Urology*. As in previous editions the editors have called upon both radiological and urological experts to present an up-to-date, comprehensive text detailing the clinical applications of ultrasound as it relates to imaging of the genitourinary system. The collaboration of a urologist and a radiologist has been ideal for allowing the presentation of material that emphasizes the proper use of this imaging technique for providing the most information about a specific clinical problem.

The use of ultrasound imaging in urological practices is increasing, and it has become more readily available. Over the past 4 to 5 years there have been significant technological changes that have resulted in improved imaging providing greater detail and clinical application. Real-time ultrasonography has become the standard and has greatly enhanced the diagnostic ability of ultrasonography in the assessment of disorders of the genitourinary system. In addition, there has been continued development of biopsy techniques and percutaneous procedures that can be performed most successfully under ultrasound guidance. New applications continue to arise, and we expect further improvements in the future. This has been particularly true in prostatic ultrasonography, which has undergone significant changes in a very short period of time.

The contributing authors of all chapters are recognized experts in their area. All have attempted to present the most modern and up-to-date information while emphasizing new developments and procedures that will be available in the future.

We wish to express our deep appreciation to the contributing authors who have greatly facilitated the development of this monograph. We would also like to thank our secretaries, Barbara Goldberg, JoAnn Gardner, and Suze Stewart, who assisted in correspondence and final manuscript preparation. Finally we would like to thank John N. Gardner and Vicki Vaughn of Williams & Wilkins for their encouragement and continued cooperation.

Martin I. Resnick, M.D.
Matthew D. Rifkin, M.D.

Contributors

Robert E. Bechtold, M.D.
Department of Radiology
The Bowman Gray School of Medicine
Wake Forest University
Winston-Salem, North Carolina

Donald R. Bodner
Assistant Professor of Urology
Case Western Reserve University
Cleveland, Ohio

Patrick J. Bryan, M.D.
Department of Radiology
University Hospital of Cleveland
Cleveland, Ohio

Peter N. Burns, Ph.D.
Associate Professor of Radiology
Director, Ultrasound Physics
Thomas Jefferson University Hospital
Philadelphia, Pennsylvania

Steven M. Cohen, M.D.
Assistant Professor of Radiology
Thomas Jefferson University Hospital
Philadelphia, Pennsylvania

Jerome J. Cunningham, M.D.
Professor of Radiology
Ohio State University Medical Center
Columbus, Ohio

Joseph R. Drago, M.D.
Department of Surgery
Ohio State University Hospitals
Columbus, Ohio

Gerald W. Friedland, M.D.
Professor of Radiology
Stanford University
Chief, Radiology Service
Palo Alto Veterans Administration Medical Center
Palo Alto, California

Hedvig Hricak, M.D.
Department of Urology and Radiology
University of California School of Medicine
San Francisco, California

R. Brooke Jeffrey Jr., M.D.
Department of Radiology
San Francisco General Hospital
San Francisco, California

Tom F. Lue, M.D.
Departments of Urology and Radiology
University of California School of Medicine
San Francisco, California

Laurence Needleman, M.D.
Department of Radiology
Division of Ultrasound
Thomas Jefferson University Hospital
Philadelphia, Pennsylvania

Ellen M. O'Mara, D.O.
Department of Radiology
Ephrata Community Hospital
Ephrata, Pennsylvania

Inder Perkash, M.D.
Division of Urology
Palo Alto Veterans Administration Medical Center
Palo Alto, California

Bhaskara K. Rao, M.D.
Department of Radiology and Radiological Sciences
Vanderbilt University School of Medicine
Nashville, Tennessee

Martin I. Resnick, M.D.
Lester Persky Professor and Chairman
Division of Urology
Case Western Reserve University
Cleveland, Ohio

Matthew D. Rifkin, M.D.
Professor of Radiology and Urology
Director, Division of Magnetic Resonance Imaging
Thomas Jefferson University Hospital
Philadelphia, Pennsylvania

Carson D. Schneck, M.D., Ph.D.
Professor of Anatomy and Diagnostic Imaging
Temple University School of Medicine
Philadelphia, Pennsylvania

Thomas E. Sumner, M.D.
Professor of Radiology and Pediatrics
The Bowman Gray School of Medicine
Wake Forest University
Winston-Salem, North Carolina

Nat E. Watson, M.D.
Department of Radiology
The Bowman Gray School of Medicine
Wake Forest University
Winston-Salem, North Carolina

Neil T. Wolfman, M.D.
Department of Radiology
The Bowman Gray School of Medicine
Wake Forest University
Winston-Salem, North Carolina

Hsu-Chong Yeh, M.D.
Professor of Radiology
Mount Sinai School of Medicine of City University of New York
New York, New York

Color Plates

PLATE 1

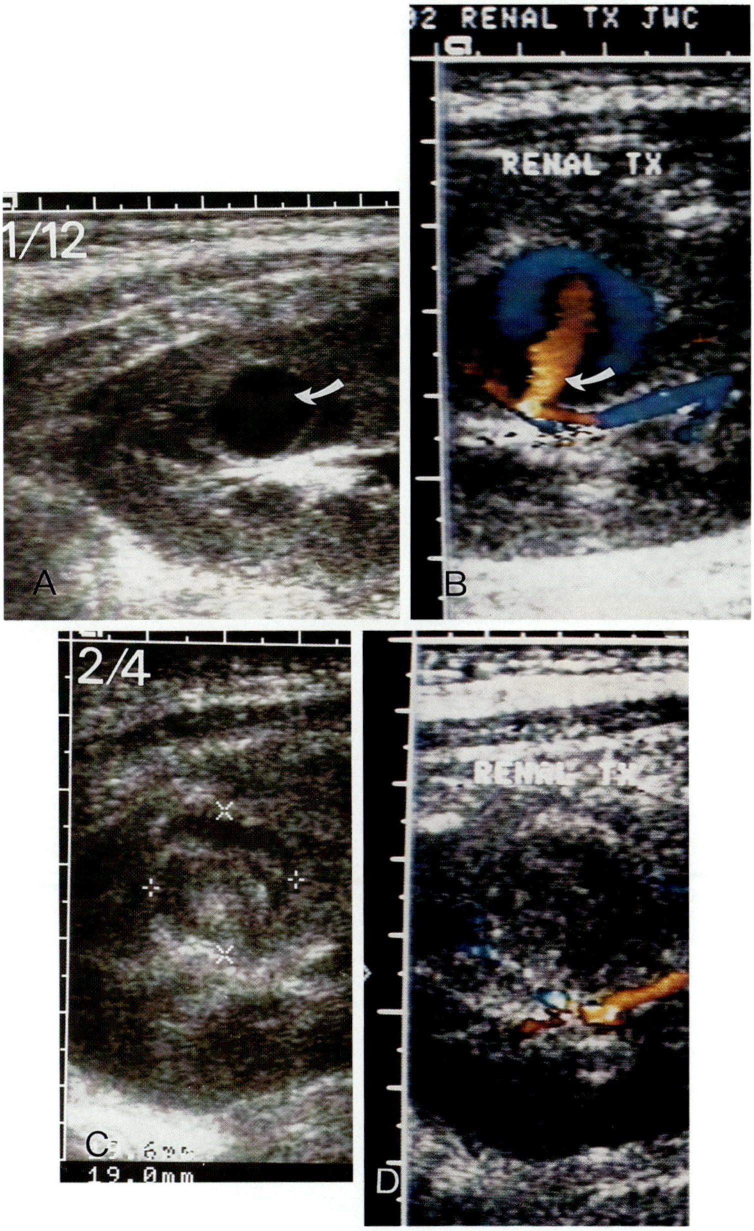

Figure 7.7.

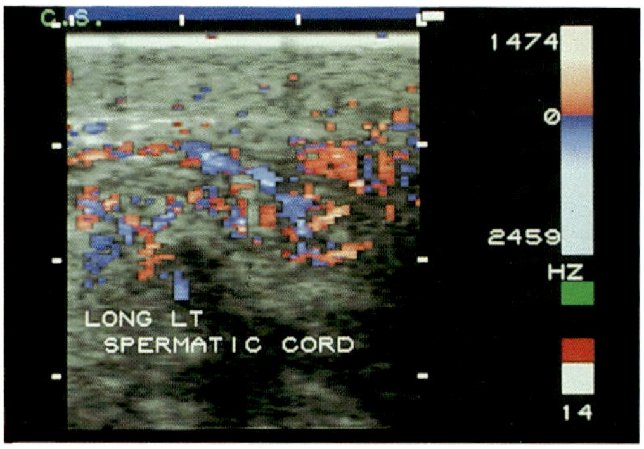

Figure 13.12.

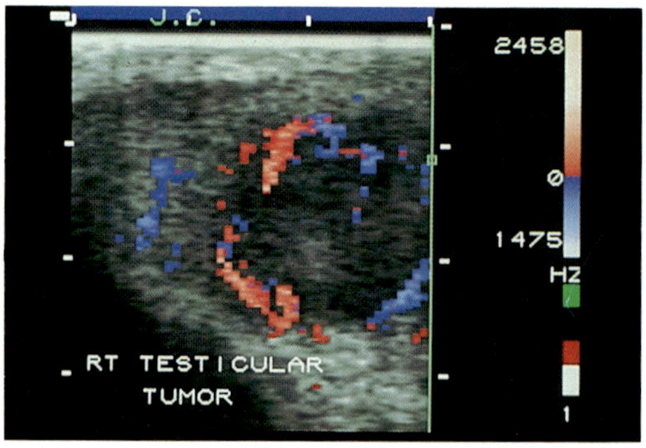

Figure 13.17F.

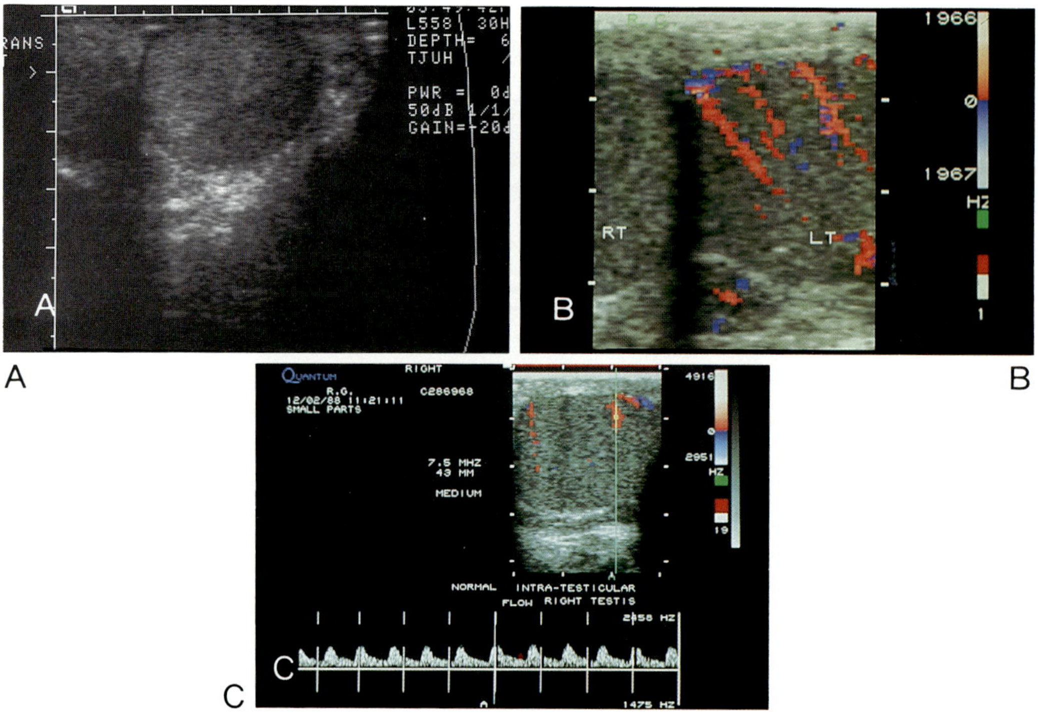

Figure 13.40, A–C.

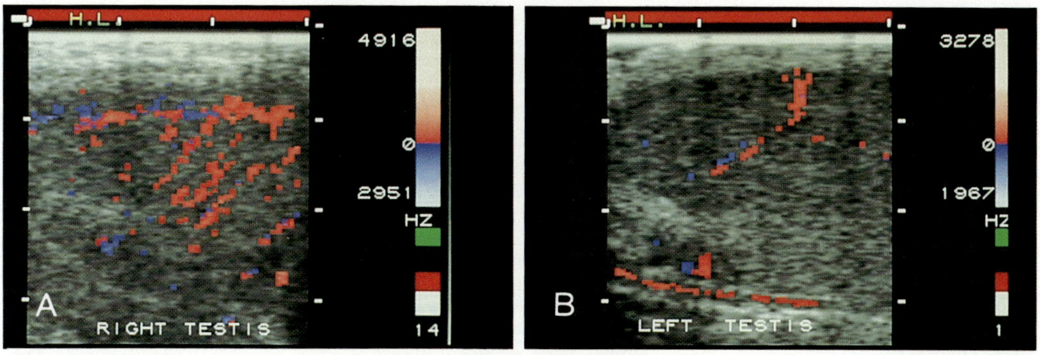

A B

Figure 13.41, A and B.

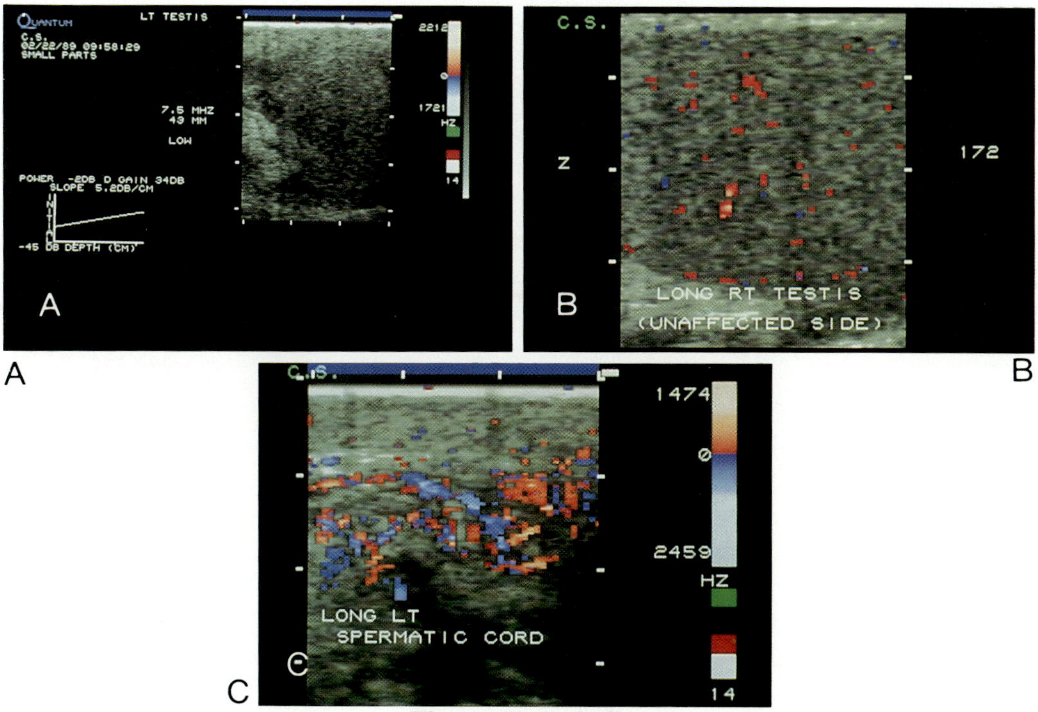

A B C

Figure 13.43, A–C.

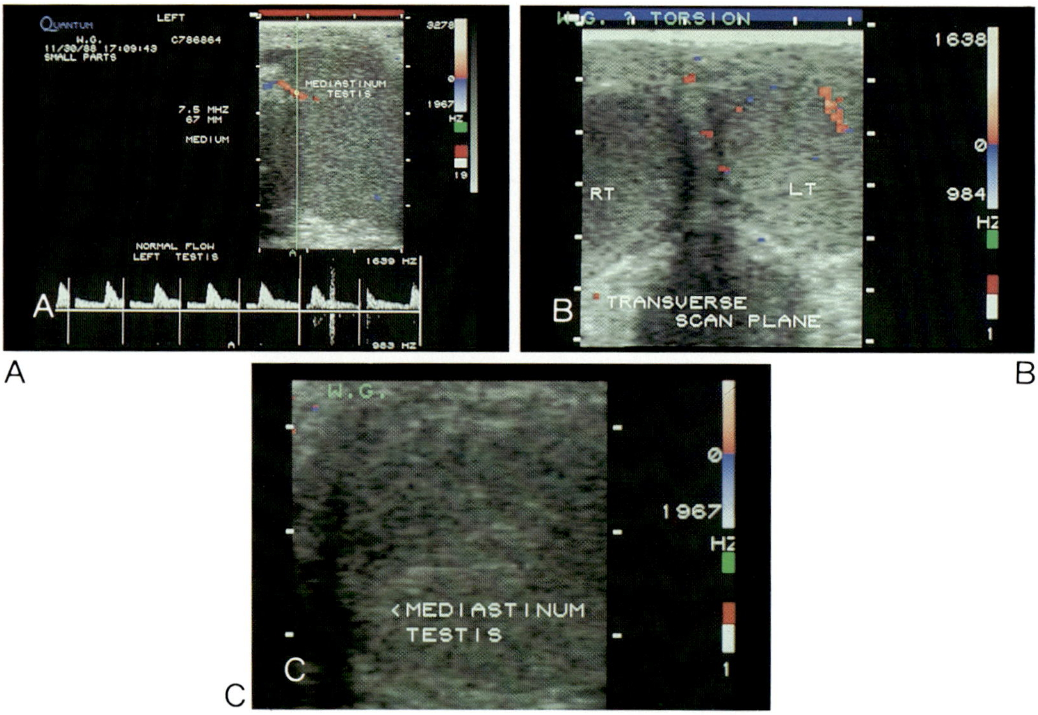

Figure 13.52, A–C.

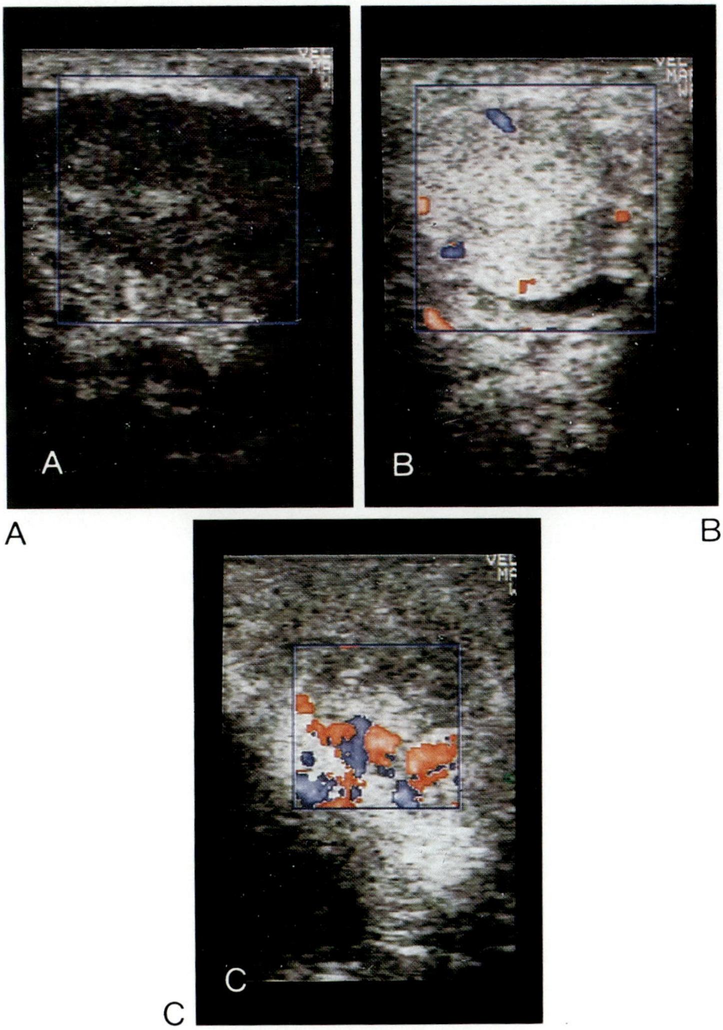

Figure 13.53, A–C.

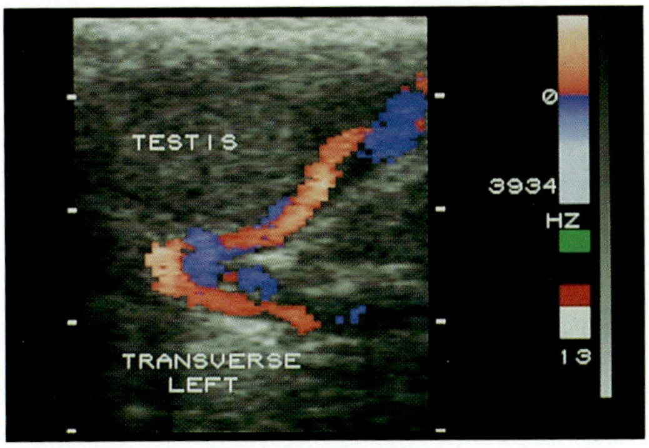

Figure 13.57.

Contents

CHAPTER 1

Ultrasound Imaging and Doppler: Principles and Instrumentation

PETER N. BURNS, Ph.D.

The rapid expansion of the use of ultrasound in genitourinary diagnosis reflects the enormous potential that noninvasive imaging and examination of blood flow offers in this area. Instruments in use range from the old static B-scanners to the most recent endo-(trans)rectal real-time imaging instruments, some with pulsed Doppler or color Doppler imaging. Although many of these technical developments have been marked by exciting new applications for the ultrasound diagnostician, they have also resulted in a rather bewildering array of new instruments, some employing techniques, such as duplex Doppler, that are still unfamiliar to many. The purpose of this chapter is to describe the common basis for all ultrasound imaging and Doppler instrumentation, thus attempting to lay a foundation for the rational interpretation of the diagnostic information it provides.

IMAGING

Ultrasound imaging is based on the "pulse-echo" principle, in which a short burst of ultrasound is emitted from a transducer and directed into tissue. Echoes are produced as a result of the interaction of sound with tissue, and some of these travel back to the transducer. By timing the period between the emission of the pulse and the reception of the echo, the distance between the transducer and the echo-producing structure can be calculated and an image formed (Fig. 1.1). In diagnostic imaging of the genitourinary system, frequencies of about 1 to 10 MHz are used, except for superficial structures such as the scrotum and penis. At these frequencies, ultrasound has a wavelength between 1.5 and 0.15 mm, a dimension that sets a fundamental limit on the potential spatial resolution of resulting image. Better resolution is associated with a higher ultrasound frequency, but attenuation of ultrasound in tissue also increases with frequency. Optimum imaging is thus obtained by choosing the highest frequency transducer that will permit adequate acoustic penetration to identify the region of interest. To this end considerable effort has been expended to develop technologies that will allow the transducer to be positioned nearer to the structure of interest and hence achieve higher resolution.

Sound consists of longitudinal vibrations that propagate through a medium such as water or soft tissue in much the same way as a compression can be seen to travel along the length of a spring. Sound consists of the repetitive (or *periodic*) production of such compressions that travel in regular succession. The number of compressions produced each second is known as the *frequency* (measured in hertz [Hz] with 1 MHz = 1,000,000 Hz), and the distance between successive compressions (which depends on the speed at which the sound travels in the medium) is known as the *wavelength.*

Ultrasound for use in diagnostic imaging instruments is generated using some form of acousto-electric transducer. Piezoelectric crystals exhibit the extraordinary physical property that, when an electrical voltage is applied across two faces, a mechanical deformation takes place. The effect is rather small, but if the voltage is reversed in polarity (that is, the positive and negative wires are transposed), the material deforms in the opposite direction. Thus, by applying an alternating voltage of the appropriate frequency (say 3 MHz), corresponding mechanical oscillations and hence ultrasound waves (in this case consisting of 3 million compressions/sec) are produced. From the point

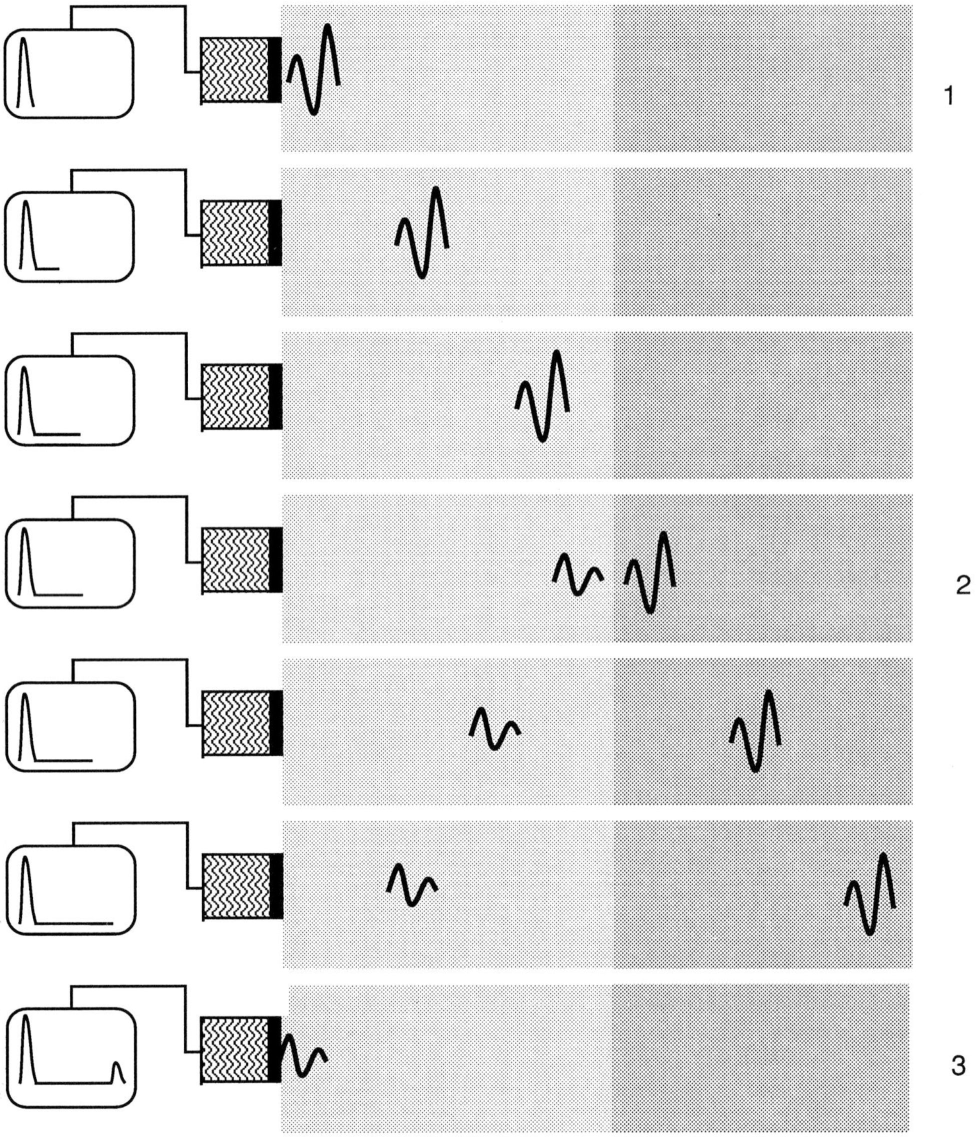

Figure 1.1. The pulse-echo principle is used to produce an ultrasound A-scan. A pulse is emitted from the transducer at the same time as a dot is set in motion from left to right on the A-scan screen. When an echo reaches the transducer, the received signal causes a vertical deflection of the trace. The distance between deflections on the A-scan corresponds to the depth of the interface from the transducer.

of view of ultrasound imaging instrumentation, it is equally significant that the piezoelectric effect works in the opposite sense, that is, varying mechanical pressure on the face of the transducer is converted into a corresponding variation in electrical potential across two faces. It is this voltage that results when the reflected portion of a pulse of ultrasound finds its way back to the transducer, and is referred to as the *echo* signal.

Echoes arise when a burst of ultrasound (which travels through tissue at about 1500 m/sec or 3500 mph) encounters an interface between structures of differing *acoustic impedance*. Acoustic impedance is a mechanical property that for bulk tissue is defined as the product of its density and the speed at which sound propagates through it. The speed of sound is itself influenced by, among other factors, the stiffness of tissue. Thus ultrasound imaging is fundamentally a modality that maps the changes in a mechanical (rather than nuclear or atomic) property of tissue. As the scale over which these mechanical properties affect ultrasound are comparable to or greater than the wavelength of sound used, it turns out that modifications to the structure of tissue at the cellular level tend to result in changes in its acoustic properties, including acoustic impedance. Thus ultrasound is an excellent method for the imaging of soft tissue structures.

Ultrasound Instrumentation

If the difference in acoustic impedance between two structures is small (as it is in most soft tissue interfaces), only a tiny proportion of the ultrasound pulse will be reflected back toward the transducer; most of it will be transmitted and continue on to the next interface. Echoes arrive back at the transducer separated in time by a period proportional to the distance between interfaces. The simplest (and in fact the most accurate) way to measure this time is by displaying the echoes as deflections on a cathode ray tube. A spot is made to traverse the screen of the cathode ray tube rapidly from left to right and the electrical signal from the transducer is arranged to cause a vertical deflection. Thus in Figure 1.1, the first deflection occurs as the electrical pulse is applied to the transducer. The acoustic pulse that results from this travels into tissue until it encounters an interface at which the acoustic impedance changes from where the reflection gives rise to an echo, which travels back to the transducer. When the echo reaches the transducer an electrical signal is produced that causes a second deflection of the spot on the cathode ray tube screen. If we assume sound to have traveled at a steady speed in the tissue, the distance between the transducer and the interface can be measured from the distance between the two deflections on the screen. A one-dimensional trace such as this with echo amplitude on the vertical axis and depth on the horizontal axis is known as an *A-mode scan* (Fig. 1.1).

The echoes can also be displayed as dots in a straight line, with brightness proportional to echo amplitude (Fig. 1.2**C**). If the transducer is then mounted on a position sensing arm, the line of view of the acoustic beam can be made to correspond to the orientation of the brightness-modulated A-scan line on the display screen. Moving the arm across the skin's surface will then produce a series of dots corresponding to the cross-section of the interface within tissue (Fig. 1.2**E**). Thus, an image of this interface is formed, known as a *B-mode* image. This cross-sectional image forms the basis for almost all those of modern ultrasound instruments. Figure 1.3 shows the major components of an ultrasound imaging system. The clock initiates the sequence that results in a single image being constructed on the screen: A pulse is created by the pulse generator and emitted by the transducer. The direction in which the transducer is oriented is registered by the coordinate computer, which feeds this information to the scan converter. As the echoes are received, they are amplified and demodulated to determine their strength. The stream of echoes is then presented to the scan converter, which is a memory capable of storing the echoes along with their time of arrival and direction. These data are then read from the memory in a television raster format and fed as a video signal to the imaging monitor. As soon as all the echoes are received, the clock initiates another, identical sequence. As the transducer is scanned over the patient, an image is formed. If the scanning process is automated at a sufficiently rapid rate, enough images can be produced every second for the motion of tissue structures to be followed in "real time."

Variations in acoustic impedance may take the form of a smooth surface (such as the bladder wall), in which case the reflection of ultrasound will be *specular* (Fig. 1.4**A**) in analogy with light striking a glass interface. Echoes will only be seen if the beam is nearly perpendicular to the surface (Fig. 1.4**B**). Older "bistable" ultrasound equipment was able to demonstrate only these strong, specular echoes. They are seen at interfaces of organs as well as from brightly reflecting smooth areas such as the walls of major vessels. Other interfaces may be irregular, in which case reflection will take place over many angles within the ultrasound beam (which is on the order of millimeters in width) and echoes are produced in many directions. Such *scattering* gives rise to echoes, some of which travel back to the transducer if the angle of incidence is one of a range of values (Fig. 1.5**A**). Because the geometry of the imaging process allows only relatively few structures to give rise to specular reflections that are

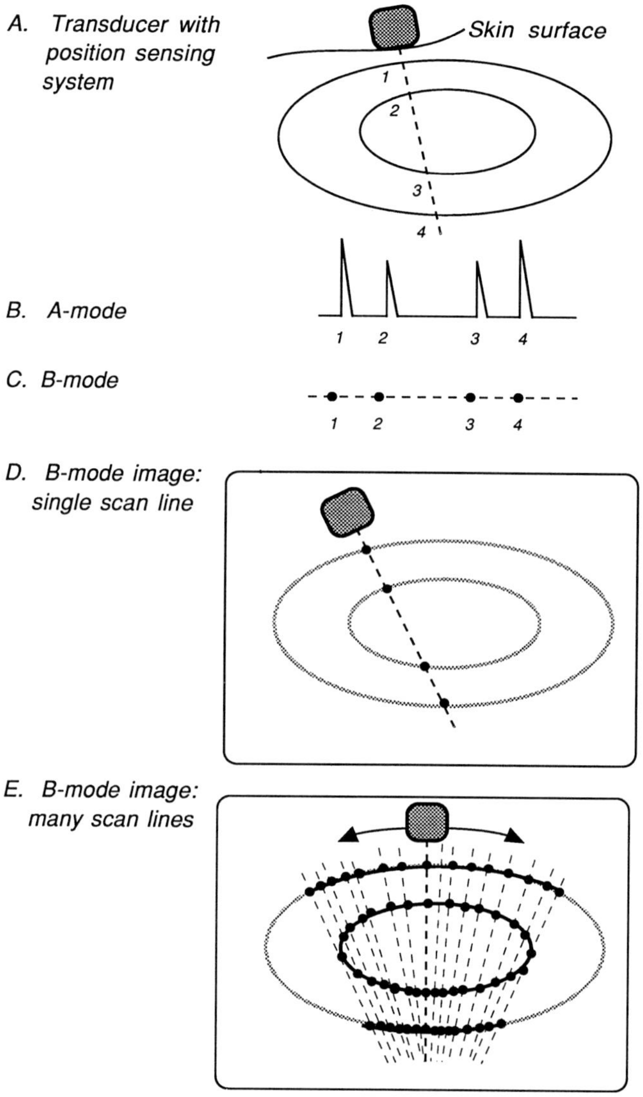

Figure 1.2. The ultrasound B-mode scanner. **A,** A transducer connected to a position sensing system is moved over the skin surface. **B,** An A-mode display is created of the four tissue interfaces lying within the beam. **C,** The echoes displayed by the A-scan line are encoded as brightness-modulated dots. **D,** The line is displayed on the image screen with the same orientation on the screen as the beam takes in the patient. **E,** The transducer is scanned across the skin surface, resulting in a series of echoes being written on the screen, thus forming a tomographic image of the tissue interfaces.

directed toward the transducer, scattering from uneven interfaces is the principal mechanism for the visualization of tissue margins using ultrasound. The diaphragm is an example of such a structure in the body. Finally, small variations in acoustic impedance are present within the tissue parenchyma itself, and these give rise to low-level isotropic scattering (Fig. 1.5**B**). The small proportion of this echo that is *backscattered* is received by the transducer. If these weak echoes are displayed by the gray scale of the ultrasound imaging system, the parenchyma of an organ is characterized by a distinct shade of gray. The structure and intensity of backscattered parenchymal echoes form the basis of gray-scale ultrasonography. In fact, such backscattered echoes are coherent in phase and interfere with each other in just the

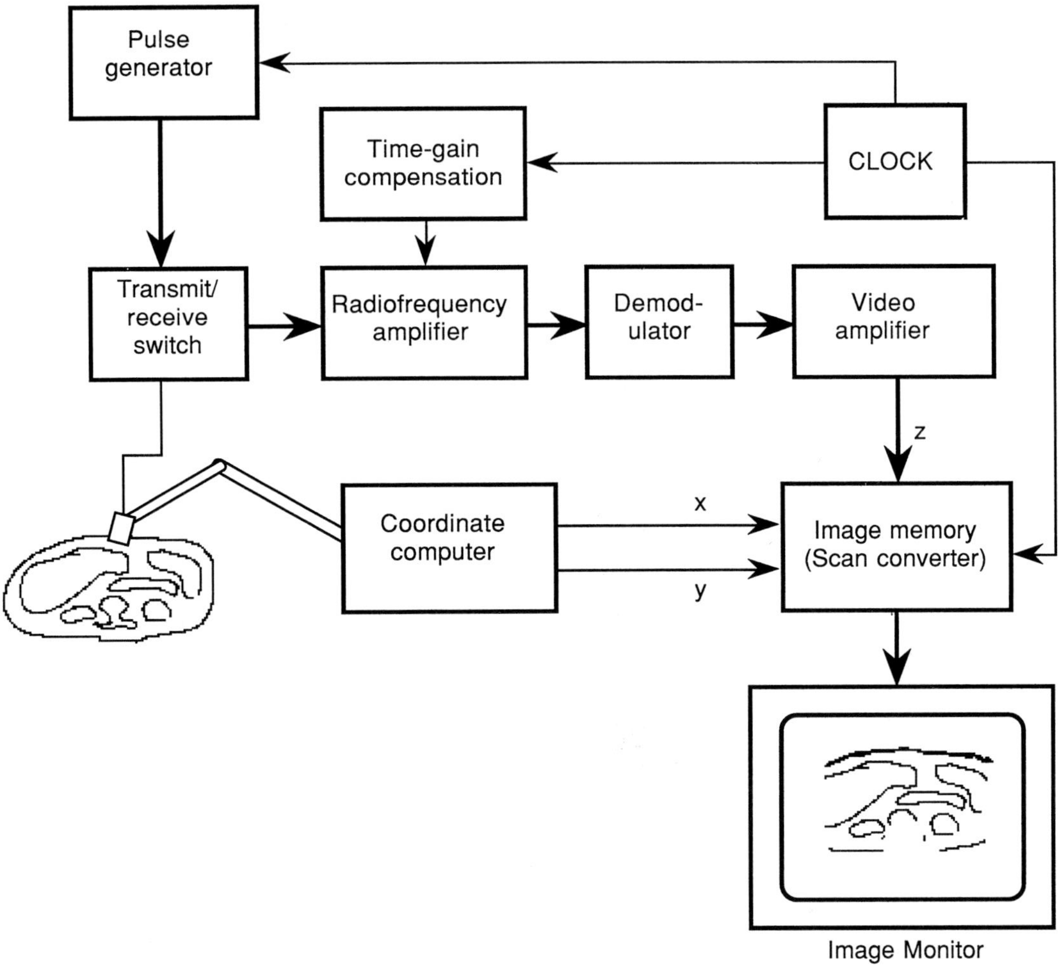

Figure 1.3. The major components of an ultrasound imaging system. A pulse is issued by the pulse generator and emitted by the transducer. The direction of orientation of the transducer is registered by the coordinate computer and fed to the scan converter. As the echoes are received from tissue, they are amplified and demodulated to determine their strength. Individual streams of echoes are then represented as lines in the appropriate direction, brightness modulated on the image monitor. As the transducer is moved, an image is produced on the monitor.

same way as ripples on water caused by many small disturbances will combine to form a pattern of crests and troughs. In ultrasound this stationary interference pattern gives rise to the speckle of a gray-scale image, a factor that determines the apparent texture of an organ imaged with ultrasound. Different organs have characteristic textures. Although the absolute intensity (or *echogenicity*) and texture from a given region cannot be used to obtain tissue-characterizing information since texture is determined primarily by a combination of the acoustic characteristics of the ultrasound beam and the mechanical structure of tissue, the relative appearance of different organs will be constant, thus allowing the diagnosis of abnormality. The normal cortex of the kidney, for example, is characterized by less intense parenchymal echoes than those of the contiguous liver, spleen, and pancreas. The parenchymal texture of these organs is also different. In addition, specular echoes from the renal sinus in the adult are more intense than those from within the cortex.

Attenuation of the ultrasound beam in normal tissue is primarily a result of the absorption of the acoustic wave motion by tissue, converting its energy to what is generally an

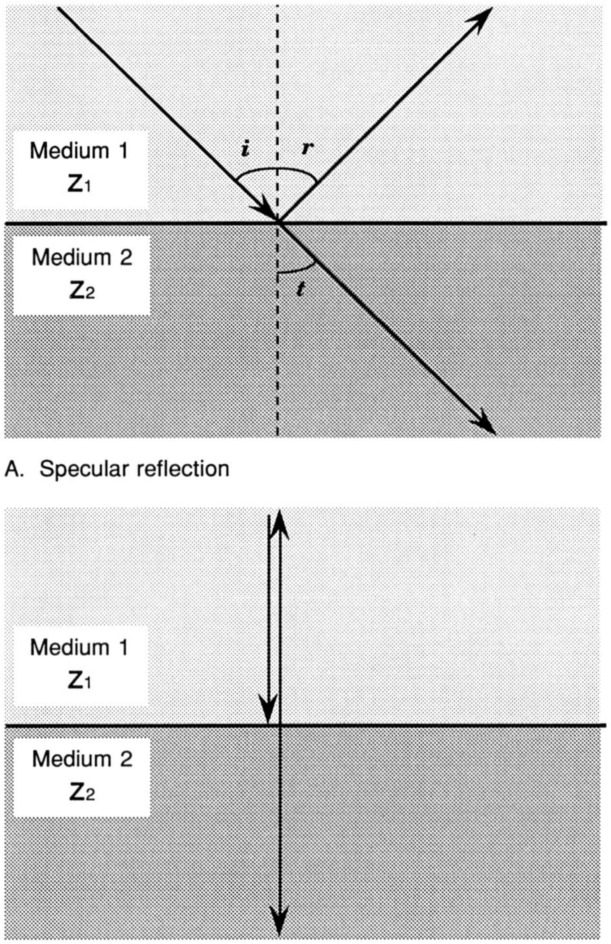

Figure 1.4. An ultrasound pulse encounters an interface between soft tissues of differing acoustic impedance. **A,** Specular reflection. A small portion of the ultrasound beam is reflected but most passes across the interface undeviated. The angle of incidence (i), the angle of reflection (r), and the angle of transmission (t) are all equal. **B,** Normal incidence. In this special case of specular reflection the angle of incidence is zero and the echo is received by the transmitting transducer.

immeasurably small quantity of heat. In practice, scattering is thought to contribute a negligible amount of attenuation. Attenuation is strongly dependent on frequency and reduces the intensity of the beam logarithmically as it travels through tissue. For example, the intensity of a 5-MHz beam is reduced to half its initial value by 6 mm of liver, 2 mm of muscle, or 0.3 mm of bone. Gas and bone attenuate ultrasound rapidly; in addition, their acoustic impedance results in almost total reflection from interfaces with soft tissue. The effect of attenuation on returning echoes is seen as a dramatic reduction in the intensity of echoes from deeper structures. To compensate for this, the gain of the receiver is increased logarithmically as echoes arrive from progressively deeper structures. When the last echo has arrived the next pulse of ultrasound is emitted from the transducer and the gain is reset to its lowest level for reception of the first echo. The gain is automatically increased throughout the subsequent period in which echoes from deeper structures arrive. In this way, echoes of equal strength from different depths are displayed with the same intensity on the screen. The control of this time gain compensation (TGC) is at the operator's disposal and must be set properly

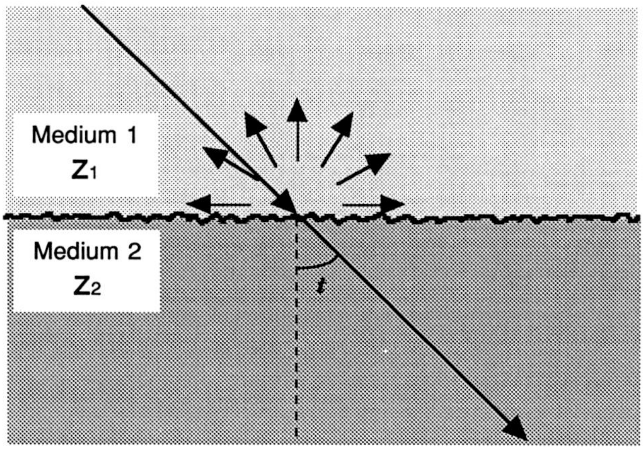

A. Rough interface

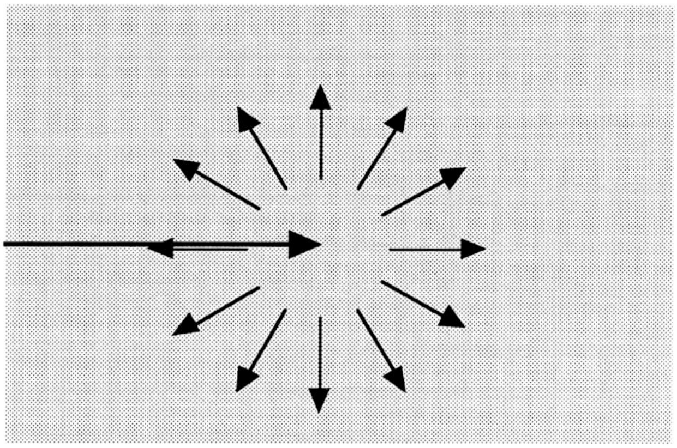

B. Inhomogeneous medium

Figure 1.5. Scattering of ultrasound. **A,** Specular reflections from a multiplicity of irregularly oriented interfaces gives rise to echoes over a range of angles. **B,** As sound propagates through the parenchyma of an organ that contains microscopic fluctuations in acoustic impedance, small quantities of ultrasound are scattered in all directions, including back toward the transducer. This is responsible for the gray-scale appearance of the organ.

if the relative echogenicity of organs at differing depths is to be assessed. Inappropriate setting of the TGC curves can lead to the appearance of artifactual lesions; conversely, real lesions may be obscured by incorrect TGC settings in the area of the abnormality.

Since the difference in echo intensity between the bright specular reflector and the weakest parenchymal scatter might be as much as 60 dB and a television screen is capable of displaying no more than about 30 dB, some compression of the range of echo amplitudes is necessary. This is achieved by amplifying the low-level echoes linearly but the high-level echoes in a manner that compresses them into a narrow dynamic range (Fig. 1.6). This characteristic (known as the display compression or post-processing curve) may be adjusted to enhance the contrast between a lesion and surrounding tissue of almost similar echo intensity. Thus, in Figure 1.6, the intensity ratios between echoes *A* and *B* and between echoes *C* and *D* are similar, but on the display the contrast between echoes *A* and *B* is greater than that between echoes *C* and *D*. Employing a different post-processing characteristic, such as that of curve *1* in Figure 1.6, will cause the display contrast to vary. In many instruments, post-processing characteristics may be adjusted after the image has been acquired and held in the scan converter. Additional enhancement of edges may be provided by electronic

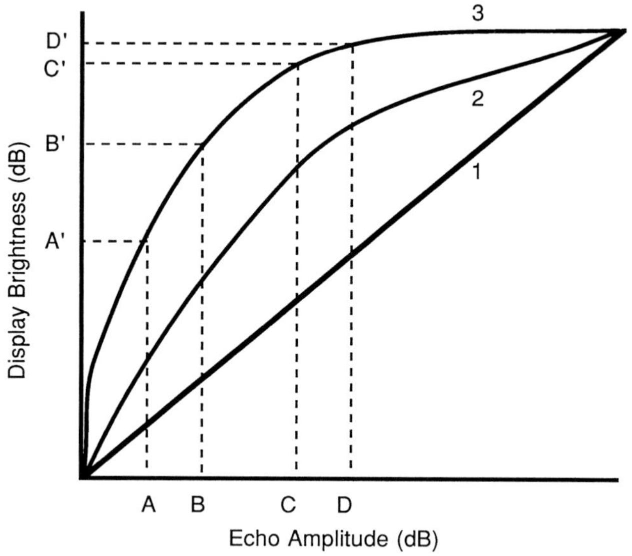

Figure 1.6. The compression amplification (or *post-processing*) curve demonstrates the relationship between the echo amplitude returning to the transducer and the display brightness. Note that there is a constant difference in echo amplitude between echoes *A* and *B* and echoes *C* and *D*. With post-processing curve *1* these would result in an equal difference between the display brightness of these two sets of echoes. With post-processing curve *3*, however, the contrast between echoes *A* and *B* is greater than the contrast between echoes *C* and *D*.

differentiation of the demodulated signal, a processing facility built into many modern abdominal scanners. In selecting post-processing characteristics, one should attempt to optimize the contrast between structures of interest without sacrificing the dynamic range (that is, the range of gray shades) in the display.

Real-Time Ultrasound Imaging

The process of moving a transducer attached to an arm has been largely replaced in modern *real-time* scanners by the movement of a transducer using a mechanical rotator or translator, driven under servo control so that the display of the scan line is moved in exact correspondence with the position of the beam (Fig. 1.7). The beam is swept with sufficient speed that an entire image can be produced in a fraction of a second, so that independent images may be acquired at a rapid rate. The display of these images in quick succession and the elimination of flicker by switching between image memories creates a device capable of visualizing structures that are moving in real time. The assessment of the movement of tissue in the abdomen yields additional diagnostic information unique to ultrasound imaging. Movement of a lesion during respiration can identify it as arising from the peritoneal or retroperitoneal space. For example, fluid-filled structures that pulsate may be identified as arteries, and ureteric jets may be visualized directly with real-time ultrasound as they empty into the bladder. Dynamic information may be recorded on videotape or "frozen" by an operator control and stored in an image memory. Review of a real-time ultrasound examination of the abdomen can, however, be difficult because the hand-eye coordination of the scanning process is impossible to record, and an appreciation of the precise plane of visualization is often difficult to gather in retrospect. Multiple views in standard planes, although lending predictability to the images produced, result in the sacrifice of many of the qualities unique to real-time ultrasound imaging.

A variety of techniques may be used to move the ultrasound beam in a real-time scanner. In the *mechanical sector* scanner (Fig. 1.7**A**), the beam from a single transducer is moved by the rotation of the ceramic element itself or of acoustic mirrors within the beam. In the *linear array* a large number of small, discrete transducer elements are arranged in a line (Fig. 1.7 **C**) and a small number are excited together to form a beam. When all the echoes have been

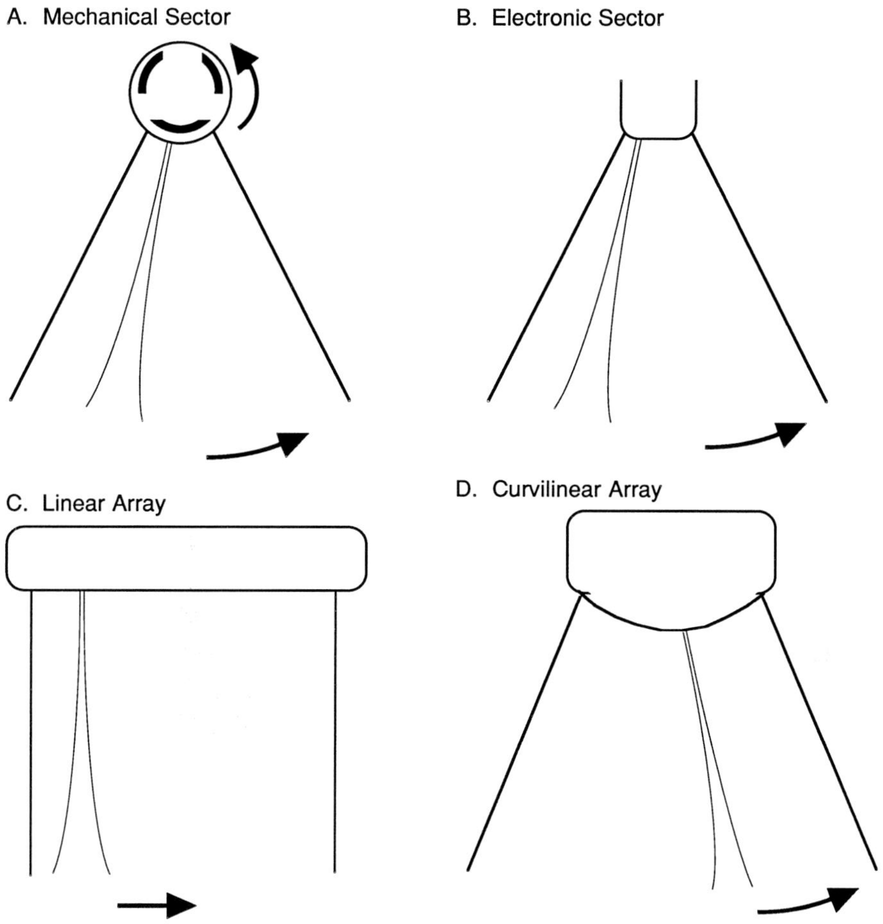

Figure 1.7. Real-time scanners. Four configurations of ultrasound transducer assemblies that permit the echoes to be collected at a sufficient speed to produce real-time images.

received along the resulting line of sight, the next pulse is issued from the adjacent series of elements, and so on. The beam is swept rapidly from one end of the transducer array to the other, forming an image. The frame rate of such an image is determined by a combination of the number of lines within the field of view (this is related to the image resolution), and the time taken for the last echo to return to the transducer once the pulse has been transmitted (this is related to the maximum depth of the field of view). Thus, the size of the field of view, the frame-rate, and the resolution of the image are all related in a real-time scanner. The optimum choice of these parameters is inevitably a matter of compromise. Electronic switching precludes the need for moving parts in the linear array scanner. One of the limitations of this configuration is that it requires a relatively large transducer and therefore cannot be applied to intercostal scanning or scanning through other small acoustic windows (a window refers to a superficial area through which deeper structures can be visualized and which is not composed of structures such as gas or bone that attenuate the ultrasound beam). On the other hand, the linear array has proved to be ideal for scanning areas with large windows and a smooth abdominal surface such as the pregnant uterus. The curvilinear array (Fig. 1.7**D**) creates a trapezoidal field of view with a somewhat smaller acoustic footprint than the linear array, but shares many of its advantages.

Finally, in the electronically steered or *phased* array scanner (Fig. 1.7**B**) the sector format is produced by precise control of the instant at which each element in a small rectangular array of transducers is excited. Here all the elements (typically there may be 48, 64, 96, or 128) are excited together but with a small, progressive time (or *phase*) difference from one side to the other. The size and direction of this difference determines the direction in which the main lobe of the ultrasound beam will emerge. By controlling this phase between successive bursts, the beam may be "steered" electronically (Fig. 1.8). Control is achieved by the implementation of small, independent electronic delay circuits in the path of each transducer element, which are controlled by common high-speed computer logic. Applying delays to the signal received by each element in the array also enables the beam to be manipulated so as to receive in the same direction as it transmits. The advantages of the electronically steered arrays are their lack of moving parts, the relatively small size of the transducer footprint (perhaps 2 cm square), and their particular ability to produce beams whose focus may be controlled electronically. Figure 1.9 illustrates the method used to achieve this. As will be seen presently, the lateral resolution of an ultrasound image depends mainly on the width of the ultrasound beam. Although it is easy to focus the ultrasound beam so that it is narrow at a particular depth (for example, by the use of an acoustic lens attached to the surface of the probe), the resulting improvement in resolution at the focal depth is at the expense of image quality of shallower and deeper structures. *Swept focusing* exploits the ability of a phased array to emulate a lens. A lens focuses a beam simply by delaying the passage of sound at its center relative to that at its edge. The delays used to steer the beam can also impose programmed delays that specify a focal distance for the beam. This creates a desired focal depth for the transmitted pulse (Fig. 1.9). However, the main benefit from swept focusing is during reception. Because echoes from each depth arrive at a different time, the period elapsed after the transmission of the pulse can be used to determine the depth from which the received echoes are originating at any one time. The array may then be instructed to focus at that depth. A moment later, the array will be focused at a slightly greater depth, and so on (Fig. 1.10). Control (at quite high speed) of elements in either a linear or phased array when receiv-

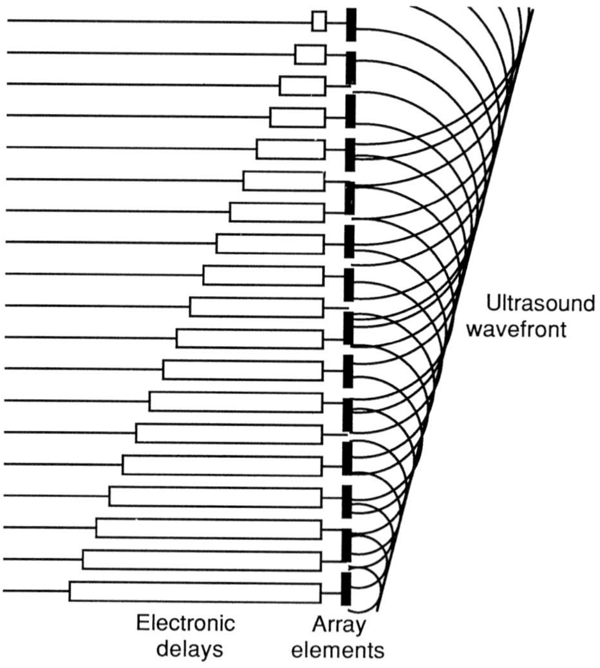

Figure 1.8. The principle of the phased array. A similar transmit pulse is fed to each of the array elements but after a delay that increases progressively from one end of the array to the other. The result is an ultrasound wavefront whose direction of motion is at an angle to the axis of the probe. Such "steering" of the ultrasound beam can be achieved very rapidly by the phased array system.

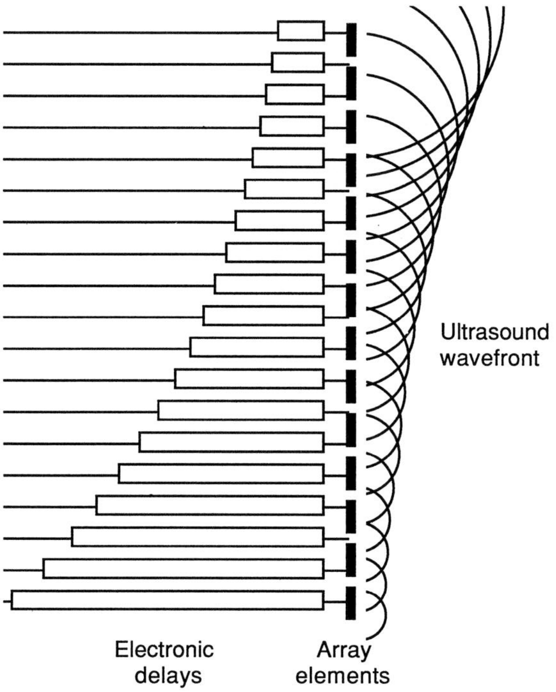

Figure 1.9. The electronically focused "steering" phased array. Precise control of the individual delays of the transmitted pulse applied to each of the array elements results in a wavefront that is oriented in the desired direction and that also has a radius of curvature creating a focus at the desired axial distance from the array phase. The array may be thought of as having synthesized the effect of a single curved-disk transducer oriented in the desired direction.

ing allows an electronic focus to be formed whose position sweeps downward as echoes arrive from progressively deeper structures. Use of electronically focused beams improves the uniformity of image quality at different depths, especially enhancing visualization of structures near the transducer face.

A hybrid of the mechanical sector scanner and the phased array, the annular array system, allows the electronic focusing of mechanically manipulated transducer elements. Here the ultrasound beam is moved mechanically, but the focal depth is determined by electronic delays (Fig. 1.11). An annular array might typically be composed of five rings. Note that the effect of this configuration is to control the focus in two dimensions (that defined by the image plane and that of the scan thickness) compared to the phased array, which controls the focus in the image plane only.

Annular arrays may be used at higher ultrasound frequencies, for which it might be difficult to create multiple small-element, phased array systems that perform as well. High frequencies are usually chosen when high-resolution imaging of superficial structures is required, such as in the testes, and here the annular array mechanical sector scanner or the high-frequency, swept focus, linear array scanner may be particularly advantageous.

Imaging Transducers

Ultrasound transducers based on the mechanical sector, the phased sector, and the linear and curvilinear array have been produced in a wide variety of sizes and shapes. Transducers designed for transrectal scanning have been built using linear array or rotating mechanical sector designs. These are used routinely for prostate and bladder imaging. Transurethral transducers are available for the examination of, for example, the walls of the bladder. Finally, small electronically steered sector scanners and high-frequency linear array systems have been designed for intraoperative use. Transducers of all types are also available with attachments to guide a biopsy needle under ultrasound imaging control.

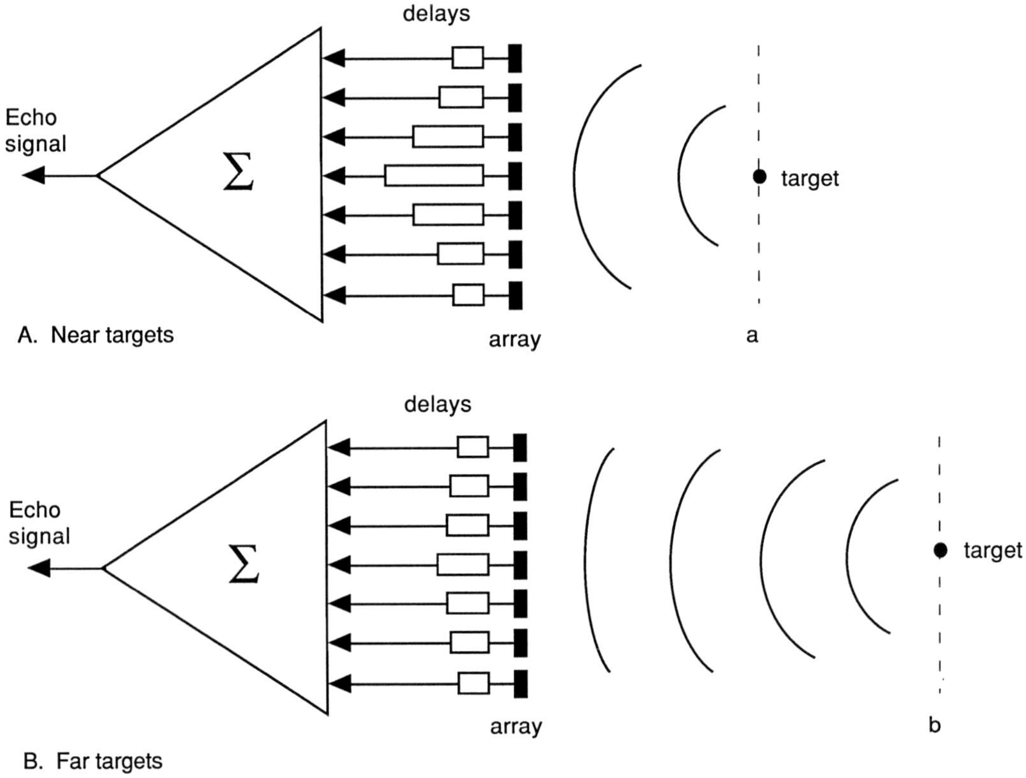

Figure 1.10. The principle of the swept focus array. The echo received by each of the array elements is delayed so as to emulate the time of arrival of the echo at different points on a curved surface. The delayed received signals are then summed together and fed to the ultrasound receiver. **A,** When echoes are being received from a distance *a* from the array phase, large delays are imposed that emulate a single transducer focused at the axial distance *a*. **B,** A short time later, echoes are being received from the greater distance *b* within tissue. Delays are imposed on the array elements that create a focus at the farther distance.

Figure 1.12 shows a sample of intracavity probe configurations that employ mechanically translated ultrasound beams. In Figure 1.12**A,** a single transducer rotates so as to produce a 360° radial scan, whose plane lies at right angles to that of the probe. Figure 1.12**B** shows a mechanical sector scanner whose plane contains the axis of the probe (an *axial* plane). In Figure 1.12**C** the 115 ° sector can be adjusted so that, while lying in an axial plane, it can be oriented to face angles from forward to perpendicular to the probe. Figure 1.12**D** shows a similar arrangement, but in which the plane of the sector, while fixed at 90° to the probe axis, can be rotated from an axial to a radial direction. In all of these systems, the motor driving the transducer motion is housed within the probe handle. Electronic arrays have the advantage for intracavity imaging that they require no moving parts and so can be made smaller. Also, linear or curvilinear arrays offer a larger field of view, which may make anatomic orientation of the operator less difficult. Figure 1.13**A** shows an axial phased array sector, Figure 1.13**B** an axial linear array with a rectangular field of view. In Figure 1.13**C** two phased sector arrays are providing images in the axial and radial directions, and Figure 1.13**D** typifies the many hybrids available, in this case of an axial linear array with a radial sector phased array. The mounting of separate transducer assemblies on the same probe allows visualization of different anatomic planes without exchanging the probe itself during the examination. In most machines, simultaneous imaging of the two fields of view is not possible. Mechanical/array hybrids are becoming more common, and might comprise, for example, a linear array

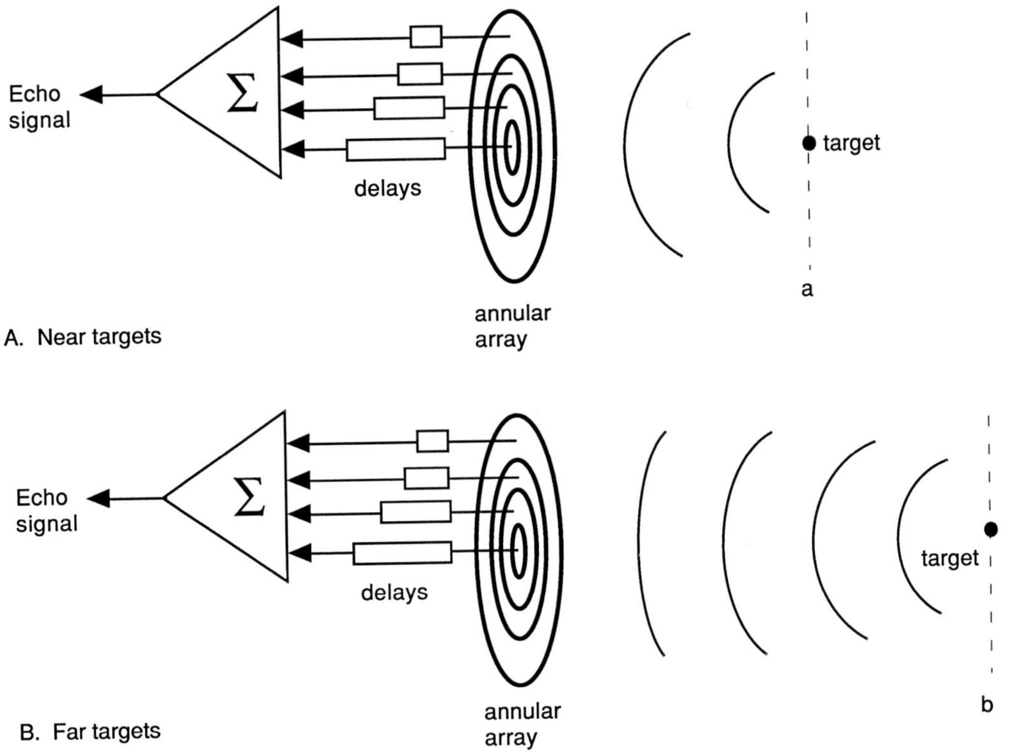

Figure 1.11. The annular array. The annular array is, like the phased array, capable of synthesizing a focus at the desired distance from the transducer, whose axial location can then be swept during the reception of each train of echoes. Note that the annular array, unlike the linear phased array, is capable of focusing the ultrasound beam in two dimensions.

axial scanner and a 360° mechanical radial scanner.

Artifacts in Ultrasound Imaging

Ultrasound images are prone to several sources of artifact. When recognized and properly understood, many artifacts are useful in diagnosis. Thus the "shadowing" distal to a stone identifies it as a highly attenuating (and thus usually calcified) lesion. Conversely, the enhancement of the ultrasound echoes distal to a cystic region, for example, identifies the contents of the cyst as having a lower attenuation than that of surrounding tissue, suggesting that it is filled with a watery fluid. A foaming fluid-gas mixture, such as that found in the bowel, contains many highly reflecting interfaces (Fig. 1.14). The pulse of sound traveling from the transducer will be reflected many times back and forth within the foam before all its energy has been lost. The result is a series of reflections that, because of the varying lengths of the ultrasound path, take differing amounts of time to reach the transducer. As the scanner assumes that echoes arriving after a longer interval originate from deeper in tissue, the image shows a "comet tail" of bright echoes distal to the foam, extending deep into the image. This "comet tail" artifact can be used to distinguish bowel containing gas from, for example, a solid tumor.

Another artifact can result from the assumption made in the imaging process that sound travels at the same speed through all tissue. Virtually all ultrasound instruments are calibrated to an average speed of ultrasound in human soft tissue (usually 1540 m/sec). There is, however, a significant variation between velocities in different soft tissues. The more dense and rigid tissues have a higher velocity, while fluids have a lower velocity than the average. The largest difference encountered clinically is that between fat and collagen, which can be as much as 12%. The effects of a region of tissue that has a different velocity all influence measurement: first, the axial extent of the region

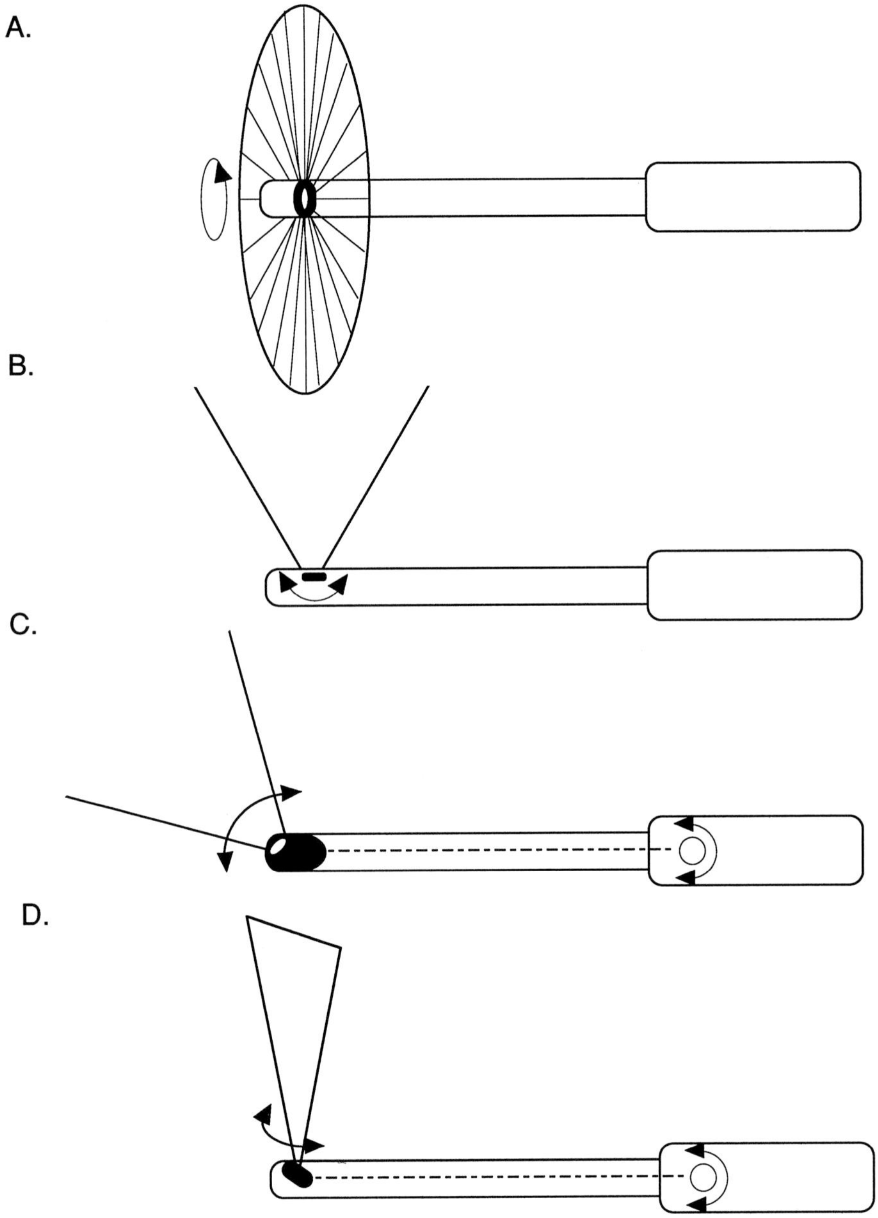

Figure 1.12. Some configurations of mechanical real-time scanners used for transrectal scanning. **A,** The 360° radial scanner. **B,** The axial sector scanner. **C,** An axial sector scanner with adjustable scan plane. **D,** A mechanical sector scanner whose scan plane may be adjusted between axial and radial planes.

itself will be misrepresented because of the incorrect velocity. Thus a fatty tumor with a velocity of 5% below the calibration velocity will be overestimated in axial length by 5%. Second, any tissue interfaces distal to the tumor will be depicted in the wrong location, because of the transit time of the pulse having been lengthened by the region (Fig. 1.15**A**).

Finally, the assumption implicit in instrument design that the ultrasound travels in a straight line may be breached by the phenomenon of *refraction* (Fig. 1.16). Among the factors

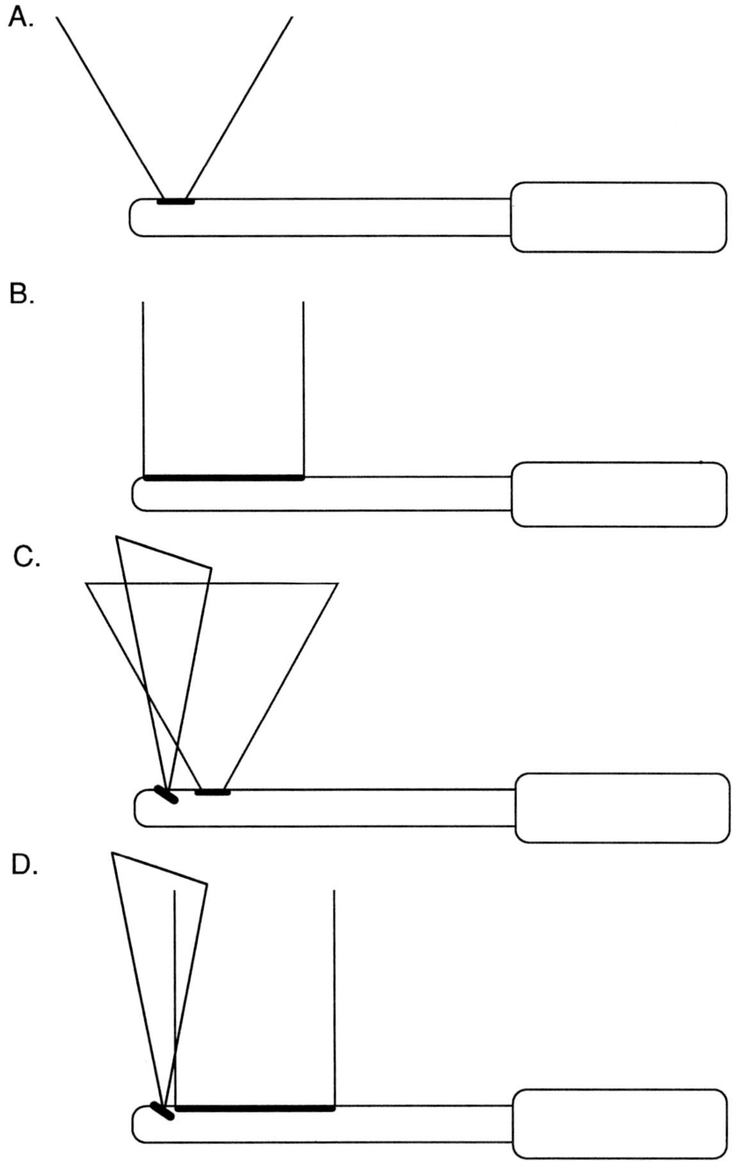

Figure 1.13. Some configurations of electronic array scanners used for transrectal scanning. **A,** The axial phased array sector scanner. **B,** Axial linear array scanner with a rectangular field of view. **C,** Two phased array sector scanners, one having an axial and one with a radial orientation. **D,** A phased array linear array hybrid, with the linear array providing the axial scan plane.

that influence the acoustic impedance of a given tissue is the velocity at which sound travels in it. Thus, an interface between two tissues of differing velocity will give rise to an echo by reflection. However, as the transmitted portion of the pulse continues into the deeper tissue, its path is deviated at the interface. The degree of deviation from a straight line depends on the difference in velocities across the interface: this may be negligible between, say, renal cortex and sinus, but can be significant between fat and collagen. As the scanner assumes ultrasound to travel in a straight line, and as the echoes return along the same path as the transmitted pulse, all structures distal to the refracting interface will be shown in the wrong

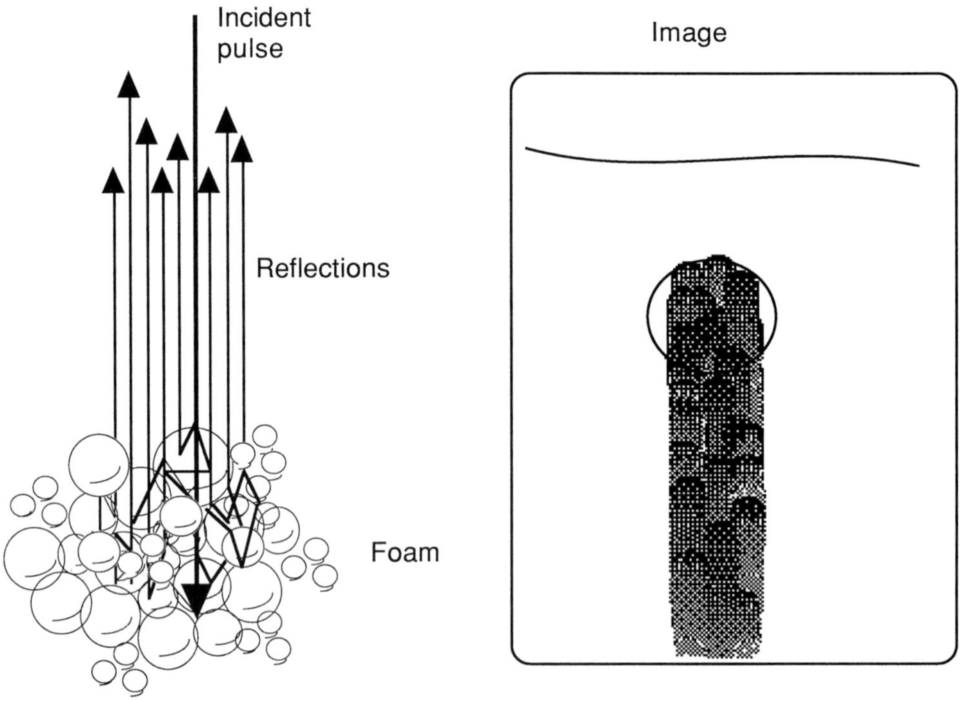

Figure 1.14. The reverberation artifact. Multiple path lengths of echoes reflected many times within a foaming air-fluid mixture results in a high-intensity vertical streak in the image.

location, and their spatial relationship to nearby structures that were imaged without refraction will be distorted (Fig. 1.15**B**).

Measurements Using Ultrasound

In many instances, ultrasound is used to make anatomic measurements of an organ or a lesion. Certain limitations to the precision of such measurements are a fundamental consequence of the physics of the image itself: no amount of care on the part of the operator will alleviate these constraints. In particular, the resolution of the image determines the best precision of any measurement made from it. In ultrasound images, the resolution varies within each image and between the three directions defined by the scan plane.

AXIAL RESOLUTION

Axial resolution is defined as the minimum separation of two targets in tissue in a direction parallel to the beam that results in their being imaged as two distinct structures. Figure 1.17 shows that the main factor that determines axial resolution is the length of the ultrasound pulse. Transducers have a tendency to "ring" after being excited by an electrical impulse, creating an acoustic pulse that has an extended length in space. The result is that even a point target produces an echo that is sustained in time. This is interpreted by the ultrasound scanner as a structure that is extended in axial length, and the result is an image that is "smeared" in the direction of the ultrasound beam. Highly dampened transducers are capable of producing pulses with a shorter spatial length, but require a more powerful impulse to achieve the same level of average acoustical energy in tissue. Moreover, shortening the length of an ultrasound pulse while keeping the total energy of the pulse constant results in a higher peak acoustic intensity. Thus a compromise is reached between the peak pressure to which tissue is exposed and the effective axial resolution of the ultrasound image.

Looking at Figure 1.17, it is clear that if the shortest pulse achievable was one solitary cycle, the length of this pulse, and hence the axial resolution, would be equal to the wavelength. In fact, the wavelength specifies the *best* resolution with which a pulse echo system is capable of defining an echo-producing structure in ax-

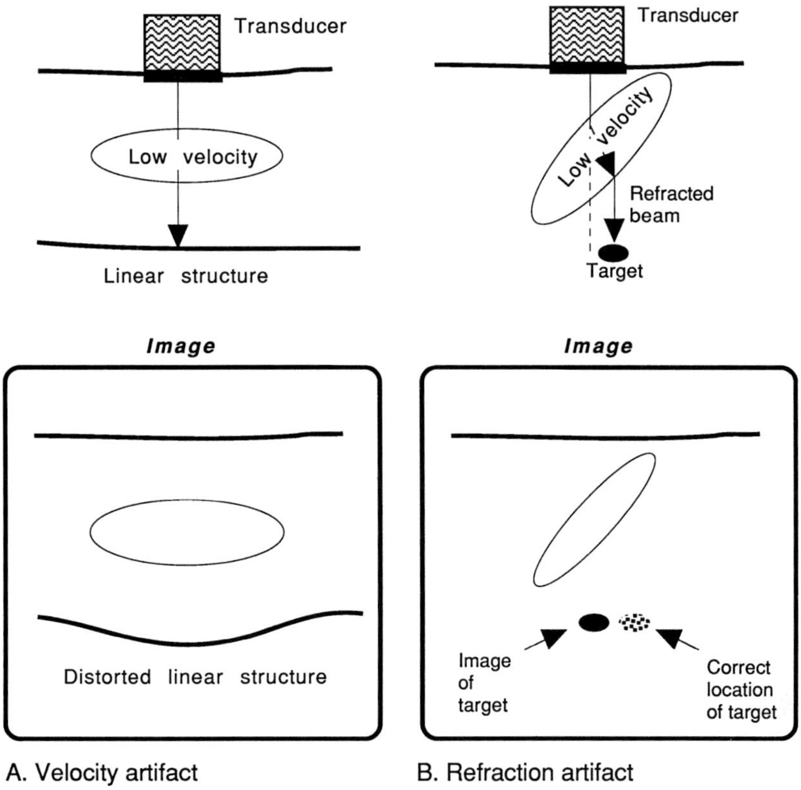

Figure 1.15. Two effects of varying velocity within the imaging field. **A,** Normal incidence of the ultrasound beam on the velocity interface. The different transit time of the ultrasound pulse through the low-velocity region causes axial distortion of the registration of structures distal to the region. **B,** Nonnormal incidence on the region of different velocity. Here, refraction causes lateral misregistration of targets distal to the low-velocity area.

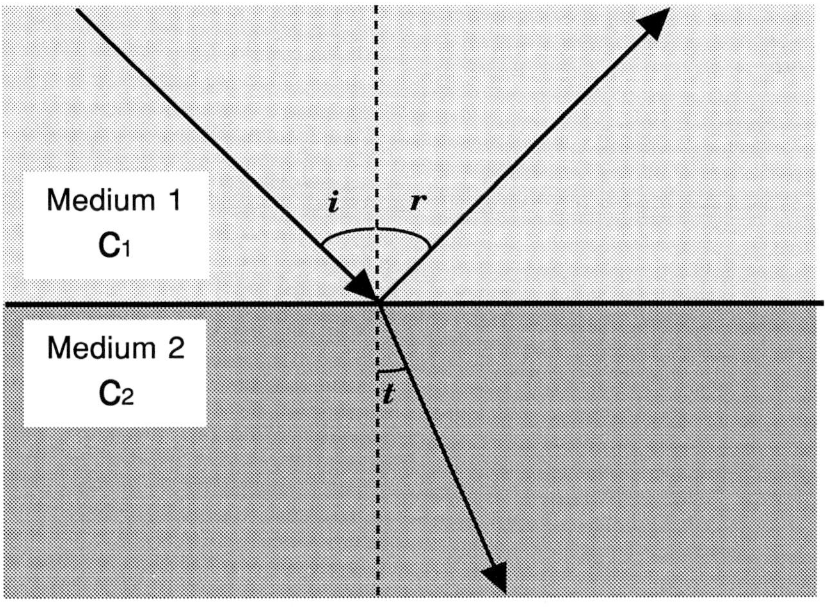

Figure 1.16. Refraction. If the velocity of sound c is different between two media, and the beam is incident at a nonperpendicular angle, the angle of transmission will be different than the angle of incidence.

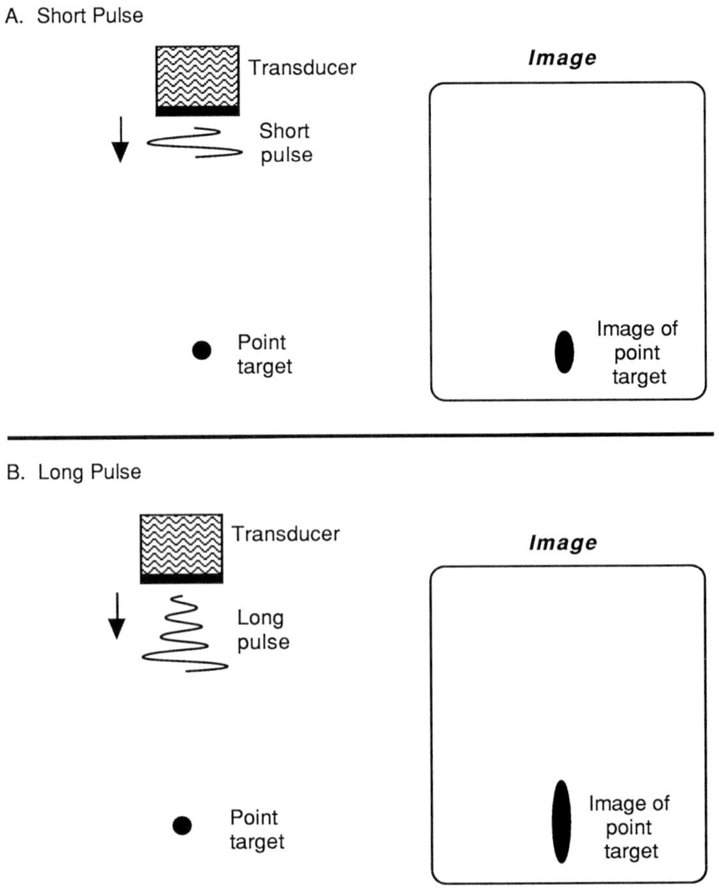

Figure 1.17. Axial resolution. The axial length of the image of a point target depends on the length of the pulse imaged from the ultrasound transducer. This varies with transducer construction and size, as well as frequency.

ial, lateral, and slice thickness directions. The wavelength of ultrasound at 3 MHz (typical of that used in abdominal imaging) is about 0.5 mm; at 10 MHz it is 0.15 mm.

LATERAL RESOLUTION

Lateral resolution is defined as the minimum separation of two targets in tissue, aligned along a direction perpendicular to the ultrasound beam, that results in their being imaged as two distinct structures. Figure 1.18 shows that the principal determinant of lateral resolution is the width of the ultrasound beam. In general, the lateral resolution is inferior to, or at best comparable to, the axial resolution. Highly focused beams, such as the one shown here, achieve good lateral resolution in the focal zone but poor lateral resolution in the near and far-field regions. Thus the precision of a distance measurement made in the lateral direction varies according to depth, the size of the transducer, and the degree of focusing achieved. With array transducer systems, neither the focus nor the effective size of the transducer remains fixed. As echoes from different depths are received at different times, the focus of the beam created by the transducer array can be arranged to coincide with the precise depth from which the echoes at that particular time are originating. The result of the swept focusing described earlier is an image with more uniform lateral resolution than that illustrated in Figure 1.18. In general, narrower beams are obtained from using higher-frequency transducers, so that lateral resolution improves with increasing transducer frequency. Even if swept focusing is employed, the high bandwidth of the pulse emitted from the transducer and the ten-

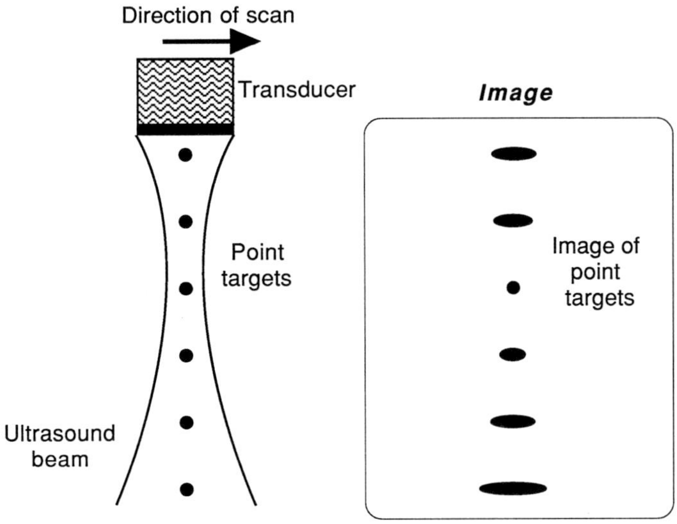

Figure 1.18. Lateral resolution. Lateral resolution of the ultrasound image is dependent on the width of the ultrasound beam. This is not usually uniform over the depth of the image. Swept focusing is one way of minimizing the inhomogeneous lateral resolution that results from such beam geometry.

dency of tissue to absorb high ultrasound frequencies more rapidly results in a lowering of the center frequency of the pulse as it traverses tissue. The result is that there is always some degradation of both axial and lateral resolution with increasing depth.

SLICE THICKNESS

The ultrasound instrument assumes that all echoes arise from the central axis of the beam. In reality, echoes are produced by the full cross-section of the beam. This leads to an inevitable uncertainty over the actual location from which an echo arises, causing what may be described as a "superimposition" effect. Echoes arising from tissues located near the edge of the beam are presented in the image as if they are located on the central axis of the beam. Therefore, any given point in the ultrasound image represents a summation of changes in tissue construction *across* a slice of tissue. When viewing the image, the observer is "looking through" a slice whose thickness is equivalent to the width of the beam that produced the image. This "slice thickness" is one source of the characteristic "fuzzy" edges of imaged spherical structures. Since most of the surfaces in the body are curved, the ultrasound image superimposes echoes from these curving surfaces, producing less well-defined margins to structures.

CONTRAST

The effective resolution with which a structure can be delineated, and thus measured, from an ultrasound image is also affected by the strength of the echo itself. Several factors are involved. First, even a strong echo may arise from tissue sufficiently deep for attenuation to render it weak by the time it returns to the transducer: it only takes about 4 mm of muscle, for example, to reduce a 2.5-MHz echo to one-half of its amplitude. A weak echo requires more amplification from the receiver, but increasing the receiver gain also increases noise. If the echo is comparable in amplitude to the noise, it will be difficult or impossible to detect it on the image, and edges will be corrupted by randomly distributed signals that have the appearance of "snow" but are in fact artifactual consequences of a low signal-to-noise ratio. Second, the ultrasound beam does not have a uniform sensitivity pattern: at greater sensitivities, the beam is effectively wider. If the gain is increased enough to detect a weak echo, stronger echoes from the same depth will be "smeared" so as to reduce lateral resolution. Thus the *contrast resolution* is affected by echo amplitude and tissue attenuation. This provokes an inevitable conflict between raising the ultrasound frequency, which results in higher spatial resolution, and lowering it, which improves signal amplitude and hence often contrast resolution. The optimum frequency with which to carry out a specific measurement is thus always a compromise.

DOPPLER

Doppler methods are unique among clinical techniques in ultrasound in that they have the potential to offer information related to the function of an organ rather than its morphology. However, they have in common with all ultrasound techniques that the information is derived from the interaction of a beam of sound with a volume of tissue and must therefore represent a combination of these two influences. Much of the interpretation of Doppler signals in clinical practice entails the extraction of information about the underlying blood flow from confounding factors related to the Doppler technique. This process has been made progressively more straightforward with the refinement of instruments for the acquisition and analysis of Doppler signals. However, the mere fact that the data cannot be presented as a conventional image can often bewilder the sonographer who relies on an intuitive interpretation of an ultrasound study. An appreciation of the physical principles of the Doppler effect not only help extend such an intuition into blood flow studies, but is an essential prerequisite for the quantitative interpretation of Doppler signals.

The Doppler Effect

When a wave is reflected from a moving target, the frequency of the wave received differs from that which is transmitted. This difference in frequency is known as the *Doppler shift* and depends on, among other things, the speed at which the target is moving and whether the motion is toward or away from the receiver. Examples of the Doppler effect abound. For example, a listener perceives the pitch of a moving source of sound to change according to whether the source is approaching or receding; an astronomer can determine the speed of rotation of the sun by measuring the difference in frequency (that is, color) of light between the advancing and receding edges; the frequency of radio waves received from a moving aircraft is shifted due to the Doppler effect. The acoustical Doppler effect occurs whenever there is relative motion between the source and the receiver of sound. Consider the case in which the source is stationary and the receiver is moving toward the source. Sound waves, comprising a series of compressions, travel toward the receiver at a steady speed determined by the medium. The frequency received is simply the number of these compressions detected per second by the receiver. In the example in which both the source and receiver are stationary, this is obviously equal to the frequency that is transmitted. If, however, the receiver moves toward the source, it will detect more compressions per second and so register a higher frequency. Conversely, if the receiver moves away from the source, fewer compressions reach the transducer per second and a lower frequency is detected. A precisely analogous effect occurs if the source moves away from a stationary receiver.

In the case of ultrasound being scattered from moving red blood cells, two successive Doppler shifts are involved (Fig. 1.19). First, the sound from the stationary transmitting transducer is received by the moving red blood cells. Second, the cells act as a moving source as they reradiate the ultrasound back toward the transducer, which is now a stationary receiver. To a first approximation, these two Doppler shifts are equal and simply add to each other. They account for the factor 2 appearing in the Doppler equation,

$$f_D = \frac{2fv \cos \theta}{c}$$

This equation relates the Doppler shift frequency f_D (measured in hertz) to the velocity of the moving blood v (in meters per second), the frequency of the ultrasound f (in hertz), the velocity of sound c in the medium (in meters per second), and the cosine of the angle θ between the direction of motion and the axis of the ultrasound beam. This angle θ enters the equation because it is seldom that a target, such as blood within a vessel, is moving directly toward or away from the transducer. More generally, it will be moving in a direction at some angle θ to the line between it and the transducer. The Doppler effect is a consequence only of motion along this line. It is therefore necessary to calculate the *component* of the velocity v along the direction of the ultrasound beam: this is given by $v \cos \theta$. In the extreme case in which the motion is aligned precisely with the beam, the angle θ is equal to 0, and cos 0 is equal to 1, so that the component of velocity responsible for the Doppler shift is simply v. Conversely, if the

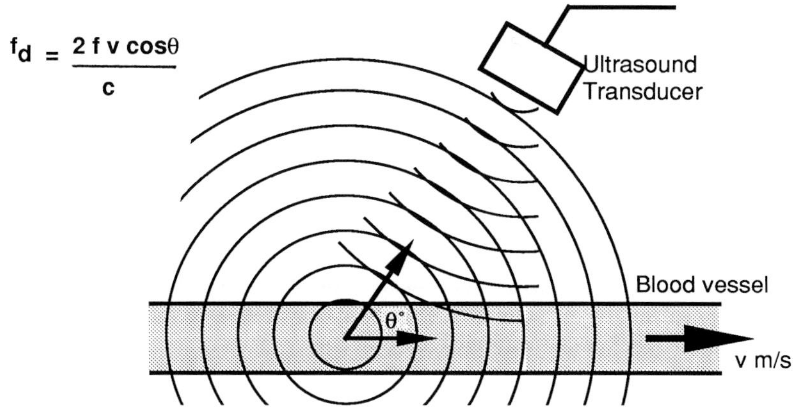

Figure 1.19. The Doppler effect. An incident ultrasound beam of frequency *f* is scattered by moving red bloods cells. As a result of the Doppler effect, the backscattered echo has a center frequency that is higher by an amount f_D.

motion is perpendicular to the beam, θ is equal to 90° and cos 90° is equal to 0, so that there is no component of velocity along the beam and hence no Doppler shift. In physical terms, it is easy to see that the target is neither approaching nor receding from the transducer in this case.

It is a purely fortuitous coincidence that, for the range of ultrasound frequencies used clinically (2 to 10 MHz), the range of tissue velocities encountered physiologically (0 to 5 m/sec), and the velocity of sound in blood, the range of Doppler shift frequencies f_D happens to lie within the audible range of frequencies up to about 15 kHz. It is both convenient and customary, then, for a Doppler flowmeter to convert the shift frequency into an audible signal that can be monitored by the operator through a loudspeaker or a pair of headphones. In spite of the fact that quantitation of the Doppler signal is not possible without further processing of this signal, it should be noted that the ear is capable of quite subtle discrimination of such noises and that the seasoned Doppler practitioner still derives benefit from listening carefully to the sounds themselves.

The Scattering of Ultrasound by Blood

The composition of blood is responsible for some important aspects of the Doppler signal. Blood consists of a suspension of erythrocytes (red blood cells), leukocytes (white blood cells), and platelets in a liquid plasma. Because of the relatively low numbers of leukocytes and the small size of platelets, it is generally assumed that the erythrocytes are responsible for the scattering of ultrasound by blood. The mean diameter of an erythrocyte is 7 μm, much less than the wavelength of the ultrasound, which is about 0.2 to 0.5 mm. Therefore, individual erythrocytes act as point scatterers, whose combined effect is referred to as *Rayleigh-Tyndall scattering*. The size of the echo from blood is small compared to that produced by specular reflection from solid tissue interfaces, as is apparent from the echo-free appearance of blood-filled structures on ultrasound images. One consequence of the Rayleigh-Tyndall process is that the intensity of the scattered wave increases with the fourth power of frequency ($I \sim f^4$). Thus, doubling the ultrasonic frequency results in an echo from blood that is 16 times stronger. This is partly responsible for a dramatic difference in performance between Doppler instruments detecting blood flow using different ultrasonic frequencies. Of course, attenuation in soft tissue also rises with frequency, tending to offset the advantage of the increased efficiency of scattering at higher frequencies. The choice of the optimum ultrasonic frequency with which to perform a Doppler examination is thus an inevitable compromise based on the frequency employed and the depth of the structure of interest. In general, the optimum frequency for a Doppler examination lies below that which is likely to be chosen for imaging the same structure; this places an additional demand on the design of duplex scanners and their transducer assemblies (see below).

Another important effect that the composition of blood has on the nature of the Doppler signal arises from the combination of many individual scattered waves produced by the erythrocytes. As long as the erythrocytes are not too close together, each behaves as though it were an independent receiver and scatterer of the sound. The wavelets resulting from these interactions spread out from their many sources much as ripples do from small stones falling onto the surface of a pond. As these waves meet each other, they combine according to their phase at the point of interception with, for example, two maxima combining to form a maximum, a maximum and a minimum combining to form zero, and so on. The resulting *interference* pattern extends back to the receiving transducer face and moves along with the moving blood. This gives rise to fluctuations in the strength of the Doppler signal both in space and with time, and accounts for the distinctive noise-like character of Doppler blood flow signals. It also allows a prediction to be made about the average strength of the signal. In fact, theory predicts that the intensity of the Doppler signal is related to the quantity of blood lying within the sensitive volume of the Doppler beam. This forms the basis of the most common method for volume flow estimation using Doppler ultrasound.

Instrumentation

The simplest Doppler instrument is the continuous-wave (CW) Doppler shift detector. Figure 1.20 shows a schematic diagram. The transducer assembly houses two elements: one to transmit, the other to receive. Their beams are arranged to overlap so as to form a sensitive volume defined by their spatial product. The oscillator produces an electrical voltage varying at the resonant frequency of the transducer (because the transmitter is operating continuously, a narrow-band transducer is used, perhaps with only air backing, which has the effect of increasing the overall sensitivity of the system). A continuous stream of echoes arrives at the receiving transducer, whose output is amplified and fed to the demodulator. The function of the demodulator is to compare the frequency of the received echoes to that of the oscillator and to derive a signal whose frequency is equal to their difference—this is the Doppler shift signal. Stationary interfaces give rise to echoes whose frequency is identical to that of the oscillator: these are rejected by the demodulator. Most demodulators employ a technique known as *phase quadrature* detection, which is capable of distinguishing between signals whose frequency is higher and those whose frequency is lower than that of the transmitted signal, corresponding to Doppler shifts toward or away from the transducer. Such a *directional* demodulator produces two outputs that, after filtering, have a phase relationship determined by the direction of flow. Further, minor processing can be used to produce a stereo audio signal to feed to the headphones, where the sounds in one ear are the Doppler shifts corresponding to motion toward the transducer and the sounds in the other corresponding to shifts away from the transducer.

The overlapping volume of the two ultrasound beams used in a typical CW system begins a short distance from the transducer face and extends to the limit of the beams due to attenuation. The detector will be sensitive to any moving target within this volume that produces an echo. Should there be moving solid structures as well as blood (for example, from the pulsation of an arterial wall), low-frequency Doppler shifts are obtained whose strength is much greater than that of the blood flow itself. This may be more than an inconvenience: if the dynamic range of the receiver is limited, overloading of the demodulator can occur, with the result that part of the blood flow signal itself is lost. For this reason most instruments incorporate high-pass filters that help eliminate Doppler signals below a certain predetermined frequency (typically 100 to 250 Hz). Even where clutter is not a problem, the presence of several vessels within the sensitive volume gives rise to a superposition of several Doppler signals. If these are simply an artery-vein pair (say the carotid artery and jugular vein), the directional resolution of the spectral display and the distinct characteristics of arterial and venous flow allow their identification. In the upper abdomen, however, there are usually too many vessels present to allow continuous-wave systems to be very helpful. The usual solution is to confine continuous-wave techniques to the examination of superficial structures and to employ a sufficiently high ultrasound frequency so that attenuation limits the penetration of the beam and hence the extent of the sensitive volume. Thus, 7- to 10-MHz systems are often used without imaging for the examination of the carotid and superficial vessels of the limbs. Many configura-

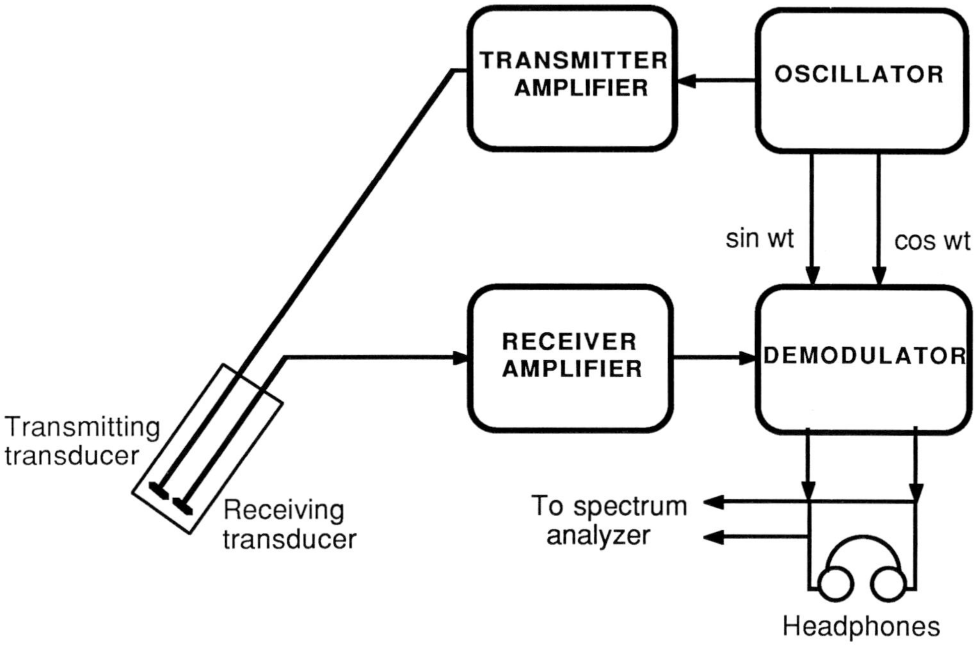

Figure 1.20. The continuous-wave Doppler system. Signals from the receiving transducers are compared in frequency to those transmitted, using a scheme known as coherent demodulation. The output of the demodulator is the audible Doppler shift signal.

tions of the continuous-wave transducer assembly have been made, allowing, for example, probes to be clipped onto vessels at surgery. The continuous-wave method is also capable of very high sensitivity to weak signals, so that it is preferred for the examination of smaller vessels such as the ophthalmic and supraorbital arteries and those supplying the female breast.

Pulsed Doppler

Pulsed Doppler ultrasound combines the velocity detection of a CW Doppler system with the range discrimination of a pulse-echo system. Short bursts of ultrasound are transmitted at regular intervals and the echoes are demodulated as they return (Fig. 1.21). If the pulses are received in sufficiently rapid succession, the output of the demodulator (which compares the phase of the received pulse with that of the oscillator) consists of a sequence of samples from which the Doppler signal can be synthesized. The same transducer is generally used for transmitting and receiving. The range in tissue at which Doppler signals are detected can be controlled simply by changing the length of time the system waits after sending a pulse before opening the gate that allows it to receive. The axial length of the sensitive volume thus produced is determined by the length of time for which the gate is open. Figure 1.21 shows that the electronic gate is generally placed after the demodulator and is governed by these two delays, which are under the control of the operator. A master clock ensures synchrony between the emission of pulses and the operation of the delays and gates. Quadrature detection, as before, produces a directional Doppler signal as the output of the system. In practice, although the range of the sample volume from the transducer is under the control of the operator, the form of the sensitive volume itself is influenced by a variety of factors. The length of time for which the received gate is open determines its axial extent, which may be varied between about 1.5 and 15 mm. The lateral dimensions, however, depend on the ultrasound beam width and are consequently affected by the position of the sample volume in the beam as well as the transducer frequency and design. Some scanners using electronic beam focusing are capable of adjusting the focus of the beam to coincide with the location of the sample volume, thus influencing its lateral extent.

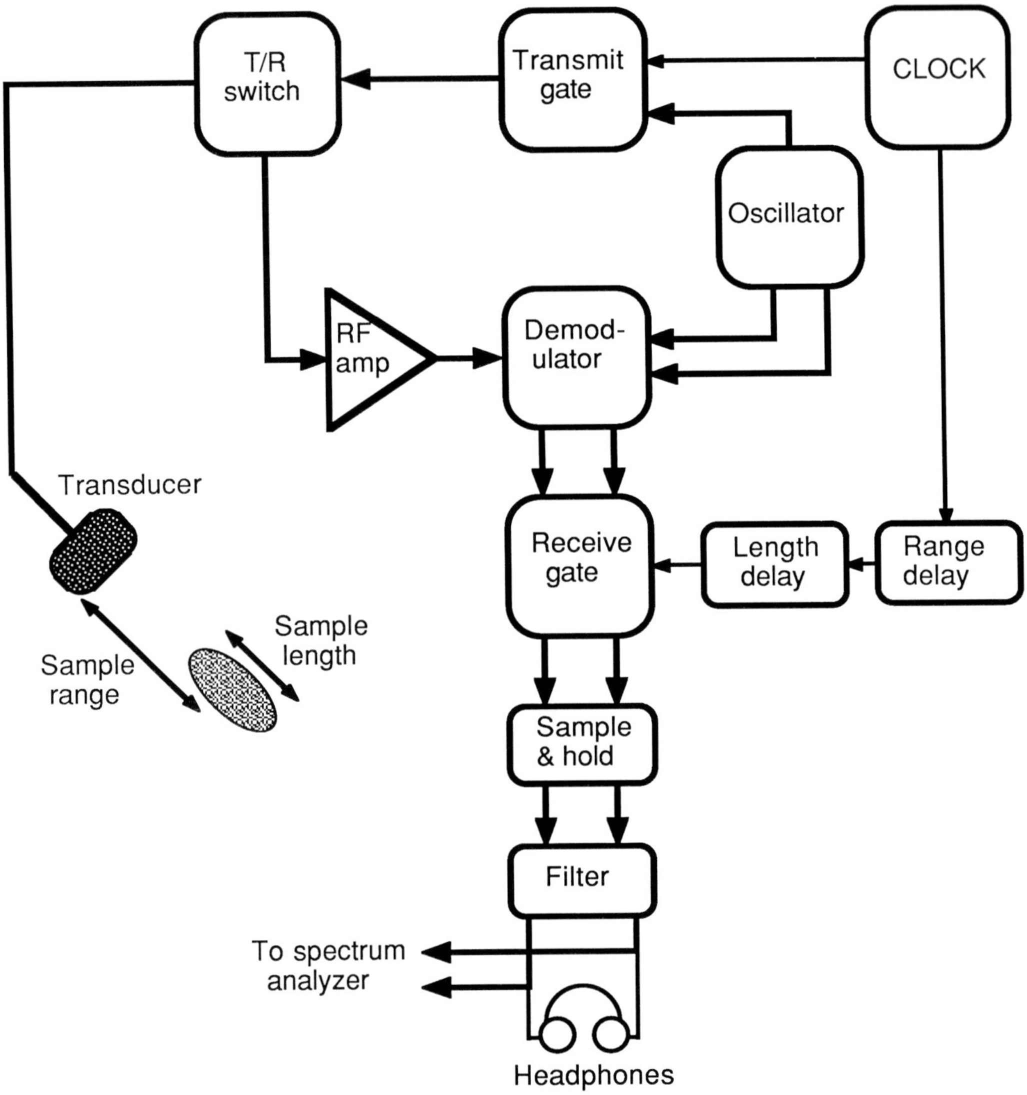

Figure 1.21. The single-gate pulsed Doppler system. The range of the flow-sensitive volume is determined by the transit time of the pulse in tissue. By controlling the range of time over which echoes from the transducer are applied to the demodulator and Doppler shifts detected, the range and length of the sensitive volume can be controlled.

One fundamental shortcoming of the pulsed Doppler system arises from the way in which the audible Doppler shift is in fact made from a large number of discrete samples, one of which is created each time an ultrasound pulse is received by the transducer. Samples that are created rapidly when compared with the rate of variation of the Doppler shift signal itself have no problems: a perfectly good representation, for example, of a 1-kHz Doppler shift signal can be made with 5000 samples per second obtained using a 5-kHz pulse repetition frequency. In fact, sampling theory shows that a signal can be reconstructed unambiguously from a sequence of samples as long as the frequency of the signal is no greater than half the sampling rate (this is known as the Nyquist limit). However, the depth of the target being interrogated for motion imposes a limit on the pulse repetition frequency: an ultrasound pulse cannot normally be emitted before the last echo caused by the preceding pulse has been received. Thus, occasions arise when the Doppler shift frequency of the moving blood is above the Nyquist limit for the depth. The result is that the system produces an incorrect, or *aliased,* Doppler shift frequency, seen as a "folding over" of the spectral display, which now shows an ambiguous relationship between velocity of motion and the displayed Doppler shift frequency. Aliasing creates a set of absolute maximum velocities that it is possible to detect unambiguously using pulsed Doppler, which depend on the ultrasound frequency, the angle of insonation, and the depth (Fig. 1.22). Various methods are available for overcoming this problem. One is simply to increase the pulse repetition rate above the limit imposed by the transit time of the ultrasonic pulse to the target and back. This may remedy the aliasing of the Doppler signal but creates a new ambiguity as to the location of echoes received when the gate is open. In effect, a second sensitive volume is created, located somewhere along the ultrasound beam. Signals are not obtained simultaneously from both locations. Judicious operation can manipulate this second sensitive volume into a region from which no Doppler signals are anticipated to arise. Other, more straightforward, solutions to the problem of aliasing are to lower the ultrasound frequency (hence lowering the Doppler shift frequencies themselves) or to resort to continuous-wave Doppler, which does not suffer from the aliasing limitation.

Less obviously, pulsed Doppler instruments tend to emit pulses of a higher average intensity than their continuous-wave counterparts. The signal-to-noise ratio of a pulsed system is inherently poorer than that of a continuous-wave system because of its higher bandwidth; that is, the pulses transmitted contain a wider range of ultrasound frequencies. Narrowing this range improves signal-to-noise performance but degrades spatial resolution. At comparable intensities, then, pulsed Doppler systems generally offer a poorer signal-to-noise ratio. Manufacturers often address this problem by increasing the power of the transmitted pulse. The practical implication of this is that the highest spatial peak temporal average (SPTA) exposure intensities used in diagnos-

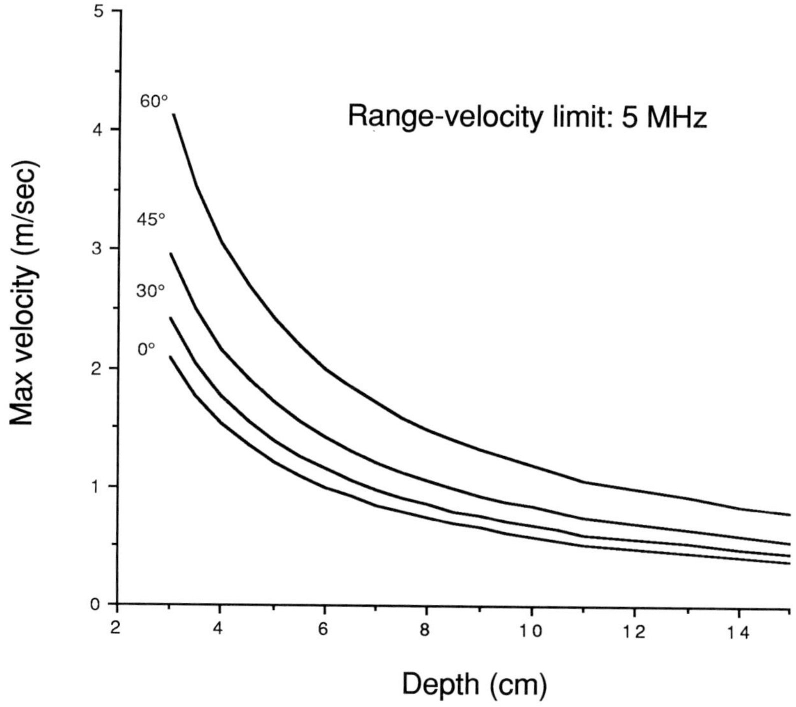

Figure 1.22. Aliasing and the range velocity limit. Shown in this graph are the maximum velocities that it is possible to detect unambiguously using a pulsed Doppler system at a given depth. Note that this velocity is dependent on both the beam flow velocity angle and the operating frequency of the transducer.

tic ultrasound are generally associated with pulsed Doppler systems. These levels can be as great as 1 W/cm^2. It is the general experience, however, that virtually all Doppler examinations, including those of small deep-lying vessels in the abdomen, can be performed successfully with modern instruments at considerably lower exposure intensities.

The Duplex Scanner

Control of the location of the sensitive volume in tissue is of little use without some form of guidance to the structures in the region of the sample volume. It is natural to contemplate the use of real-time ultrasound imaging for such guidance; the combination of real-time imaging and Doppler techniques is referred to as *duplex* scanning. Most commonly, duplex scanners consist of a combination of real-time sector imaging and a pulsed Doppler.

Whereas the ultrasound beam moves rapidly to create a real-time image, it must dwell for a much longer period in one orientation to obtain Doppler information: a duplex scanner rarely performs imaging and Doppler simultaneously, in spite of the implication of its name. Generally, the real-time image is used to select the location for interrogation with the Doppler system and then the scanner is switched to operate in Doppler mode, during which the machine aligns the beam in the appropriate direction and sets the range delays accordingly. Figure 1.23 shows some typical configurations of real-time scanners with which Doppler methods have been combined. Because of rotational inertia in mechanically steered systems such as that of Figure 1.23**A**, it is not possible to switch between imaging and Doppler modes very rapidly; the image is usually "frozen" on the screen while the Doppler signal is acquired. Because many mechanical scanners employ more than one transducer for imaging, some of them are able to use different transducers, and possibly different frequencies, for the two functions of Doppler interrogation and imaging. These might exploit the superior performance of a swept-focus annular array for imaging and a single disk or dual-element (for continuous wave) transducer for Doppler. Typical combinations might be 7 to 10 MHz for imaging and 5 MHz for Doppler in the carotid, or 5-MHz imaging together with 3-MHz Doppler in the abdomen. Electronic sector scanners are capable of switching between imaging and Doppler modes at a sufficiently high rate to permit real-time "duplex" imaging at a somewhat reduced frame rate. Although this is sometimes at the expense of signal-to-noise performance of the Doppler system, the facility of simultaneous imaging and Doppler is useful where there are slow movements (such as those of respiration or of a fetus) that can make the positioning of the Doppler volume difficult.

The linear array configuration with an offset Doppler is particularly useful when low angles of insonation are desired for vessels lying parallel to the transducer face. One ingenious approach to the implementation of such a method is to employ a number of elements within the linear array as a "phased" system, delivering the transmit pulse to each of the elements in the group with very small successive delays, which has the effect of steering the Doppler beam in a direction that differs from that of the beams used for imaging (Fig. 1.23**C**). Such systems may be used in the examination of the carotid and other superficial vessels lying parallel to the skin surface. Electronic arrays may also address the problem of the different optimum imaging and Doppler frequencies by employing sufficiently broadband transducers so that the two functions can be served by the same array operating at different frequencies. The agility of the beam produced by such arrays is capable of providing imaging, Doppler, and M-mode functions at such rapid alternations as to allow real-time examination of the heart. The curvilinear array of Figure 1.23**D** is a useful compromise between the relative advantages of the electronic sector scanner and the linear array duplex scanner. Using an array for the pulsed Doppler system allows electronic control of the lateral extent of the beam in the direction of the array elements but places quite heavy demands on aspects of the performance (such as the dynamic range) of the beam-forming electronics. High-performance Doppler systems using such arrays have only become available relatively recently.

A powerful advantage of the duplex system is that it allows estimation of the velocity of flow from the Doppler shift frequency. As has already been explained, the Doppler shift frequency depends not only on the velocity of flow, but also on the ultrasound frequency, the velocity of sound, and the angle between the ultrasound beam and the direction of flow. Many duplex systems are equipped to calculate velocity from Doppler shift frequency and hence allow for these factors. The velocity of sound and

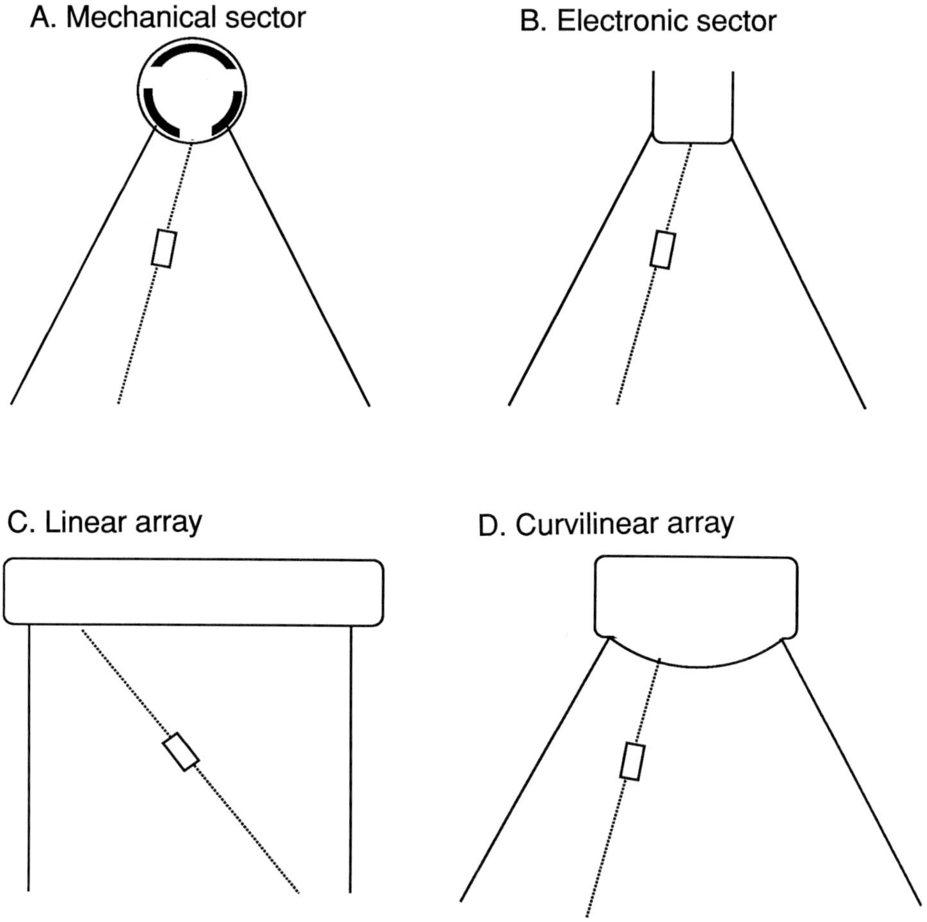

Figure 1.23. Four common configurations of the duplex scanner. **A,** The mechanical sector scanner. **B,** The electronically steered sector scanner. **C,** The linear array with electronically steered Doppler beam. **D,** The curvilinear array.

the frequency of the scanner are known and may be programmed into the machine. The Doppler angle, however, must be measured. Assuming that flow is parallel to the wall of the vessel (that there are not, for example, substantial helical components to flow), this angle may be measured directly from the ultrasound image. Inevitably, errors are associated with the measurement: the vessel axis may not lie exactly within the scanned plane, the vessel may be curved, or the flow may not be aligned with the axis of the vessel. As discussed below, the error in velocity estimation resulting from such an inaccuracy is strongly dependent on the beam-vessel angle itself. Velocity should not be estimated when this angle is above 60°. In correcting for the operating frequency of the Doppler system, velocity estimates eliminate one factor that may vary between individual duplex instruments. Thus, even if a constant value of insonation is used in the examination, the estimated velocity is a better parameter to report than Doppler shift frequency.

The Multigate Pulsed System

The signal range-gate system of Figure 1.21 is only capable of detecting Doppler signals from one sample volume at a time. If, however, several parallel channels are connected to the output of the demodulator, each with its own receive gate controlled by a different range delay, it is possible to produce a large number of Doppler signals simultaneously from different selected points along the ultrasound beam. In a typical configuration for such a *multigate* system (Fig. 1.24), the range cells are arranged to

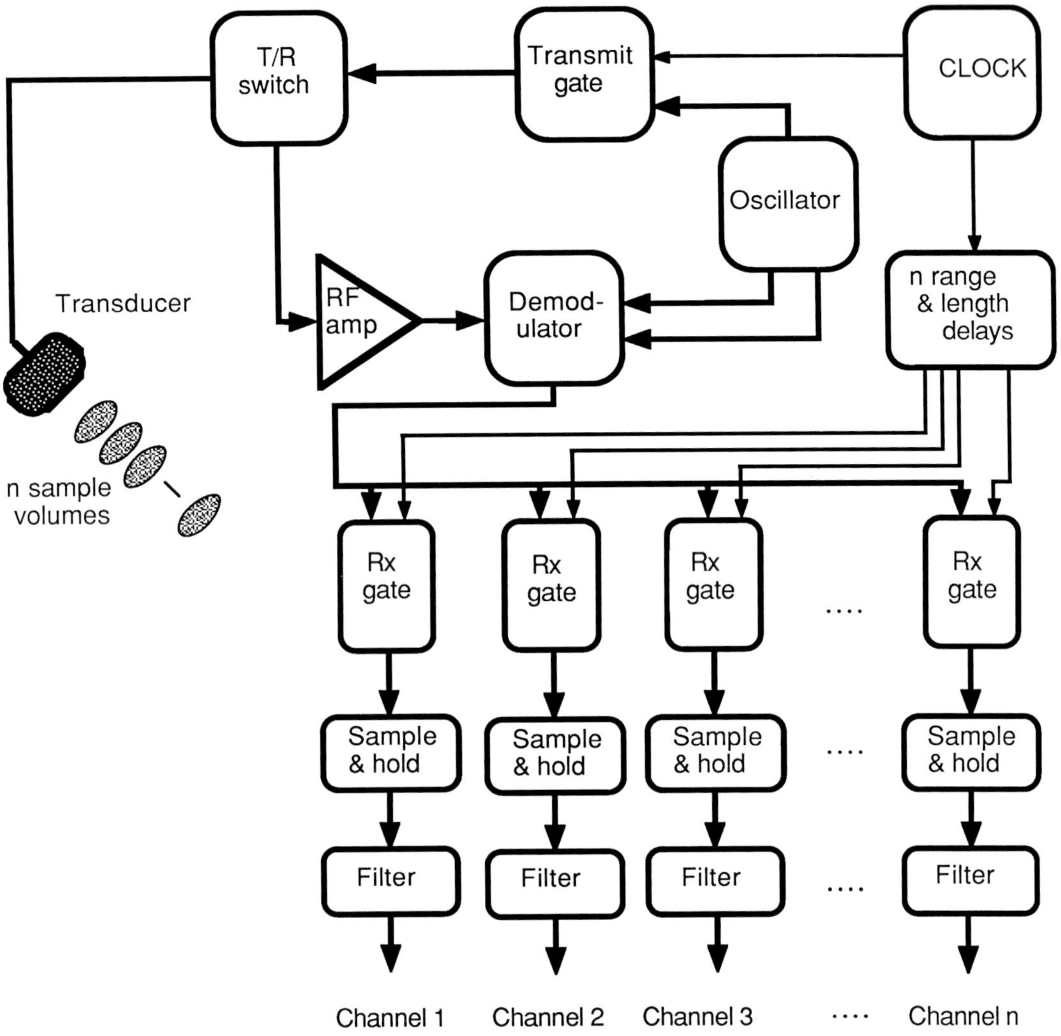

Figure 1.24. The multigate Doppler system. The basic configuration of the pulsed Doppler is supplemented by a number of parallel channels, each with an independent control of the sample range and length, providing a number of parallel Doppler outputs corresponding to a series of discrete depths.

be close to each other within the lumen of a single large blood vessel. The Doppler signal from each gate is then fed into some form of *velocity estimator*—a device that, for example, gives the instantaneous average Doppler shift frequency—whose output consists of a single number, varying with that sample volume. The outputs from all the channels may be combined to yield an instantaneous estimate of the variation of flow velocity across the diameter of the vessel lumen—the *velocity profile.* A typical system for measuring the velocity profile in a carotid artery might operate at 5 MHz and contain 16 or 32 gates, each approximately 1 mm in axial length.

Color Flow Imaging

Looking at Figure 1.24, it is easy to see how the information from a multigate system could be used in another way: to map the extent of Doppler signals obtained over an entire cross-sectional image. All that would be required is a scanning arrangement capable of steering the Doppler beam and registering its direction, and a sufficient number of range gates to map a single Doppler parameter (for example, the average Doppler shift frequency) from near the transducer face to the deepest point in each scan line. If a duplex system were to be used, the Doppler information could be superimposed on the real-time image, with the different velocities encoded using a color scale. This is the principle of color flow mapping, but its implementation using such a system, although possible, would not be practical.

The problem is time. As has been stated, the ultrasound beam must remain stationary for an appreciable length of time (typically about 10 msec) while Doppler information is collected and the signal constituted from the series of sample phase measurements made by the demodulator. A number of parallel channels in a multigate system is, of course, capable of obtaining this information from each of its range gates in the same period of time. However, to obtain Doppler information along a large number of scan lines so as to form an image rapidly enough to be part of a real-time system, a very large number of parallel channels must be used. It is prohibitively expensive in hardware and software to manufacture the, say, 128 channels required to obtain Doppler signals from the entire length of the scan line simultaneously. Even if this were possible, a simple calculation shows that the beam could not dwell for 10 msec on each line and still produce a real-time Doppler image. What is required is a method for obtaining not necessarily the Doppler signal itself, but an estimate of a Doppler parameter such as the instantaneous average Doppler shift frequency, from the entire length of the scan line quickly and simultaneously without the use of parallel channels. The autocorrelation detector serves precisely this function.

The autocorrelation processor is a form of Doppler detector that is capable of processing an entire line of echo data derived from the quadrature-demodulator echoes of one pulse with that derived from the previous pulse, where the latter has been delayed by a length of time equal to the interval between the two pulses. The result is that the two streams of echoes are "compared" for changes in phase due to the Doppler shift. If there are no moving structures giving rise to the echoes, the output from the autocorrelation detector is zero. For this reason, the method is sometimes referred to as a "moving target indicator." Although such a device is capable in principle of yielding the instantaneous Doppler shift along a whole scan line after only three pulses (i.e., less than 1 msec at a pulse repetition frequency of 4 kHz), generally between four and eight pulses might be used. The problem of clutter is crucial in such a system because the very large echoes from solid structures moving slowly can inhibit the detection of the weaker Doppler-shifted echoes from moving blood. Color flow mapping systems employ digitally controlled filters designed to eliminate the effect of clutter.

One requirement of a color flow mapping system is that the beam remains stationary for a brief time, moves to the next scan line and remains stationary there, and so on. In addition, the flow mapping function must be alternated with conventional imaging. The agility of the electronically switched beam of a linear array (or a hybrid of the two) is therefore ideally suited to color flow mapping (Fig. 1.25).

The superposition of flow information as colors on a gray-scale real-time image presents the Doppler information in a novel and appealing way. These systems are clearly well suited to identifying the location of high-velocity flow (such as in a stenosis) or of mapping the extent of flow in a certain region. However, the Doppler information presented is that of a single parameter encoded in color, a parameter whose value is changing rapidly and is derived from, but does not describe, the full Doppler frequency spectrum. Therefore, it seems likely that spectral analysis should remain an essential component of most Doppler examinations, whether or not color flow mapping is included. Indeed, present color instruments offer the flow mapping facility as an addition to, rather than a replacement of, conventional duplex scanning and spectral analysis.

Analysis of the Doppler Spectrum: The Spectral Display

Although the movement of the single target gives rise to a Doppler shift signal of one frequency whose pitch is proportional to the target velocity, the sample volume of a pulsed Doppler (or the sensitive region of a continuous-wave Doppler) usually insonates blood cells moving at a large number of differing velocities, sometimes even in opposite directions within the same vessel. Therefore, the Doppler signal is perceived by the operator as a complex and changing set of sounds. The successful application of quantitative techniques in a clinical setting relies to a great extent on the appropriate choice of subsequent processing and measure-

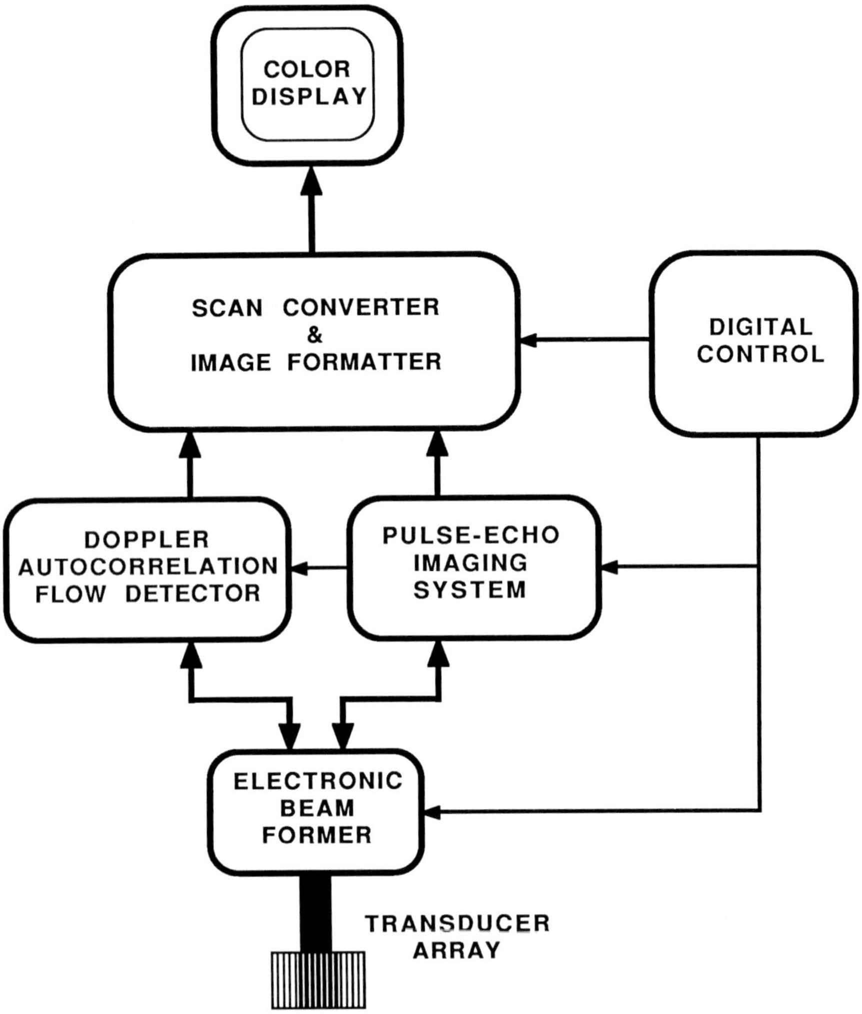

Figure 1.25. The major components of a color flow mapping system. The array imaging system produces a gray-scale real-time display by manipulating the beam electronically over the field of view. At the same time, the autocorrelation detector produces Doppler information with which to encode the image in color. In a typical display, flow toward the probe is represented in hues of red and flow away from the probe in hues of blue.

ment made on this signal. To this end a variety of signal processing methods are available, some of which are now incorporated routinely in commercial instruments.

As the basis for the information contained within the signal lies in the combination of different Doppler shift frequencies of which it is composed, it is natural that the fundamental tool for the processing of Doppler signals should be the frequency (or spectrum) analyzer. This instrument is capable of determining the relative powers of the various frequency components present in the signal at a given time. Although there are several methods for implementing spectral analysis, the most common uses the digital fast Fourier transform (FFT). Short periods of the signal are digitized and analyzed mathematically for their frequency components. Dedicated arithmetic processors can perform the necessary calculations at sufficient speed to be able to accept the next period for analysis as it arrives, thus producing a series of spectra in real time. These spectra are simply graphs showing the relative amplitude of each of the frequency components constituting the Doppler signal. If the target is blood flowing in a single vessel uniformly insonated by the ultrasound beam, the power at a given frequency relates to the quantity of blood flowing at the corresponding velocity. The spectrum at a specific point in the vessel is usually displayed as a *sonogram,* in which a single spectrum is depicted as a vertical line on whose axis lies frequency, brightness modulated at each point to represent amplitude. Subsequent spectra are displayed as vertical lines at a fixed distance apart, creating an image that scrolls from left to right with time. The three variables—time, frequency, and amplitude—are thus shown in real time as the signal is heard. With *in vivo* signals the power spectrum changes with time and the *sonogram* becomes the most useful display format.

Interpretation of the Doppler Spectrum

QUALITATIVE METHODS

Presence of Flow

Determining whether or not flow is present is one of the simplest but perhaps most useful applications of Doppler. It may be used to exclude occlusion by thrombosis, for example, or to determine the point of occlusion of a limb vessel during a pressure measurement. Confirming the absence of flow is, by its nature, a little more difficult. It is necessary to be certain that the lack of Doppler signal is a consequence of lack of flow, rather than the acoustical or electrical parameters of the system. It is prudent to check that normal flow signals can be obtained with the same machine settings from comparable structures at comparable depths before concluding that flow is absent at a particular location.

Direction of Flow

The directional resolution of the Doppler system is best when the beam-vessel angle is relatively small and the signal lies in the middle of the dynamic range of the receiver. If a mirror image of the signal is seen in the reverse-flow sideband of the display, care should be taken with the adjustment of angle and receiver gain so as to obtain a trace showing an unambiguous direction.

Identification of Characteristic Flow

It is apparent that normal flow in various pats of the arterial circulation shows distinct characteristics according to its precise location. Those characteristics of waveform shape and spectral distribution are often consequences of hemodynamic factors unique to each vessel. These allow the identification of the origin of a flow signal from the spectral display (and the aural quality of the sound) alone and are particularly useful in circumstances where the image may be ambivalent.

SEMIQUANTITATIVE METHODS

Disturbed Flow

The characteristics that distinguish disturbed and turbulent flow from laminar flow are reflected in the content of their respective Doppler signals. In a vessel with a flat velocity profile, the spectral display shows a narrow range of Doppler shift frequencies, especially in systole. This is the origin of the "window" below the spectral trace in systole—a Doppler sign of laminar flow with a blunt profile. Slower moving laminae are found toward the edge of the vessel, so the size of the window (and with it the contrast between laminar and disturbed flow signals) can be increased by employing a small sample volume situated toward the center of the vessel. Flow disturbance produces velocity vectors whose direction varies. This means that the components of velocity along the direction of the Doppler beam change with time. The combination of many such components results in a wide range of Doppler shifts, seen as a broadening of the spectral display and a reduction in the size of the window. As the velocity increases, vortices form and the Doppler sample volume encounters rotating flow elements. Velocities, and hence Doppler shifts, are noticeably higher. The vortices contain simultaneous forward and reverse flow in a range of velocities. Vortex formation is time dependent in arteries; they will be apparent on a Doppler trace at the point at which the critical point is attained in the upstroke of systole. Suddenly, laminar flow will give way to rotating flow, and the Doppler spectrum shows simultaneous forward and reverse velocities together with a broad range of Doppler shifts. Laminar flow reappears in diastole as the Reynolds number is reduced.

As flow velocities increase, vortices are shed and travel downstream. As they move through a Doppler sample volume, they are responsible for fluctuation of Doppler shift frequency with time. These rotational components can also have their origin in geometry: a quite normal, but tortuous, splenic artery will often show a broad spectrum with dramatic fluctuations of maximum Doppler shift frequency. At high Reynolds numbers, turbulence ensues and may be sustained throughout the cardiac cycle. The time-velocity waveform produced by a tight stenosis is very much less pulsatile than its normal counterpart. Simultaneous, disorganized, forward and reverse Doppler shifts are seen and velocities remain high throughout the cardiac cycle.

Vascular Impedance and Pulsatility

The maximum Doppler shift frequency is a single value quantity which, in an artery, varies over the cardiac cycle with the velocity of the fastest moving blood flowing within the sample volume. Characterization of the variation of this quantity with time can yield information relating to both the condition of the proximal circulation and the impedance of the distal receiving bed. With a given pressure waveform at the entrance of an arterial segment the relative diastolic flow velocity will change with the impedance of the receiving circulation. Thus, time-velocity waveforms with high flow in diastole (or high diastolic "runoff") accompany a low downstream impedance, whereas waveforms with little or reverse flow during diastole are seen when the impedance downstream is high. This effect is a direct consequence of pressure wave propagation in a compliant vessel, and is independent of volume flow rate. As the Doppler shift frequency is proportional to flow velocity, with the constant of proportionality determined by the beam vessel angle, the ratio of two Doppler shift frequencies is independent of angle. Such ratios may be used to define an index of pulsatility to the waveform that is independent of probe vessel angle and that can be used as an indicator of distal impedance. The higher the distal impedance, the more pulsatile the waveform.

Referring to Figure 1.26, at least three ratios have been used to describe placental time-velocity waveforms (each of which have been called the "pulsatility index" by their various proponents):

Pulsatility index: $PI = \frac{A - B}{\text{mean}}$

(Gosling and King, 1975)

Pourcelot (resistance) index: $RI = \frac{A - B}{A}$

(Planiol and Pourcelot, 1974)

A/B (or S-D) ratio: $\frac{A}{B}$ (Stewart et al., 1980)

Although each of these indices is independent of probe vessel angle, the pulsatility index (PI) is less susceptible to variation due to heart rate and the setting of the high-pass filter characteristic of the flowmeter, has the greatest number of degrees of freedom, and might be considered the most robust of the indices. This is, however, the only quantity of the three that requires the digitizing of the entire time-velocity waveform, making it the least convenient to measure. If the instrument used does not offer this analysis facility, it is a simple matter to employ a microcomputer to digitize a hard copy of the trace offline.

Deep Doppler

The relatively recent availability of high-quality duplex Doppler instruments that operate at ultrasonic frequencies suitable for abdominal scanning has brought several exciting new areas of clinical diagnosis into view. These include the assessment of blood flow in the heart and great vessels of the fetus as well as the adult and the assessment of flow in the vessels and organs of the upper abdomen and pelvis. In many cases the addition of information related to blood flow complements the role of conventional abdominal ultrasound imaging. Particular problems associated with abdominal Doppler examinations include signal-to-noise ratio (the depth and small size of the vessels places their blood flow signals at the limit of detectability with current systems) and *clutter* (the intrusion of high-amplitude, low–Doppler-shift elements in the signal that have their origin in moving solid tissue).

The most simple applications of Doppler in the abdomen and pelvis may also be the most useful clinically. The inaccessibility of the splanchnic venous system to other forms of investigation render it a particularly profitable object of Doppler study. The clinical documentation of the presence and direction of blood flow in, for example, the renal, hepatic, splenic and superior mesenteric circulations might allow the exclusion of vascular compromise, including thrombosis and stenosis. The suitability of

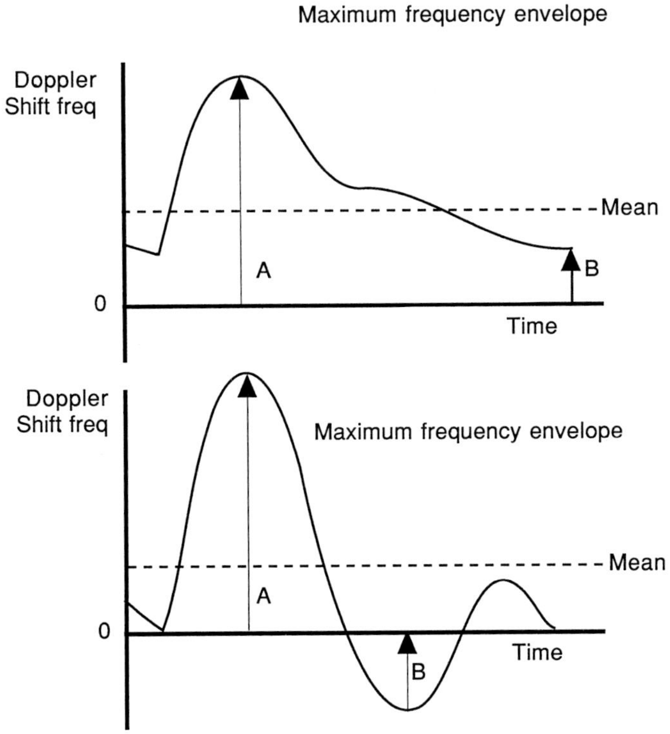

Figure 1.26. Typical time-velocity waveforms when the distal impedance is low (*top*) and high (*bottom*). The maximum peak systolic Doppler shift *A* and the minimum value of the maximum frequency Doppler shift *B* and the mean of the maximum frequency Doppler shift (*mean*) are used to define indices of pulsatility.

the Doppler method for repeated and portable use makes it particularly appropriate for patients who have undergone recent surgery such as organ transplantation.

Doppler can also be used to assess flow disturbance due to stenosis in deep vessels, though the diagnostic criteria differ somewhat from those used in the carotid circulation. Signals show changes following, for example, successful renal artery angioplasty and can be used to document functional improvement. Finally, and perhaps most speculatively, Doppler may be used to help characterize the functional state of tissue itself. Characteristic blood flow signals that accompany neovascularization of a developing malignant tumor have been described and exemplify the prospect that Doppler offers as a complement to the ultrasound image in the differentiation of solid tissues.

Suggested Readings

Atkinson P, Berry MV. Random noise in ultrasonic echoes diffracted by blood. J Physiol (Lond) 1974; 11:1293–1301.

Burns PN. Physical principles of Doppler ultrasound and spectral analysis. J Clin Ultrasound 1987;15: 567–590.

Burns PN. Interpretation of Doppler signals. *In:* Taylor KJW, Burns PN, Wells PNT. Clinical applications of Doppler ultrasound. New York: Raven Press, 1987.

Lafortune M, Patriquin H, Burns PN. Doppler ultrasound in the evaluation of portal and splanchnic blood flow. In: Ferrucci J, ed. New methods of liver imaging. St Louis: CV Mosby, in press.

McDonald DA. Blood flow in arteries. 2nd ed. London: Edward Arnold, 1974:64–69.

Namekawa K, Kasai C, Omoto R. Real-time two-dimensional bloodflow imaging using ultrasound Doppler. J Ultrasound Med 1983;2:10–15.

Wells PNT. Biomedical ultrasonics. London: Academic Press, 1977.

CHAPTER 2

Sectional Anatomy of the Genitourinary System

CARSON D. SCHNECK, M.D., Ph.D.

Ultrasound imaging of the organs of the genitourinary system requires a thorough comprehension of their three-dimensional orientation, relationships, and internal tissue characteristics. Because ultrasound images can be acquired from many directions and in an infinite variety of planes, an appreciation of the geometry and orientation of each organ is vital both for planning optimum imaging planes and for interpreting the images. Hence, emphasis is placed on developing an understanding of the causative factors that determine the three-dimensional characteristics of each organ. Relationships of a given organ to adjacent structures are also stressed, since these can be useful both for locating the normal organ and in interpreting pathological displacements and extensions. The internal features of genitourinary organs are also described as these relate to the organ's ultrasound tissue characteristics. The transverse (axial) sections and sagittal sections through the abdominal portion of the urinary tract are arranged in an atlas form at the end of the abdominal portion of the genitourinary system in Figures 2.6 to 2.21. The transverse and coronal sections of the male pelvis are also arranged in atlas form at the end of the pelvic part of the genitourinary system in Figures 2.24 to 2.40.

KIDNEYS

The orientation of the kidneys and their related structures is determined by the geography of the posterior abdominal wall upon which they lie (1). The posterior wall of the abdomen is deeply indented by a longitudinal midline ridgeline formed by the lordosis of the lumbar spine, the psoas major muscles on either side of the spine, and the aorta and inferior vena cava, which course along the apex of this ridgeline (Fig. 2.1). On either side of the ridgeline there are deep paravertebral gutters formed by the diaphragm, quadratus lumborum, transversus abdominus, and iliacus muscles. These gutters slope substantially forward as they descend from the diaphragm to the paired, obliquely placed ridgelines of the pelvic inlet, which in turn are formed by the bony pelvic inlet, the diverging psoas major muscles, and the common and external iliac vessels.

Because of the geography of the posterior abdominal wall the kidneys show three degrees of obliquity with respect to the standard anatomic planes (2). Since each kidney is suspended into the paravertebral gutter by its vascular pedicle, its hilus is directed anteromedially rather than medially. Likewise, its convex antihilar border is directed posterolaterally instead of laterally. The usually named anterior surface faces anterolaterally and the posterior surface faces posteromedially.

The second obliquity of the kidney is that its inferior pole is normally farther from the midline than its superior pole (Fig. 2.2). This is caused by the widening of the lower part of the midline ridgeline because of the increasing size of the lower lumbar vertebral bodies and the increasing volume of the psoas major muscles.

The third obliquity of the kidney is that the inferior pole is anterior to the superior pole because of the forward slope of the paravertebral gutters as they descend toward the pelvic inlet (see Figs. 2.16 and 2.17).

An appreciation of the three-dimensional obliquity of the kidney's major and minor axes clarifies why it is usually necessary to acquire oblique ultrasound images to determine its maximum dimensions. Although kidney size varies with the size, sex, and age of an individual, the average dimensions are 12 cm in length, 7 cm width (from hilus to antihilar border), and 3 cm in thickness (3). A long-axis view of the right kidney from the anterior axillary line uses the liver as a window and shows its

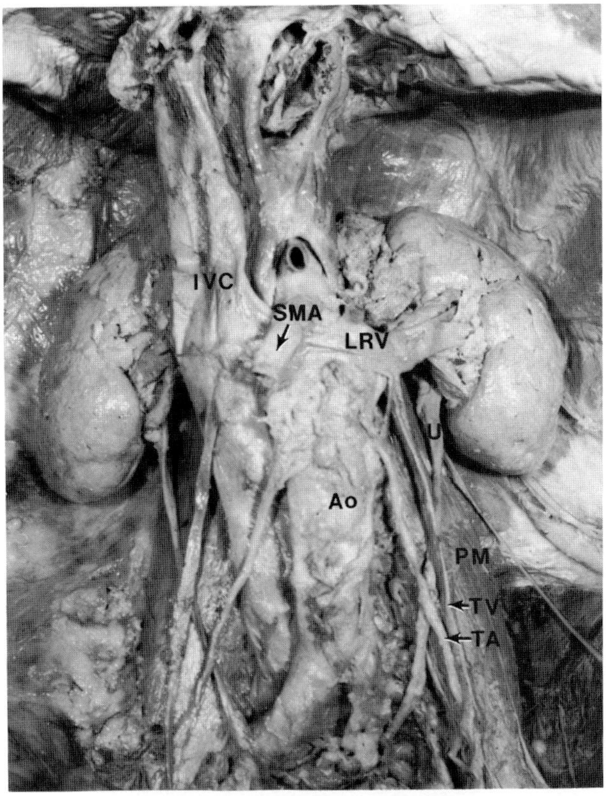

Figure 2.1. Anterior view of the posterior abdominal wall with all organs removed except the kidneys and adrenals. The aorta (*Ao*) and inferior vena cava (*IVC*) descend the posterior abdominal wall along the midline ridgeline formed by the lumbar spine. The left renal vein (*LRV*) courses posterior to the superior mesenteric artery (*SMA*). The testicular artery (*TA*) and vein (*TV*) cross anterior to the ureter (*U*) on the surface of the psoas major (*PM*).

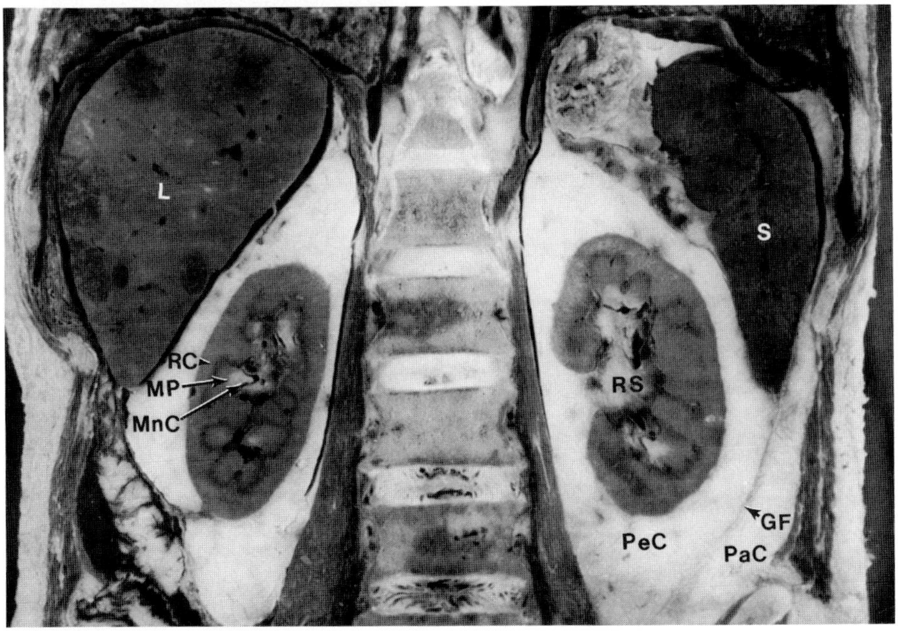

Figure 2.2. Coronal section through the hilus of the left kidney and just posterior to the hilus of the right kidney. The renal cortex (*RC*), medullary pyramids (*MP*), and minor calices (*MnC*) are well visualized. Gerota's fascia (*GF*) separates the perirenal (*PeC*) and pararenal compartments (*PaC*) of the retroperitoneum. Perirenal fat is continuous through the hilus with that in the renal sinus (*RS*). The lateral relationships of the liver (*L*) and spleen (*S*) to the kidneys illustrate why they provide good renal acoustic windows.

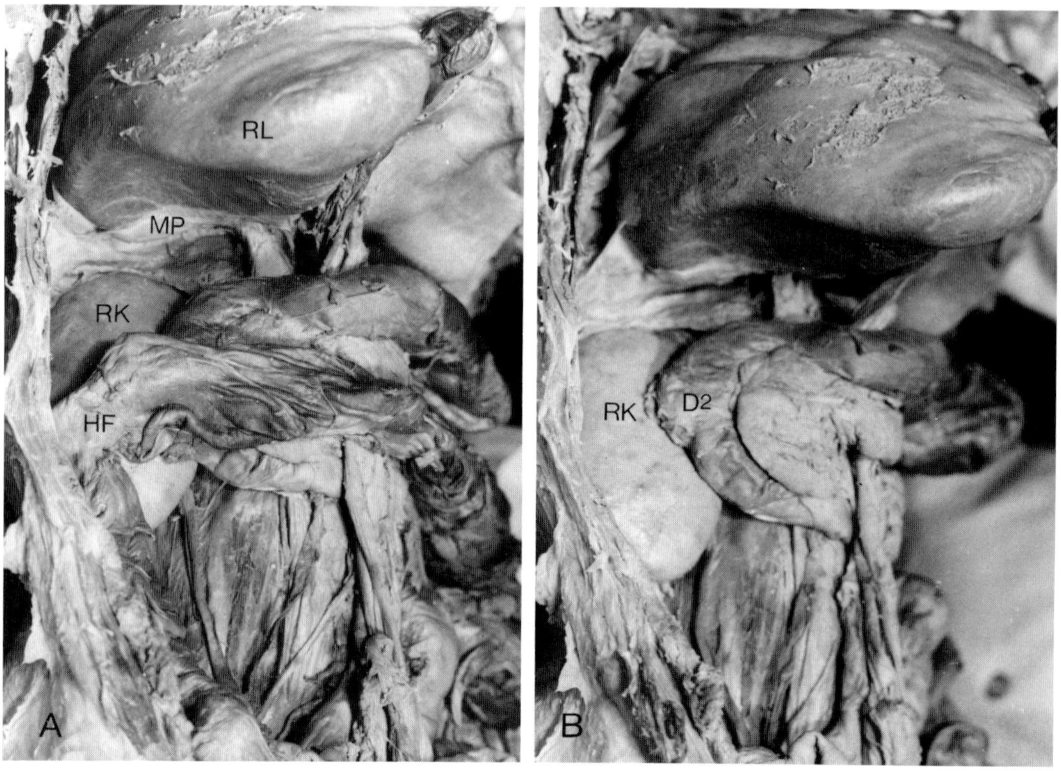

Figure 2.3. Staged dissection of the right kidney (*RK*) viewed from the right. **A** shows its relationships to the hepatic flexure of the colon (*HF*), right lobe of liver (*RL*), and Morrison's pouch (*MP*). **B** demonstrates its relationships to the second part of the duodenum (*D2*). In **C** the duodenum is retracted to display the kidney's relations to the adrenal (*Ad*), inferior vena cava (*IVC*), and psoas major (*PM*). **D** shows the right testicular artery (*TA*) and vein (*TV*) crossing the right ureter (*U*) and the right renal artery (*RRA*) passing behind the inferior vena cava. (**B** and **D** are modified from Schneck CD. The anatomical basis of abdominopelvic sectional imaging. Clin Diagn Ultrasound. Churchill Livingstone, New York, 1983;11:32–33.)

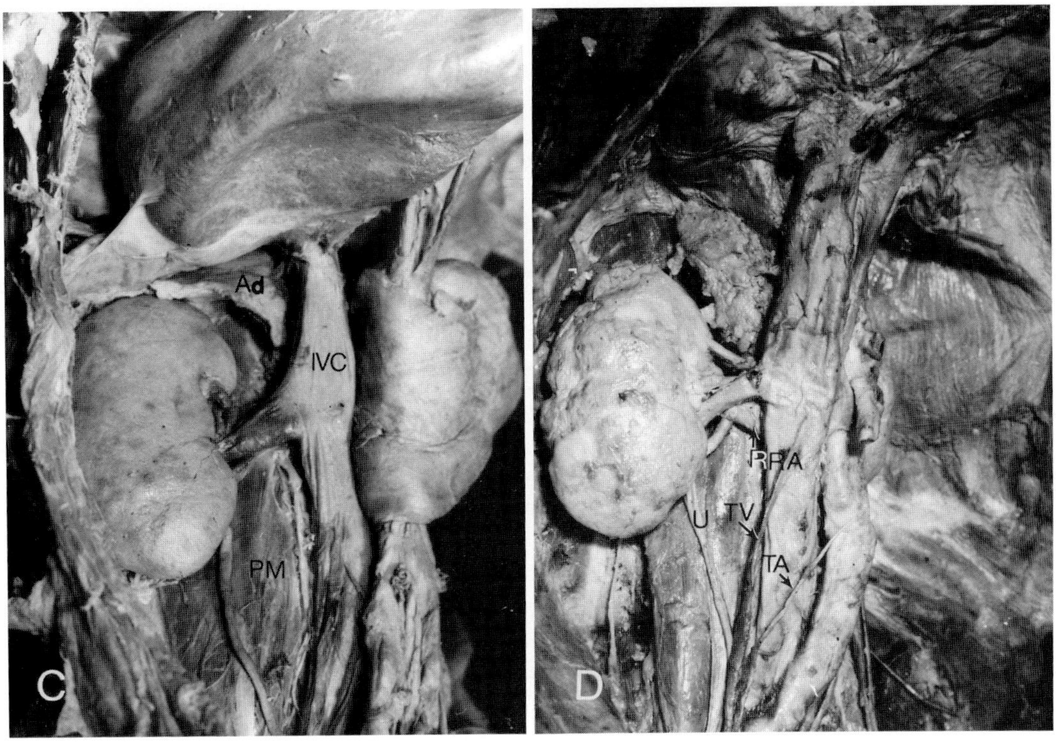

Figure 2.3. C and **D.**

length and thickness (Fig. 2.2). A long-axis view of the left kidney from the posterior axillary line uses the spleen as a window and displays its length and width (4). Transverse views of the kidneys provide width and thickness information.

The right kidney is typically, though not invariably, a centimeter or two lower than the left kidney, because of the larger volume of its superincumbent liver in comparison to the smaller normal spleen. In a supine position the kidneys usually lie at the level of the second lumbar vertebra where their vascular pedicle arises. In spite of their retroperitoneal position the kidneys are quite mobile and can descend a vertebral level or two in the upright position.

The right kidney has the right adrenal gland situated largely superiorly, though it usually descends a few centimeters down the kidney's upper anteromedial border (Figs. 2.3, 2.7, and 2.8). The upper part of its anterolateral surface is related to the right lobe of the liver across the hepatorenal pouch of Morrison (see Figs. 2.8 to 2.10 and 2.16 to 2.17). In the supine position Morrison's pouch is the most gravitationally dependent portion of the right side of the greater peritoneal sac. Hence, it is a common site of abscess formation within the greater peritoneal cavity. Since the duodenal loop usually droops posteriorly into the right paravertebral border, the second or descending part of the duodenum typically has an intimate relationship to the hilus of the right kidney and its vascular pedicle (Figs. 2.3 and 2.11 to 2.13). The lower anterolateral surface of the right kidney is related to the ascending colon and hepatic flexure (Figs. 2.3**A**, 2.11, and 2.12).

The left kidney has the left adrenal gland related more to its upper anteromedial border than to its superior aspect (Figs. 2.4, 2.5**A**, 2.7, and 2.8). The upper medial portion of its anterolateral surface is in the posterior wall of the omental bursa (lesser sac) (see Fig. 2.20) and is typically crossed by the pancreatic body and its associated splenic vessels (Figs. 2.4, 2.7, 2.8, and 2.20). The upper lateral portion of the kidney's anterolateral surface is related to the spleen across the greater peritoneal cavity (Figs. 2.4, 2.7, 2.8, and 2.20). The splenorenal ligament separates the lesser and greater peritoneal sacs at this point. The lower portion of the anterolateral surface of the left kidney is related to the splenic flexure and descending colon (see Figs. 2.8 to 2.12 and 2.21).

The muscular bed of both kidneys is formed by the diaphragm superiorly. Below it is formed from medial to lateral by the psoas major, quadratus lumborum, and transversus abdominus (see Figs. 2.1, 2.4**D**, 2.12, 2.16, and 2.17). The higher left kidney has a greater relationship to the diaphragm and often rises up to the tenth intercostal space. The right kidney more commonly ascends only to the eleventh intercostal space. Across the diaphragm the upper poles of non-ptotic kidneys are usually related to the costodiaphragmatic recess of the pleural cavity. The subcostal, iliohypogastric, and ilioinguinal nerves cross the kidney bed at lower levels (Fig. 2.4**D**).

The renal arteries arise from the aorta and the renal veins end in the inferior vena cava at the level of the upper part of the second lumbar vertebra (see Figs. 2.1, 2.3, and 2.4). The renal veins are usually anterior to the arteries until they break up into segmental branches as they approach the renal hilus. The right renal artery passes posterior to the inferior vena cava (see Figs. 2.3**D** and 2.18). The left renal vein courses anterior to the aorta within the "nutcracker" formed by the aorta behind and the superior mesenteric artery in front (Figs. 2.4 and 2.10). The left renal vein receives the left adrenal, left gonadal, and a communication from the second lumbar vein (Fig. 2.4). All of these veins typically enter the inferior vena cava on the right. Ultrasound evaluation of the renal vessels can detect occlusive phenomena and intravascular extension of renal carcinoma. At the renal hilus there is a continuing deep indentation into the kidney called the renal sinus. It contains the segmental branches of the renal vessels, the collecting system, and fat. The acoustic impedance differences between the diverse structures in the renal sinus produce a dense central echo complex on ultrasound images (see Figs. 2.8**B**, 2.10**B**, and 2.17**B**).

The renal parenchyma surrounds the renal sinus on all sides except at the hilus (see Figs. 2.2, 2.11, and 2.17). It is composed of an outer cortex that surrounds the more internally situated cone-shaped medullary pyramids (see Figs. 2.2, 2.9, and 2.16). The bases on the medullary pyramids face peripherally and their apices form renal papillae, which protrude into minor calices within the renal sinus. The cortex extends between the medullary pyramids to the renal sinus as the so-called renal columns of Bertin. However, to call these extensions columns is a misnomer, since they surround the medullary pyramids on all sides much like an egg carton surrounds its eggs (Fig. 2.7). A medullary pyramid and its surrounding cortex form a functional lobe of the kidney, since all of the urine produced in the surrounding cortex drains into that medullary pyramid. Each medullary pyramid has a grossly visible grain converging toward its papilla. This grain is produced by the parallel collecting ducts, the straight segments of Henle's loop, and interposed parallel vessels. Because of the homogeneity of the geometry of the tissues in the medullary pyramid they frequently appear quite sonolucent by ultrasound (see Fig. 2.16**B**). Their surrounding cortex has an echogenicity intermediate between the strong, dense echoes of the renal sinus and the sonolucent medullary pyramids. The closely spaced low-level echoes of the renal cortex are probably produced by the geometric heterogeneity of its renal and vascular structures, which include glomeruli, convoluted tubules, straight tubules, and arched and straight collecting ducts. The renal cortex is usually less echogenic than the adjacent liver or spleen parenchyma (4). The sonolucency of the medullary pyramids could be confused with a distended collecting system within the renal sinus. They can be differentiated from distended calices by the cortex between the pyramids and by the sometimes visualized arcuate arteries that arch over the base of the medullary pyramids and appear ultrasonically as bright specular echoes (see Fig. 2.16**B**).

As the ureter approaches the renal hilus it dilates to become the renal pelvis. This enters the renal sinus where it usually divides into two or three major calices. Each major calix divides into two to four minor calices whose expanded ends are indented by the renal papillae.

ABDOMINAL PORTION OF THE URETERS

A few centimeters outside of the hilus the renal pelvis narrows to form the ureter. Initially the ureters lie on the lateral aspect of the psoas major. As they descend toward the pelvis they gradually move onto the anterior aspect of the psoas major (see Figs. 2.1, 2.3, 2.4, and 2.13). At any level the left ureter may be more anterior than the right, because it originated higher and had an earlier opportunity to move forward (Fig. 2.13). The ureters typically cross the pelvic inlet anterior to the bifurcation of the common iliac artery. All other major vessels to which they are related tend to cross anterior to them. These can include an accessory renal artery, which commonly crosses the junction of the renal pelvis and ureter. Accessory renal arteries are frequently an inferior segmental branch that has an independent origin from the aorta. The ureters are also crossed on their anterior aspect by the right and left colic vessels and the gonadal vessels (Figs. 2.3 and 2.4). The ureters typically have three natural points of narrowing, which may retard the passage of calculi: the renal pelvis–ureter junction, where they cross the bifurcation of the common iliac artery, and as they pass through the bladder wall. The ureters can receive blood supply from any of their related arteries, from the renal arteries down to the inferior vesical arteries. The pelvic course of the ureter is described with the pelvis.

ADRENAL GLANDS

The adrenal glands are relatively flat organs with an outer cortex and an inner medulla. The left adrenal is semilunar in outline since it is molded over the superior and upper anteromedial aspects of the left kidney (Figs. 2.4**C** and 2.5**A**). The right adrenal is more triangular in outline because its anterior edge is flattened where it abuts the posterior aspect of the inferior vena cava (Fig. 2.3**C**). Both adrenal glands usually have a relatively sagittal orientation since they are situated on the side slopes of the longitudinal midline ridgeline of the posterior abdominal wall. They receive multiple arterial branches that enter their periphery, including superior branches from the inferior phrenic artery, a middle branch from the aorta, and inferior branches from the renal arteries. They are drained by a single vein, which leaves the adrenal gland at its hilus. The adrenal glands have a hilus which is a slit-like indentation running longitudinally down its lateral surface (Fig. 2.5**A** and **B**). The hilar indentation into this flat gland raises a ridge on the medial side of the gland (Fig. 2.5**C**). Hence in transverse section the adrenal glands can have a V-, K-, Y-, or X-shaped appearance on transverse sections through its hilus (Fig. 2.5**D**). In cuts above or

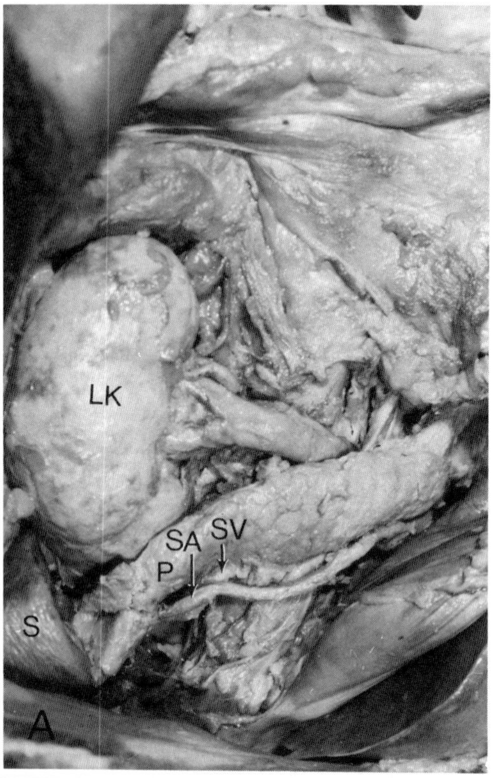

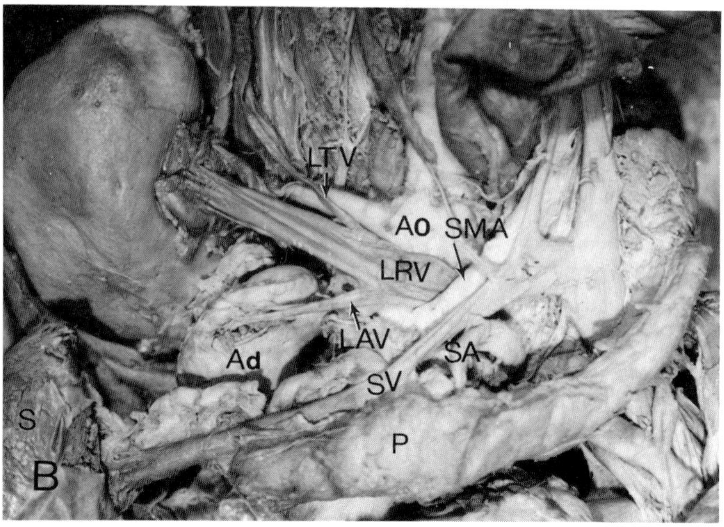

Figure 2.4. Staged dissection of the left kidney (*LK*) viewed from the left. **A** shows its relationships to the pancreas (*P*), spleen (*S*), and splenic artery (*SA*) and vein (*SV*). In **B** the pancreas and splenic vessels are elevated to reveal the kidney's left adrenal (*Ad*) relationships. In **B** and **C** the left renal vein (*LRV*) receives the left adrenal (*LAV*) and left testicular veins (*LTV*) and then passes through the nutcracker between the superior mesenteric artery (*SMA*) and aorta (*Ao*). The splenic vein passes anterior to the superior mesenteric artery. **D** shows the kidney bed relationships to the diaphragm (*D*), psoas major (*PM*), quadratus lumborum (*QL*), transversus abdominus (*TA*), subcostal nerve (*SN*), iliohypogastric nerve (*IHN*), and its ilioinguinal nerve (*IIN*). (**B** and **C** are modified from Schneck CD. The anatomical basis of abdominopelvic sectional imaging. Clin Diagn Ultrasound. Churchill Livingstone, New York, 1983;11:30.)

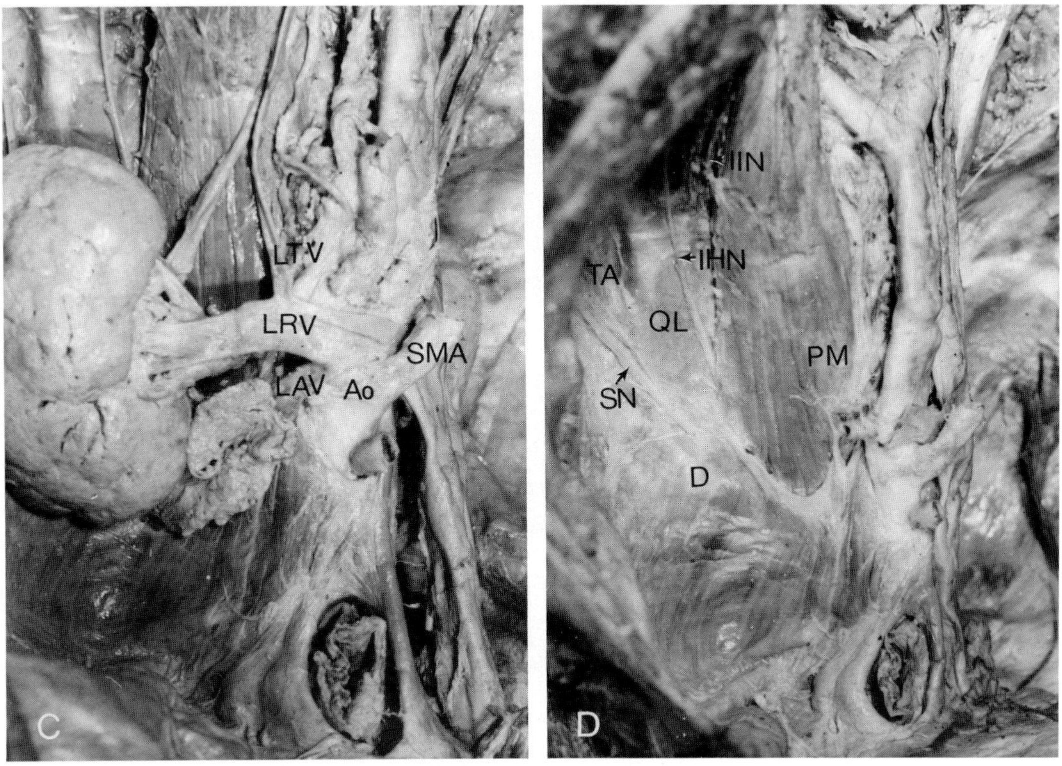

Figure 2.4. C and **D.**

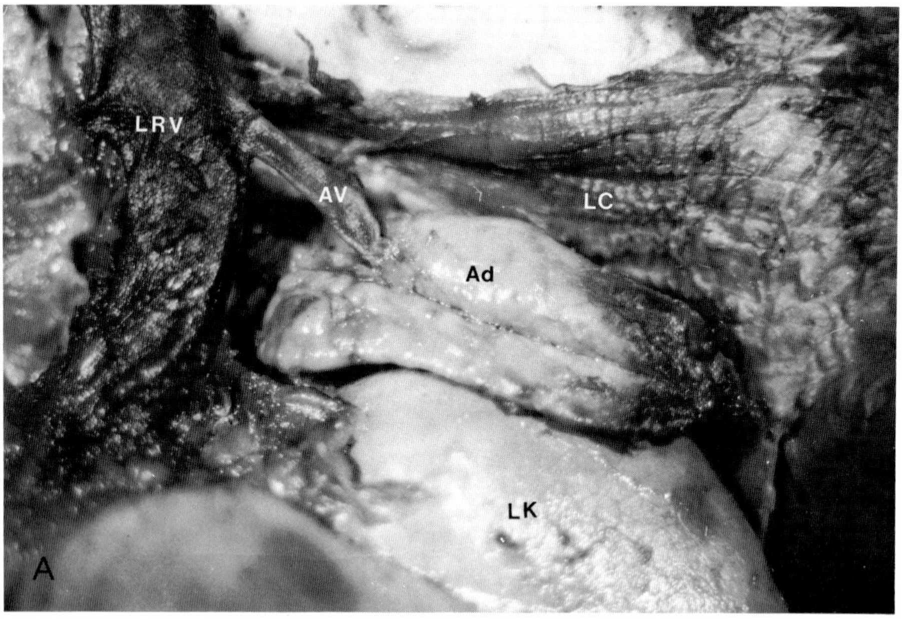

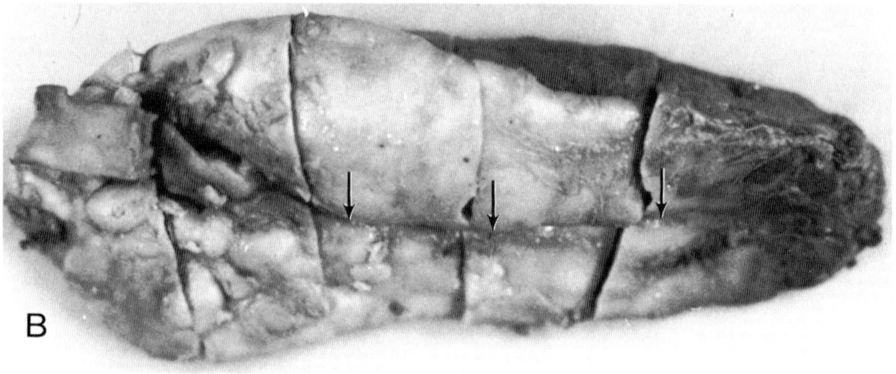

Figure 2.5. **A,** Lateral view of the left adrenal (*Ad*) gland in contact with the left kidney (*LK*) and left crus of the diaphragm (*LC*). Note the adrenal vein (*AV*) emerging from the lower part of its hilus and entering the left renal vein (*LRV*). **B,** Close-up view of the lateral aspect of the left adrenal after five axial cuts have been made. Note the longitudinally running hilus (*arrows*). **C,** Close-up view of the medial aspect of the left adrenal gland after sectioning. Note the longitudinally running medial ridge produced by the lateral hilar indentation. **D,** Transverse view of sections of left adrenal gland showing its changing axial geometry at different levels. Note that the infolded adrenal vein (*arrows*) produces the hilus.

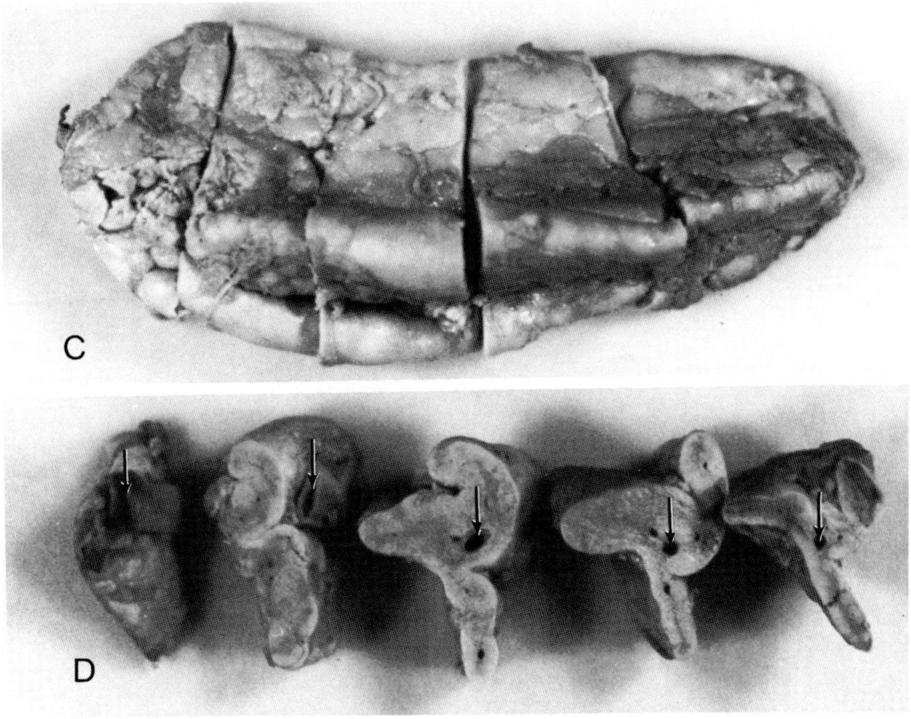

Figure 2.5. **C** and **D.**

below the hilus it usually has a linear or slightly wavy appearance.

The right adrenal gland is bounded medially by the right crus of the diaphragm, laterally by the right lobe of the liver, anteriorly by the inferior vena cava, and inferiorly and posteriorly by the right kidney (see Figs. 2.3, 2.7, 2.8, and 2.18). The upper part of the right adrenal is in contact with the bare area of the liver, while its lower portion is covered by the peritoneum over the posteromedial wall of Morrison's pouch. By ultrasound the right adrenal can be visualized posterior to the inferior vena cava at the level where it is crossed by the portal vein (see Fig. 2.18**B**). It is situated about 2 cm above the point where the right renal artery passes behind the inferior vena cava.

The left adrenal lies in the posterior wall of the omental bursa, where it is usually covered anterolaterally by the distal end of the pancreatic body and the associated splenic artery and vein (see Figs. 2.4, 2.7, and 2.8). This adrenal is related medially to the left crus of the diaphragm, posteriorly to the left kidney, and inferiorly to the left renal vein, to which it is tethered by the left adrenal vein.

ORGANIZATION OF THE RETROPERITONEUM

The retroperitoneum is situated between the parietal peritoneum covering the posterior abdominal wall and the fascia covering the inner aspect of the muscles of the posterior abdominal wall. It is divided into three compartments or spaces by the two layers of the renal (Gerota's) fascia. The anterior pararenal compartment is situated between the parietal peritoneum and the anterior layer of Gerota's fascia (Figs. 2.11 and 2.12). It contains the ascending colon, second through fourth parts of the duodenum, pancreas, descending colon, celiac trunk and its branches, superior mesenteric vessels, splenic vein, and their surrounding fat.

The perirenal compartment is situated between the anterior and posterior layers of Gerota's fascia. These fuse lateral to the kidney to become continuous with a layer of fascia called the lateroconal fascia that extends to the parietal peritoneum of the lateral paracolic gutter. The lateroconal fascia completes the separation of the anterior and posterior pararenal spaces laterally. Medially the renal fasciae blend with the renal vessels so that the perire-

Figure 2.6. The planes of the transverse (axial) sections of Figures 2.7 through 2.14.

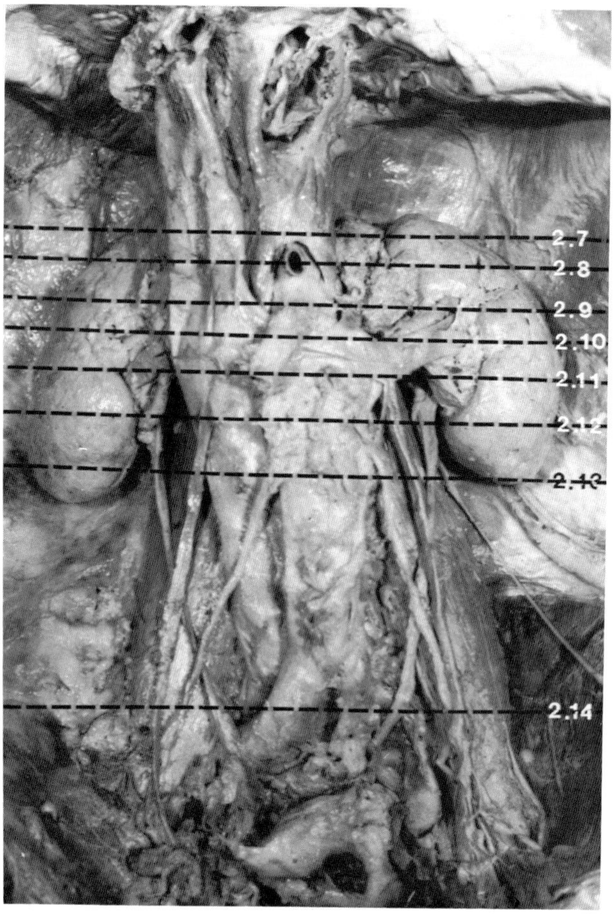

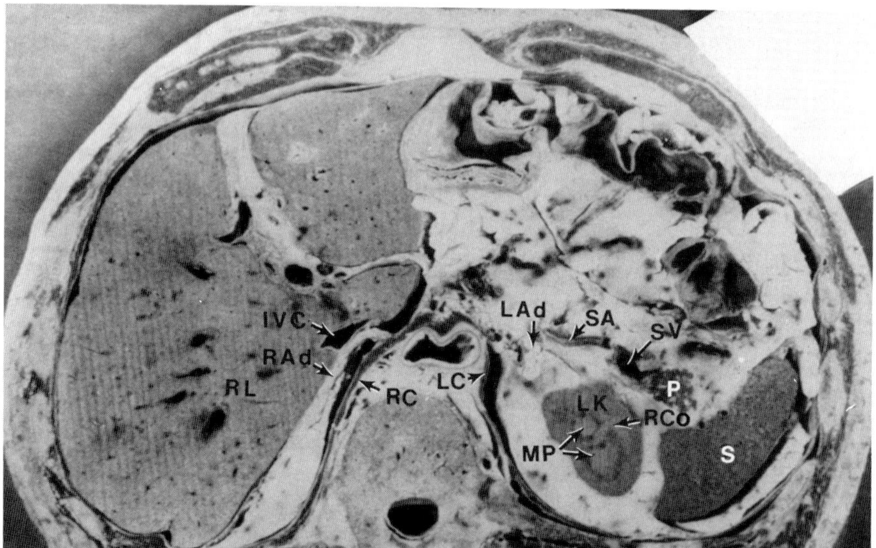

Figure 2.7. Transverse section through the right adrenal (*RAd*), left adrenal (*LAd*), and upper pole of the left kidney. The right adrenal's relationship to the right lobe of the liver (*RL*), inferior vena cava (*IVC*), and right crus of the diaphragm (*RCo*) are seen. The relationships of the spleen (*S*), pancreas (*P*), splenic artery (*SA*) and vein (*SV*), and left crus of diaphragm (*LC*) to the left kidney and left adrenal are shown. Note that the renal cortex (*RCo*) completely surrounds two medullary pyramids (*MP*) of the left kidney.

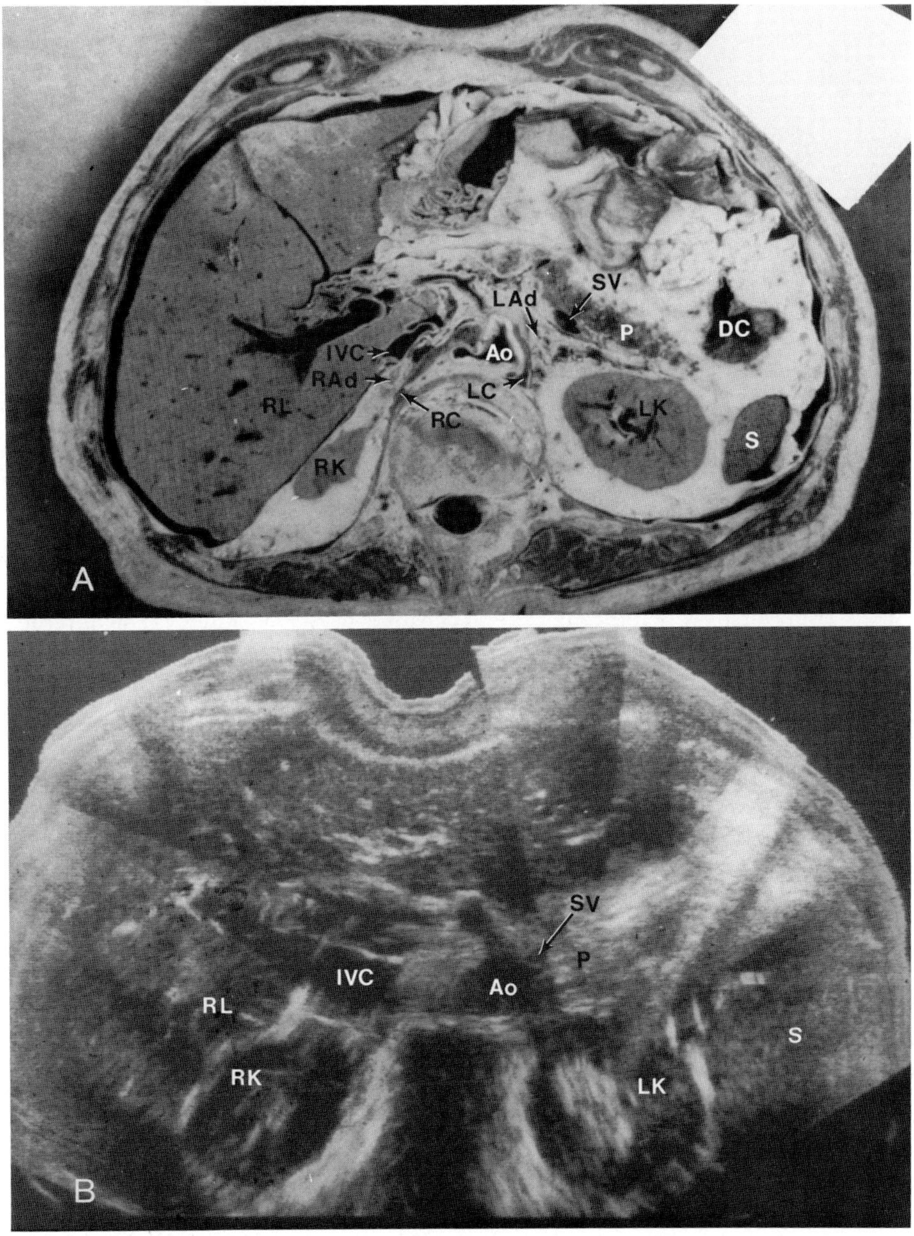

Figure 2.8. **A,** Transverse section through the upper pole of the right kidney. The relationships of the right adrenal (*RAd*) and right kidney (*RK*) to the right lobe of the liver (*RL*), inferior vena cava (*IVC*), and right crus of the diaphragm (*RC*) are shown. Also visible are the relations of the left adrenal (*LAd*) and left kidney (*LK*) to the spleen (*S*), pancreas (*P*), descending colon (*DC*), splenic vein (*SV*), aorta (*Ao*), and left crus of the diaphragm (*LC*). (Modified from Schneck CD. The anatomical basis of abdominopelvic sectional imaging. Clin Diagn Ultrasound. Churchill Livingstone, New York, 1983;11:15.) **B,** Transverse ultrasound at a level similar to **A** displaying many of the same relations.

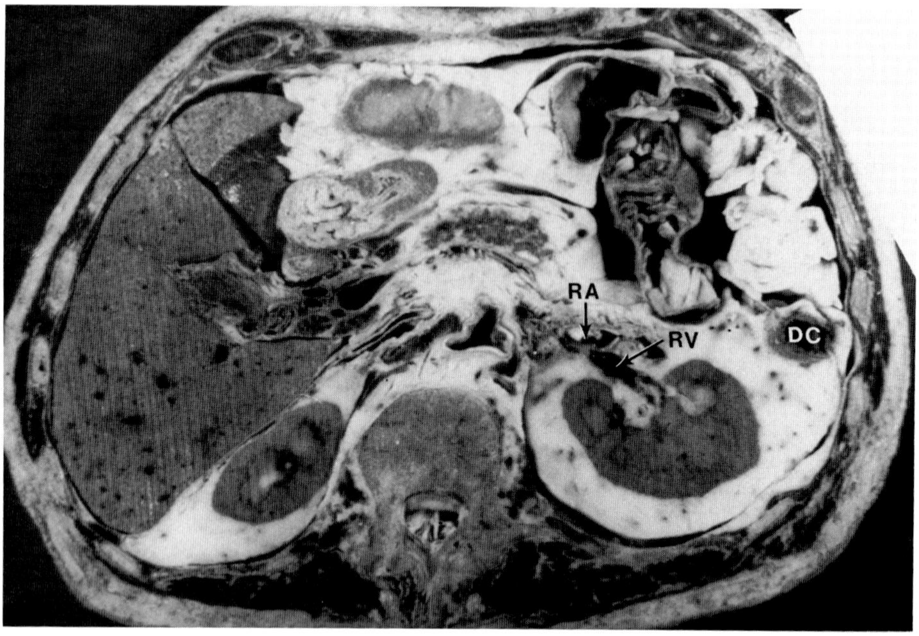

Figure 2.9. Transverse section through the upper hilus of the left kidney. The anteromedially directed hilus of the left kidney displays the renal artery (*RA*) and vein (*RV*). The relationship of the descending colon (*DC*) to the left kidney is shown. (Modified from Schneck CD. The anatomical basis of the abdominopelvic sectional imaging. Clin Diagn Ultrasound. Churchill Livingstone, New York, 1983;11:16.)

nal compartments of the two sides typically do not communicate. The perirenal compartment of each side contains the kidney, ureter, adrenal, the renal end of the renal vessels, and the perirenal fat, which is continuous with the fat in the renal sinus.

The posterior pararenal compartment is located between the posterior layer of Gerota's fascia and the fascia on the inner aspect of the muscles of the posterior abdominal wall. It contains only fat. It is continuous anteriorly with the extraperitoneal tissues of the anterolateral abdominal wall, which are sometimes called the properitoneal connective tissues. While the three compartments tend not to communicate with each other through most of the length of the abdomen, they have been described as having some continuities below at the level of the iliac fossae (5). The clinical significance of these three subdivisions of the retroperitoneum is that disease processes developing within one of the compartments tends to stay confined to that compartment. Hence, pathological findings localized within a given compartment (e.g., edema or hemorrhage) typically limit the differential diagnosis to pathology involving organs of that compartment.

PELVIC WALLS

The muscles lining the bony pelvis are frequently observed by ultrasound as relatively homogeneous structures with low echogenicity. They are commonly separated or surrounded by hyperechoic fascial planes. Recognition of these muscles can be useful in identifying important adjacent vascular and visceral structures. Further, pathological processes can occasionally originate in these muscles or more commonly invade them from adjacent structures. The muscles of greatest interest are the iliopsoas, piriformis, obturator internus, and the levator ani and coccygeus portions of the pelvic diaphragm.

The iliacus lines the inside of the ala of the ilium. The psoas major runs obliquely downward, forward, and laterally along the bony pelvic inlet (Fig. 2.22). They join to form the iliopsoas before they pass under the lateral part of the inguinal ligament. At lower levels the psoas major develops a dense tendon within its center. Hence, by ultrasound the iliopsoas muscle has a characteristic sonolucent periphery and a highly echogenic center. On descending transverse sections the iliopsoas gradually moves forward into the anterolateral pelvic walls (see Figs. 2.25 to 2.27). The common iliac and external iliac vessels lie along the medial aspect of the psoas and iliopsoas muscles. The vein typically lies behind its respective artery. On real-time ultrasonography these vessels appear anechoic. They can be differentiated by the pulsation of the artery and the distention of the vein during a Valsalva maneuver. Intimately related to these vessels are the common and external iliac lymph nodes, which can receive drainage from both bladder and prostate (Fig. 2.22**B**). The bifurcation of the common iliac artery serves as a landmark for locating the ureter as it enters the pelvis.

The obturator internus muscle arises from the inner aspect of the circumference of the obturator foramen. On transverse sections it is visible in the lateral pelvic walls throughout most of their superior-inferior extent (see Figs. 2.27 to 2.32). This muscle serves as a landmark for locating many pelvic vascular and visceral structures on sectional images. At higher pelvic levels the obturator neurovascular bundle lies along this muscle's anterior border (Figs. 2.22 and 2.27 to 2.29). These vessels are accompanied by the obturator lymph nodes, which receive some of the lymphatic drainage of the bladder and the prostate. The ureter and mainstem of the anterior divisions of the internal iliac artery and vein course along the inner aspect of the posterior part of the obturator internus (Figs. 2.22**B** and 2.27). The vas deferens runs along the medial aspect of the most anteroinferior portion of the muscle (Fig. 2.23**C**).

The piriformis muscle occupies the posterolateral pelvic side walls at high pelvic levels (Figs. 2.22**A** and 2.27). It originates from the front of the middle sacral segments and courses anterolaterally to exit the pelvis through the greater sciatic foramen. The sacral plexus, the posterior division of the internal iliac vessels, and the pelvic autonomic plexus are situated on its inner aspect. Therefore, any pelvic tumors extending to the piriformis muscles can produce lower-limb sensory and motor deficits and disruption of bowel, bladder, and genital function.

The pelvic diaphragm separates the pelvis above from the perineum below. It is composed of the levator ani and coccygeus muscles, which are enclosed by superior and inferior fasciae. It is shaped like an elliptical funnel with its apex directed posteroinferiorly (Figs. 2.22**A**, 2.31, 2.32, 2.37, and 2.38). The levator ani muscle forms the major part of the pelvic diaphragm. It originates anteriorly from the pubis on either side of the symphysis and posteriorly from the ischial spine. Between these two bony points of attachment it arises from the fascia over the obturator internus, which it converts into a tendinous arch. It separates the upper pelvic portion of the obturator internus from the lower perineal part. A major component of the levator ani is its pubococcygeus portion. These fibers sweep posteriorly from the pubis toward an anococcygeal raphe, which is stretched between the anal canal and coccyx. This part of the muscle is most intimately related to the prostate and anal canal (see Figs. 2.31 and 2.32). It is frequently seen ultrasonically as a sonolucent bounding structure for these organs (Fig. 2.32**B**). It has an elliptical outline with a major axis in the anteroposterior direction. The coccygeus is the smaller posterosuperior part of the pelvic diaphragm. It extends from the ischial spine to the sacrococcygeal junction (Figs. 2.22**A** and 2.29**A**).

PELVIC PORTION OF THE URETERS

After crossing the bifurcation of the common iliac artery the ureter descends along the posterior part of the obturator internus lying on the anterior aspect of the internal iliac artery (Figs. 2.22**B**, 2.23**C**, 2.26, and 2.27). The ureter then diverges medially where it is crossed on its anterosuperior surface by the ductus (vas) deferens as it approaches the bladder (Figs. 2.23**C**, 2.23**D**, and 2.29**A**). It typically enters the bladder wall just anterior to the fundus of the seminal vesicle. The intramural course of the ureter is very oblique. Hence, the intramural ureter is much longer than the thickness of the bladder wall.

BLADDER

The bladder apex lies posterosuperior to the pubis and commonly contacts the lower abdominal wall (Figs. 2.23 and 2.36). The superior aspect of the body of the bladder (bladder dome) is peritonealized as is its posterosuperiorly situated fundus (Fig. 2.23). These are usually in contact with loops of bowel that fill the rectovesical pouch (Figs. 2.27 and 2.28). The posteroinferior aspect is its base. It is situated be-

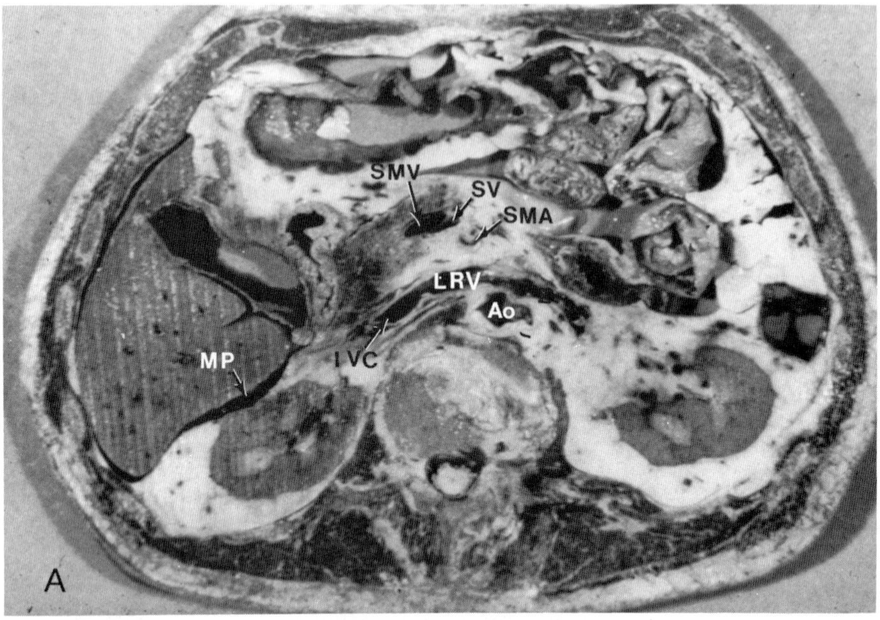

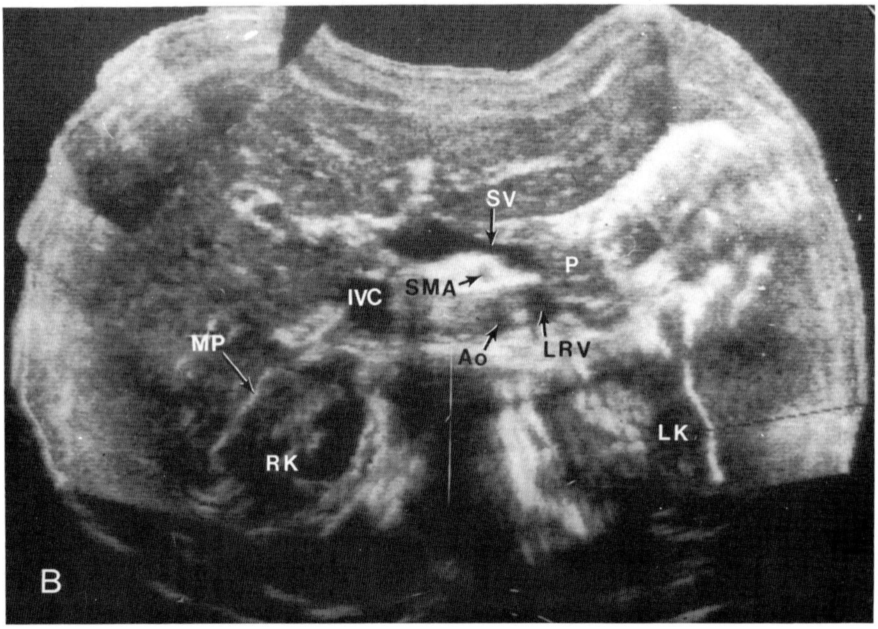

Figure 2.10. **A** is a transverse section through the hilus of both kidneys where the left renal vein (*LRV*) passes through the nutcracker formed by the aorta (*Ao*) and superior mesenteric artery (*SMA*) and enters the inferior vena cava (*IVC*). The splenic vein (*SV*) crosses anterior to the superior mesenteric artery and joins the superior mesenteric vein (*SMV*) to form the portal vein. Morrison's pouch (*MP*) is well visualized between the right lobe of the liver and right kidney. (Modified from Schneck CD. The anatomical basis of abdominopelvic sectional imaging. Clin Diagn Ultrasound. Churchill Livingstone, New York, 1983;11:16.) **B,** Transverse ultrasound at a level similar to **A** demonstrating many of the same relationships. *RK,* right kidney; *LK,* left kidney; *P,* pancreas. **C,** Transverse ultrasound demonstrating the left renal vein passing through the nutcracker of the superior mesenteric artery and aorta.

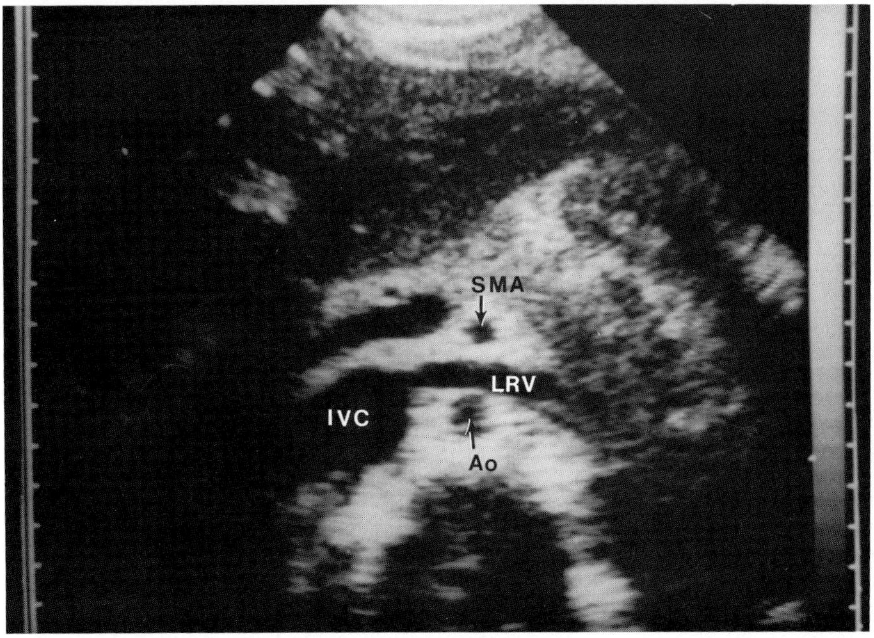

Figure 2.10 C.

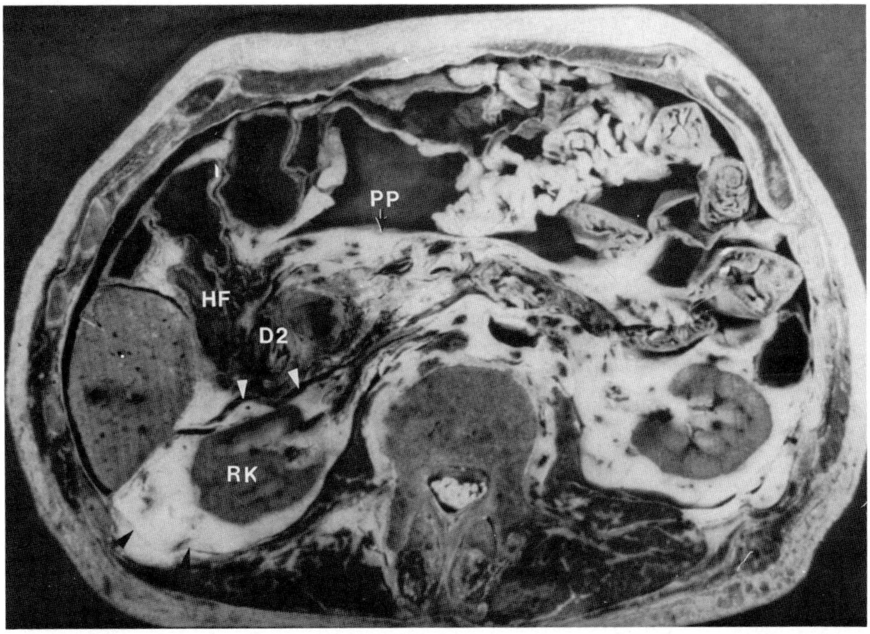

Figure 2.11. Transverse section through the lower hilus of both kidneys. It shows relationships of right kidney (*RK*) to the hepatic flexure (*HF*) and second part of the duodenum (*D2*). Both anterior (*white arrowheads*) and posterior layers (*black arrowheads*) of Gerota's fascia are seen on the right, as is the parietal peritoneum (*PP*) over the posterior abdominal wall.

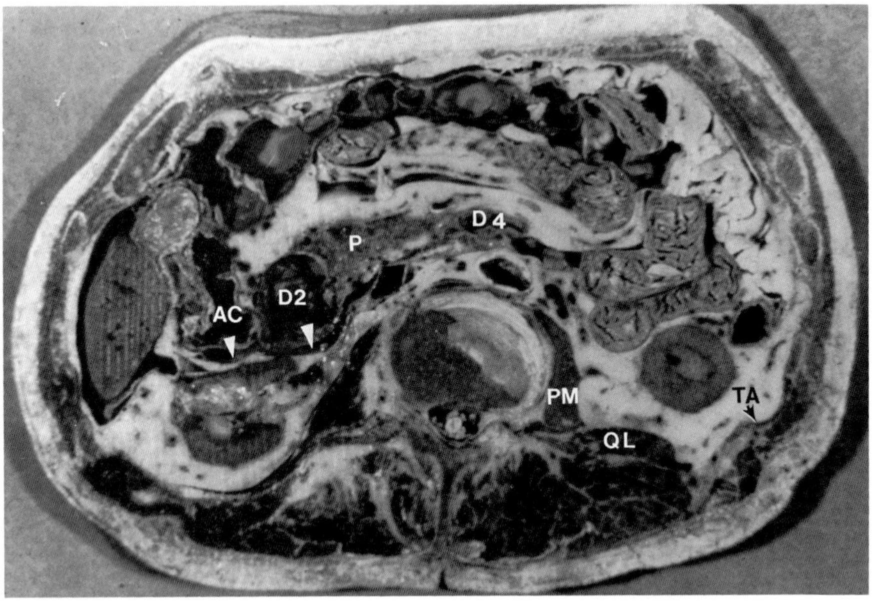

Figure 2.12. Transverse section through the lower pole of the left kidney. The anterior layer of Gerota's fascia (*white arrowheads*) appears as a fascial cleft. The ascending colon (*AC*), second (*D2*) and fourth (*D4*) parts of the duodenum, and the pancreatic head (*P*) are seen as contents of the anterior pararenal compartment. At this level the bed of the left kidney is formed by the psoas major (*PM*), quadratus lumborum (*QL*), and transversus abdominus (*TA*) muscles. (Modified from Schneck CD. The anatomical basis of abdominopelvic sectional imaging. Clin Diagn Ultrasound. Churchill Livingstone, New York, 1983;11:17.)

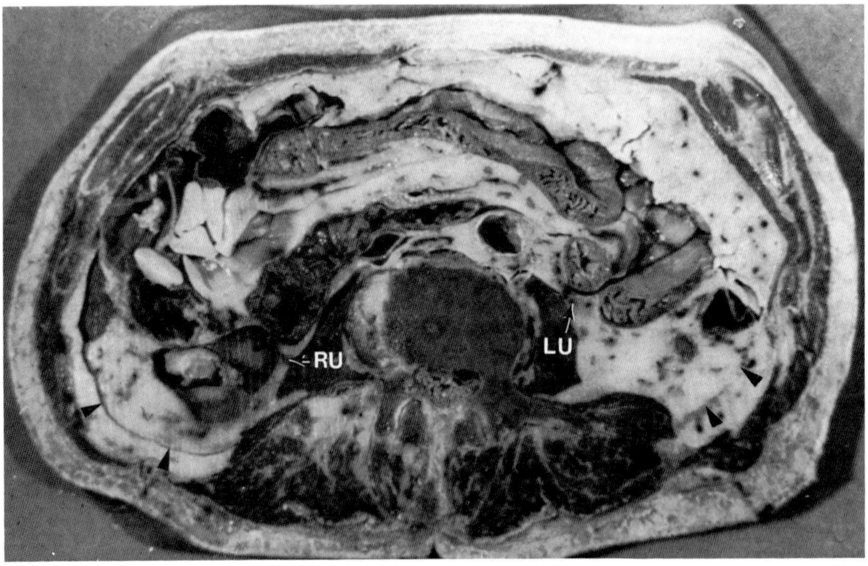

Figure 2.13. Transverse section through the lower pole of the right kidney, which contains a solitary cyst. The posterior layer of Gerota's fascia is shown on both sides (*black arrowheads*). Note that the posterior pararenal compartment is fat filled. The right ureter (*RU*) is lateral to the psoas major muscle, while the left ureter (*LU*) has moved farther anteriorly. (Modified from Schneck CD. The anatomical basis of abdominopelvic sectional imaging. Clin Diagn Ultrasound. Churchill Livingstone, New York, 1983;11:17.)

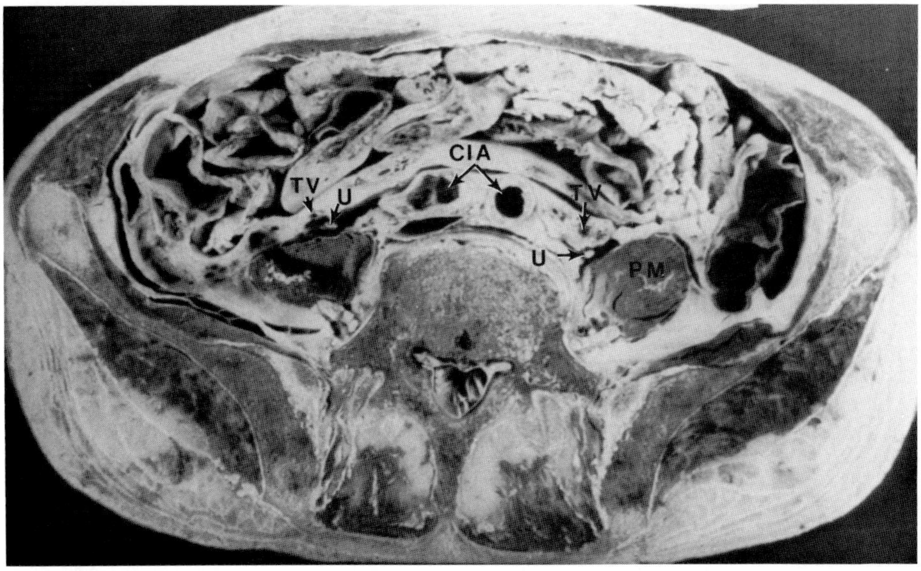

Figure 2.14. Transverse section just below the bifurcation of the aorta into common iliac arteries (*CIA*). Both ureters (*U*) are now on the anterior aspect of the psoas major muscles (*PM*). The testicular vessels (*TV*) cross the anterior surface of both ureters.

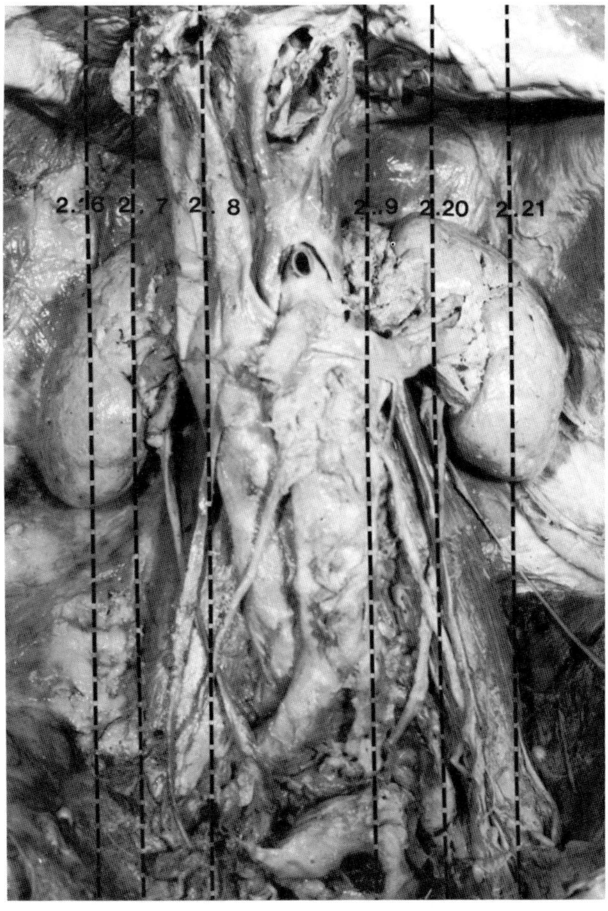

Figure 2.15. The planes of the sagittal sections of Figures 2.16 through 2.21.

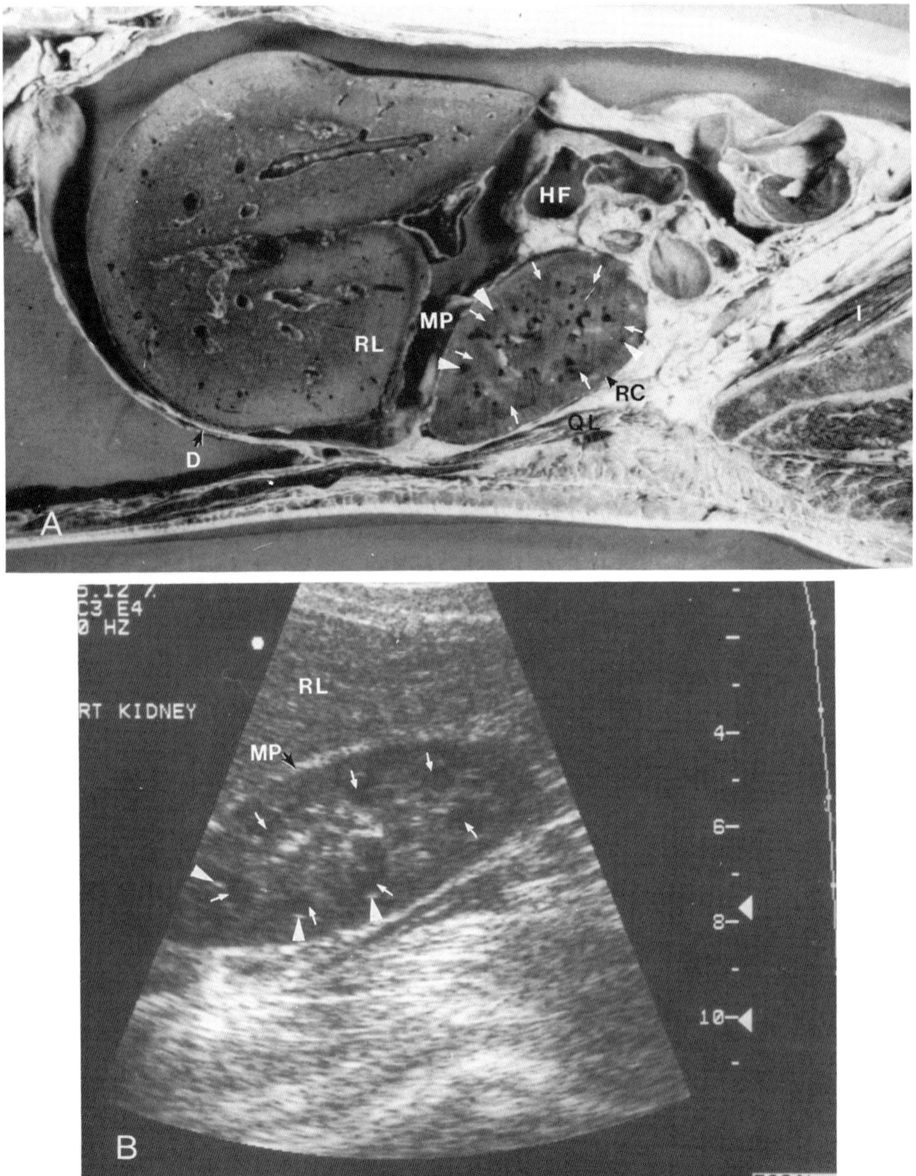

Figure 2.16. **A,** Sagittal section through the lateral part of the right kidney showing its cortex (*RC*), medullary pyramids (*small white arrows*), and some arcuate arteries at the base of the pyramids (*white arrowheads*). The right kidney's anterosuperior relationship with the right lobe of the liver (*RL*) across Morrison's pouch (*MP*) is demonstrated. The hepatic flexure contacts the kidney's lower anterior surface. The diaphragm (*D*), quadratus lumborum (*QL*), and iliacus (*I*) form the posterior abdominal wall. (Modified from Schneck CD. The anatomical basis of abdominopelvic sectional imaging. Clin Diagn Ultrasound. Churchill Livingstone, New York, 1983;11:18.) **B,** Sagittal ultrasound at a similar level to **A** showing many of the same features. Note especially the sonolucent medullary pyramids, the moderately echogenic renal cortex, and the bright specular echoes of the arcuate arteries.

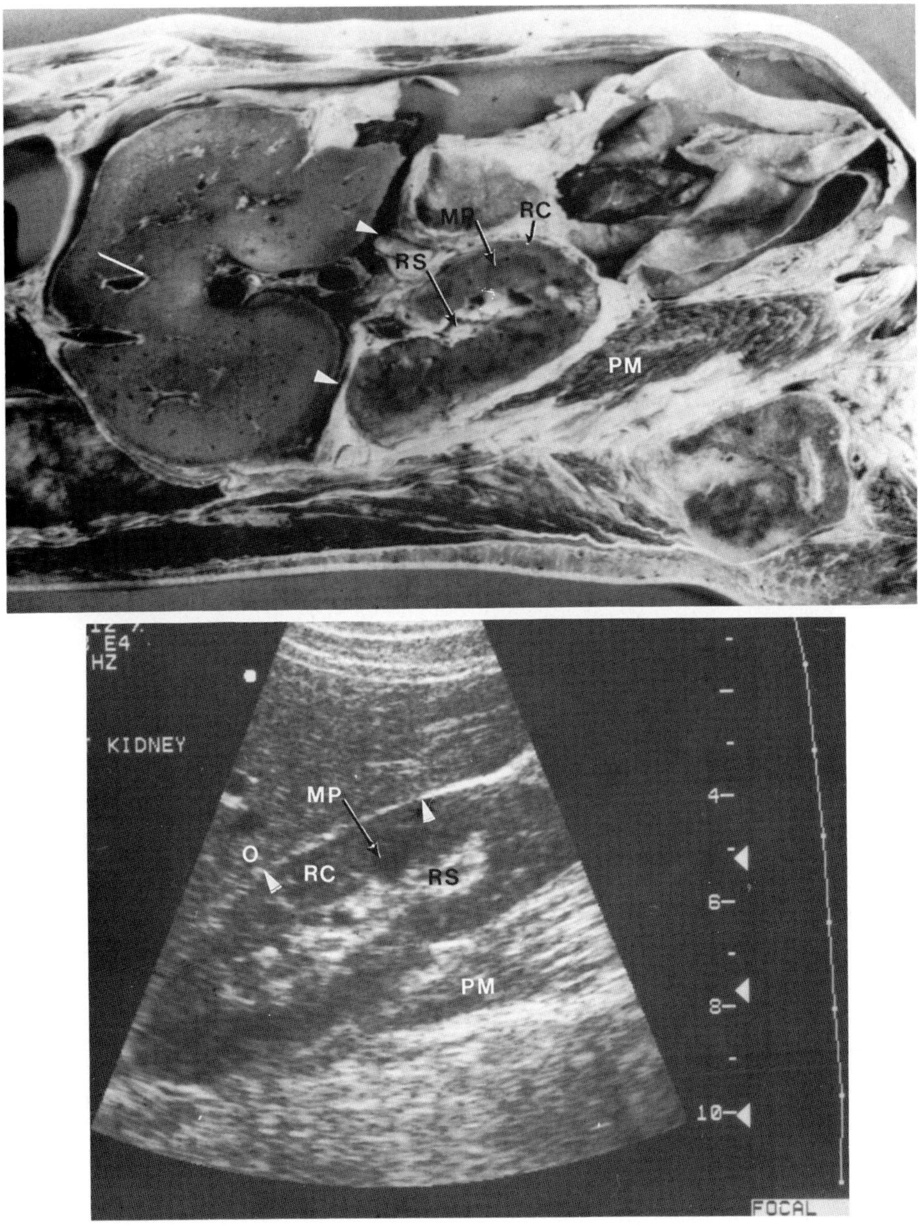

Figure 2.17. **A,** Sagittal section through renal sinus (*RS*) at the renal hilus displaying renal cortex (*RC*) and medullary pyramids (*MP*). *White arrowheads* indicate Morrison's pouch. The psoas major (*PM*) forms much of the medial part of the kidney bed. (Modified from Schneck CD. The anatomical basis of abdominopelvic sectional imaging. Clin Diagn Ultrasound. Churchill Livingstone, New York, 1983;11:18.) **B,** Sagittal ultrasound at about the same level as **A** showing many similar features.

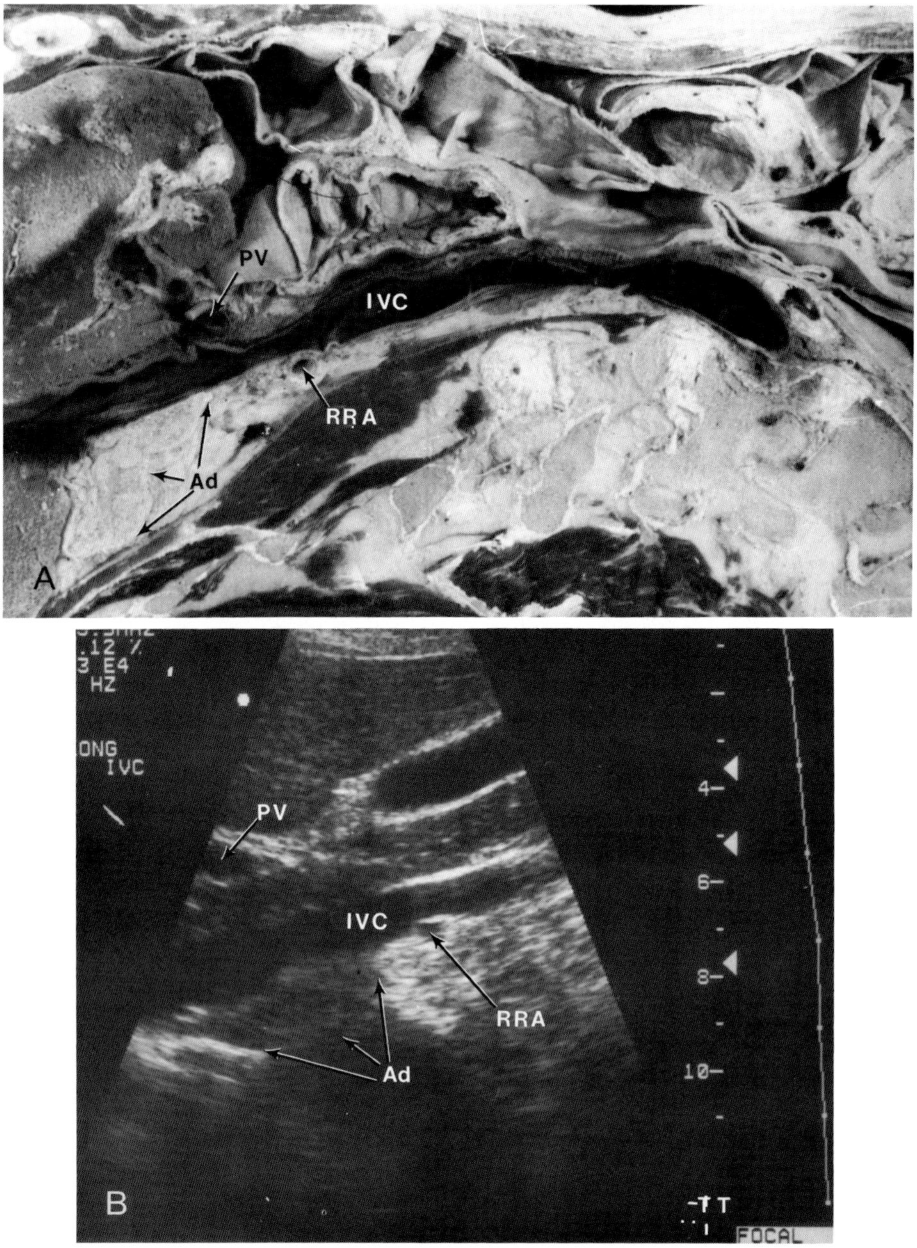

Figure 2.18. **A**, Sagittal section through the inferior vena cava (*IVC*) and right adrenal (*Ad*). Note portal vein (*PV*) crossing in front of the cava at the same level as the adrenal. The right renal artery (*RRA*) courses behind the cava about 2 cm below the adrenal. (Modified from Schneck CD. The anatomical basis of abdominopelvic sectional imaging. Clin Diagn Imaging. Churchill Livingstone, New York, 1983;11:19.) **B,** Sagittal ultrasound at the same level as **A** showing similar relationships.

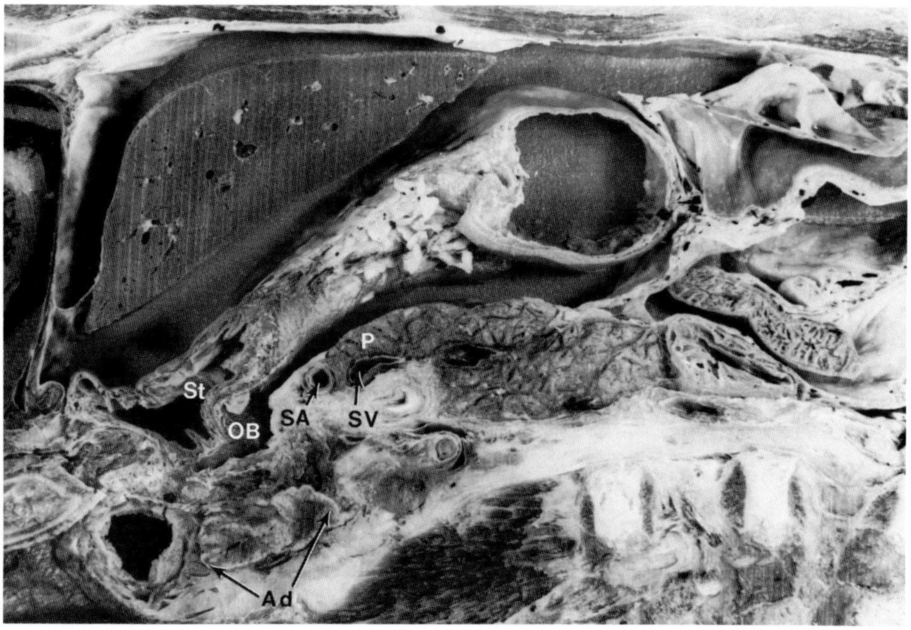

Figure 2.19. Sagittal section through the left adrenal (*Ad*). Note that it is related anteriorly to the stomach (*St*) across the omental bursa (*OB*) and to other retroperitoneal structures, including the pancreas (*P*) and the splenic artery (*SA*) and vein (*SV*). (Modified from Schneck CD. The anatomical basis of abdominopelvic sectional imaging. Clin Diagn Imaging. Churchill Livingstone, New York, 1983;11:19.)

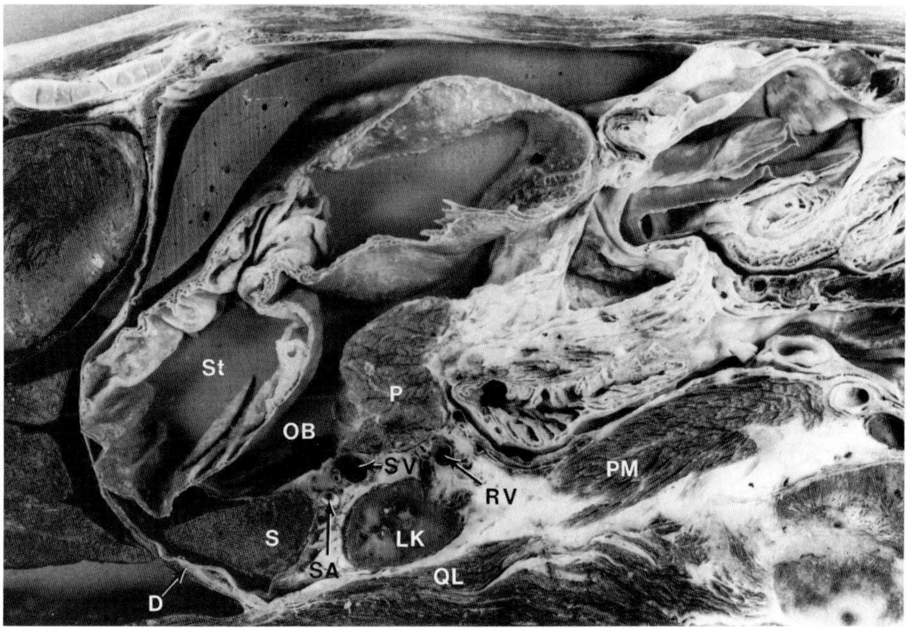

Figure 2.20. Sagittal section through only the medially situated upper pole of the left kidney (*LK*) with the renal vessels (*RV*) appearing to be inferior to the kidney. The kidney is related anterosuperiorly to the spleen (*S*), splenic artery (*SA*) and vein (*SV*), and pancreas (*P*). It is only indirectly related to the stomach (*St*) across the omental bursa (*OB*). Posterior to the kidney the diaphragm (*D*), quadratus lumborum (*QL*), and psoas major (*PM*) can be seen. (Modified from Schneck CD. The anatomical basis of abdominopelvic sectional imaging. Clin Diagn Imaging. Churchill Livingstone, New York, 1983;11:19.)

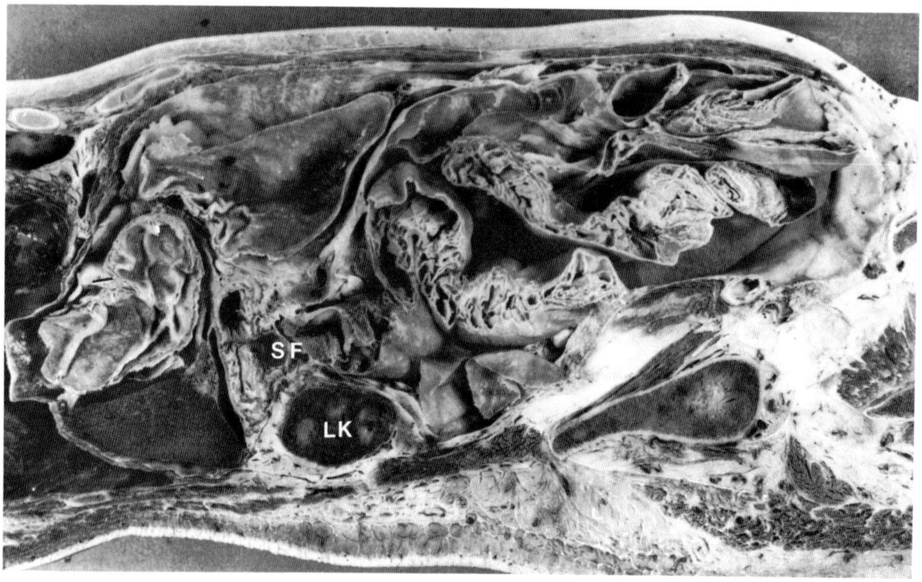

Figure 2.21. Sagittal section through the lateral portion of the left kidney (*LK*). It is now related anteriorly to the splenic flexure (*SF*) of the colon.

tween the intramural ureters and the urethra. It corresponds to the trigone region of the bladder interior. This part of the bladder is subperitoneal. It is related posteriorly to the seminal vesicles and ampullae of the vas deferens (Figs. 2.23, 2.29, and 2.30). The bladder neck surrounds the internal urethral orifice. It is related below to the base of the prostate gland. The anteroinferior aspect of the bladder is separated from the pubis by the loose connective tissue and fat of the retropubic space of Retzius (Figs. 2.23, 2.30, and 2.36).

The size, shape, and relationships of the bladder vary with its degree of filling. When it is empty it is very thick-walled and flattened against the posterosuperior aspect of the pubis, and thereby confined to the true pelvis (Fig. 2.23). As the bladder fills it becomes more round or ovoid and expands posterosuperiorly to fill more of the true pelvis and also expands anterosuperiorly to cross the pelvic inlet into the lower abdomen (see Figs. 2.27 and 2.28). It can then gain an anterior relationship to the rectus abdominus and a lateral relationship to the obturator internus, external iliac vessels, and iliopsoas. The distended bladder can produce a supravesical or prevesical peritoneal pouch between the bladder dome and the anterior abdominal wall (Fig. 2.28). As the filling bladder narrows the rectovesical pouch it displaces the contained bowel loops up into the abdominal cavity. This removes possible contained gas from the pelvis and facilitates ultrasound examination of the more posterior pelvic structures.

The bladder wall is formed by a narrow inner mucosa of transitional epithelium backed by the loose connective tissue, an intermediate detrusor layer of smooth muscle, and an outer connective tissue fibrosa that becomes a serosa on its peritonealized surfaces. In the contracted bladder the detrusor musculature throws the mucosa into folds except over the trigone region, where it is typically smooth. The trigone is the small triangular region bounded superolaterally by the internal ureteral orifice and inferiorly by the internal urethral orifice (Fig. 2.37). On a sagittal 3.5-MHz linear array sonogram the bladder wall appears as a single thin echogenic line surrounding the anechoic bladder cavity (Fig. 2.28**B**) (6). But with a 5.0-MHz scan three layers of the bladder wall can be resolved as a pair of echogenic lines flanking a sonolucent strip (Fig. 2.28**C**).

The bladder's arterial supply comes from superior vesical branches of the umbilical artery and from inferior vesical and occasional middle vesical branches of the internal iliac artery. Venous return drains into a perivesical plexus that is tributary to the internal iliac veins. Lymphatic drainage from the anterior bladder can reach the external iliac nodes and that from the lateral bladder can go directly to the obturator nodes. From the posterior bladder

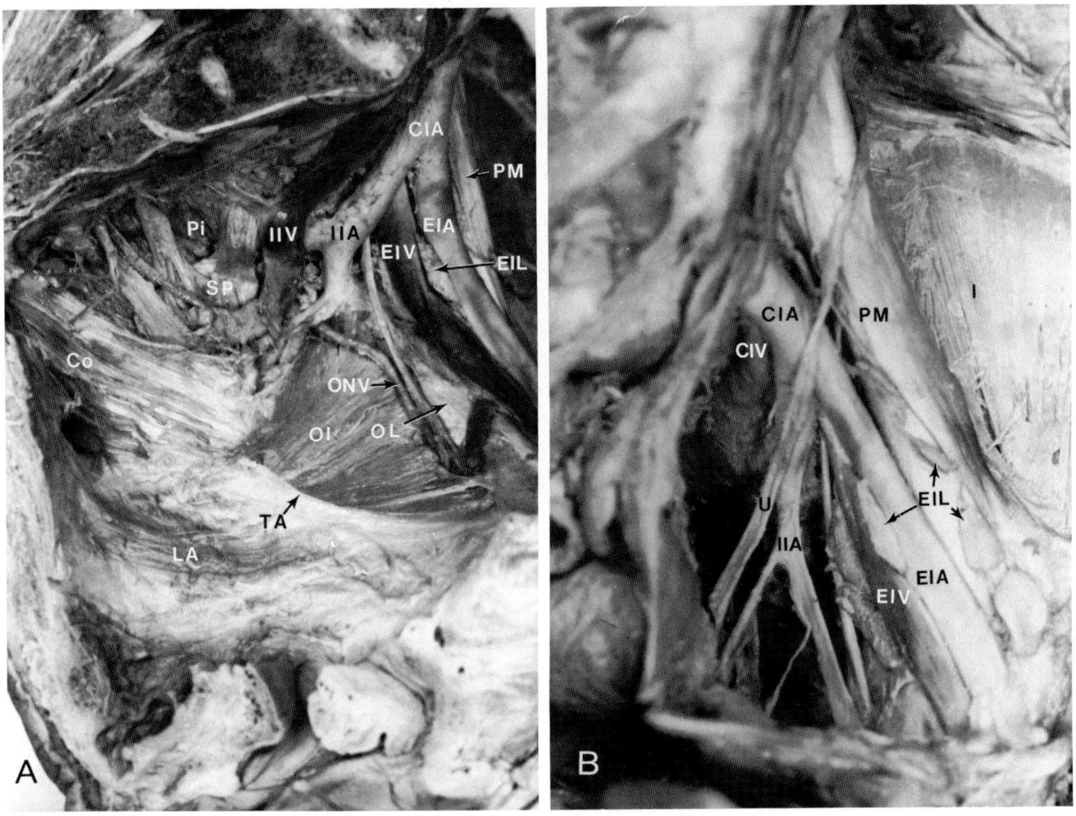

Figure 2.22. Pelvic walls. **A,** Midsagittal view of the pelvic sidewalls after removal of all organs. The psoas major (*PM*), common iliac artery (*CIA*), and external iliac artery (*EIA*) and vein (*EIV*) descend along the pelvic inlet. Accompanying these vessels are some external iliac lymph nodes (*EIL*). The obturator internus muscle (*OI*) has the internal iliac artery (*IIA*) and vein (*IIV*) coursing along its posterior border and the obturator neurovascular bundle (*ONV*) and obturator lymph nodes (*OL*) lying along its anterior border. The piriformis muscle (*Pi*) underlies the ventral rami of sacral plexus (*SP*). The coccygeus (*Co*) and levator ani (*LA*) portions of the pelvic diaphragm are displayed, as is its tendinous arch (*TA*) over the obturator internus. **B,** Anterior view of the left side of the pelvis demonstrating the iliacus (*I*), psoas major (*PM*), common iliac artery (*CIA*) and vein (*CIV*), and the external iliac artery (*EIA*) and vein (*EIV*) and their accompanying lymph nodes (*EIL*). The ureter (*U*) crosses the bifurcation of the common iliac artery and then runs along the anterior aspect of the internal iliac artery (*IIA*). (Modified by permission from Schneck CD et al. Embryology, anatomy, and histology. In: Friedman AC et al., eds. Clinical pelvic imaging. St. Louis: CV Mosby, 1990:9.)

drainage is into the internal iliac and occasionally the presacral nodes.

PROSTATE GLAND, PROSTATIC URETHRA, AND EJACULATORY DUCTS

The prostate gland is molded by the laterally related funnel-shaped levator ani into an inverted cone (Figs. 2.23 and 2.37). It has a flattened posterior surface that has a shallow median sulcus or furrow (Figs. 2.23**D** and 2.31). The flat prostate base is related above to the bladder neck. It typically slopes downward from behind forward, so on some axial images the lower bladder can project anterior to the prostate base (Fig. 2.23). The inferiorly directed prostate apex rests below on the urogenital diaphragm. At its base the prostate gland's mediolateral dimension is 4 cm and its anteroposterior dimension is 3 cm (7, 8). It measures 3.4 cm cephalocaudally. The convex anterior surface of the prostate is separated from the pubis by the fat-filled retropubic space of Retzius, sometimes called the anterior prostatic fascia. The flatter posterior surface of the prostate is typically separated from the rectum only by a relatively thin fascial layer called Denonvillier's fascia (Fig. 2.31). The posterosuperior aspect of the prostate is related to the duct of the seminal vesicle and vas deferens as they converge to form the ejaculatory duct. The prostate gland receives most of its arterial supply

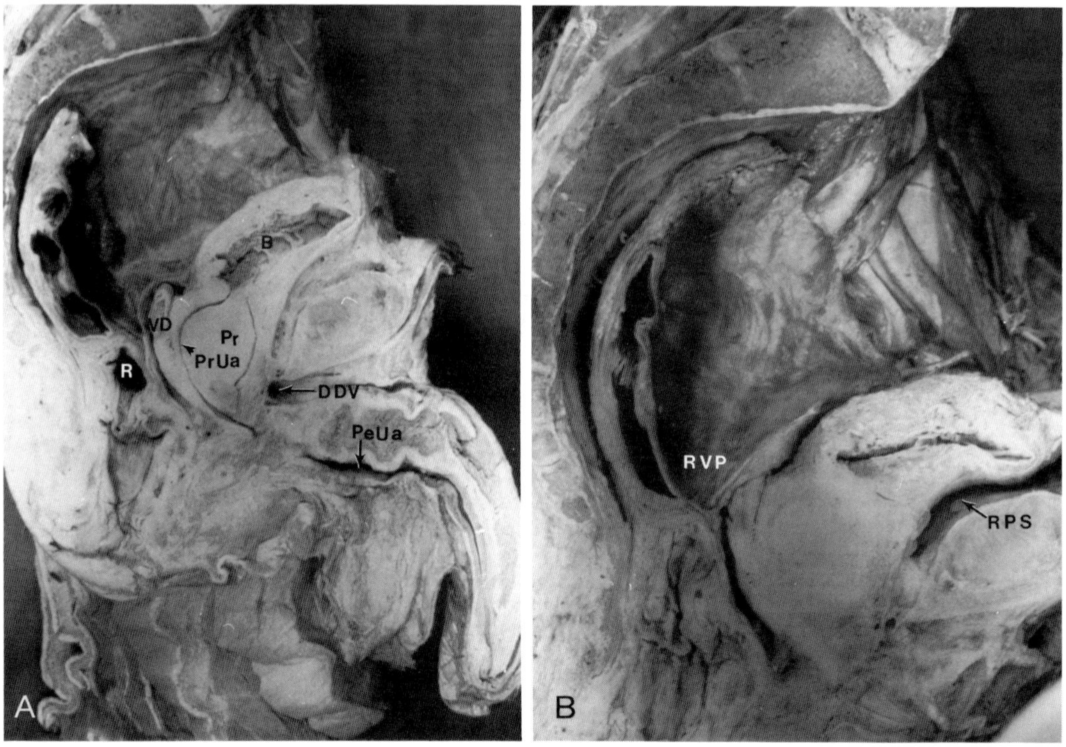

Figure 2.23. Dissections of the male pelvis. **A,** Midsagittal section of the male pelvis and perineum. Shown are the bladder (*B*), prostate (*Pr*), deep dorsal vein of the penis (*DDV*), prostatic urethra (*PrUa*), penile urethra (*PeUa*), vas deferens (*VD*) and rectum (*R*). **B,** Midsagittal section of the male pelvis with the peritoneum intact. It demonstrates the rectovesical pouch (*RVP*) and retropubic space of Retzius (*RPS*). **C,** The same specimen as **B** with the peritoneum removed to demonstrate the ureter (*U*) descending anterior to the internal iliac artery (*IIA*) and being crossed anterosuperiorly by the vas deferens (*VD*). The seminal vesicle (*SV*) is just lateral to the ampulla of the vas. **D,** Posterior view of a removed prostate (*Pr*), vas deferens (*VD*), seminal vesicles (*SV*), ureter (*U*), and bladder base (*B*). (Modified by permission from Schneck CD et al. Embryology, anatomy, and histology. In: Friedman AC et al., eds. Clinical pelvic imaging. St. Louis: CV Mosby, 1990:11.)

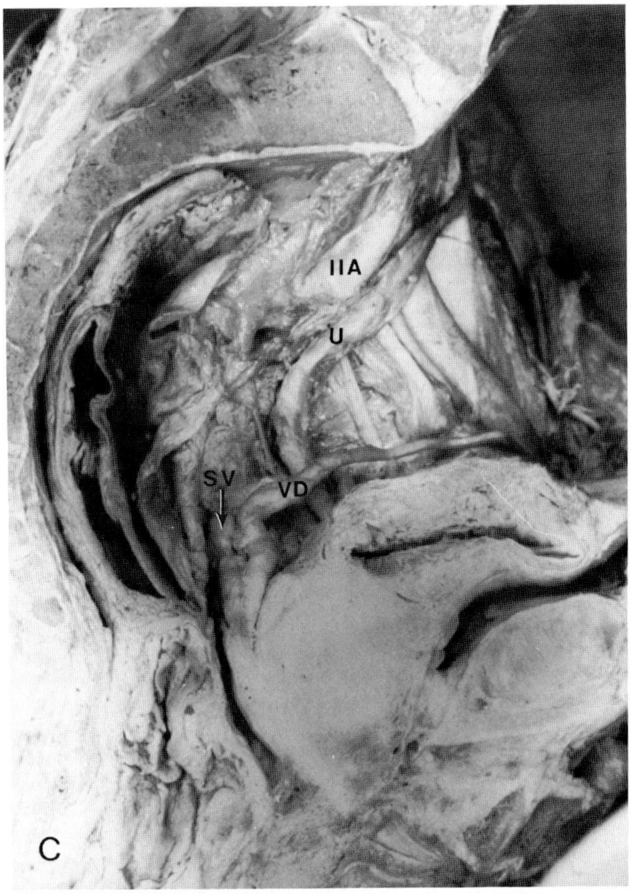

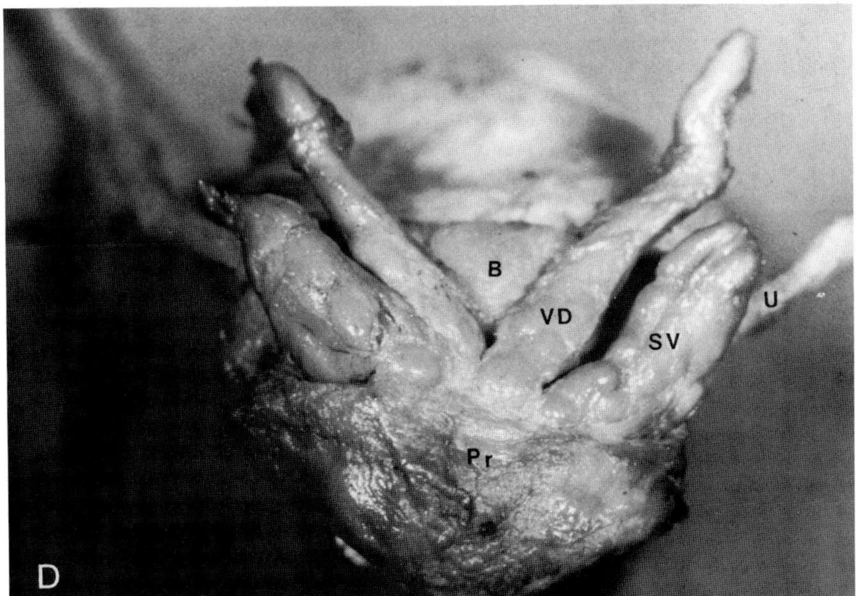

Figure 2.23. **C** and **D.**

Figure 2.24. A midsagittally sectioned and dissected male pelvis to orient the transverse (axial) planes of section of Figures 2.25 through 2.34.

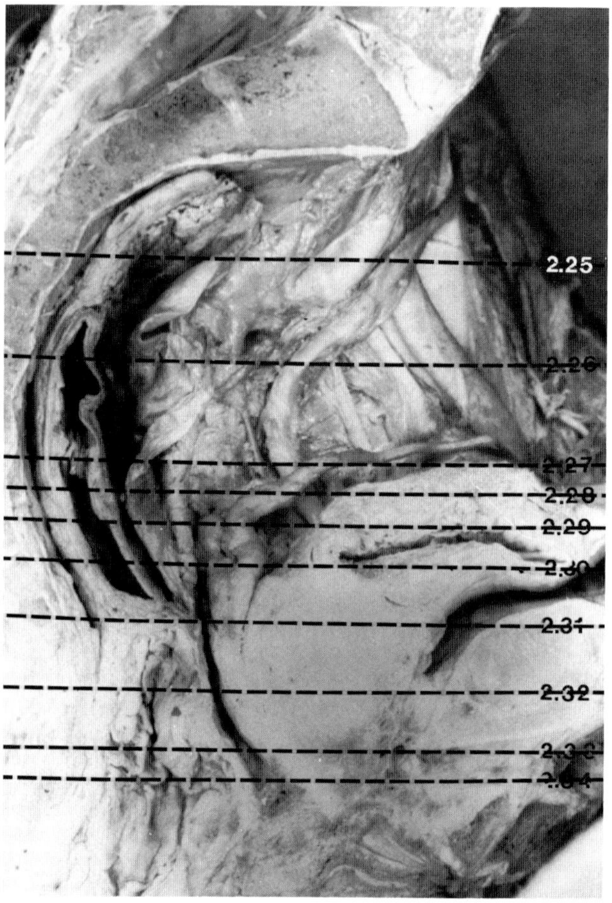

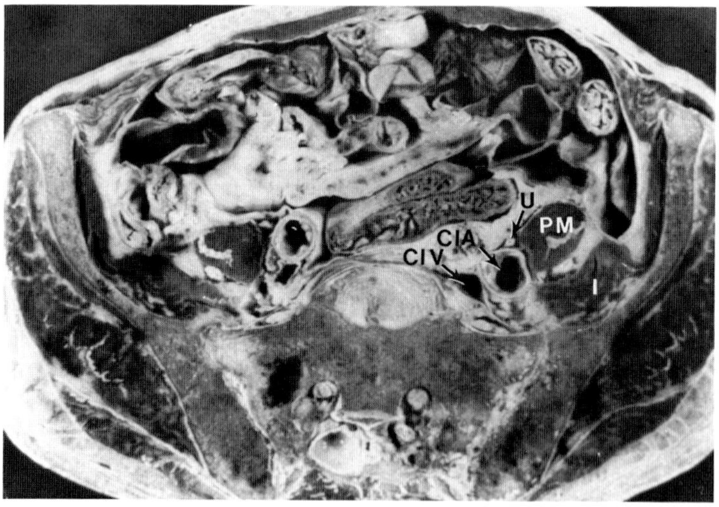

Figure 2.25. Transverse section at the level of the sacral promontory. The common iliac artery (*CIA*) and vein (*CIV*) are medial to the psoas major (*PM*). The ureters (*U*) are anterior to the common iliac artery. The iliacus (*I*) occupies the iliac fossa. (Modified by permission from Schneck CD, Friedman AC, Peterson RO. Embryology, anatomy, and histology. In: Friedman AC et al., eds. Clinical pelvic imaging. St. Louis: CV Mosby, 1990:29.)

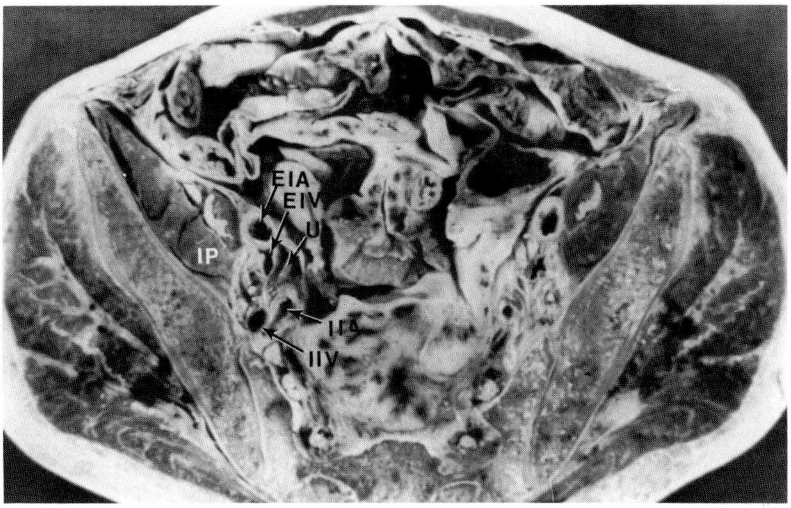

Figure 2.26. Transverse section at the level of the lower part of the sacroiliac joint. The external iliac artery (*EIA*) and vein (*EIV*) are medial to the iliopsoas muscle (*IP*). The ureter (*U*) is anterior to the internal iliac artery (*IIA*) and vein (*IIV*). (Modified by permission from Schneck CD, Friedman AC, Peterson RO. Embryology, anatomy, and histology. In: Friedman AC et al., eds. Clinical pelvic imaging. St. Louis: CV Mosby, 1990:30.)

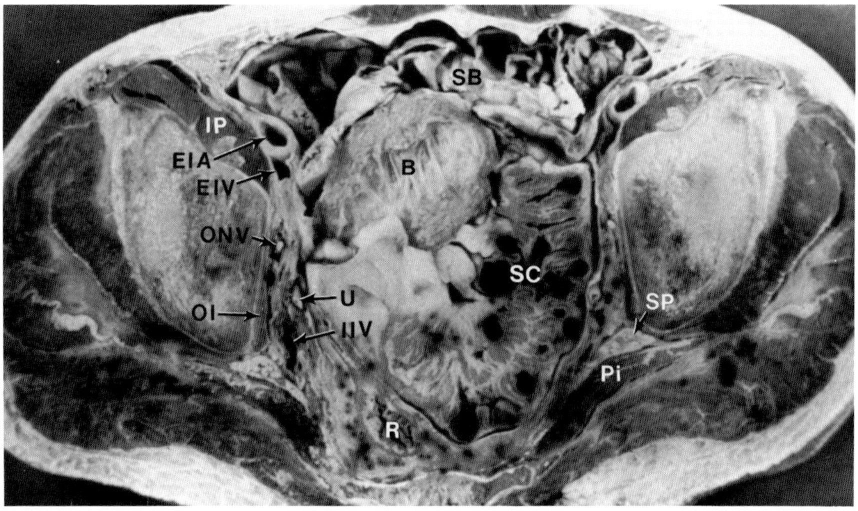

Figure 2.27. Transverse section through the bladder dome (*B*) of a distended bladder. The external iliac artery (*EIA*) and vein (*EIV*) and the iliopsoas (*IP*) course along the pelvic inlet. The obturator internus muscle (*OI*) forms the lateral pelvic side walls. It has the obturator neurovascular bundle (*ONV*) running along its anterior border and the ureter (*U*) and internal iliac vessels (*IIV*) coursing along its posterior portion. The piriformis muscle (*Pi*) forms the posterolateral pelvic sidewalls as it emerges from the greater sciatic foramen with the sacral plexus (*SP*) on its inner aspect. The rectum (*R*) lies on the anterior surface of the sacrum. Loops of sigmoid colon (*SC*) fill the rectovesical pouch and loops of small bowel (*SB*) fill the prevesical pouch. (Modified by permission from Schneck CD, Friedman AC, Peterson RO. Embryology, anatomy, and histology. In: Friedman AC et al., eds. Clinical pelvic imaging. St. Louis: CV Mosby, 1990:31.)

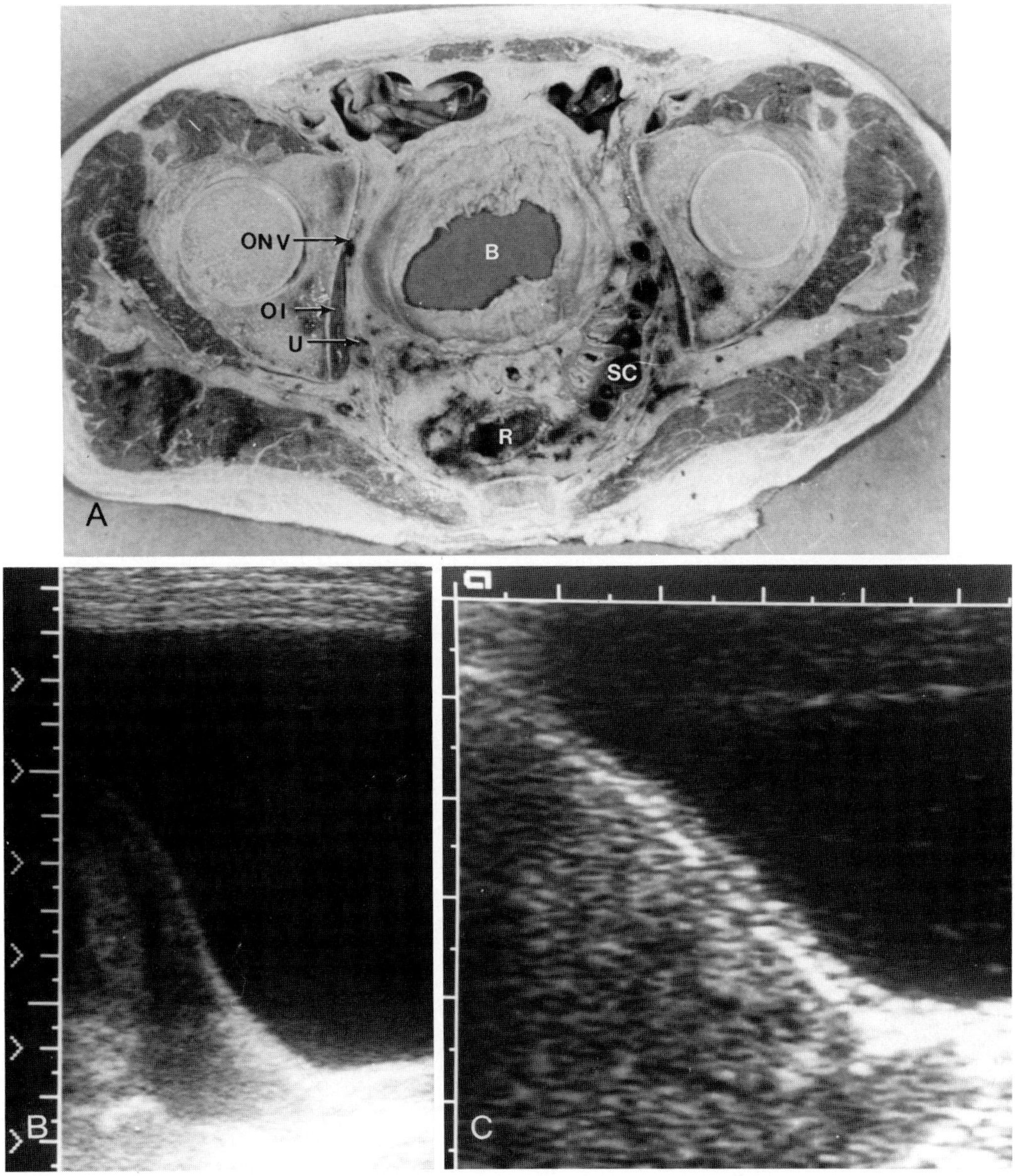

Figure 2.28. **A,** Transverse section through the upper portion of the body of a distended bladder (*B*) at the level of the upper hip joint. The obturator internus muscle (*OI*) has the obturator neurovascular bundle (*ONV*) coursing along its anterior border and has the ureter (*U*) medial to its posterior portion. Sigmoid colon (*SC*) separates the bladder (*B*) and rectum (*R*). (Modified by permission from Schneck CD, Friedman AC, Peterson RO. Embryology, anatomy, and histology. In: Friedman AC et al., eds. Clinical pelvic imaging. St. Louis: CV Mosby, 1990:32, 59.) **B,** Sagittal 3.5-MHz linear array sonogram that shows the bladder wall as a single thin echogenic line surrounding a distended anechoic bladder cavity. **C,** A 5.0-MHz scan that displays a three-layered bladder wall containing a pair of echogenic lines flanking a sonolucent strip.

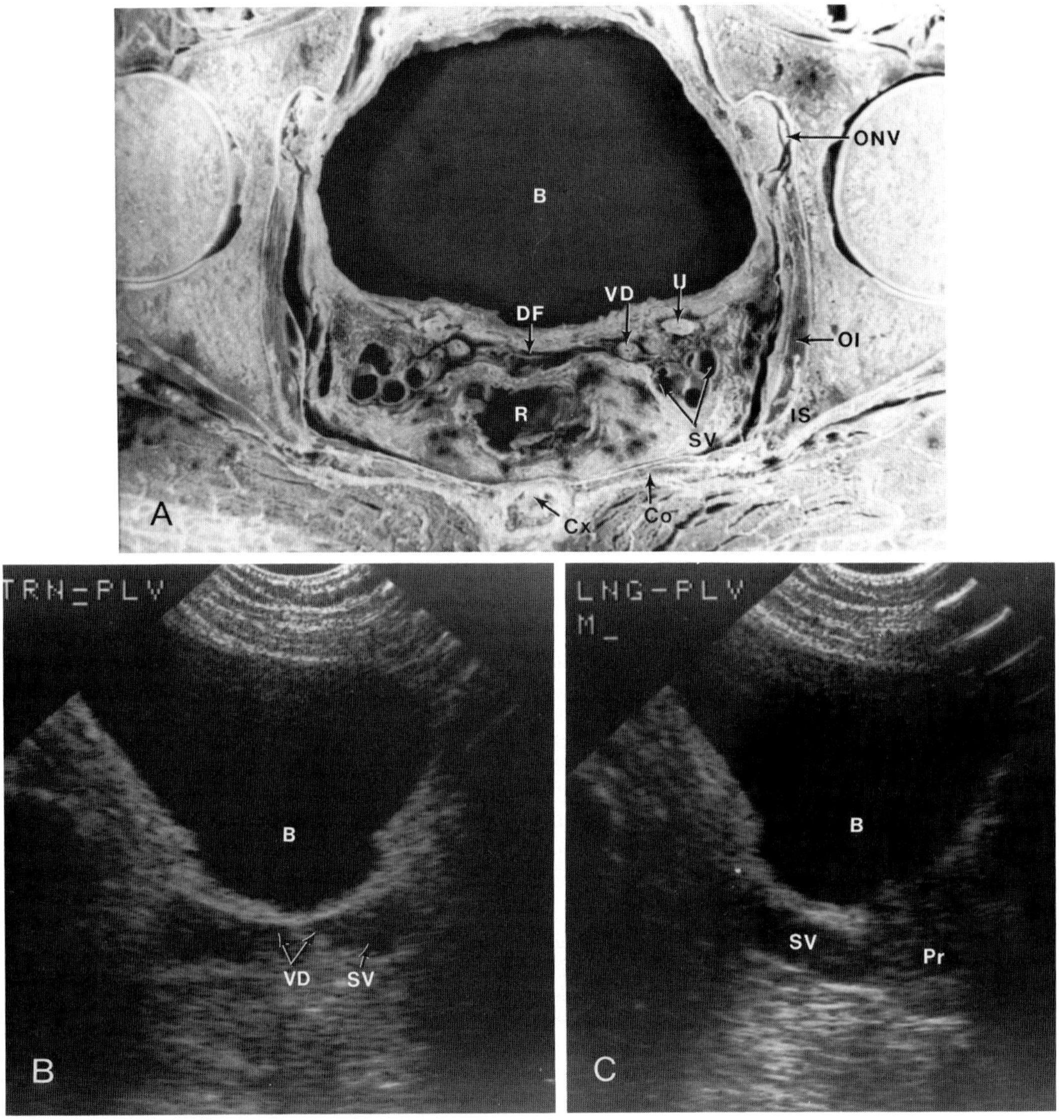

Figure 2.29. **A,** Transverse section through the midportion of a distended bladder just below the rectovesical pouch. The ureters (*U*) are just beginning their intramural course through the bladder (*B*) wall. They have the vas deferens (*VD*) medial to them and the apex of the seminal vesicles (*SV*) posterior to them. The bladder base is separated from the rectum (*R*) by a thin Denonvillier's fascia (*DF*). The coccygeus muscle (*Co*) extends from the iliac spine (*IS*) to the coccyx (*Cx*). The obturator neurovascular bundle (*ONV*) is now anterior to the obturator internus muscle (*OI*) as it is about to enter the obturator foramen. (Modified by permission from Schneck CD, Friedman AC, Peterson RO. Embryology, anatomy, and histology. In: Friedman AC et al., eds. Clinical pelvic imaging. St. Louis: CV Mosby, 1990:33.) **B,** Transverse sonogram demonstrating the bow tie appearance of the seminal vesicles (*SV*) and vas deferens (*VD*) as they lie posterior to the bladder (*B*). **C,** Parasagittal longitudinal sonogram demonstrating the long axis of the hypoechoic seminal vesicle (*SV*) posterior to the bladder (*B*) and above the more echogenic prostate gland (*Pr*). (Modified by permission from Schneck CD, Friedman AC, Peterson RO. Embryology, anatomy, and histology. In: Friedman AC et al., eds. Clinical pelvic imaging. St. Louis: CV Mosby, 1990: 33.)

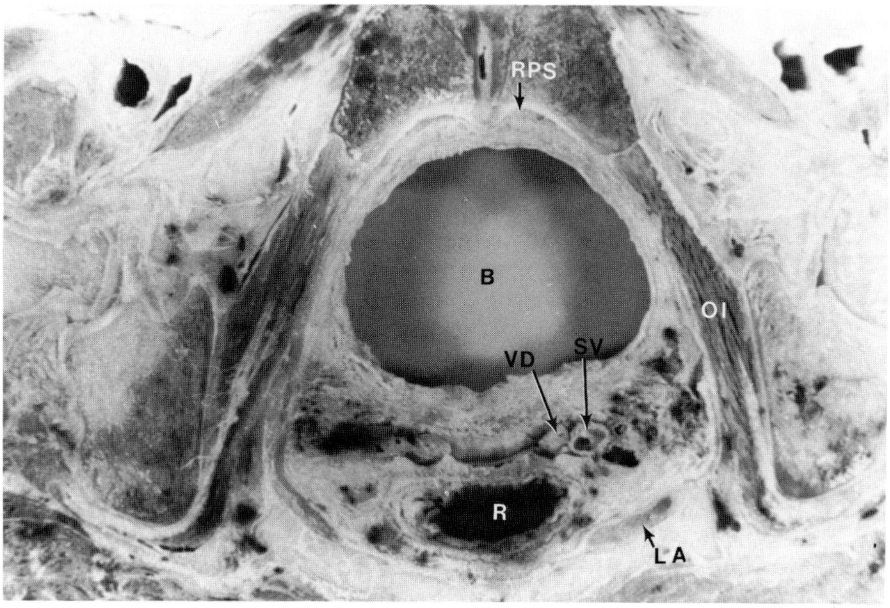

Figure 2.30. Transverse section through the bladder base. The retropubic space of Retzius (*RPS*) is anterior to the bladder (*B*). Lateral to the bladder the obturator internus (*OI*) muscles cover the inner aspect of the obturator foramen. Posterior to the bladder base the vas deferens (*VD*) and duct of the seminal vesicle (*SV*) are converging to form the ejaculatory duct. They are bounded posteriorly by the rectum (*R*). The levator ani (*LA*) portion of the pelvic diaphragm demonstrates some dehiscences as it encloses the lateral and posterior aspects of these pelvic organs. (Modified by permission from Schneck CD, Friedman AC, Peterson RO. Embryology, anatomy, and histology. In: Friedman AC et al., eds. Clinical pelvic imaging. St. Louis: CV Mosby, 1990:35.)

from the inferior vesical arteries. Its venous drainage is into the periprostatic venous plexus of Santorini, which also receives the deep dorsal vein of the penis (Figs. 2.23**A**, 2.31, and 2.32). Like the bladder, its lymphatic drainage can enter the internal iliac, external iliac, obturator, or presacral nodes.

The prostatic portion of the urethra courses through the prostate from the middle of its base to its apex (Fig. 2.23**A**). The posterior wall of the lower prostatic urethra is indented by a small rounded elevation called the seminal colliculus or verumontanum (Figs. 2.32 and 2.37). The term verumontanum means true mountain. This is a bit of an exaggeration to all but the cystoscopist. The paired ejaculatory ducts enter the posterosuperior aspect of the prostate and course downward and forward to open in the seminal colliculus (Figs. 2.23**A**, 2.31, 2.32, and 2.37). Between the openings of the ejaculatory duct there is a small midline cul-de-sac called the prostate utricle or vagina masculina (Fig. 2.32). This is a vestigial remnant of the fused müllerian ducts. The longitudinal grooves on either side of the verumontanum are the prostatic sinuses. They receive the majority of the openings of the prostatic ducts.

The prostate gland can be subdivided into five major lobes with somewhat imprecise boundaries (Figs. 2.23**A** and 2.31). The middle or median lobe is situated between the urethra and the ejaculatory ducts. It has a wedge shape in sagittal sections with a broad base that contacts the lower trigone region of the bladder and a narrow apex at the junction of the ejaculatory ducts and urethra. The posterior lobe is the relatively thin shell of tissue behind the ejaculatory ducts. Paired lateral lobes are lateral to the urethra and the anterior lobe is anterior to the urethra.

The prostate gland has a fibromuscular capsule that sends septa into its interior that separate its complex glandular elements. This stroma-parenchymal pattern occurs because the embryonic prostate gland develops as multiple epithelial ductal outgrowths from the urethra, which invade its posterior fibromuscular wall. As these ducts ramify complexly they

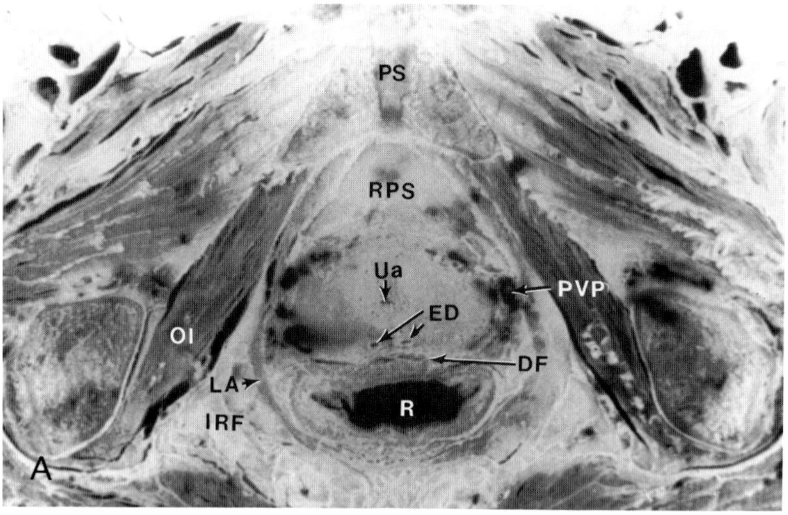

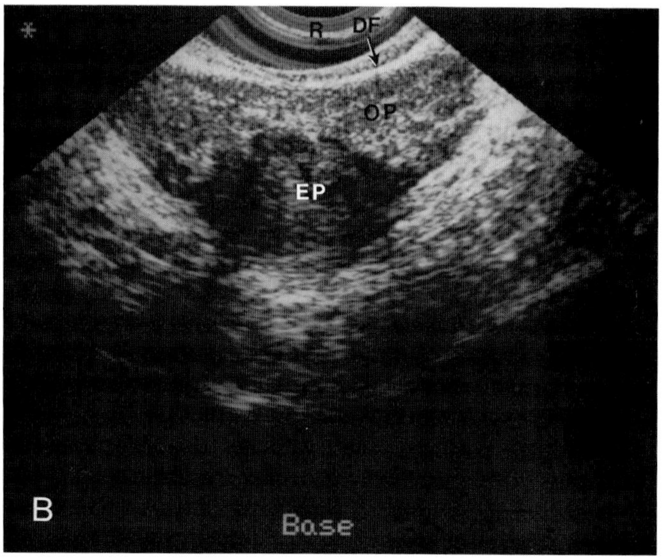

Figure 2.31. **A,** Transverse section through the prostate base that demonstrates the urethra (*Ua*) and ejaculatory ducts (*ED*) within the prostate. The prostate is related anteriorly to the pubic symphysis (*PS*) across the retropubic space of Retzius (*RPS*), laterally to the levator ani (*LA*) and posteriorly to the rectum (*R*), from which it is separated by the thin Denonvillier's fascia (*DF*). The prostate is surrounded by a substantial periprostatic venous plexus of Santorini (*PVP*). Outside the levator ani the fat-filled ischiorectal fossae (*IRF*) are seen. They are bounded laterally by the lower perineal part of the obturator internus (*OI*). (Modified by permission from Schneck CD, Friedman AC, Peterson RO. Embryology, anatomy, and histology. In: Friedman AC et al., eds. Clinical pelvic imaging. St. Louis: CV Mosby, 1990:36.) **B,** Transverse tranrectal sonogram displaying an echogenic outer prostate (*OP*) and a more anteriorly situated hypoechoic endoprostate (*EP*). Denonvillier's fascia (*DF*) provides a thin echogenic interface between the rectum (*R*) and prostate.

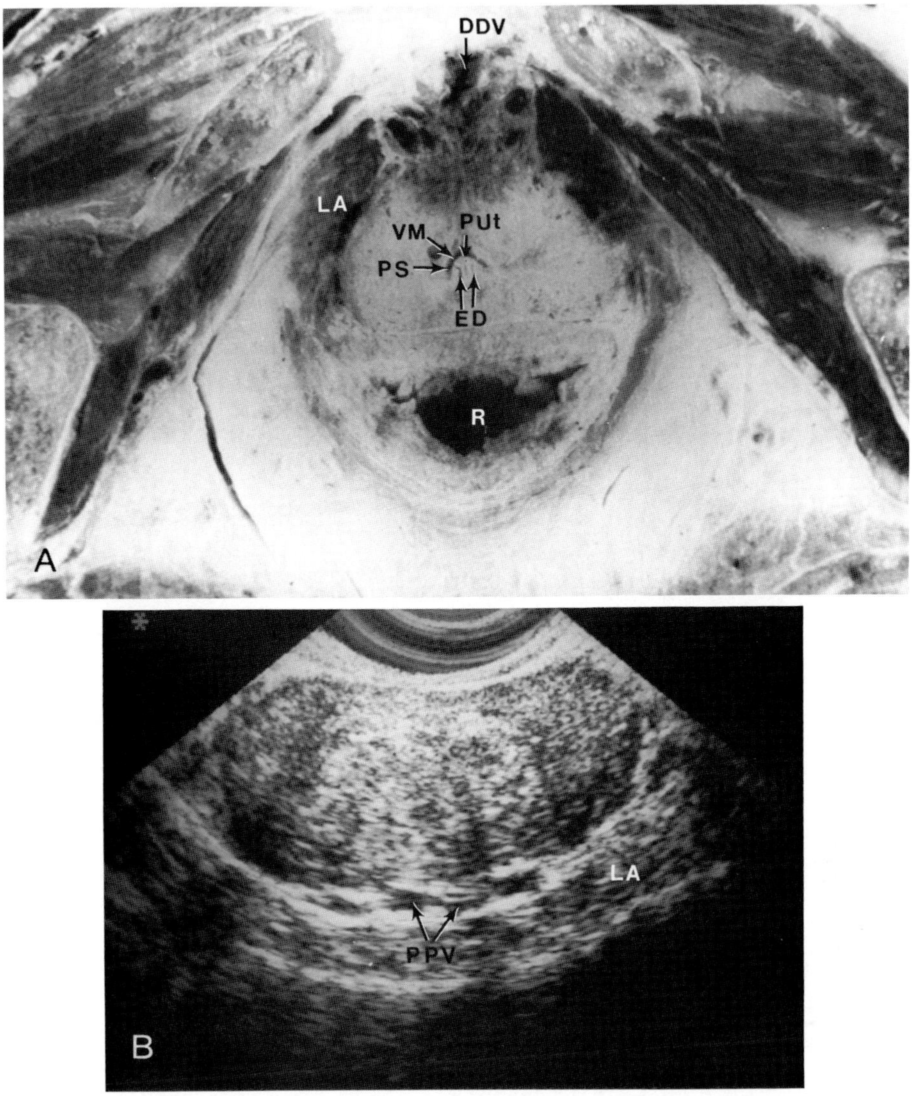

Figure 2.32. **A,** Transverse section through the prostate apex demonstrating the verumontanum (*VM*) and prostatic sinus (*PS*). The ejaculatory ducts (*ED*) and prostatic utricle (*PUt*) open on the verumontanum. The thicker lower part of the levator ani (*LA*) surrounds the prostate and rectum (*R*). The deep dorsal vein (*DDV*) of the penis is seen entering the periprostatic veins anterior to the prostate. (Modified by permission from Schneck CD, Friedman AC, Peterson RO. Embryology, anatomy, and histology. In: Friedman AC et al., eds. Clinical pelvic imaging. St. Louis: CV Mosby, 1990:38.) **B,** Transverse transrectal sonogram through the lower prostate displaying anteriorly situated periprostatic veins (*PPV*) and the levator ani (*LA*). **C, D,** and **E,** Longitudinal voiding cystourethrosonograms through the bladder (*B*), prostate (*Pr*), and prostatic urethra (*PrUa*). **C** demonstrates the upper prostatic urethra, **D** the midprostatic urethra, and **E** the lower prostatic urethra. The verumontanum (*VM*) is seen in **D** and **E.**

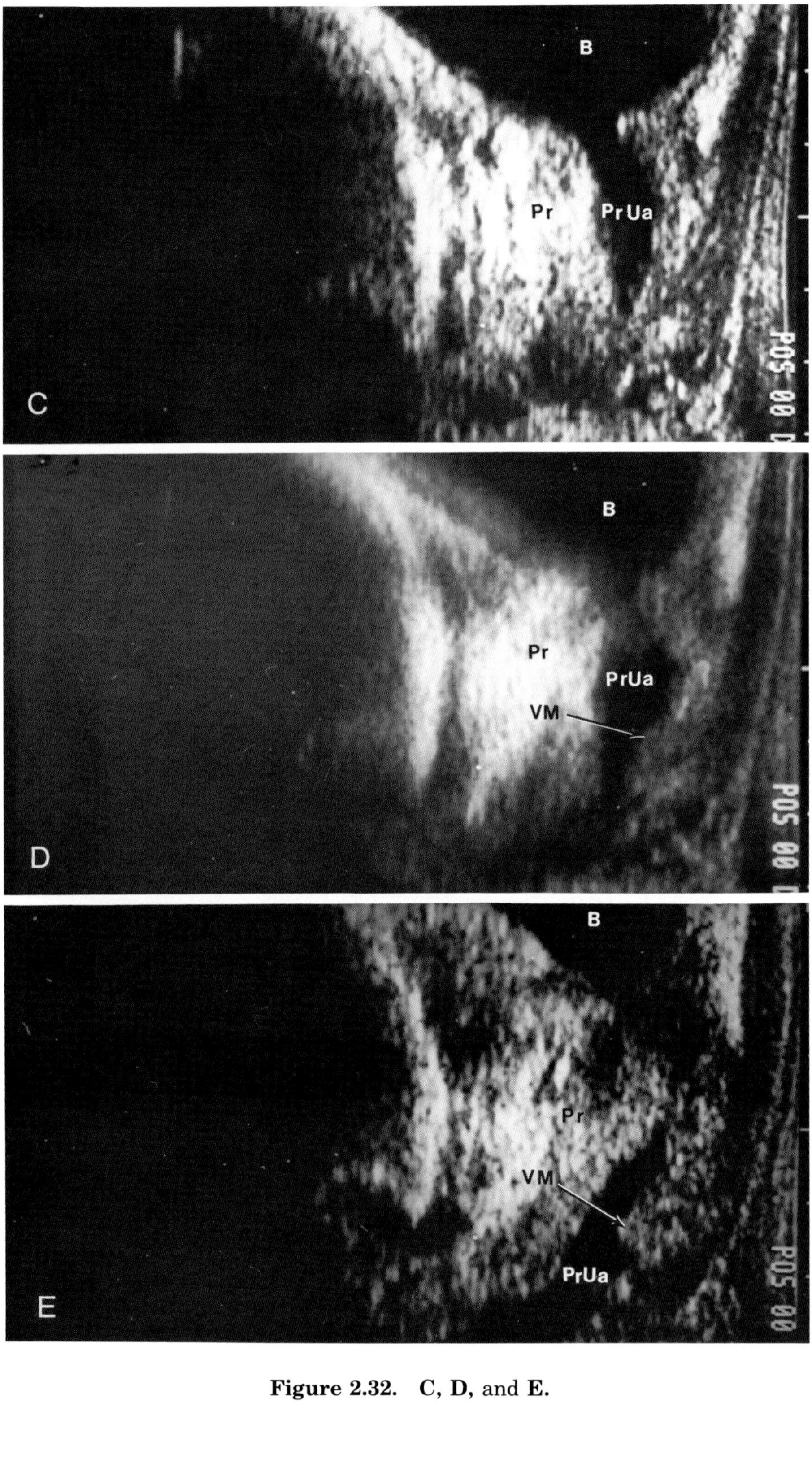

Figure 2.32. C, D, and E.

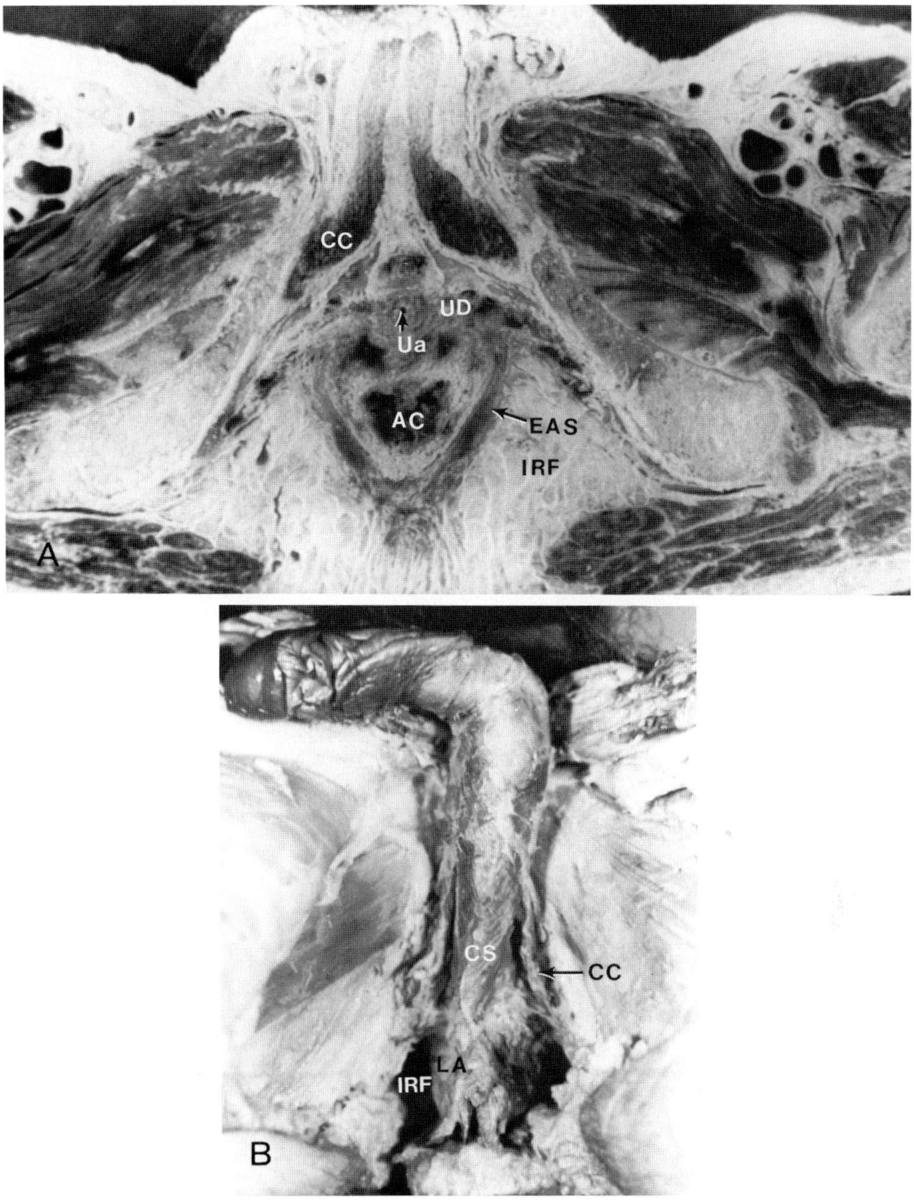

Figure 2.33. A, Transverse section through the urogenital region of the perineum. The corpora cavernosa (*CC*) arise from the ischiopubic rami. The urethra (*Ua*) is observed penetrating the urogenital diaphragm (*UD*). Posteriorly the anal canal (*AC*), external anal sphincter (*EAS*), and ischiorectal fossae (*IRF*) are shown. **B,** Dissection of the male perineum. In the urogenital region the corpus spongiosum (*CS*) is covered by the bulbospongiosus muscle and the corpora cavernosa (*CC*) are covered by the ischiocavernosus muscle. In the anal region the ischiorectal fossa (*IRF*) fat has been removed to demonstrate the funnel-shaped levator ani (*LA*) muscle in its medial wall. (Modified by permission from Schneck CD, Friedman AC, Peterson RO. Embryology, anatomy, and histology. In: Friedman AC et al., eds. Clinical pelvic imaging. St. Louis: CV Mosby, 1990:40.)

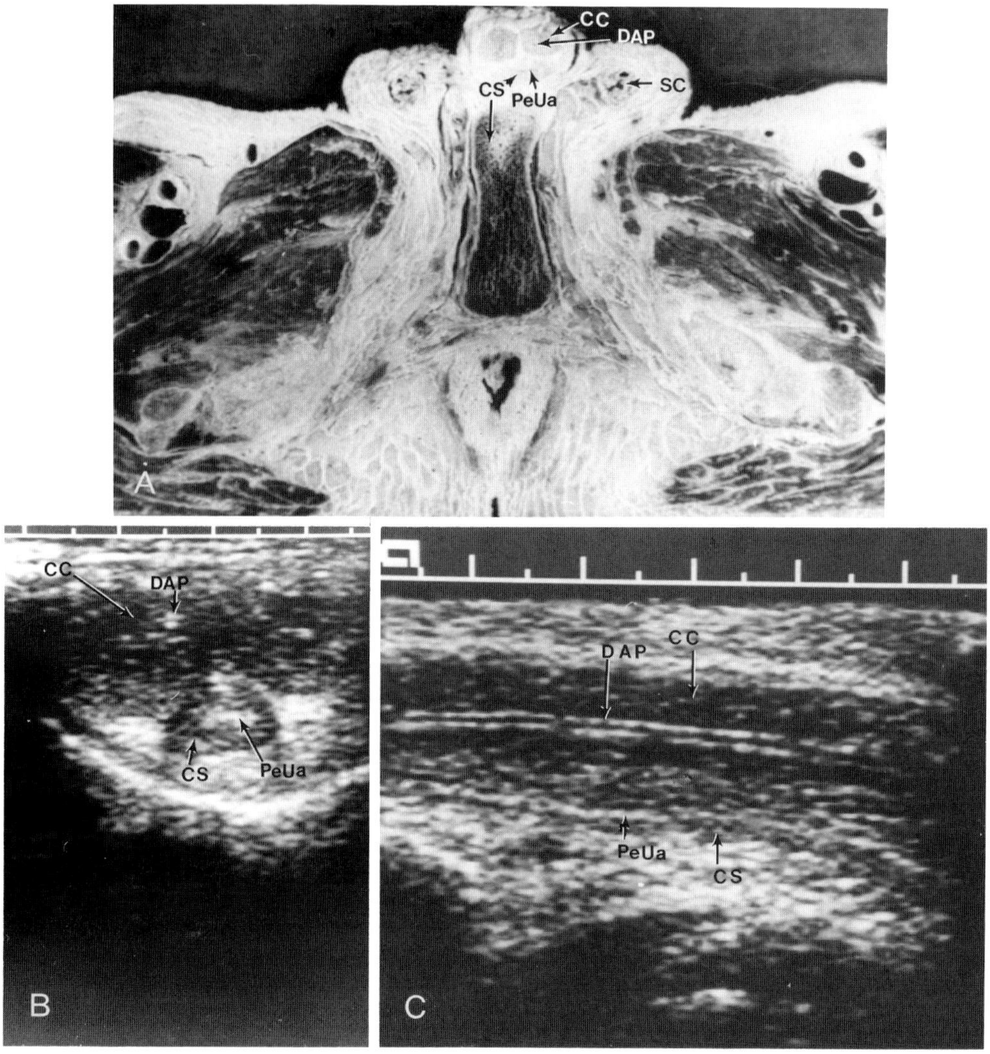

Figure 2.34. **A,** Transverse section through the corpus spongiosum. The root of the penis is cut in cross-section and shows the corpora cavernosa (*CC*), deep artery of the penis (*DAP*), corpus spongiosum (*CS*), and penile urethra (*PeUa*). The spermatic cord (*SC*) structures are seen in the subcutaneous tissues on either side of the base of the penis. **B,** Transverse sonogram of the penis displaying the corpus spongiosum (*CS*), penile urethra (*PeUa*), corpora cavernosa (*CC*), and the deep artery of the penis (*DAP*) visualized as a double echo. **C,** Longitudinal sonogram through the corpus spongiosum (*CS*), penile urethra (*PeUa*), and one corpus cavernosum (*CC*), with the deep artery of the penis (*DAP*) seen as two echogenic lines separated by a sonolucent interval. (Modified by permission from Schneck CD, Friedman AC, Peterson RO. Embryology, anatomy, and histology. In: Friedman AC et al., eds. Clinical pelvic imaging. St. Louis: CV Mosby, 1990:41.)

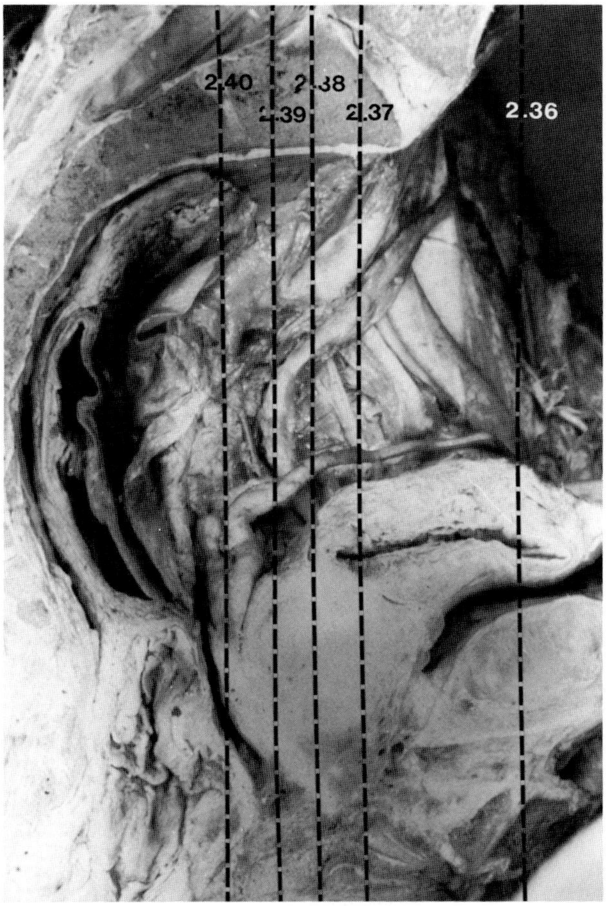

Figure 2.35. Midsagittal section of the male pelvis to demonstrate the planes of the coronal sections of Figures 2.36 though 2.40.

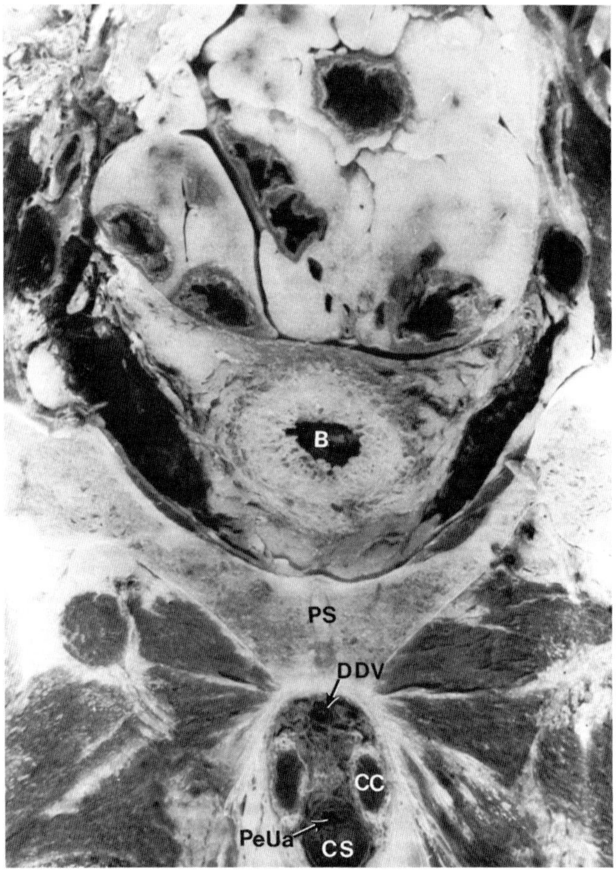

Figure 2.36. Coronal section through the bladder apex (*B*) as it rests above the pubic symphysis (*PS*). Below the symphysis the deep dorsal vein of the penis (*DDV*), corpora cavernosa (*CC*), corpus spongiosum (*CS*), and penile urethra (*PeUa*) are seen. (Modified by permission from Schneck CD, Friedman AC, Peterson RO. Embryology, anatomy, and histology. In: Friedman AC et al., eds. Clinical pelvic imaging. St. Louis: CV Mosby, 1990:54.)

grow forward to completely surround the urethral lumen. The resultant acoustical interfaces between the prostate's fibromuscular septa and these long, complex glands cause the larger peripheral or outer portion of the prostate to display moderate to low-level echoes on ultrasound examination (Fig. 2.31**B**) (7). The inner prostate or endoprostate is formed by much shorter, less complex periurethral glands. Its echo texture relative to the outer prostate varies with age. The endoprostate is located near the base of the prostate and somewhat anterior of its center. The walls of the undistended urethra are typically approximated. Hence, on a sagittal transrectal sonogram it can appear as a hyperechoic linear reflection that generally parallels the anterior rectal wall. Occasionally the ejaculatory ducts can be visualized by ultrasound in the more posterior part of the prostate. During a voiding sonourethrogram the distended urethra becomes sonolucent and the seminal colliculus may be observed as an echogenic posterior wall protrusion (Fig. 2.32**C** to **E**).

VAS DEFERENS AND SEMINAL VESICLES

The ductus or vas deferens begins in the scrotum at the tail of the epididymis as a continuation of the duct of the epididymis (Fig. 2.41). It joins the spermatic cord structures to ascend in the prepubic subcutaneous tissue to the inguinal canal (Fig. 2.34). At the deep inguinal ring it enters the extraperitoneal connective tissues medial to the anterior part of the obturator internus, where it passes posteriorly and inferiorly just internal to the anterior branches of the internal iliac vessels (Fig. 2.23**A** and **C**). As it reaches the bladder fundus it courses medially over the anterosuperior and then the medial aspect of the ureter to reach the medial aspect of the seminal vesicle (Figs. 2.23**C** and **D**, 2.29, and 2.30). Throughout most of its course the vas deferens has a thick muscular wall and a narrow lumen, giving it a cordlike feel. As it descends medial to the seminal vesicle it dilates to form its ampulla. At this point it is situated between the bladder base and the rectum. It narrows again just before it joins the duct of the seminal vesicle to form the ejaculatory duct near the base of the prostate.

The paired seminal vesicles are fusiform structures lateral to the ampullae of the vas deferens (Figs. 2.23**C** and **D**, 2.29, 2.30, 2.39, and 2.40). They are also situated between the bladder base and rectum. Their upper poles are usually closely related in front to the intramural course of the ureter. From the upper poles to their duct they incline medially at about a 45° angle. Hence, they virtually parallel the oblique anteroinferior margin of the bladder trigone. The seminal vesicle is a complexly evaginated saccular organ that has a multiloculated appearance when sectioned (Fig. 2.29). Both seminal vesicles and vas deferens receive branches of the inferior vesical vessels.

On transverse sonograms the vas deferens and seminal vesicles have a bow tie appearance (Fig. 2.29**B**). The seminal vesicles form the expanded lateral ends and the vas deferens the narrower central portion of the bow tie. The seminal vesicles can be examined in their long axis with an oblique sagittal scan (Fig. 2.29**C**). The seminal vesicles and vas deferens typically appear less echogenic than the prostate.

PENIS

The male external genitalia are situated in the urogenital region of the perineum. The perineum is the body region below the pelvic diaphragm and within the diamond-shaped boundaries of the pelvic outlet. The urogenital region is its anterior triangular area bounded by the ischiopubic rami (Figs. 2.33 and 2.37). It contains a deep and a superficial compartment. The deep compartment is the urogenital diaphragm that attaches on either side to the deep margin of the ischiopubic rami. The superficial compartment contains the roots of the erectile organs and their covering muscles. The paired crura of the corpora cavernosa arise from the ischiopubic rami. They are covered superficially by the ischiocavernosus muscles. As they run forward they converge upon the dorsolateral aspects of the corpus spongiosum at the root of the penis (Fig. 2.33). The unpaired midline corpus spongiosum is attached to the inferior aspect of the urogenital diaphragm (Figs. 2.23**A**, 2.33**B**, 2.34, and 2.37). It is covered superficially by the bulbospongiosus muscle. Its posterior dilated bulb receives the urethra after it penetrates the urogenital diaphragm. The penile or cavernous portion of the urethra then runs within the corpus spongiosum to its expanded distal glans. Each of the

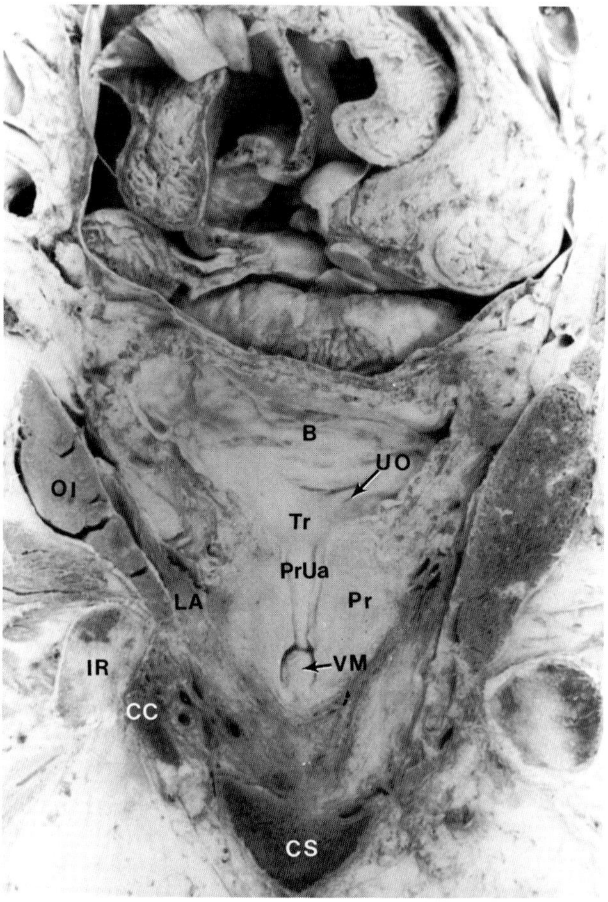

Figure 2.37. Coronal section through the posterior bladder (*B*) and prostatic urethra (*PrUa*). The internal urethral orifices (*UO*) can be seen at the upper angles of the trigone (*Tr*). The verumontanum (*VM*) bulges into the posterior wall of the lower prostatic urethra. Lateral to the prostate (*Pr*) the levator ani (*LA*) arises from the obturator internus fascia (*OI*). Below the ischiopubic rami (*IR*) the corpora cavernosa (*CC*) and corpus spongiosum (*CS*) can be seen. (Modified by permission from Schneck CD, Friedman AC, Peterson RO. Embryology, anatomy, and histology. In: Friedman AC et al., eds. Clinical pelvic imaging. St. Louis: CV Mosby, 1990:55.)

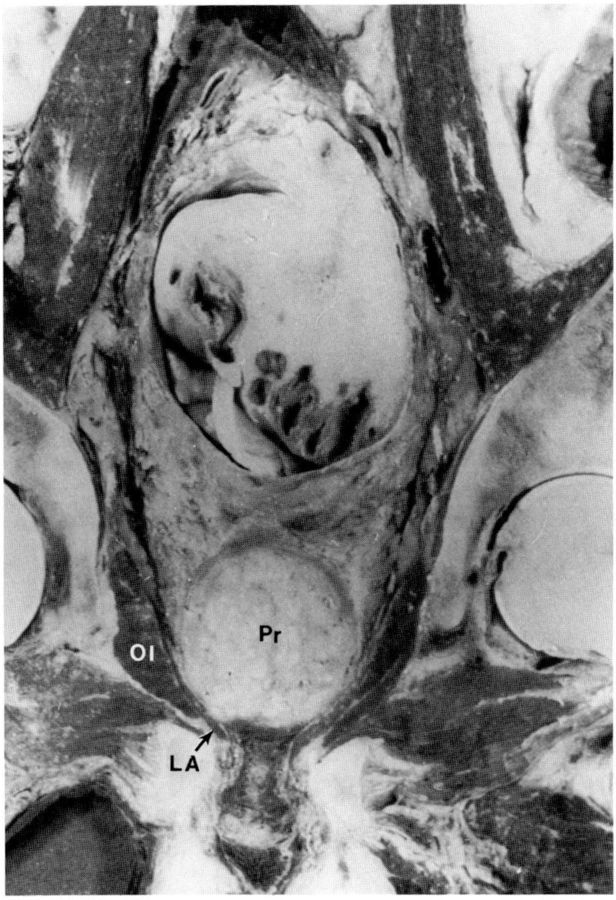

Figure 2.38. Coronal section through the posterior prostate (*Pr*) showing its lateral relationships to the levator ani (*LA*) and obturator internus (*OI*). (Modified by permission from Schneck CD, Friedman AC, Peterson RO. Embryology, anatomy, and histology. In: Friedman AC et al., eds. Clinical pelvic imaging. St. Louis: CV Mosby, 1990:58.)

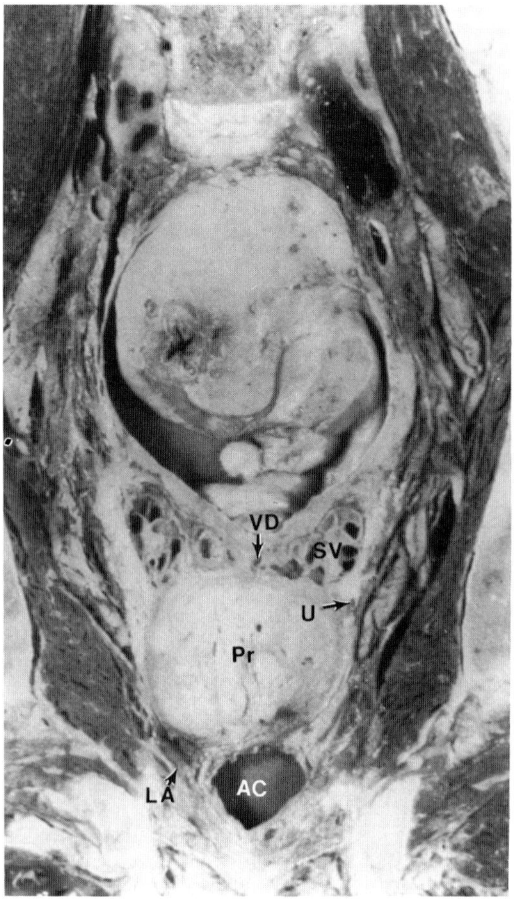

Figure 2.39. Coronal section through the posterior prostate (*Pr*) showing the ureter (*U*), seminal vesicles (*SV*), and vas deferens (*VD*) projecting above the prostate base and the levator ani (*LA*) and anal canal (*AC*) projecting below the prostate apex. (Modified by permission from Schneck CD, Friedman AC, Peterson RO. Embryology, anatomy, and histology. In: Friedman AC et al., eds. Clinical pelvic imaging. St. Louis: CV Mosby, 1990:56.)

three erectile structures of the penis is enclosed within a dense fibrous capsule, the tunica albuginea. This is particularly thick around the corpora cavernosa. Their interior is composed of dilated venous sinusoids separated by connective tissue septae. The corpora cavernosa contain a longitudinally running deep or central artery of the penis (Fig. 2.34). As the erectile structures converge at the root of the penis they are all enclosed by Buck's fascia and their tunica albuginea tend to fuse. The paired corpora cavernosa are situated dorsolaterally and their fused tunica form a dense midline penile septum. The corpus spongiosum is situated ventromedial to the corpora cavernosa.

On ultrasound examination the corpora cavernosa and spongiosum appear relatively hypoechoic (Fig. 2.34**B** and **C**). On a transverse scan the nondistended urethra is sometimes visualized as a short, transversely oriented, linear or double linear reflection (Fig. 2.34**B**). The central arteries of the penis are seen within the center of the corpora cavernosa as two bright

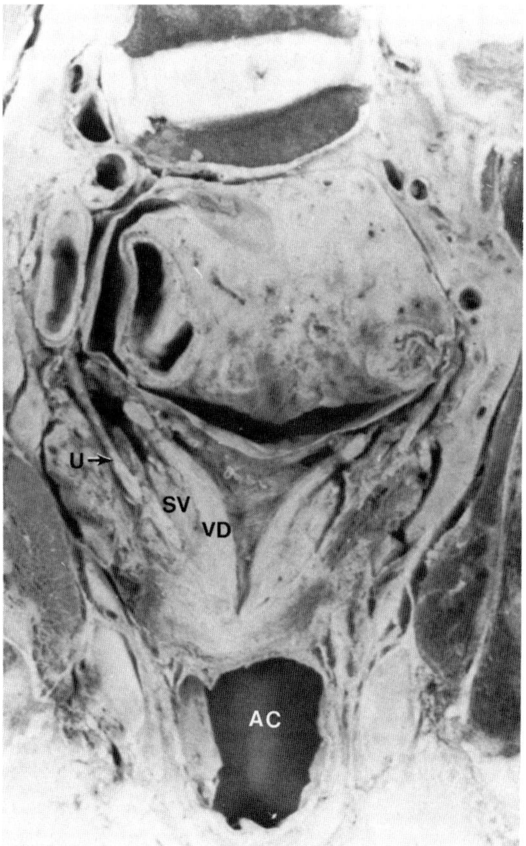

Figure 2.40. Coronal section just posterior to the prostate displaying the ureter (*U*), vas deferens (*VD*), and seminal vesicles (*SV*) bounded below by the anal canal (*AC*). (Modified by permission from Schneck CD, Friedman AC, Peterson RO. Embryology, anatomy, and histology. In: Friedman AC et al., eds. Clinical pelvic imaging. St. Louis: CV Mosby, 1990:56.)

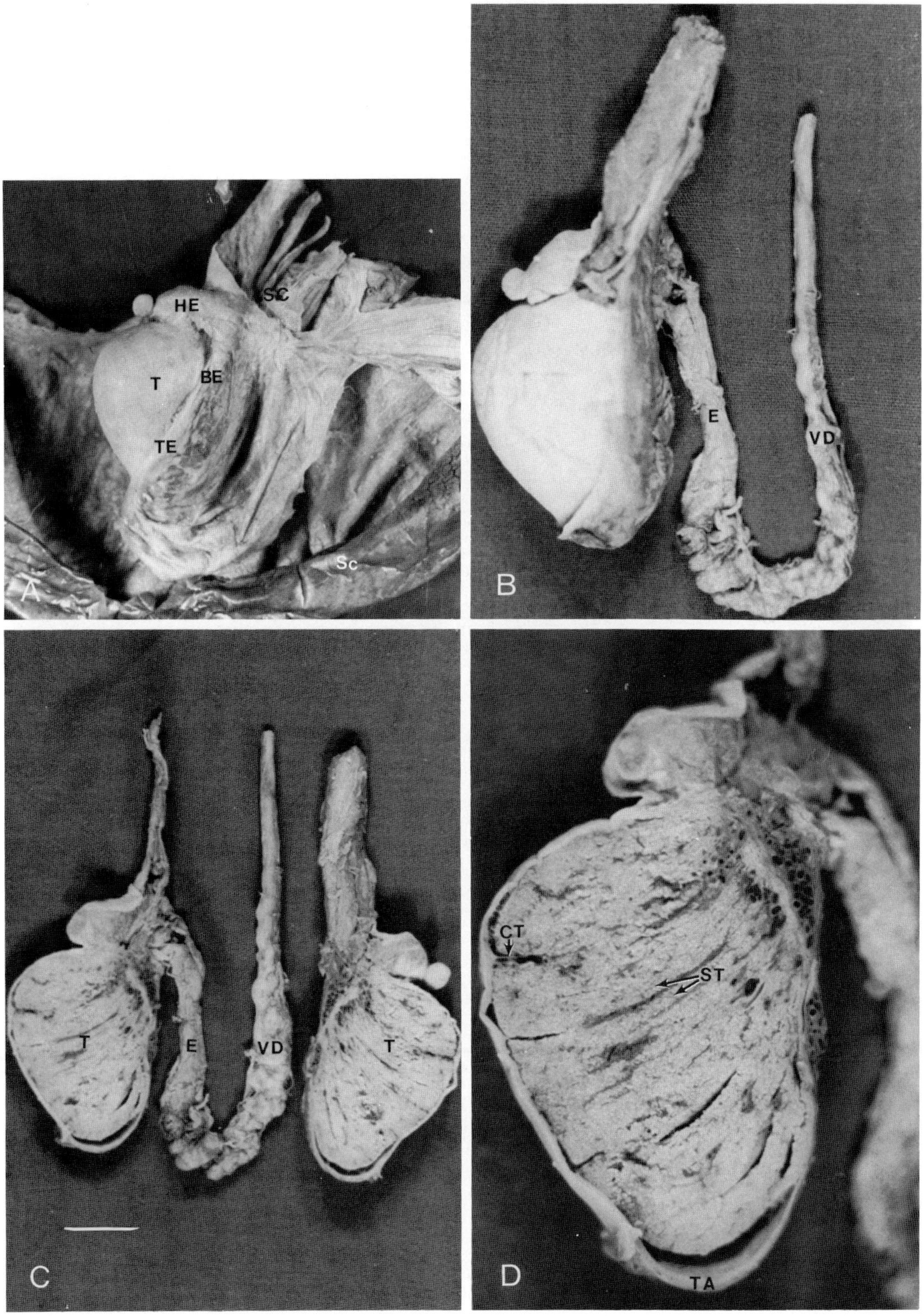

Figure 2.41. In **A** the scrotum (*Sc*) has been reflected to expose a medial view of the right testis (*T*). The head (*HE*), body (*BE*), and tail (*TE*) of the epididymis are seen, as is the spermatic cord (*SC*). In **B** the epididymis (*E*) has been dissected to show its continuity with the vas deferens (*VD*). In **C** the testis has been sagittally sectioned. **D** is a close-up view that displays the tunica albuginea (*TA*), the seminiferous tubules (*ST*), and their separating connective tissue septa (*CT*).

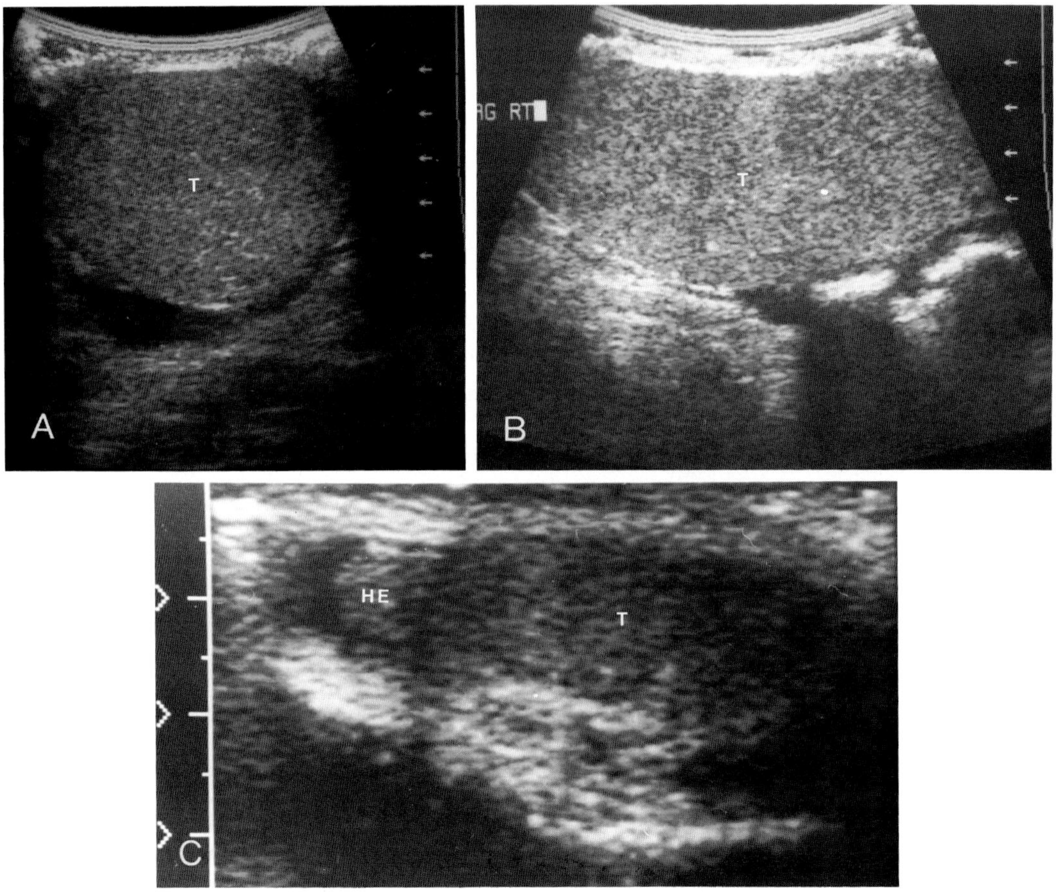

Figure 2.42. **A,** Transverse sonogram of the testis (*T*) demonstrating its fine echo pattern. **B,** Sagittal longitudinal sonogram displaying the fine echo pattern of the testis (*T*). **C,** Longitudinal scan showing both testis (*T*) and the head of the epididymis (*HE*). (C is modified by permission from Schneck CD, Friedman AC, Peterson RO. Embryology, anatomy, and histology. In: Friedman AC et al., eds. Clinical pelvic imaging. St. Louis: CV Mosby, 1990:42.)

echoes separated by a sonolucent interval. On longitudinal sonograms these arteries appear as long, double linear reflections separated by a sonolucent interval (Fig. 2.34**C**).

SCROTUM, TESTIS, AND EPIDIDYMIS

The scrotal wall is formed of skin, subcutaneous tissue, dartos tunic, and the three sheaths of the spermatic cord. The fibromuscular dartos tunic gives rise to a midline scrotal septum. A serous cavity, the tunica vaginalis, separates the scrotal wall structures from the testis and epididymis on all sides except posteriorly (Fig. 2.41). The tunica vaginalis is normally a closed serous sac that is derived from the embryonic evagination of the peritoneal cavity, the processus vaginalis, which precedes the descent of the testis. The tunica vaginalis has a parietal layer adherent to the inside of the scrotal wall and a visceral layer that covers all but the posterior aspect of the testis and epididymis. Its cavity normally contains only a small amount of serous fluid, which can increase in hydrocele.

The testis is an ovoid organ with its major axis oriented superoinferiorly. It is surrounded by a dense capsule that is also called a tunica albuginea (Fig. 2.41). There is a longitudinal invagination of the tunica into the testis about the efferent ductules, which exit the posterosuperior aspect of the testis. This is called the mediastinum testis. The tunica also sends many smaller septa into the interior of the testis. They divide the testis into lobules, which contain the much-coiled seminiferous tubules (Fig. 2.41**C** and **D**). The seminiferous tubules converge posteriorly toward the mediastinum to form a tubular network called the rete testis. This, in turn, gives rise to the efferent ductules that empty into the duct of the epididymis within its head.

The epididymis is draped along the superior and posterior aspects of the testis (Fig. 2.41**A** and **B**). It has a superiorly expanded head, an intermediate tapering body, and a narrow inferior tail. It is only partially separated from the testis by a laterally located, narrow slit-like recess of the cavity of the tunica vaginalis. It is formed of the greatly coiled duct of the epididymis, which at its tail becomes continuous with the vas deferens. As the vas ascends the posterior aspect of the epididymis, to which it is bound by connective tissue, it is joined by the other structures of the spermatic cord. These include the testicular artery, pampiniform plexus of veins, lymphatics, autonomic nerves, and their surrounding fascial sheaths. The gravitational dependence of the testis predisposes the pampiniform plexus to the development of varices, which here are called varicocele.

On ultrasound examination the testis and epididymis display a fine homogeneous echo pattern of moderate to low echo intensity (Fig. 2.42). This is consistent with the interfaces between the highly coiled seminiferous tubules and the fine separating septa and the coiled duct of the epididymis and its surrounding connecting tissue. At times the greater connective tissue of the mediastinum testis is seen as a linear reflection within the testis. The head of the epididymis is more commonly discriminated from the testis than is the rest of the epididymis (Fig. 2.42**C**).

References

1. Schneck CD. The anatomical basis of abdominopelvic sectional imaging. Clin Diagn Ultrasound 1983;11:13–41.
2. Stein BS, Schneck CD, Kendall AR. Surgical anatomy of the upper genitourinary tract. In: Practice of surgery. Philadelphia: Harper & Row, 1983.
3. Olssum CA. Anatomy of the upper urinary tract. In: Walsh PC, Gittes RF, Perlmutter AD, Stamey TA, eds. Campbell's urology. Philadelphia: WB Saunders, 1986.
4. Finberg H. Renal ultrasound: anatomy and technique. Semin Ultrasound 1981;2:7–20.
5. Koenigsberg M, Hoffman JC, Schnur MJ. Sonographic evaluation of the retroperitoneum. Semin Ultrasound 1982;3:79–96.
6. Schneck CD, Friedman AC, Peterson RO. Embryology, anatomy and histology. In: Friedman AC, Radeck PD, Lev-Toaft AS, Hilpert PL, eds. Clinical pelvic imaging. St. Louis: CV Mosby, 1990.
7. Rifkin MD. Diagnostic imaging of the lower genitourinary tract. New York: Raven Press, 1985.
8. Clemente CD. Gray's anatomy of the human body. Philadelphia: Lea & Febiger, 1985.

CHAPTER 3

Ultrasonography of the Adrenal Glands

HSU-CHONG YEH, M.D.

The normal adrenal glands are a pair of thin organs, high and deep in the rib cage near the vertebrae. Therefore, delineation of the normal adrenal glands and small adrenal lesions has been one of the most difficult techniques in ultrasonography (1–10). They are easily obscured by the ribs and transverse process of the spine on both sides, and also by the stomach and bowel gas on the left side. With the advent of the high-resolution, real-time scanner (especially the sector scanner, which can be readily applied to the intercostal spaces), examination of the adrenal glands has become much easier than before. Successful scanning, however, requires understanding of the anatomy of both the adrenal glands per se and their surrounding structures, as well as a proper approach and technique (11, 12). High-resolution equipment is not absolutely essential for delineating normal glands and small masses (11), but they are certainly helpful, especially in delineating fine details (e.g., adrenal medulla). Since many functioning adrenal tumors are small and surgical resection of such tumors may result in permanent cure of the serious diseases, detection of such small masses is very important. When such tumors are multiple, every one should be detected. Delineation of large adrenal masses by ultrasonography is usually easy from any approach. However, when the mass is huge, its origin may be difficult to determine.

NORMAL ADRENAL GLANDS AND THEIR SURROUNDINGS

The adrenal glands are usually confined to the areas surrounded by ultrasonographically well-defined landmark structures. Although normal adrenal glands are not always visible by ultrasonography, if the adrenal area is carefully scanned from the appropriate angle and no mass lesion is seen, one may practically exclude an adrenal mass. Therefore, for a successful examination one should not only be familiar with normal adrenal anatomy but also with its surroundings. The incidence of visualization of normal adrenal glands depends on the equipment, the scanning approach, the skill of the ultrasonographer, and the effort of scanning. The normal right and left adrenal glands are visualized by manual scanning in 78 and 44% of cases respectively (11) and by real-time scanning between 92 and 97% and between 71 and 90% respectively (13, 14). In newborn infants with a high-frequency scanner, the incidences are between 97 and 100% and 83 and 96% respectively (15, 16).

The normal adrenal glands are a pair of flat organs that consist of an anteromedial ridge and two wings that open posterolaterally (Figs. 3.1 and 3.2) (11, 12, 17). The two wings are also called "limbs" in the computed tomographic (CT) literature (18, 19), since they appear as thin, elongated structures on cross-sectional imaging of CT (similarly seen on ultrasonography). The term "wing" is more appropriate, since it indicates a flat structure. The right gland is somewhat triangular and the left gland is semilunar (20, 21). Due to their flat shape, the glands are characteristically thin, only 0.3 to 0.6 cm in thickness, although they are 4 to 6 cm in length and 2 to 3 cm in width (21). The normal adrenal gland usually appears somewhat smaller when seen on ultrasonography than on CT (22).

The two wings of the adrenal gland are not symmetric. The medial wing is more prominent superiorly and small or absent inferiorly, and vice versa for the lateral wing (Fig. 3.2). Due to this specific configuration, a series of cross sections from above downward will demonstrate the following: (*a*) On the superior section only the anteromedial ridge and the medial wing are seen. This results in a linear or curvilinear structure that is oriented in anteroposterior di-

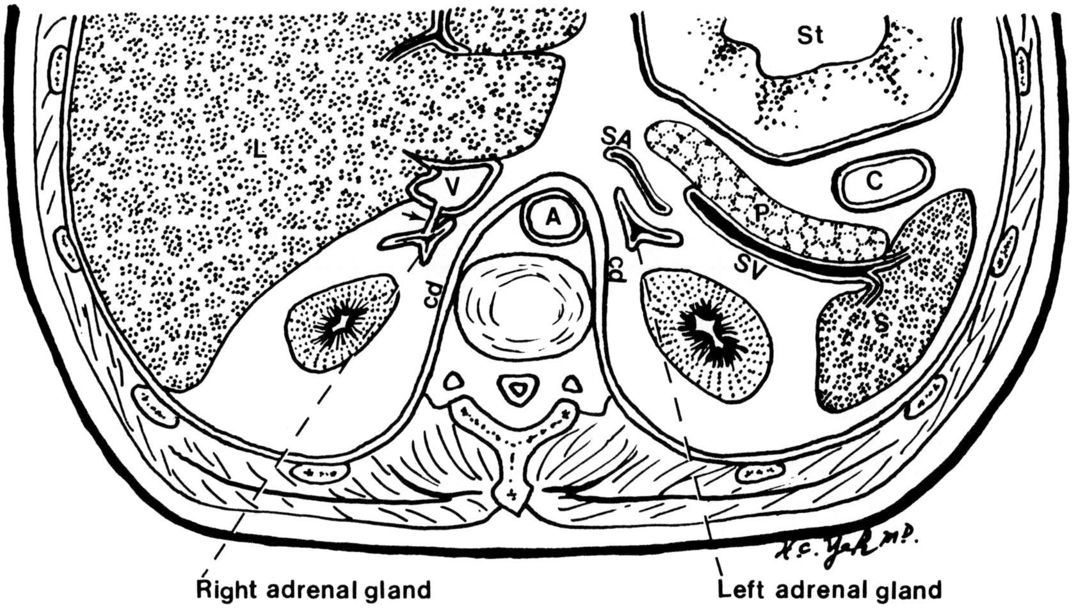

Figure 3.1. Drawing of transverse section of the upper abdomen showing both adrenal glands and their relation to the surrounding structures. *Arrow,* right adrenal vein; *P,* pancreas; *V,* inferior vena cava; *A,* aorta; *cd,* crus of diaphragm; *SA,* splenic artery; *SV,* splenic vein; *St,* stomach; *C,* colon; *L,* liver; *S,* spleen.

rection. (*b*) On the middle section, both wings are seen simultaneously. The two wings open posterolaterally straddling the medial edge of the kidney. The two wings and the anteromedial ridge form an inverted Y-shaped structure or, when the anteromedial ridge is small or absent, an inverted V-shaped structure. (*c*) On the lower section the medial wing may be small or absent, whereas the lateral wing is long. This together with the anteromedial ridge form an L-shaped structure for the left gland, but a reverse L-shaped structure for the right gland (Fig. 3.3) (11). Therefore, the features of cross-sectional images (e.g., ultrasonography and CT) of a single adrenal gland vary in different planes of sections, and one should not classify the shape of normal adrenal gland according to the appearance in a single section as in the literature (19, 22). Furthermore, due to the characteristic features in different planes of section, one can determine the level of section on any transverse adrenal image. The echogenic medulla may be seen in normal (Figs. 3.4 and 3.5) and hyperplastic adrenal glands (Fig. 3.6).

The glands are located anteromedial to the upper pole of the kidneys, only partly extending above the kidneys (Fig. 3.2), and therefore they are not really suprarenal in location. Usually, a larger portion of the right gland extends above the kidney than does the left gland. The left gland frequently extends more inferiorly; 10% of a normal left gland extends down to the renal hilum (18). The right gland is located immediately posterior to the inferior vena cava. The anteromedial ridge of the gland is contiguous with the posterior wall of the vena cava in most individuals. The right gland is lateral to the crus of the diaphragm and medial to the right lobe of the liver. The left gland is lateral to the crus of the diaphragm and medial to the right lobe of the liver. The left gland is located lateral or slightly posterolateral to the aorta, lateral to the crus of the diaphragm, posterior to the lesser omental sac superiorly, and posterior to the pancreas inferiorly. Since the lesser omental sac is usually collapsed and located behind the stomach, the superior portion of the left adrenal gland is practically posterior to the stomach. Both glands are adhered to the anteromedial roof of Gerota's fascia, i.e., at the top of the perirenal space. They are therefore less movable than the kidneys (Fig. 3.7). They are usually surrounded by varying amounts of fat

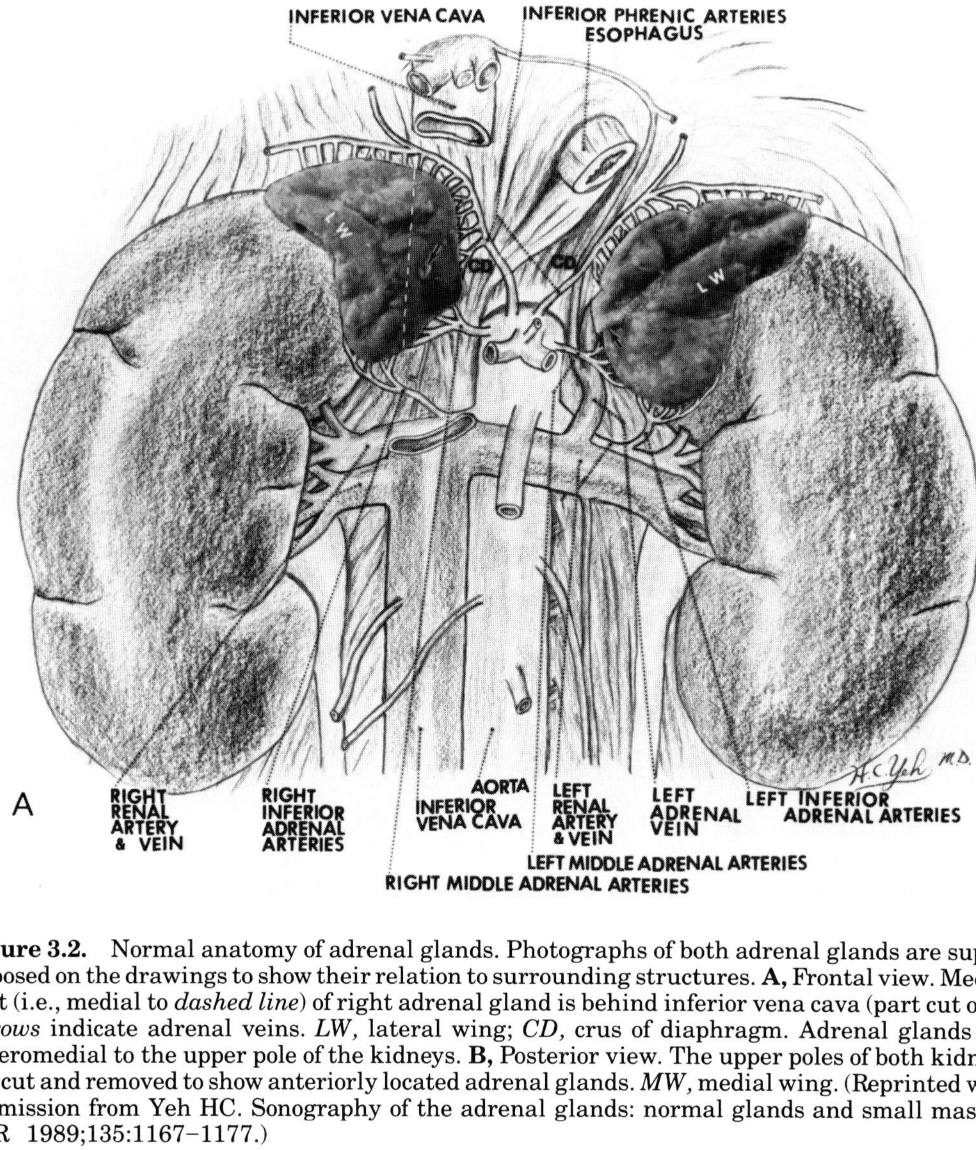

Figure 3.2. Normal anatomy of adrenal glands. Photographs of both adrenal glands are superimposed on the drawings to show their relation to surrounding structures. **A,** Frontal view. Medial part (i.e., medial to *dashed line*) of right adrenal gland is behind inferior vena cava (part cut out). *Arrows* indicate adrenal veins. *LW,* lateral wing; *CD,* crus of diaphragm. Adrenal glands are anteromedial to the upper pole of the kidneys. **B,** Posterior view. The upper poles of both kidneys are cut and removed to show anteriorly located adrenal glands. *MW,* medial wing. (Reprinted with permission from Yeh HC. Sonography of the adrenal glands: normal glands and small masses. AJR 1989;135:1167–1177.)

Figure 3.3. Ultrasonographic and CT features of normal right adrenal gland. **A,** Transverse sector scan from right upper flank shows the superior section of the right adrenal gland (*arrow*) to be a thick linear structure posterior to the inferior vena cava (*V*) and lateral to the crus of diaphragm (*arrowhead*). *H,* liver; *K,* kidney. **B,** Scanned slightly inferiorly, the middle section of the right adrenal gland becomes an inverted V-shaped structure. **C,** Scanned further inferiorly, the base of the adrenal gland appears as a reversed L-shaped structure. (Reprinted with permission from Yeh HC. Ultrasonography of the adrenals. Semin Roentgenol 1988;23:250–258.) **D** through **F,** Corresponding CT scans in a different individual show similar features of the right adrenal gland (*arrows*) at different levels. All labels are the same as on the ultrasonographs except *S,* spleen; *black arrowhead,* splenic artery. (Reprinted with permission from Yeh HC. Sonography of the adrenal glands: normal glands and small masses. AJR 1989;135:1167–1177.)

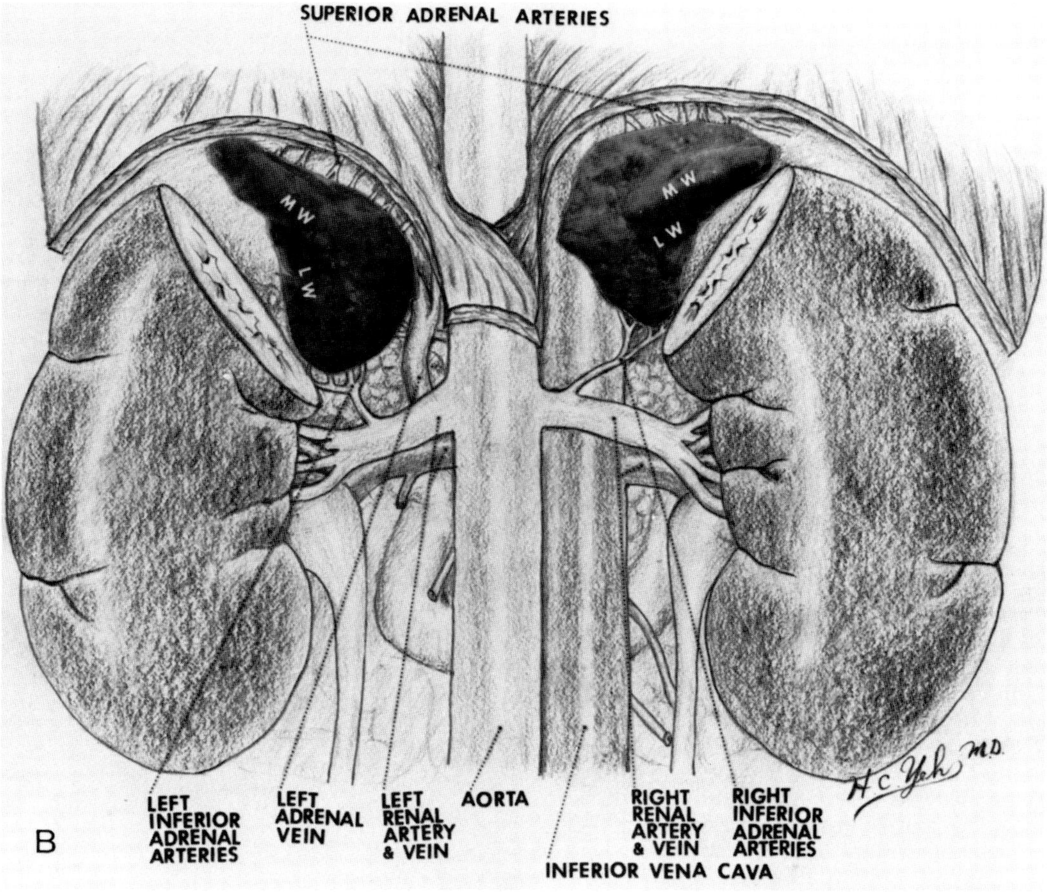
SUPERIOR ADRENAL ARTERIES
M W
L W
M W
L W
LEFT INFERIOR ADRENAL ARTERIES
LEFT ADRENAL VEIN
LEFT RENAL ARTERY & VEIN
AORTA
RIGHT RENAL ARTERY & VEIN
RIGHT INFERIOR ADRENAL ARTERIES
INFERIOR VENA CAVA
B

Figure 3.2. B.

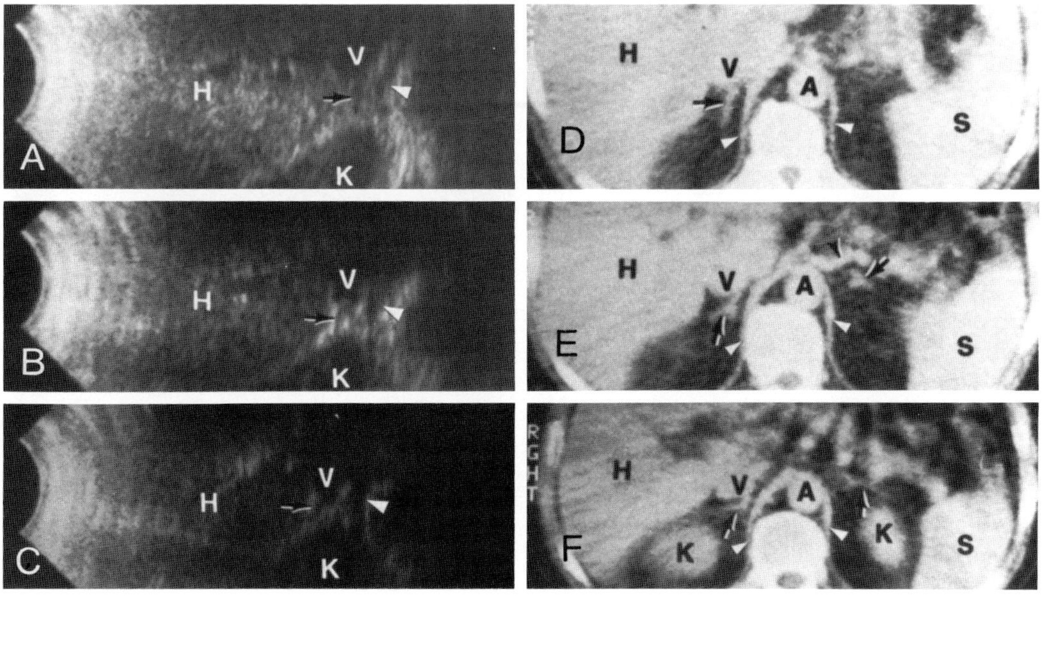
A
H
V
K
B
H
V
K
C
H
V
K
D
H
V
A
S
E
H
V
A
S
F
H
V
A
K
K
S

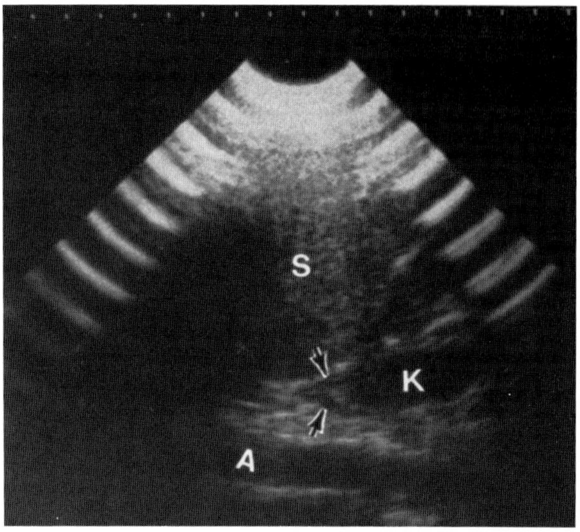

Figure 3.4. Normal left adrenal gland on longitudinal oblique scan from left flank region. The adrenal gland (*arrows*) is a horizontal Y-shape and not a triangular shape. Note the echogenic medulla within the gland. *S*, spleen; *A*, aorta; *K*, kidney.

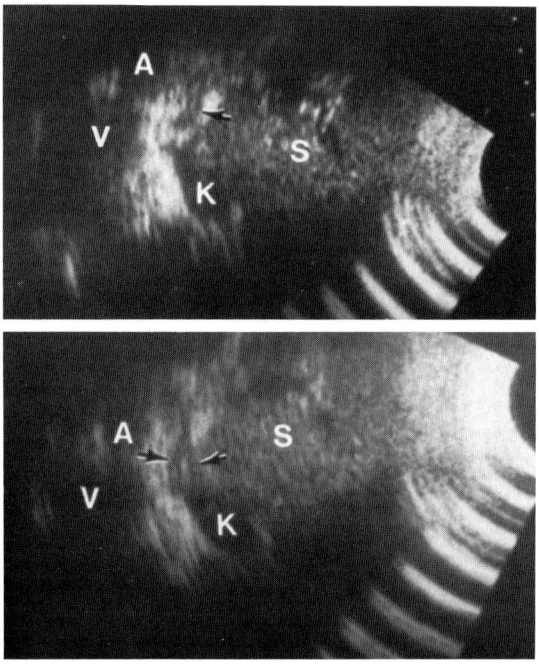

Figure 3.5. Normal left adrenal gland on transverse scan from left upper flank region *Top,* Superior section of the gland (*arrow*) appears as a thick curvilinear structure. *Bottom,* Middle section of the gland (*arrows*) appears as an inverted Y-shaped structure. *A*, aorta; *S*, spleen; *K*, kidney; *V*, vertebral body. Note the echogenic medulla within the gland in both sections. (Reprinted with permission from Yeh HC. Adrenal gland non-renal retroperitoneum. Urol Radiol 1987;9:127–140.)

except between the anteromedial ridge and the inferior vena cava.

The fetal adrenal gland is relatively large. The large fetal adrenal gland may appear triangular in shape on coronal scan (Fig. 3.8). The adrenal gland is larger than the kidney at the third to fourth fetal month and is one-third the size of the kidney at birth. In adults, it is only one-thirtieth of the kidney in size, only slightly larger than the gland of a newborn. In the fetus with renal agenesis or ectopic kidney, the adrenal gland appears more elliptical. This in association with echogenic central medullar echoes may be easily mistaken for a normal kidney on ultrasonograph (23).

SCANNING METHOD

The adrenal glands are located deep in the rib cage posteriorly and medially. Posterior scanning is usually unsuccessful unless the mass is large, since the gland is easily obscured by the rib or transverse process of the spine.

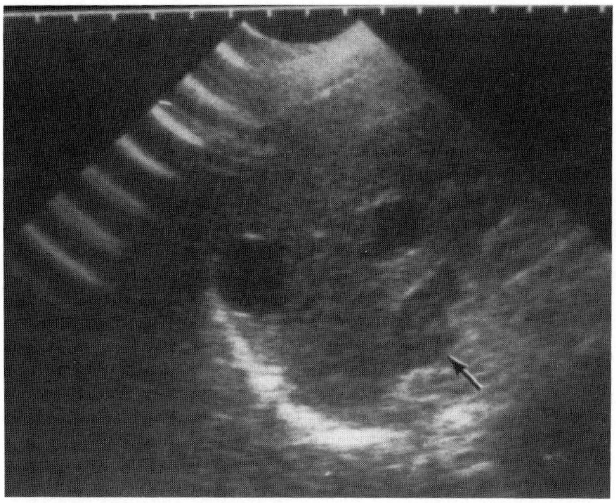

Figure 3.6. Adrenal hyperplasia. Oblique longitudinal scan of the right upper abdomen shows a "fat" horizontal V-shaped adrenal gland (*arrow*). The thickness of the lateral wing is 1.2 cm, more than twice normal. Note the echogenic medulla within the gland, indicating a hyperplastic gland rather than an infiltrating process. (Reprinted with permission from Yeh HC. Adrenal gland non-renal retroperitoneum. Urol Radiol 1987;9:127–140.)

The best approach for scanning the right adrenal gland is from the right flank region through an intercostal space (Fig. 3.9) (11). Using the liver or the right kidney as an acoustic window, one should aim the transducer toward the inferior vena cava. The crus of the diaphragm usually can be seen as a poorly echogenic curvilinear structure adjacent to the lateral margin of the vertebral body. The crus of the diaphragm sometimes may be quite thickened due to hypertrophic muscles. The adrenal gland is located within the echogenic fat space between the liver and the crus of the diaphragm immediately posterior to the inferior vena cava. The configuration of the gland is, as previously mentioned, a linear or curvilinear structure superiorly, an inverted Y or inverted V shape in the middle section, and a reverse L shape inferiorly. Since the echo pattern of the adrenal gland may be similar to that of the surrounding fat and may be difficult to discern, one should carefully adjust the gain setting to best visualize the tissue contrast in that area. The gland is usually confined to a well-defined area surrounded by the inferior vena cava, the medial liver margin, the crus of the diaphragm, and the upper pole of the kidney. Therefore, if one scans carefully and sweeps the area with the transducer slowly up and down repeatedly, from 3 to 5 cm above the kidney down to the renal hilum, the adrenal area can be thoroughly examined.

The scanning technique for the left adrenal gland is similar to that for the right adrenal gland except that the transducer may have to be placed more posteriorly (i.e., at the posterior axillary line). The spleen or the left kidney is used as an acoustic window. Since the spleen is usually smaller than the liver and the gas in the stomach and colon in the left upper quadrant of the abdomen may easily obscure the adrenal gland, the left adrenal gland is usually much more difficult to examine than the right gland. The spleen is frequently located posterolaterally rather than laterally. Therefore, it is necessary to place the transducer posterolaterally with the patient in the semidecubitus position to scan the left adrenal (11). When the stomach content mimics an adrenal mass lesion, drinking of water may clarify the anatomy because the mass-like structure becomes fluid filled, or echogenic food particles or small gas bubbles moving within the stomach may be observed. The left adrenal gland that was once obscured by large gastric bubbles may sometimes become visible through a water-filled stomach.

Anterior longitudinal scanning may delineate the medial portion of the adrenal gland, which is seen posterior to the inferior vena cava (Fig. 3.10) (11). The adrenal gland is usually seen at the level of the porta hepatis (11), but when the liver is enlarged, the porta hepatis is displaced inferiorly and, therefore, the adrenal gland becomes superior to the level of the porta hepatis (Fig. 3.10). The adrenal gland assumes a horizontal Y or V shape, with the two wings open inferiorly. The "anterior" wing in this scan actually represents the lateral wing and the "posterior" wing represents the medial wing. Scanning medially one may see a long horizontal linear or band-like structure poste-

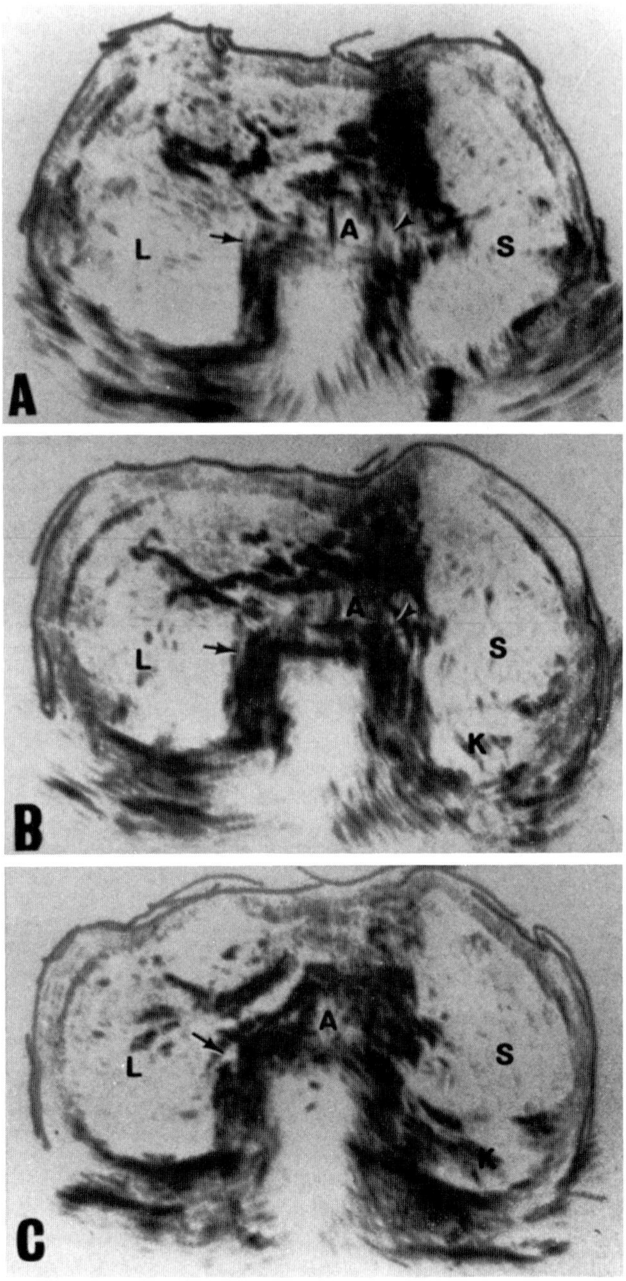

Figure 3.7. Normal adrenal glands in a patient with a markedly enlarged spleen (*S*). *A*, aorta; *L*, liver; *K*, left kidney. **A,** Transverse scan 15 cm above the umbilicus. The superior section of the right adrenal gland (*arrow*) is an anteroposteriorly oriented, linear structure. The middle section of the left adrenal (*arrowhead*) is an inverted Y-shaped structure in the usual location in spite of the inferior displacement of the left kidney (seen in next scan) due to the large spleen. **B,** Transverse scan 13 cm above the umbilicus. The left kidney is displaced both inferiorly and posteriorly, becoming quite separate from the left adrenal gland (*arrowhead*). **C,** Transverse scan 12 dm above the umbilicus. The inferior section of the right adrenal gland (*arrow*) is an inverted V shape. (Reprinted with permission from Mitty HA, Yeh HC. Radiology of the adrenals with sonography and CT. Philadelphia: WB Saunders, 1982.)

rior to the inferior vena cava (Fig. 3.10). This represents the crus of the diaphragm and should not be mistaken for a normal or enlarged adrenal gland. A right adrenal mass frequently indents the inferior vena cava from posteriorly. This is most evident on the anterior longitudinal scan.

The left adrenal gland is not usually visualized on the anterior longitudinal scan. It is usually obscured by the gas in the stomach. It may occasionally be seen posterior to the pancreas. The feature is similar to that of the right adrenal gland (11).

Transverse scanning from epigastrium usually does not clearly delineate a normal adrenal gland or a small adrenal mass, although a relatively large mass may be seen on this scanning plane.

Sample (12) developed a longitudinal oblique scanning technique specially for visualizing

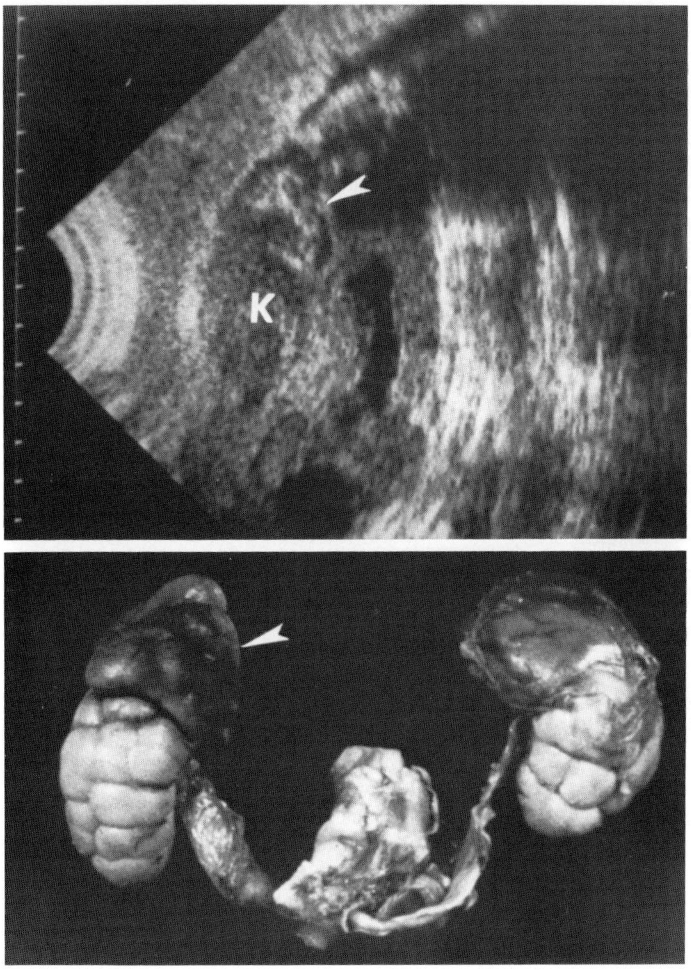

Figure 3.8. A normal fetal adrenal gland at 31 weeks' gestation. *Top,* Ultrasonograph shows coronal section of the right kidney (*K*) of the fetus. The adrenal gland (*arrowhead*) is relatively large compared to the kidney and
is triangular, the echogenic medulla is clearly seen within it. *Bottom,* Autopsy specimen of a pair of adrenal glands and kidneys of another fetus shows similar findings.

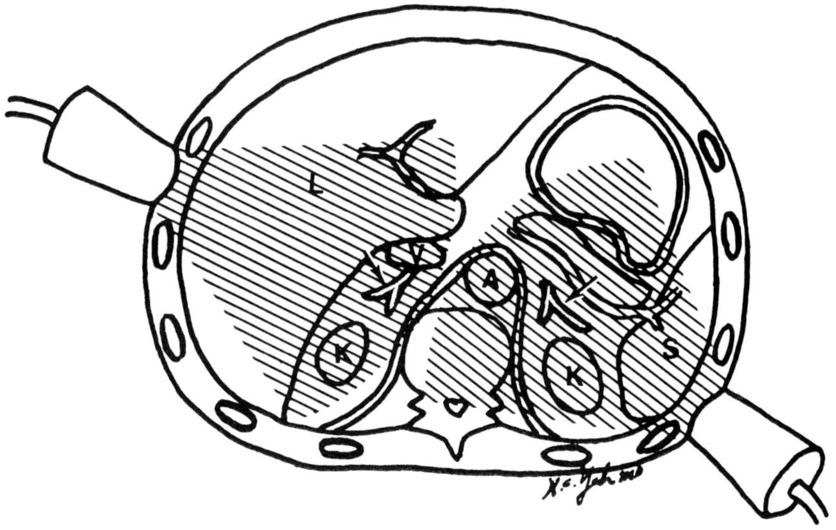

Figure 3.9. Scanning approaches for adrenal glands. Drawing shows transverse section of upper abdomen. With a sector real-time transducer placed at the right lateral flank region and scanning through the intercostal space, the right adrenal area can be examined. For the left adrenal gland, one may have to place the transducer more posteriorly (e.g., to avoid gas in the stomach or bowel). *L,* liver; *S,* spleen; *K,* kidney; *V,* inferior vena cava; *A,* aorta; *arrows,* adrenal glands. (Modified from Yeh HC. Ultrasonography of the adrenals. Semin Roentgenol 1988;23:250–258.

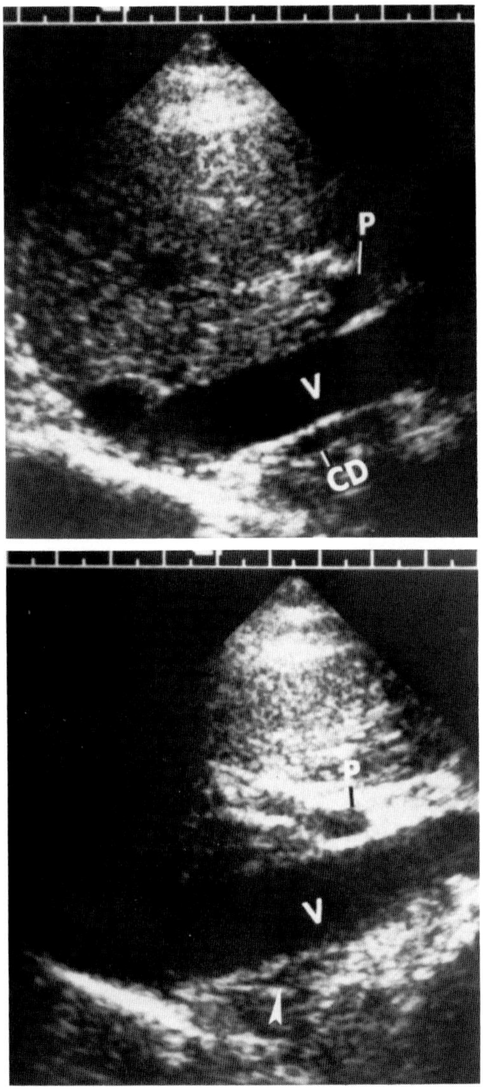

Figure 3.10. Normal adrenal gland on longitudinal scan. *Top,* Right parasagittal scan shows a thick linear structure (*CD*) posterior to the inferior vena cava (*V*) representing crus of diaphragm. *P,* portal vein. *Bottom,* Scan slightly more laterally shows a horizontal Y-shaped normal adrenal gland (*white arrowhead*) posterior to the inferior vena cava. Note that the portal vein (*P*) is below the level of the adrenal gland because of hepatomegaly.

normal adrenal glands in coronal section. The plane connecting the long axis of the kidney and aorta (or inferior vena cava for the right adrenal gland) is plotted out from a series of transverse manual scans. The plane intersecting the skin is marked on the skin and a scan is done along the plotted line on the predetermined plane with the patient in the decubitus position. The normal adrenal gland is said to appear as a triangular structure between the spleen, aorta, and upper pole of the kidney on the left and between the liver, inferior vena cava, and upper pole of the kidney on the right. Although a high success rate in visualizing the "normal gland" has been attained by this method, the triangular structure in fact does not really represent the normal adrenal gland but perirenal fat (24). The adrenal gland is always a thin horizontal Y- (Fig. 3.11) or V-shaped (Fig. 3.4), linear or curvilinear structure on this scanning plane. It is never triangular unless the gland is markedly enlarged or thickened or during the fetal or neonatal stage.

With the advent of the high-resolution real-time scanner, any scanning plane can be easily obtained. A longitudinal scan of the adrenal gland can be easily performed from the upper flank region through the intercostal space, similar to the transverse scan as mentioned above except that the transducer is turned 90° so that the transverse scan becomes a longitudinal scan. Since the orientation of the adrenal area is better with the transverse scan, one should do the transverse scan first then supplement it with a longitudinal scan either for searching for an adrenal mass or for obtaining the third dimension of the mass.

The normal adrenal glands and small adrenal masses are usually not seen on posterior scanning. A mass of less than 2 cm is only occasionally seen on posterior scanning (11, 25). A large adrenal mass can be seen on any scanning plane.

ADRENAL TUMORS

Focal Tumor

The adrenal gland may be involved in disease processes focally or diffusely. Except for bilateral hyperplasia, focal lesions are much more common than the diffuse disease. The ultrasonographic features of a focal mass lesion are usually different from that of diffuse disease unless the mass is huge and irregular. In the latter instance both focal and diffuse lesions may appear similar.

The focal tumors usually present as a round or oval mass but may become irregular in shape when large. They may be located in any part of the gland. When the mass is relatively small, the uninvolved part of the adrenal gland may also be visualized. Therefore, the diagnosis of an adrenal mass can be certain in such cases and the precise location of the lesion in the adrenal gland can be determined. When the mass is located at the tip of one of the wings and grows outward, the mass may appear to arise outside the gland.

SMALL ADRENAL MASSES

A small adrenal mass less than 3 cm in diameter used to be difficult to delineate by ultrasonography. With proper technique, however, most of the small masses can be delineated and the rate of detection may be as high as 97% (11). A mass as small as 0.6 cm can be seen (Fig. 3.11) (24). Since the diameter of a small adrenal mass is usually larger than the thickness of a normal adrenal gland and the mass is usually less echogenic than the surrounding fat, a small adrenal mass is easier to delineate than a normal adrenal gland. Therefore, when the adrenal areas are thoroughly examined and no mass is seen, an adrenal mass can be practically excluded even though the normal glands are not visualized (11). The adrenal areas are within well-defined anatomical landmarks as previously mentioned. By following these landmarks one can be certain that the adrenal areas are thoroughly examined.

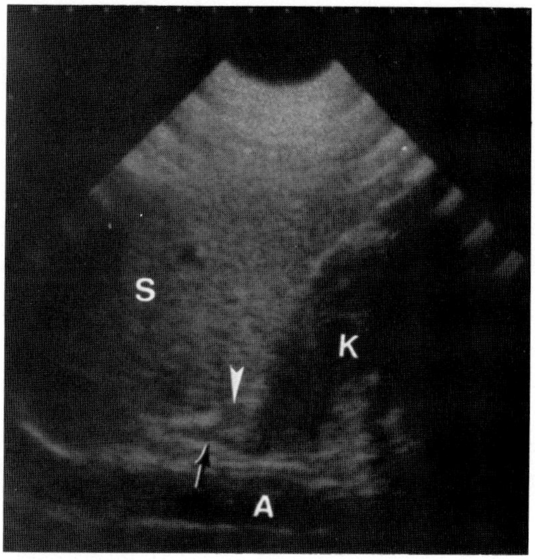

Figure 3.11. A small adrenal adenoma. Coronal scan from left upper flank shows a small nodule (*arrowhead*) 0.6 cm in diameter in the tip of the lateral wing of the left adrenal gland, which is horizontally Y-shaped (*arrow*). *S*, spleen; *K*, kidney; *A*, aorta. (Reprinted with permission from Yeh HC. Adrenal gland and non-renal retroperitoneum. Urol Radiol 1987; 9:127–140.)

Although the rate of detection of small adrenal masses by ultrasonography is slightly less than by CT (11), some masses are better visualized by ultrasonography than by CT, especially the right adrenal mass in thin patients and in infants and children. This is because the liver is an excellent acoustic window for ultrasound scanning. In thin patients and the pediatric population the fat surrounding the adrenal gland is scanty, especially on the right. This improves penetration of the sound beam. In obese patients or patients with Cushing's syndrome, on the contrary, abundance of perirenal and periadrenal fat help to visualize adrenal lesions by CT because of the low attenuation number of fat, which serves as a natural contrast on CT but prevents good visualization of the adrenal lesion by ultrasonography. The large size of patients also prevents sound beams from penetrating and reaching the adrenal area. Some adrenal neoplasms, especially those originating from the adrenal cortex, may contain relatively large amounts of lipids, resulting in low attenuation numbers in CT (26). When the attenuation number is as low as that of water, the mass may simulate a cyst (Fig. 3.12). If the attenuation number is very low, a small mass may be difficult to visualize by CT since the mass has little density contrast to the surrounding fat and the small mass does not cause deformity of the surrounding structures (i.e., no mass effect). Ultrasonography will clearly demonstrate the former as a solid mass and the latter as a well-demarcated mass.

The nonfunctioning adrenal adenoma and the functioning aldosteronoma are usually small (Figs. 3.12 and 3.13). The adenoma of Cushing's syndrome are also not uncommonly small. Contrary to the common belief that pheochromocytomas are large (27), small masses are found in 20% of the cases in any experience (28).

The most common small adrenal malignant masses are metastatic tumors, most commonly from bronchogenic carcinoma. Tumors from breast, kidneys, lymphoma, and melanoma are also not uncommon. Differentiation between small benign and malignant tumors is usually impossible by ultrasonography or CT. They are usually round or oval and hypoechoic compared to the surrounding fat tissue. On magnetic resonance imaging (MRI), when the intensity of

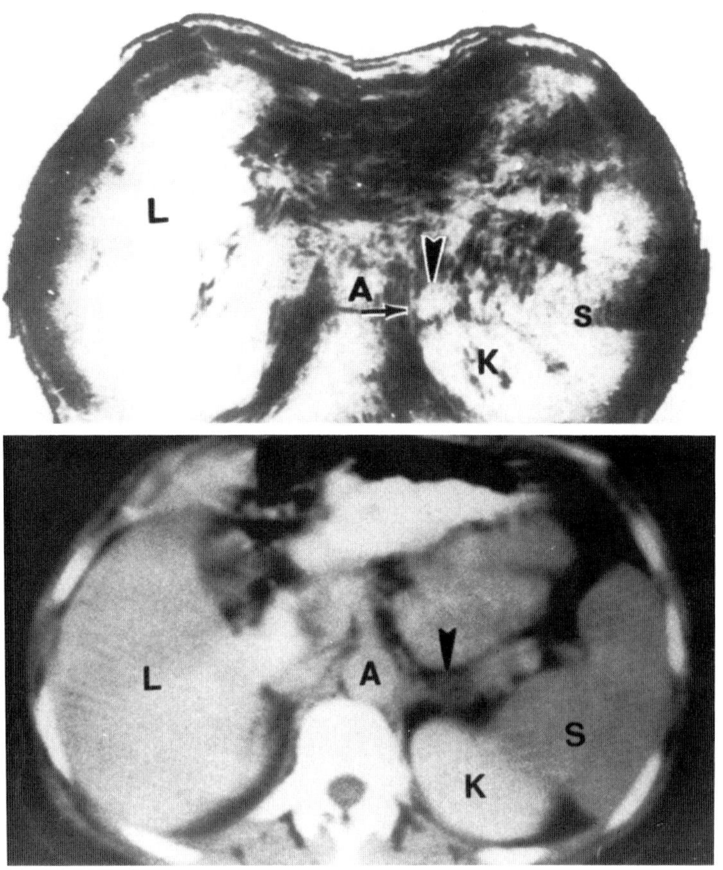

Figure 3.12. A small aldosteronoma in the left adrenal gland with low attenuation value on CT, simulating a cyst. *Top,* Transverse manual scan shows a solid mass (*arrowhead*) to be located in the lateral wing of the left adrenal gland. *Arrow,* medial wing of adrenal gland; *A,* aorta; *K,* kidney; *S,* spleen; *L,* liver. *Bottom,* Corresponding CT scan shows the adrenal mass (*arrowhead*) to be the density of water, similar to a cyst.

the adrenal mass is similar to that of uninvolved normal parts of the adrenal gland or liver on both T_1- and T_2-weighted scanning, or when the intensity ratio of adrenal mass to fat on T_2-weighted scanning is less than 0.6, a nonfunctioning (benign) adenoma is suggested. There are, however, 21 to 31% of benign and malignant masses sharing the same intensity range on T_1- or T_2-weighted scanning (29, 30).

A small nodule or nodules may be seen in bilateral adrenal hyperplasia causing various adrenal hyperfunctions (e.g., Cushing's syndrome, hyperaldosteronism). Differentiation of such nodules from a small functioning adrenal adenoma is also important, since the latter requires surgical removal whereas the bilateral hyperplasia (with or without nodules) may need only conservative treatment unless a pituitary tumor or some other ACTH-producing tumor is found. In bilateral hyperplasia, the nodule may be single or multiple and micronodular (smaller than 0.8 cm) or occasionally macronodular (0.8 cm to 7 cm), and the adrenal gland may be diffusely enlarged (31). The enlarged adrenal gland is manifested mainly by an increase in its thickness. However, in bilateral adrenal hyperplasia, the adrenal glands are frequently normal in size (thickness) and, therefore, hyperplasia may be difficult to detect. The functioning adenomas are usually single except pheochromocytoma, which may be multiple. Complete clinical and laboratory workup usually differentiates pheochromocytomas from other adrenal hyperfunction. When differentiating between a functioning and a hyperplastic nodule is difficult by ultrasonography, CT, or MRI, then adrenal venography and venous blood sampling may be necessary. In bilateral hyperplasia high hormone levels in the sampled blood may be obtained from both sides.

Most nonfunctioning adrenal adenomas are less than 3 cm in size (Figs. 3.11 and 3.14) (32, 33), although occasionally they may be up to 10 cm (Fig. 3.15) (30). The internal echoes are usually homogeneous but may sometimes be heterogeneous (Fig. 3.15) due to focal necrosis or hemorrhage. When an adrenal mass of less

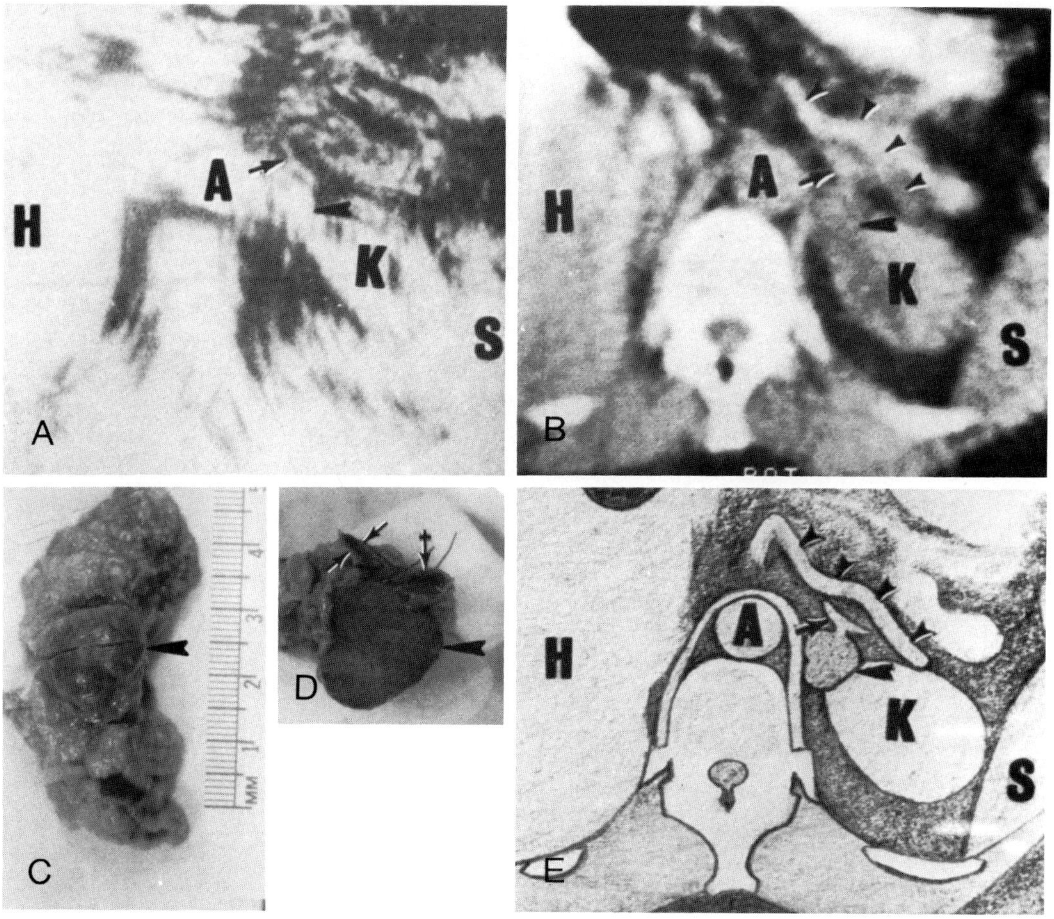

Figure 3.13. Aldosteronoma (1.8 cm) in the middle of the left adrenal gland. Anterior ridge (*arrow*) and lateral wing of gland are intact. **A** and **B,** Anterior transverse scan and corresponding CT scan. A mass (*large arrowhead*) is in the posterior edge of the medial wing of the left adrenal gland. The splenic artery (*small arrowheads*) is anterior to the adrenal gland. **C,** Surgical specimen viewed from posterior. Mass (*arrowhead*) protrudes posteriorly from the middle part of the gland. Adipose tissue around the normal part of the gland has not been removed. **D,** Transverse section of a specimen corresponding to findings on sonogram and CT scan. The normal adrenal gland (*between arrows*) is thin (3 mm). The lateral wing (*crossed arrow*) of the gland appears thicker because tissue has been split open. **E,** Drawing of CT scan. *H,* liver; *A,* aorta; *K,* kidney; *S,* spleen. (Reprinted with permission from Yeh HC. Sonography of the adrenal glands: normal glands and small masses. AJR 1989;135:1167–1177.

than 3 cm is incidentally found in an ultrasonogram for some other purpose, if the patient had no known malignant tumor elsewhere in the body and normal workup shows no suspicion of functional adrenal tumor, the adrenal mass may be considered a nonfunctioning adenoma (30). Follow-up examination may be done in 6 months to 1 year, depending on the clinical condition (30), but if the patient is considered to be of slightly higher risk of having cancer, follow-up may be done in 2 months, 3 months, and 18 months (34). When a mass is larger than 5 cm in size, the operation is advisable (30) because of higher incidence of carcinoma in such cases, although the surgery is not absolutely indicated.

LARGER ADRENAL MASSES

Moderate (3.5 cm to 5 cm in diameter) and large (larger than 5 cm) adrenal masses are usually easy to delineate by ultrasonography. They can be visualized from many scanning

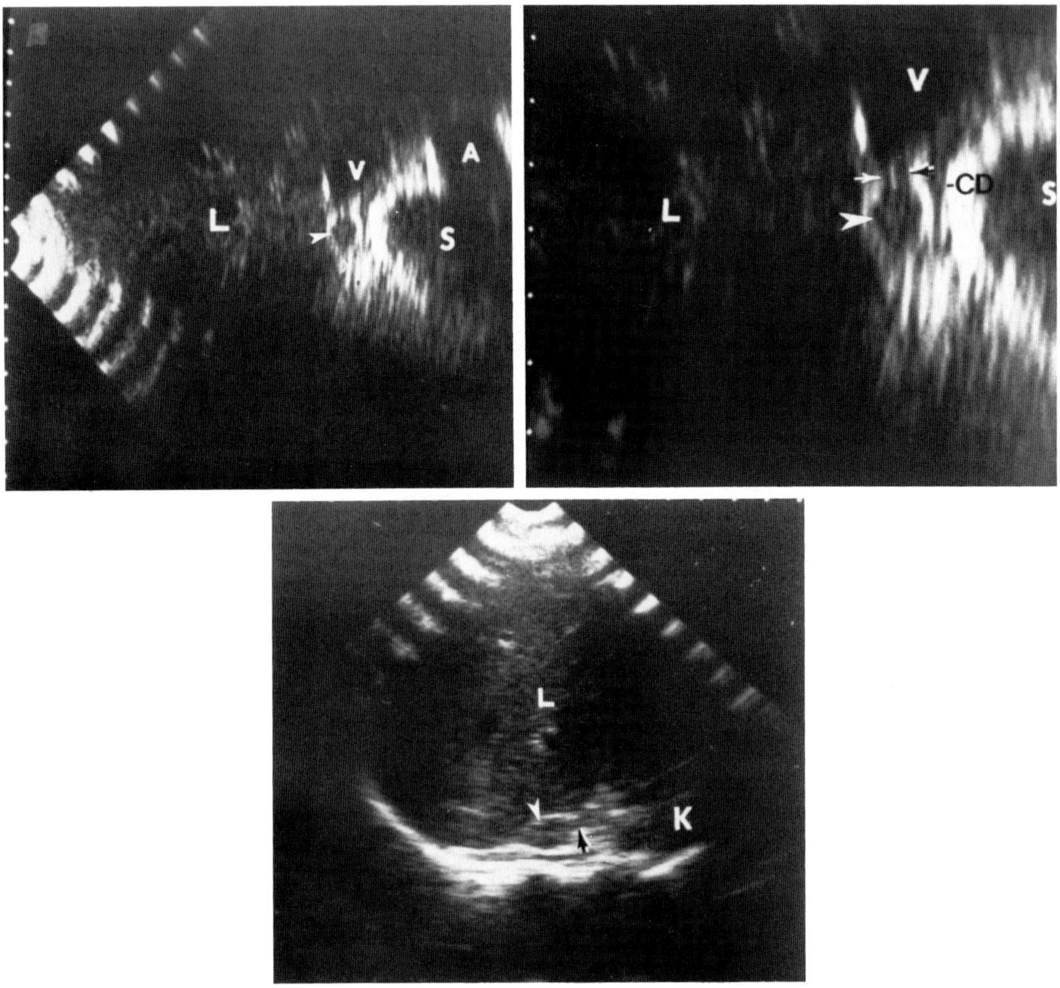

Figure 3.14. A small adenoma in the posterior aspect of the medial wing of the apical portion of right adrenal gland. *Upper left,* Transverse scan from right upper flank region. A small mass (*white arrowhead*) is seen in the right adrenal gland. *V,* inferior vena cava; *A,* aorta; *S,* vertebral body; *L,* liver. *Upper right,* Zoom up view of the same shows the mass (*white arrowhead*) to be in the posterior aspect of the medial wing of the apical portion of adrenal gland. *Black arrow,* uninvolved portion of normal adrenal; *White arrow,* adrenal vein that drains directly into inferior vena cava (*V*); *CD,* crus of diaphragm; *S,* vertebral body; *L,* liver. *Bottom,* Longitudinal scan from right upper flank region shows the adrenal mass (*white arrowhead*) in the apical portion of adrenal gland (*black arrow*). *K,* kidney; *L,* liver.

approaches (i.e., anteriorly, laterally, or posteriorly). They may be round, but the larger masses are frequently oval because of relative restriction in the narrow fat space. The right adrenal mass usually indents or displaces the inferior vena cava anteriorly. This may occur even with a relatively small mass if it is located in the anteromedial ridge of the gland, which is in direct contact with the inferior vena cava. Occasionally, the mass protrudes anteriorly between the inferior vena cava and aorta, displacing the cava laterally.

A moderately sized adrenal mass is typically located anteromedial to the upper pole of the kidney. A large adrenal mass may displace the upper pole of the kidney laterally or the entire kidney inferiorly (Fig. 3.16). When the mass is huge, the entire kidney may be displaced downward, or the upper pole of the kidney may rotate extremely laterally so that the kidney becomes

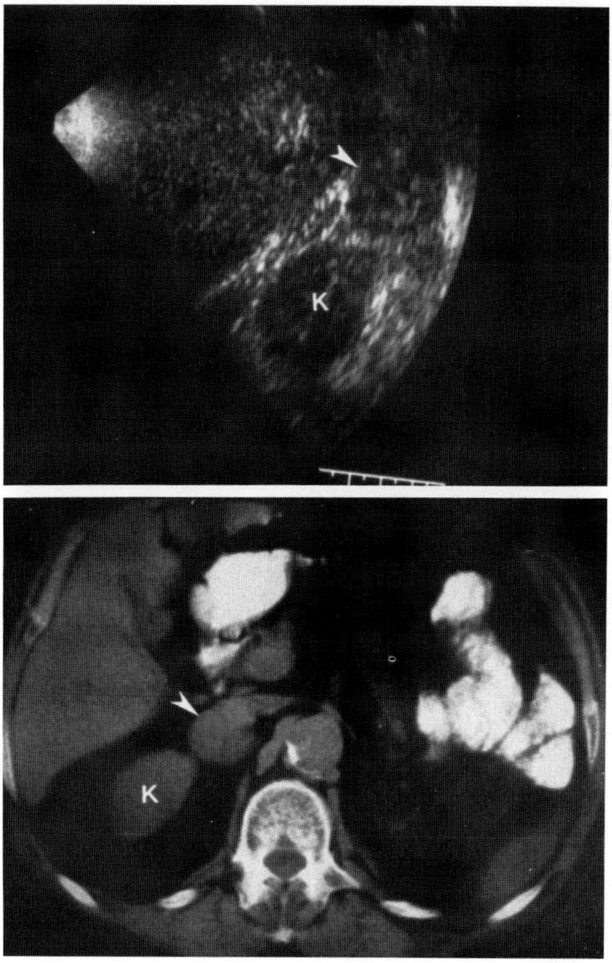

Figure 3.15. Right adrenal adenoma. *Top,* Transverse scan from right upper flank region shows a mass (*arrowhead*) anteromedial to the upper pole of the kidney (*K*). The mass contains multiple hypoechoic areas possibly due to necrosis or hemorrhage. The mass has not changed its size for 3 years and the patient has no known malignancy. *Bottom,* Corresponding CT scan shows the adrenal mass (*arrowhead*) anteromedial to the upper pole of the right kidney (*K*).

horizontal in position. Occasionally, a large adrenal mass may extend inferiorly along the anterior surface of the kidney without causing significant downward displacement of the kidney (35). This occurs more frequently on the left side (Fig. 3.16).

A large left adrenal mass may also displace the pancreas and stomach anteriorly since the left adrenal gland is located posterior to these two organs. The proximal abdominal aorta is more firmly fixed and less likely displaced by the adrenal masses. Occasionally the aorta may be partially surrounded (encased) by the left adrenal malignant tumor, causing difficulty in complete resection of the tumor (35).

The liver may be indented by a large right adrenal mass. When more than half of the mass protrudes outside the liver, the mass is probably from the adrenal gland rather than the liver and vice versa (Fig. 3.17). Occasionally more than half of the adrenal mass may be embedded in the liver so the mass appears intrahepatic. A huge adrenal tumor may greatly displace the right lobe of the liver superiorly and occupy a large part of the liver bed (Fig. 3.18). The mass then conforms to the shape of the right lobe of the liver on transverse section to simulate a large liver mass (17, 36). In such instances, one should carefully scan the liver-mass junction, which may be located high up in the rib cage. The transducer should be placed in the high lateral intercostal space. A notch presenting at the outer margin of the liver-mass demarcation line indicates an extrahepatic or adrenal mass. The demarcation line between the liver and the mass may be highly echogenic or thickened due to interposition of fat when the mass is extrahepatic or adrenal. The echogenic or thickened demarcation may not be seen throughout the entire liver-mass border. Dur-

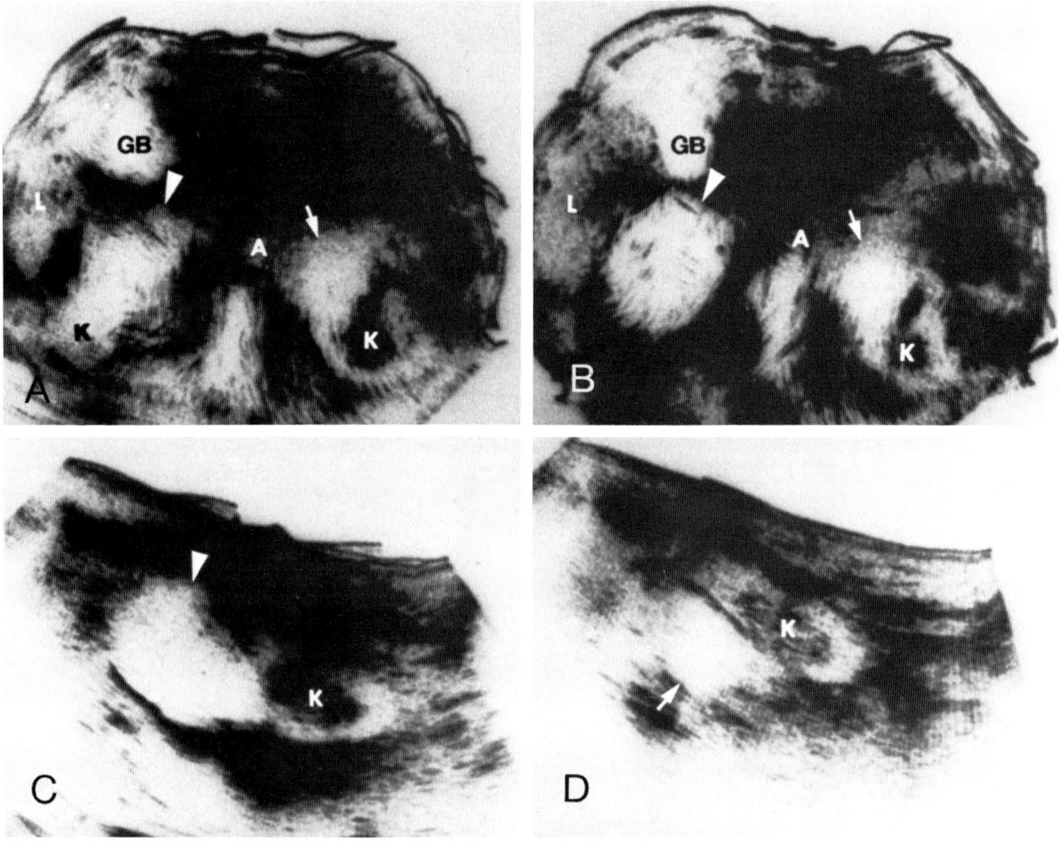

Figure 3.16. Adrenal insufficiency due to metastatic pulmonary carcinoma to both adrenals. **A,** Transverse scan 13 cm above umbilicus. There is a mass in each adrenal gland. *Arrowhead,* right adrenal mass; *arrow,* left adrenal mass; *A,* aorta; *K,* kidney; *L,* liver; *GB,* gallbladder. **B,** Transverse scan 14 cm above umbilicus. The main portion of the right adrenal mass (*arrowhead*) is above the right kidney, which is not seen in this scan. **C,** Right posterior longitudinal scan. The right adrenal mass (*arrowhead*) is mainly superior to the kidney except the inferior portion, which is anterior to the upper pole of the kidney. The kidney is displaced inferiorly by the mass. **D,** Left posterior longitudinal scan. The left adrenal mass (*arrow*) is anterior to the kidney (*K*). The kidney is not significantly displaced inferiorly by the mass. (**A** and **B** reprinted with permission from Mitty HA, Yeh HC. Radiology of the adrenals with sonography and CT. Philadelphia: WB Saunders, 1982.)

ing deep inspiration, if the liver slides over the mass (i.e., the mass does not move with the liver), the mass is extrahepatic or adrenal.

A moderately sized or large adrenal mass may similarly indent or compress the upper pole of the kidney, and questions of whether the mass is renal or adrenal in origin may also arise in such instances. When the larger portion of the mass protrudes outside the expected contour of the kidney, the mass is more likely to be of extrarenal or adrenal origin (17). A thin demarcation line between the kidney and the mass may be seen in both renal and extrarenal masses (17), although a thick echogenic demarcation line (or band) will be more suggestive of extrarenal origin. During deep inspiration, demonstration of relative motion between the mass and the kidney indicates that the mass is of extrarenal or adrenal origin.

A larger adrenal mass is more likely to contain areas of necrosis of hemorrhage except pheochromocytoma, which may become totally hemorrhagic even at a relatively small size (Fig. 3.19). Ultrasonographic features of both focal necrosis and hemorrhage are quite similar. When not liquefied, focal necrosis may

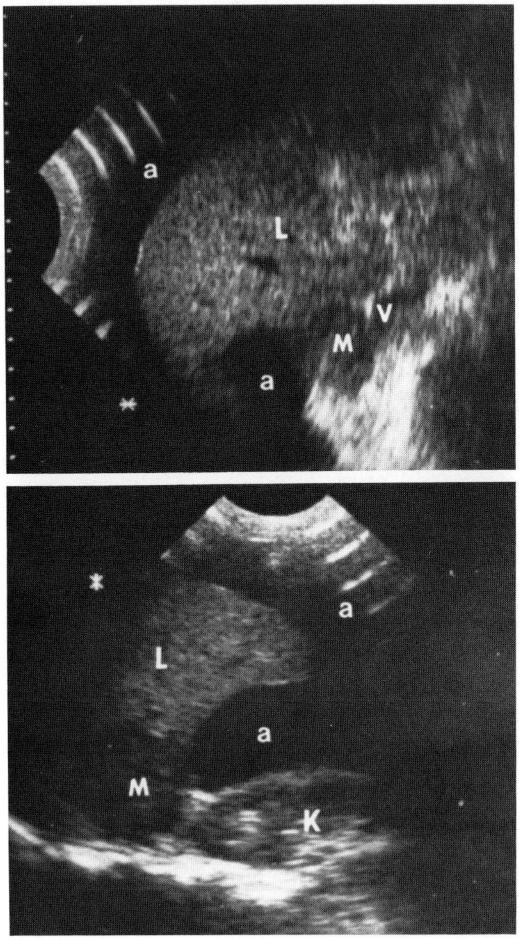

Figure 3.17. A liver mass simulating an adrenal tumor. *Top,* Transverse scan from right upper flank region shows a mass (*M*) in the right adrenal region. The mass is partly within the liver (*L*). *V,* inferior vena cava; *a,* ascites. *Bottom,* Longitudinal scan from the right upper flank region shows the mass (*M*) to be superior to the kidney (*K*), but most of the mass is within the liver and therefore it is more likely to be a liver mass than an adrenal mass. *a,* ascites. The mass was proven to be a hepatocellular carcinoma and not an adrenal mass.

show areas of high echogenicity. Focal hemorrhage or blood may also be highly echogenic. Liquefied necrosis and hematomas are poorly echogenic or anechoic, similar to a cyst. Both nonliquefied necrosis with marked edema and completely clotted hematoma may also appear echo free to simulate a cystic lesion (Fig. 3.19) (35). Therefore, an echo-free focus within an adrenal mass may represent necrosis that is liquefied or nonliquefied, or a hematoma that is solid or liquid. The wall of a necrotic or hemorrhagic adrenal tumor may be thick or thin and may be shaggy or smooth (35).

Large primary adrenal tumors are usually malignant except pheochromocytomas. Adrenal carcinomas are usually discovered when large (larger than 5 cm, the same in children) (33, 37, 38), because the tumors grow quickly or the symptoms appear late even when the tumors are functional. The production of hormones by a functional carcinoma is usually not as profuse as by a functional adenoma. Some benign pheochromocytomas, on the other hand, may grow to a huge size to markedly compress and displace the liver and may contain extensive necrosis and hemorrhage.

Tumor metastases to the adrenal glands are not uncommon, especially from the lungs. They range from a very small size, undiscernible by ultrasonography or CT (39), to a huge size. They are single or multiple, and the latter may be unilateral or bilateral. Diffuse involvement of the adrenal gland may occasionally be seen (29). Bilateral involvement of the adrenal gland may cause adrenal insufficiency (Fig. 3.16) (40).

MULTIPLE ADRENAL MASSES

Multiple adrenal masses, either unilateral or bilateral (Figs. 3.20 and 3.21), are not uncommon. They occur in (*a*) metastasis from some other primary malignancy, especially bronchogenic carcinoma (Fig. 3.16), renal cell carcinoma, and melanoma (41, 42); (*b*) pheochromocytoma, mostly with familial history and benign, but may be malignant; (*c*) lymphoma, mainly of non-Hodgkin's type, may be primary in the adrenals or secondary; (*d*) bilateral adrenal hyperplasia with multiple hyperplastic nodules, usually less than 1 cm in size, but may be larger in macronodular hyperplasia.

Small, unilateral, multiple adrenal masses may be seen as discrete nodules in different parts of the adrenal gland. When they are larger, the adjacent masses may partly fuse to form a dumbbell shape (Fig. 3.20). If such masses are aligned in craniocaudal orientation, they may appear as a single mass on CT scans (Fig. 3.20) unless a sagittal or coronal scan is done. Ultrasonography will clearly show dumbbell-shaped masses (Fig. 3.20). When the masses are on the right side they may cause double indentation on the posterior wall of the inferior vena cava. A small mass on a larger

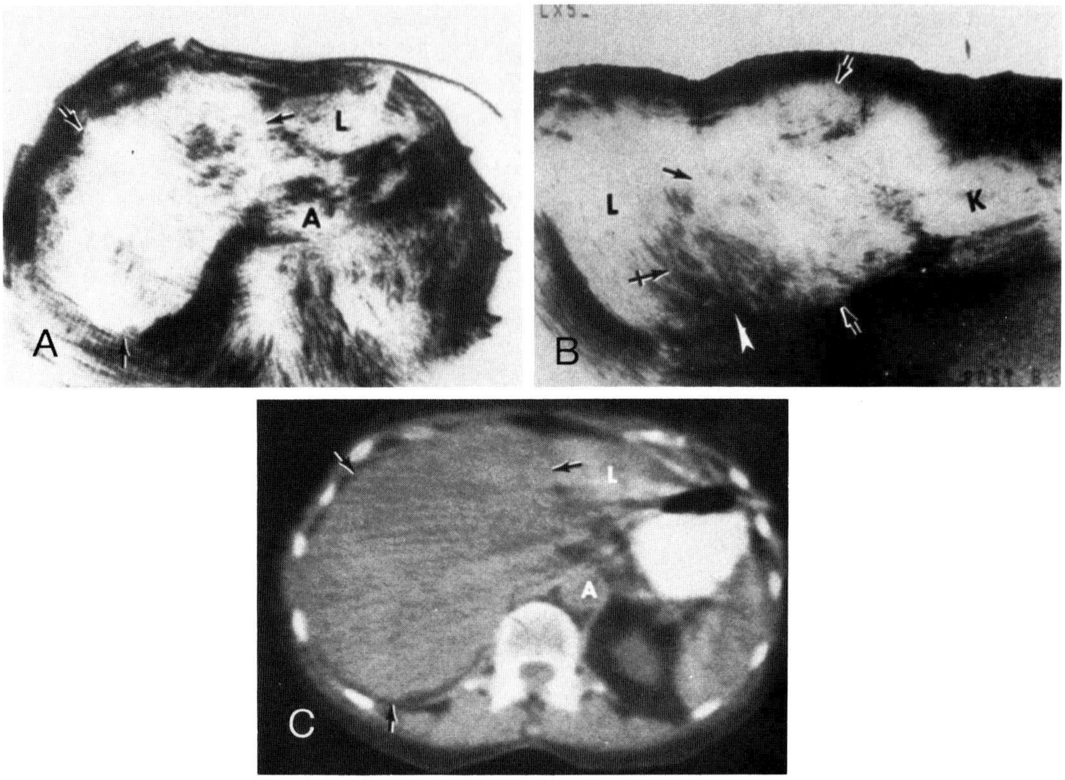

Figure 3.18. Large adrenal carcinoma simulating a liver mass. This 73-year-old woman had been previously admitted to another hospital where the diagnosis of liver tumor was made on the basis of ultrasonography, CT, and celiac arteriography. Needle biopsy showed cancer cells probably of hepatic origin. Ultrasonography was repeated after the patient's admission to Mount Sinai Hospital, and an adrenal tumor was diagnosed. Adrenal venography confirmed the diagnosis, and the adrenal carcinoma was surgically proven. There was no tumor in the liver. **A,** Transverse scan of the upper abdomen shows a large mass (*arrows*) that appears to involve the entire right lobe of the liver. *L,* normal left lobe of the liver; *A,* aorta. **B,** Longitudinal scan 5 cm to the right of the midline. The liver (*L*), high in the rib cage, was scanned through multiple intercostal spaces. The mass (*arrows*) is located inferior to the liver and above the kidney (*K*). A thick echogenic demarcation (*crossed arrow*) is seen between the liver and the mass, and a notch (*white arrowhead*) is present at the posterior end of the demarcation. **C,** CT scan corresponding to **A.** The tumor location is easily mistaken to be the liver. (Reprinted with permission from Yeh HC. Ultrasonography of the adrenals. Semin Reontgenol 1988;23:250–258.)

mass will show a budding appearance. Finding all masses, especially if they are bilateral, may be important for diseases (e.g., pheochromocytomas) in which only complete excision will constitute a cure. Therefore, careful scanning for both the adrenal glands should be done.

Diffusely Enlarged Adrenal Glands

The adrenal gland may become diffusely enlarged due to a variety of causes:

1. Bilateral adrenal hyperplasia. The adrenal gland may become enlarged in response to stress. Bilateral adrenal hyperplasia also occurs in various endocrine hyperfunctions (e.g., Cushing's syndrome, hyperaldosteronism, adrenogenital syndrome). It may also be seen after administration of ACTH or in ectopic ACTH syndrome. In ectopic ACTH syndrome, ACTH is produced by neoplasms not arising from the pituitary gland but from elsewhere in the body. As adrenal glands enlarge, they become thickened. The adrenal glands may become greatly enlarged in ectopic ACTH syndrome. However, this is more easily discerned on CT than on

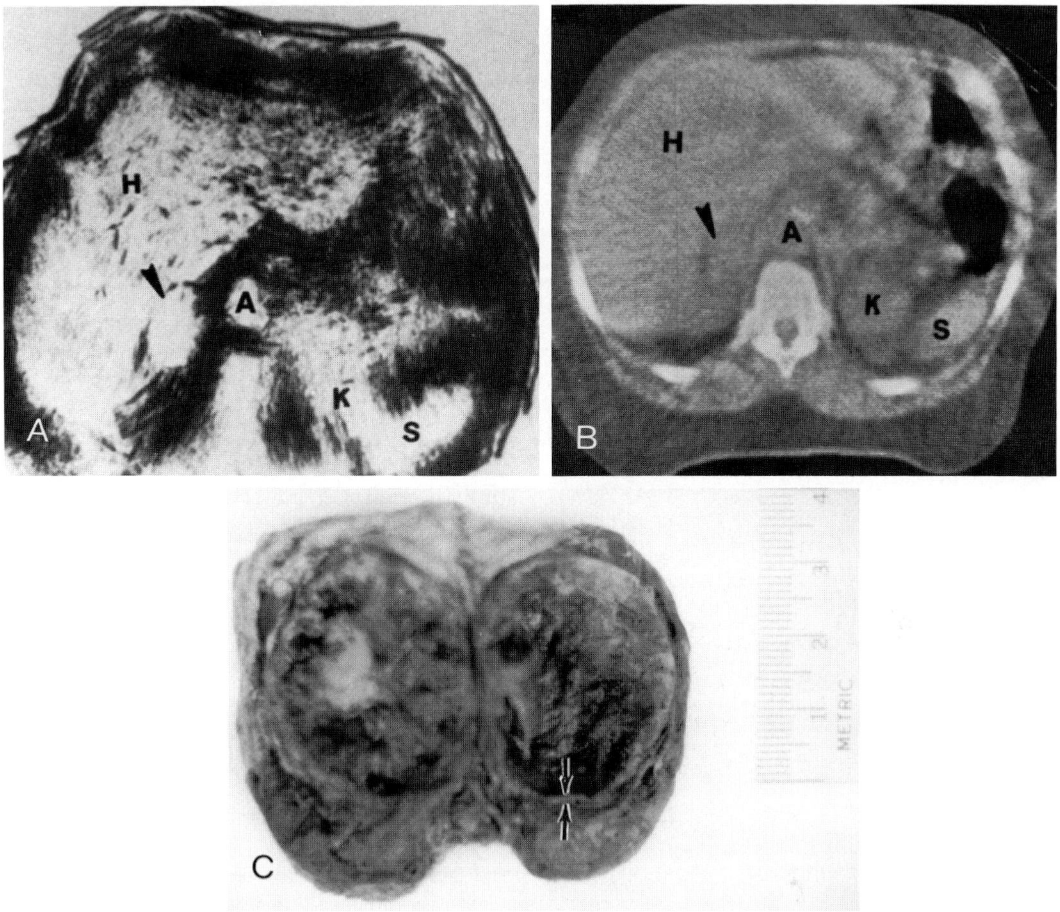

Figure 3.19. A small hemorrhagic pheochromocytoma. **A,** Transverse scan of upper abdomen shows a cystic lesion (*arrowhead*) in the right adrenal gland. *A,* aorta; *K,* upper pole of left kidney; *H,* liver; *S,* spleen. **B,** Corresponding CT scan shows the cystic lesion (*arrowhead*) to have soft tissue density. **C,** Pathology specimen shows the lesion to be a pheochromocytoma filled with a blood clot but with only a thin rim (between *arrows*) of viable tumor tissue in the wall. (Reprinted with permission from Yeh HC, Mitty HA, Rose J, Wolf BS, Gabrilove JL. Ultrasonography of adrenal masses: unusual manifestations. Radiology 1978;127:475–483.)

ultrasonography. This is especially true in patients with Cushing's syndrome due to an abundance of perirenal fat, which degrades the images in ultrasonography but improves the visualization of the gland on CT., Furthermore, while the normal adrenal gland is quite variable in size, only about 50% of patients with bilateral hyperplasia have grossly enlarged adrenal glands. Although the convex contour of the gland on radiographs (e.g., retroperitoneal pneumograph) (43) and on longitudinal oblique sonograms (44) has been considered to indicate hyperplasia, in fact a convex contour is frequently seen in normal glands on gas insufflation and venographic studies in vitro (45) as well as on anatomical specimens (Fig. 3.2). The convex contour is most frequently seen on the medial border of the right gland and the superior medial border of the left gland (45). In general, bilateral hyperplasia cannot be diagnosed with certainty by ultrasonography or CT unless the glands are markedly thickened or multiple hyperplastic nodules are seen. The convex border of adrenal hyperplasia reported on longitudinal oblique sonography (44) may simply represent perirenal fat and not the adrenal gland per se.

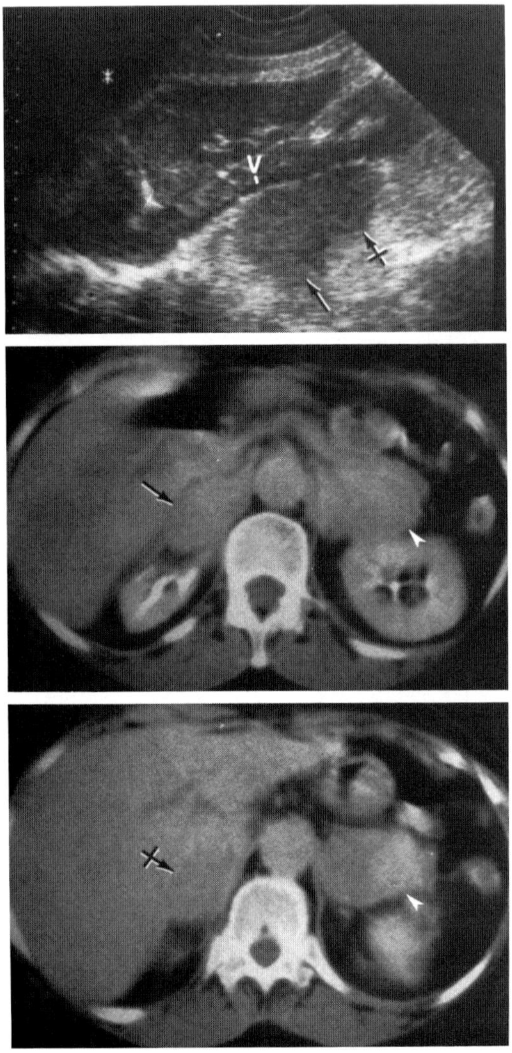

Figure 3.20. Double metastatic adrenal masses from lung cancer. *Top,* Right paramedian longitudinal scan of upper abdomen shows two masses (*arrow* and *crossed arrow*) forming a dumbbell shape. The masses cause double indentations on the inferior vena cava (*V*). *Middle,* CT scan of upper abdomen shows a mass (*arrow*) in the right adrenal gland. Another mass (*white arrowhead*) is seen in the left adrenal gland. *Bottom,* CT scan 3 cm inferior to the above section shows the right adrenal mass (*crossed arrow*) appearing as the same mass as the one in the above image.

When the adrenal glands are diffusely enlarged, the echogenic medullae become more easily seen. Visualization of an intact adrenal medulla indicates hyperplasia (Fig. 3.6) rather than a diffuse infiltrative process; in the latter case the medulla will not be seen.

2. Neoplastic diseases. Most commonly lymphoma of non-Hodgkin's variety (24, 46, 47), but also bronchogenic and renal cell carcinoma may diffusely involve the adrenal glands.
3. Inflammatory disease. Tuberculosis (49), histoplasmosis (48, 50), etc.

As the adrenal glands diffusely enlarge, they maintain the basic form of a normal adrenal gland as previously mentioned; that is, a vertical linear shape on the upper section of the gland, an inverted Y or V shape on the middle section, and an L (left) or reverse L (right) shape on the inferior section. As the adrenal gland is greatly enlarged, however, the characteristic features are modified. A vertical oval structure may be seen in the upper section, a triangular structure in the middle section, and a wedge-shaped structure in the lower section (24). Therefore, one may easily mistake it as a focal mass lesion based on a single sectional image. In fact, a diffusely enlarged adrenal gland was said to be indistinguishable from a focal mass lesion in CT literature (51). Diffuse enlargement of the adrenal gland can be diagnosed, however, by finding the characteristic features on serial sections (24). Occasionally, when a diffusely enlarged adrenal gland is huge, it may become irregular in shape and may be difficult to differentiate from a huge focal mass (24). Following chemotherapy or radiation treatment, as the mass decreases in size, the gland becomes normal in shape even though it is still enlarged. Recognition of diffuse enlargement is of diagnostic importance because there is a high incidence of lymphoma when the adrenal glands are markedly, diffusely enlarged bilaterally. Occasionally a focal mass lesion may be seen superimposed on a diffusely enlarged adrenal gland.

Functioning Adrenal Lesions

Since the adrenal gland provides multiple endocrine functions due to various hormones secreted from the cortex or medulla of the gland, there are a variety of functioning lesions, each presenting with different clinical features, corresponding to the type of excessive hormone the lesion excretes.

ADRENAL CORTICAL HYPERFUNCTIONS

There are three distinct clinical syndromes due to hyperfunction of the adrenal cortex:

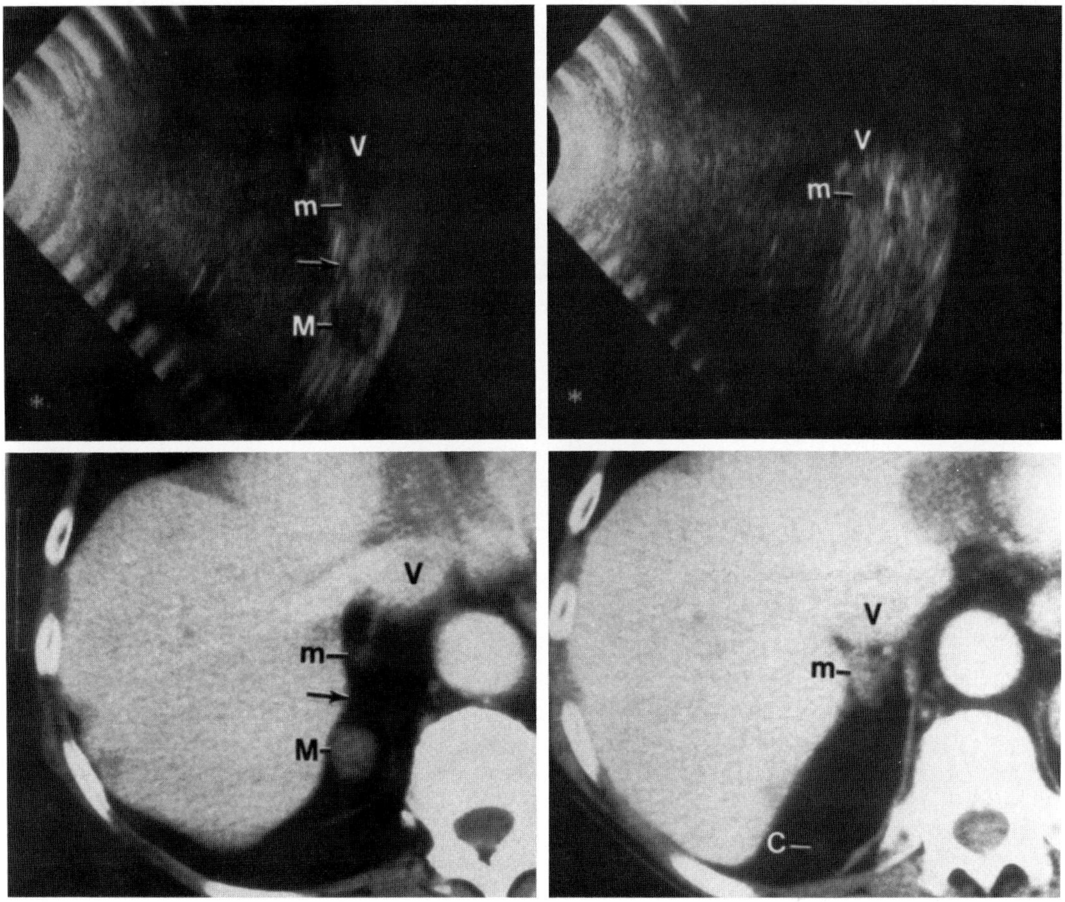

Figure 3.21. Double masses in the right adrenal gland due to lymphoma. *Upper left,* Transverse sector scan from right upper flank region shows two masses in the right adrenal gland. The posterior mass (*M*) is at the posterior tip of the medial wing of the gland and the anterior mass (*m*) is at the anteromedial ridge of the gland, i.e., posterior to the inferior vena cava (*V*). Note the uninvolved normal portion (*arrow*) of the adrenal gland. *Upper right,* Scanning slightly inferiorly, the anterior mass (*m*) is more clearly seen. *Lower left,* CT scan corresponding to upper left panel shows the masses (*M, m*). The uninvolved portion of the adrenal gland is only vaguely seen. *V,* inferior vena cava. *Lower right,* CT scan corresponding to upper right panel shows the anterior mass (*m*). *C,* a cyst in the upper pole of the right kidney.

1. *Cushing's syndrome.* Due to excessive secretion of cortisol, which has glucocorticoid activity. This results in the clinical features of moon face, buffalo hump, purple abdominal striae, muscle wasting, hirsutism, acne, hypertension, etc.
2. *Hyperaldosteronism.* Caused by hypersecretion of aldosterone, a mineralocorticoid, manifested by hyperkalemia, decrease in plasma renin concentration, and hypertension.
3. *Adrenogenital syndrome.* Excessive secretion of androgen causes pseudohermaphroditism in female infants (girls), enlarges external genitalia in boys (precocious puberty), and causes virilization of adult females. On the other hand, on rare instances, feminizing tumors of the adrenal cortex, mostly carcinomas, may be seen in men.

These syndromes may be caused by bilateral adrenal hyperplasia, adenoma, or carcinoma, although the incidence of each pathological entity may be different in each syndrome and the cause of bilateral hyperplasia may also vary. In Cushing's syndrome there is a high incidence

(80%) of adrenal hyperplasia and many of these cases are due to basophilic adenoma (or microadenoma) of the pituitary gland (i.e., Cushing's disease) that can be treated surgically.

In hyperaldosteronism, only 10% is caused by diffuse hyperplasia, which is best treated medically. In the adrenogenital syndrome, hyperplasia may be caused congenitally, but some patients may have late onset at adulthood. Congenital deficiency of 21-hydroxylase or 11β-hydroxylase prevents the conversion of cortical precursors. This results in little or no production of cortisol and ACTH continues to stimulate the adrenal glands. The adrenal glands become hyperplastic and the hyperplastic adrenal gland secretes excessive androgen.

As previously mentioned, the adrenal glands are normal in size in many patients (less than 50% of patients in one series) (33) with bilateral hyperplasia. This has led to the use of the term "non-tumorous adrenocortical hyperfunction" or "Cushing's syndrome without adrenal tumor" rather than bilateral adrenal hyperplasia (33).

In hyperaldosteronism, the majority of cases are caused by adenomas that are usually small (smaller than 3 cm) and therefore require careful scanning with ultrasonography to detect the lesion.

ADRENAL MEDULLARY HYPERFUNCTION

Pheochromocytoma

The tumor arises from adrenal medullary cells, the pheochromocytes, which secrete epinephrine or norepinephrine or both. Since these are potent hormones, the tumors are almost invariably lethal if untreated. The tumor can be removed and the patient can be cured. Therefore, diagnosis of this disease is important. Clinical features are extremely variable, hence pheochromocytoma is a great mimic. However, the most common presenting feature is hypertension that is characteristically paroxysmal. Other symptoms are headache, sweating, pallor, tachycardia, postural hypotension, and a raised basal metabolism.

The majority (90%) of the tumors arise from the adrenal medulla, and about 10% are of extraadrenal origin. Approximately 10% of the tumors are malignant and about 10% of patients have multiple masses. Although large adrenal masses tend to be malignant, benign pheochromocytomas may grow to larger size (e.g., 22 cm in our institution). Unlike other tumors which, when multiple, are frequently malignant due to metastases, multiple pheochromocytomas are often benign. Furthermore, other malignant tumors in general tend to outgrow their blood supply and cause necrosis or hemorrhage. Benign pheochromocytomas, however, also tend to necrose and hemorrhage, even at a small size (35). This causes a nonhomogeneous echo pattern or foci of hyper- or hypoechoic areas on ultrasonography and irregular enhancement on CT scan with intravenous contrast, similar to malignant tumors (28). Not uncommonly one may see a relatively small pheochromocytoma almost completely necrosed or hemorrhaged, resulting in an appearance of a cyst on ultrasonography and CT (35). When hemorrhage is relatively recent, however, a completely echo-free cystic appearing pheochromocytoma may show a mass with soft tissue density on CT (Fig. 3.19). In short, many ultrasonographic and CT features of benign pheochromocytomas are similar to malignant tumors. In fact, malignant and benign pheochromocytomas may have a similar histologic appearance, and the only absolute criteria upon which a diagnosis of malignancy can be made is the presence of distant metastases (42). One should, however, not mistake multiple benign lesions for metastases.

The extraadrenal pheochromocytomas are frequently seen in the organ of Zuckerkandl, which is usually located at the origin of the inferior mesenteric artery. The tumor may also be found elsewhere along the sympathetic nervous system or in the wall of the urinary bladder, and only rarely (1%) are pheochromocytomas located in the chest.

Pheochromocytomas may be seen as part of multiple endocrine neoplasia (MEN) syndrome, especially in type 2 (Sipple's syndrome). In MEN type 2 the pheochromocytoma is associated with medullary thyroid carcinoma and sometimes hyperparathyroidism. The disease is familial, and the pheochromocytomas are frequently bilateral or multiple.

Pheochromocytomas may also be associated with Von Hippel-Lindau disease in about 10% of cases and are associated with neurofibromatosis in less than 1% of cases.

Neuroblastoma and Ganglioneuroma

Neuroblastomas also arise from adrenal medullae (30 to 50%) or sympathetic gangliomas in the abdomen or chest, but are usually discovered in childhood. Increased catecholamine secretion may also be seen. The patients may become hypertensive. Ultrasonography frequently shows the mass to be highly echogenic (Fig. 3.22) (35) or irregularly echogenic (52) due to calcifications, necrosis, or hemorrhage (35). Calcifications may be found in 50% of patients on CT. The major differential diagnosis at this age is Wilms' tumor, which arises from the kidney. Therefore, determining whether the tumor is extrarenal in origin is very important in diagnosing neuroblastoma. This is discussed in detail elsewhere in this chapter. Metastases to paraaortic nodes and liver are frequently seen on ultrasonography.

Ganglioneuroma is a benign form of neuroblastoma. This is a rare tumor that can be seen in children or adults. Neuroblastoma may sometimes mature spontaneously into benign ganglioneuroma.

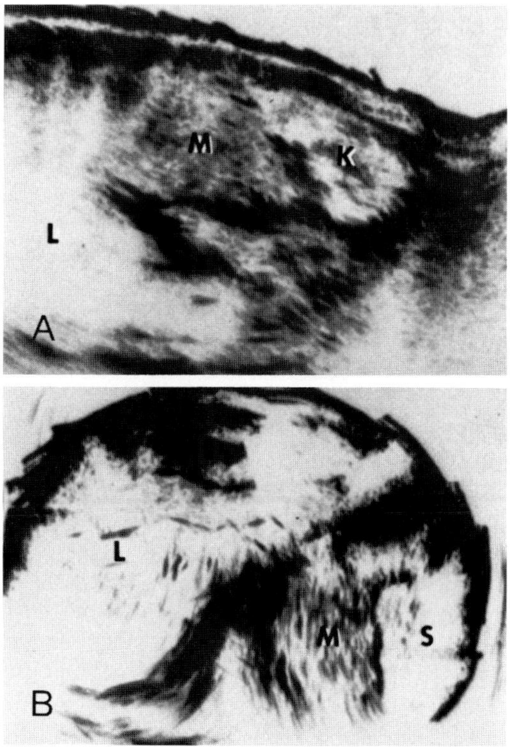

Figure 3.22. Neuroblastoma of the left adrenal gland. **A,** Posterior longitudinal scan shows a highly echogenic mass (*M*) anterosuperior to the kidney (*K*), representing neuroblastoma. The kidney is markedly indented. *L,* liver. **B,** Anterior transverse scan 12 cm above umbilicus. The adrenal mass (*M*) is medial to the spleen (*S*).

Malignant Tumors of the Adrenal Glands

PRIMARY ADRENOCORTICAL CARCINOMAS

Most adrenal carcinomas are functioning tumors; 50% are associated with Cushing's syndrome, 20% with adrenogenital syndromes, 4% with combined Cushing's and virilizing syndrome, and 4% with hyperaldosteronism. Nonfunctioning tumors constitute the remaining primary adrenal carcinomas. Both functioning and nonfunctioning carcinomas are usually large when discovered, but this is more true for nonfunctioning carcinomas. The nonfunctioning adrenal carcinomas are quite invasive; widespread metastases to the liver, lung, bone, and peritoneal cavity are frequently discovered simultaneously; and survival is frequently shorter than with functioning carcinomas.

PRIMARY MALIGNANCIES OF ADRENAL MEDULLA

These are pheochromocytomas and neuroblastomas, which have been previously mentioned.

Occasionally lymphomas, especially those of non-Hodgkin's type, may arise from adrenal glands as primary tumors and may diffusely involve the adrenal gland (46).

METASTASES TO THE ADRENAL GLANDS

These are not uncommon (27% at autopsy) (42) but may be only microscopic. In an autopsy series, 75.6% of lung cancer and 53.9% of breast cancer metastasized to the adrenal gland. Lymphoma and melanoma are also not uncommon. Ultrasonography will show a solid lesion that is indistinguishable from those of primary malignancies. Bilateral metastases may occur simultaneously or on different occasions and are not uncommonly seen (35).

ADRENAL HEMORRHAGE

The neonatal adrenal glands are proportionately much larger than adult adrenal glands. The large adrenal glands greatly decrease in size within 4 weeks of birth. As the bulk of primitive adrenal cortex undergoes atrophy immediately after birth, the already dilated vascular channels in the primitive cortex become even more engorged and the neonatal adrenal gland becomes more vulnerable to hemorrhage (Fig. 3.23). It is more so for the right gland, possibly because the right adrenal vein is short and readily transmits the increased pressure in the inferior vena cava. The neonatal adrenal veins do not contain muscle fibers in their walls and therefore cannot contract in response to increases in venous pressure as in adult adrenal veins, which contain muscle fibers. Neonatal adrenal hemorrhage may be caused by fetal distress, complicated delivery, asphyxia, coagulation disorders, or sepsis.

An echo-free lesion that is similar to a cyst (53–55) is seen in early hematoma (Fig. 3.23). Some echoes may be seen due to the presence of blood clots. The lesion is highly transonic, even though some have internal echoes, and therefore should be differentiated from a neuroblastoma. The hematoma is round, oval, elongated, or somewhat irregular in shape. As lysis of blood clots occurs, the echoes may disappear.

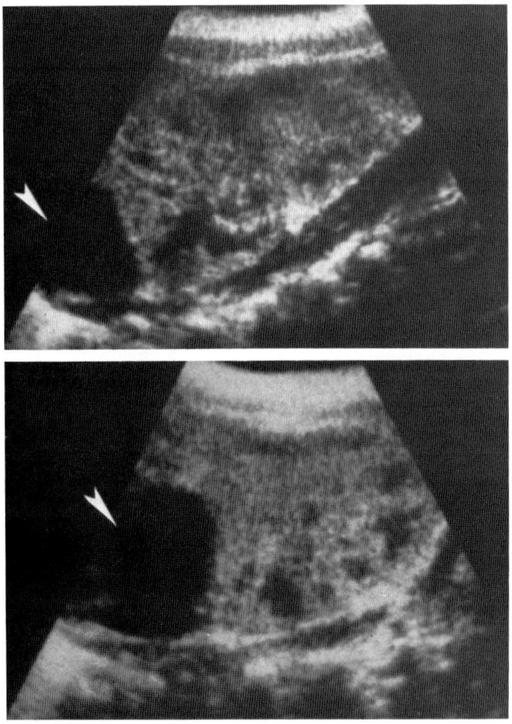

Figure 3.23. Bilateral adrenal hemorrhage in a newborn. *Top* and *bottom,* Longitudinal oblique scans show an echo-free lesion (*arrowhead*) above each kidney, representing the hematomas. (Reprinted with permission from Yeh HC. Adrenal gland and nonrenal retroperitoneum. Urol Radiol 1987;9:127–140.)

The hematoma usually decreases in size in 4 to 5 weeks, and some internal echoes may reappear due to organization of the hematoma. The hematoma may eventually disappear or become calcified. The calcification may be detected in 4 to 9 months by ultrasonography as a highly echogenic lesion with acoustic shadows (53). The ultrasonographic and clinical features and progressive changes are usually helpful in the diagnosis. A fine-needle aspiration under ultrasound guidance may be done in doubtful cases. Aspiration of the unclotted blood usually confirms the hematoma.

In both adults and children adrenal hemorrhage may occur in Waterhouse-Friderichsen syndrome, most commonly due to meningococcal infection, but also possibly due to a variety of other microorganisms. There is infection and hemorrhagic necrosis of the adrenal gland, and therefore this has also been referred to as adrenal apoplexy. In patients undergoing ACTH treatment, the hypertrophic adrenal glands are also vulnerable to hemorrhage. The hemorrhage may appear as focal hematoma similar to neonatal hemorrhage (56), or blood may infiltrate the entire adrenal gland to cause diffuse adrenal enlargement.

The diffusely enlarged adrenal glands are similar to infiltrative processes due to other causes such as neoplasm. On CT scans without intravenous injection of contrast medium, a high attenuation number seen in the glands indicates recent hemorrhage.

ADRENAL CYST

Adrenal cysts are usually seen in the fifth and sixth decades. They are of various origins, most commonly in endothelial cysts (45%) that are mostly lymphangiomata, but occasionally they may be angiomatous (57). Pseudocysts of adrenal glands are also not uncommon. The pseudocysts are caused by liquefaction of encapsulated hematomas due to trauma, sepsis, or some other acute serious illness. Other cysts include epithelial, glandular, or echinococcal cysts.

On ultrasonography, the adrenal cysts are usually echo free with a thin wall, but calcified cyst walls are highly echogenic (Fig. 3.24) and may cast an acoustic shadow (25). Calcification of an adrenal cyst occurs in about 15% of cases. In contrast to calcified renal cysts, which have a high incidence of carcinoma, the calcified adrenal cysts are usually benign.

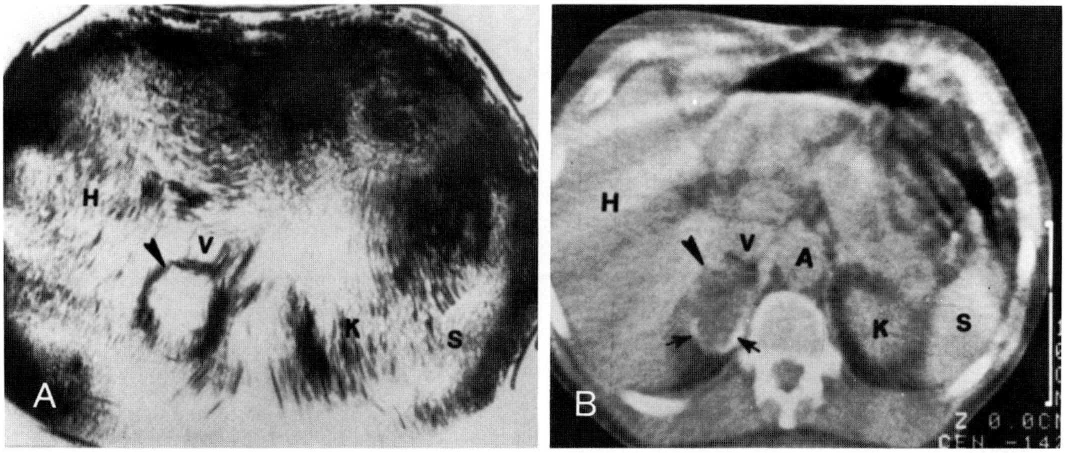

Figure 3.24. Adrenal cyst, calcified. **A,** Transverse sonographic scan 15 cm above the umbilicus. A cystic lesion *(arrowhead)* is seen behind the inferior vena cava *(V)*. *H,* liver; *K,* kidney; *S,* spleen. **B,** Corresponding CT scan., The lesion *(arrowhead)* is of water density with a calcified wall *(arrows)*. (Reprinted with permission from Yeh HC, Mitty HA, Rose J, Wolf BS, Gabrilove JL. Ultrasonography of adrenal masses: usual features. Radiology 1987;127:467.)

Fine-needle aspiration under ultrasound guidance may confirm the cyst. The fluid obtained may be clear or bloody (old blood). Cholesterol crystals may be seen within the fluid. Due to the blood content, the attenuation number on CT scanning may be higher than that of water, so the cystic nature may not be apparent unless it is scanned both before and after contrast injection to demonstrate no contrast enhancement. Ultrasonography will usually clearly show the cystic nature.

MISCELLANEOUS LESIONS

Inflammatory Disease

Adrenal glands may be involved in tuberculosis (49) or histoplasmosis (48). Both may result in Addison's disease. A mass-like lesion may be seen in the adrenal gland or the adrenal gland may be diffusely enlarged. Calcification may be seen in chronic cases.

A fibro-fatty mass of the adrenal gland may be caused by some nonspecified old inflammatory disease. An ill-defined echogenic mass may be seen by ultrasonography (35).

Myelolipoma

This is a relatively uncommon tumor, usually seen in the fourth and sixth decades. The tumor contains fat and bone marrow cells. The fat content causes high echogenicity on ultrasonography (58) and characteristic low attenuation on CT scanning. This is similar to an angiomyelipoma of the kidney, and therefore when it is relatively large it should be determined whether the mass is of adrenal or renal origin.

Varicosity of the Adrenal Vein

In patients with portal hypertension, adrenal veins may occasionally become elongated, dilated, and tortuous due to varicosity (59).

Calcification of the Adrenal Glands or Adrenal Masses

This may be seen after hemorrhage, in neuroblastoma (most common calcified masses), cysts (Fig. 3.16), cortical adenomas, carcinoma, metastasis, pheochromocytomas, tuberculosis, histoplasmosis, disseminated herpes simplex and myelolipoma, etc. (60, 61, 64).

DIFFERENTIAL DIAGNOSIS

Mass on Upper Pole of Kidney

A mass protruding from the upper pole of the kidney may simulate an adrenal mass. When the main bulk of the mass is outside the expected renal contours, and the demarcation line between the mass and the kidney is a thick, highly echogenic line and a notch is seen at the edge of demarcation, the mass is most likely of extrarenal or adrenal origin. The extrarenal origin of the mass is further confirmed when relative motion between the kidney and the mass is demonstrated on deep inspiration during real-time scanning. A thin demarcation line between the mass and the kidney may be seen in either renal or adrenal masses (35). The delineation of the demarcation line between the mass and the kidney depends on scanning angle and technique (17). By careful scanning one may sometimes see the normal thickness of the renal cortex, which is depressed by the extrarenal mass.

Accessory Spleen

This is usually a small 1- to 2-cm round structure, most frequently located at the splenic hilum. The echo pattern is homogeneous, similar to splenic parenchymal echoes. It is located more lateral to the left adrenal gland. A vessel may be seen to connect the structure to splenic artery or vein (62).

Medial Tubercle of Spleen

A medial tubercle of the spleen may simulate an adrenal mass on posterior scanning (17), except that it is located more lateral than the usual adrenal mass. It may appear oval or round. The echo pattern is the same as that of splenic parenchyma, and after careful scanning from various approaches a connection to the spleen may be found.

Protruding Liver Mass

A mass protruding from under the surface of the right lobe of the liver may simulate an adrenal tumor (Fig. 3.16). Similar to differentiating from a renal mass, if the bulk of the mass is outside the expected liver contour, a thick echogenic demarcation line is seen between the mass and the liver, a notch rather than a beak is seen at the edge of the demarcation, and there is demonstration of relative motion between the liver and mass on deep inspiration, the mass is most likely extrahepatic or adrenal in origin.

Stomach or Duplication of Stomach

Part of the stomach may occasionally simulate an adrenal mass. Its location is slightly more anterior than that of an adrenal mass, and peristalsis may be observed. Drinking of water observed under real-time scanning will clearly demonstrate the flow of water.

Duplication of the stomach may be located posterior to the stomach and simulate an adrenal cyst. It may be located more lateral to the adrenal area.

Second Portion of the Duodenum

When the second portion of the duodenum appears rather posteriorly located, it may simulate an adrenal mass (Fig. 3.11). It is, however, located lateral to the inferior vena cava and peristalsis or passage of gas bubbles may be induced by compression of the epigastrium or by giving the patient a drink of water (Fig. 3.25).

Enlarged Paraaortic or Retropancreatic Nodes

When the normal adrenal gland is seen clearly separate from the mass, an extraadrenal mass or an enlarged lymph node can be diagnosed. However, if the mass appears to be attached to the tip of an adrenal wing, it is difficult to determine whether the mass is intra- or extraadrenal in origin. An angiogram may be necessary to demonstrate feeding vessels so that the origin of the mass can be determined.

Splenic Vessels

The splenic artery is frequently tortuous and may pass by the adrenal area to simulate an enlarged adrenal gland. An aneurysm of the splenic artery may simulate an adrenal mass. These structures can be traced to connect to the splenic artery at the splenic hilum. Expansile pulsation and Doppler signals may be seen in a splenic arterial aneurysm. The splenic vein is less likely to be confused with an adrenal lesion since it is usually straighter and more anterior than the artery, located immediately posterior to the pancreas.

Lesions in the Tail of the Pancreas

A mass or pseudocyst protruding from the tail of the pancreas posteriorly may simulate an adrenal lesion. These lesions can be seen to be partly within the pancreas by scanning from the flank region or by anterior transverse scanning or anterior longitudinal scanning tilting the transducer toward the left.

On the posterior longitudinal scan or longitudinal oblique scan (11) the normal pancreatic tail may sometimes simulate an adrenal mass

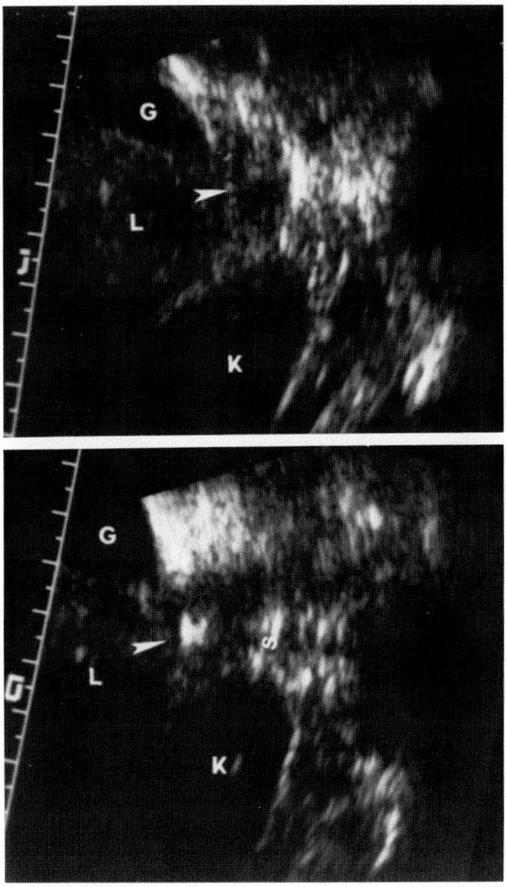

Figure 3.25. The duodenal loop simulates an adrenal mass. *Top,* A mass-like structure (*white arrowhead*) is located anterior to the upper pole of the right kidney (*K*). The structure is located slightly more lateral than the usual adrenal area. *L,* liver; *G,* gallbladder. *Bottom,* After a few minutes, rescanning of the area shows a gas bubble within the structure (*white arrowhead*). The gas bubble cast an acoustic shadow. This proved the structure to be a duodenal loop.

anterior to the upper pole of the left kidney. The anatomy can be clarified by scanning from the left upper flank as previously described.

Enlarged Retrocrural Nodes

The enlarged retrocrural node may be located adjacent to the adrenal area (Fig. 3.26). However, when the normal adrenal gland and the crus of the diaphragm are clearly delineated by ultrasonography, the retrocrural lymphadenopathy can be diagnosed.

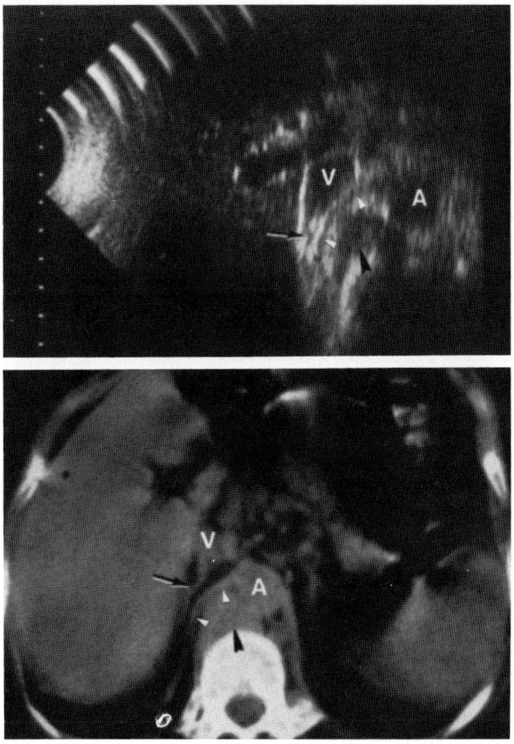

Figure 3.26. An enlarged retrocrural node due to lymphoma. *Top,* Transverse scan from right upper flank region shows a crescent-shaped mass (*black arrowhead*) posterior to the crus of diaphragm (*white arrowheads*). The adrenal gland (*black arrow*) is seen lateral to the crus of diaphragm and posterior to the inferior vena cava (*V*). *A,* aorta. *Bottom,* Corresponding CT scan confirms the retrocrural mass.

DIAGNOSTIC ACCURACY AND CLINICAL APPLICATION OF ULTRASONOGRAPHY

The success of ultrasonographic delineation of the adrenal gland and adrenal lesions greatly depends on the technique, knowledge, experience, and skill of the operator and the effort in scanning. Therefore, the accuracy of detecting adrenal lesions greatly varies, especially for small mass lesions. Although the high-resolution sector scanner has greatly facilitated scanning the adrenal lesions, success is still highly dependent on the operator. The incidence of detecting an adrenal mass can be quite high even with manual scanning with a 2.25-MHz transducer (i.e., sensitivity 97%, specificity 96.5%, and accuracy 96.6%) (11).

The masses not detected are usually small left adrenal masses in obese patients or in patients with excessive bowel gas. CT scanning may miss small masses when a close space or overlap scan is not done, when the mass is of very low density, when the patient is very thin or small (e.g., pediatric patients), or when the mass is obscured by artifacts due to respiratory motion or surgical clip artifacts, etc. These problems, however, are not present in ultrasonography, especially with a real-time scanner.

Adrenal scintigraphy with [^{131}I]19-iodocholesterol may detect functional adrenal tumors or hyperplasia (63, 64), and NP-59 scintigraphy may differentiate an adenoma from a metastatic adrenal mass (65). However, a delay of 4 to 15 days after the injection of isotope may be necessary before useful images can be obtained, and small masses may not be seen. Nevertheless, detection of hyperfunction is possible before adrenal glands become enlarged and adenomas can be distinguished from nodular hyperplasia. The increased uptake of so-called nonfunctioning adenomas on NP-59 scintigraphy also indicates that the adenoma is in fact functioning, but the function is not too excessive to cause overall hyperfunction of the entire adrenal glands. Therefore, the proper name should be "nonhyperfunctioning" adenoma rather than nonfunctioning adenoma.

Adrenal venography is useful in detecting small aldosteronomas. The mass can be localized by blood sampling and venography (66). This is particularly helpful when the findings on CT or ultrasonography are negative or equivocal.

In clinical practice, ultrasonography or CT will be the initial imaging procedure for the evaluation of patients suspected of having adrenal disease. The choice between the two modalities will depend on the patient's age and body habits, the availability of equipment, and the experience of the ultrasonographer. In children, thin adults, and pregnant women (Fig. 3.27) ultrasonography is the method of choice because of the lack of ionizing radiation. When examination of both ovaries is also required, such as in women with hirsutism, ultra-

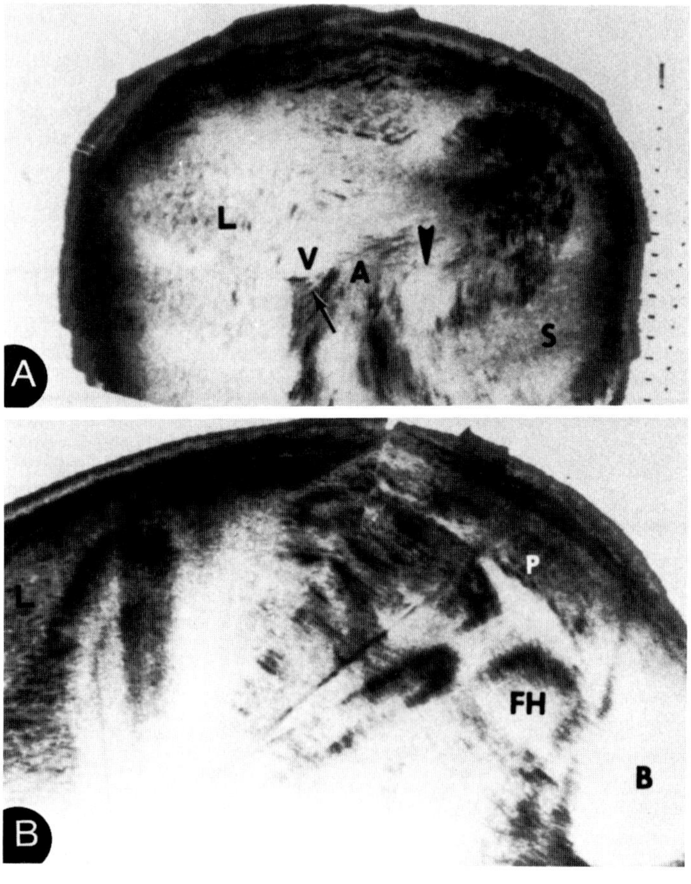

Figure 3.27. An adrenal adenoma causing Cushing's syndrome in a pregnant woman. **A,** Transverse scan 14 cm above umbilicus. A mass (*arrowhead*) is seen in the left adrenal region. The right adrenal gland (*arrow*) is normal. *L,* liver; *A,* aorta; *V,* inferior vena cava; *S,* spleen. **B,** Longitudinal scan at midline showing a fetus in the uterus. *FH,* fetal head; *P,* placenta; *B,* bladder.

sonography is also preferred since it will clearly delineate the ovaries and follicles. CT not only will not delineate all of these structures in detail, but also causes radiation to the gonads.

Acknowledgments

The author thanks Gwen Hanley and Louisa Haigler for their excellent secretarial work.

References

1. Binholtz JC. Ultrasound imaging of adrenal mass lesions. Radiology 1973;109:163–166.
2. Davidson JK, Morley P, Hurley GD, Holford NGH. Adrenal venography and ultrasound in the investigation of the adrenal gland: an analysis of 53 cases. Br J Radiol 1975;48:435–450.
3. Ghorashi B, Holmes JH. Gray scale sonographic appearance of an adrenal mass: a case report. J Clin Ultrasound 1976;4:121–123.
4. Holm HH, Kristensen JK, Rasmussen SN, Pedersen JF. Ultrasonic diagnosis of juxtarenal masses. Scand J Urol Nephrol 1972;6(suppl 15):83–88.
5. Holm HH. Ultrasonic scanning in the diagnosis of space-occupying lesions of the upper abdomen. Br J Radiol 1971;44:24–36.
6. Lyons EA, Murphy AV, Arneil GC. Sonar and its use in kidney disease in children. Arch Dis Child 1972;47:777-786.
7. Pitts WR Jr, Kazam E, Gershowitz M, Muecke EC. A review of 100 renal and perinephric sonograms with anatomic diagnosis. J Urol 1972; 114:21.
8. Brascho DJ. Clinical applications of diagnostic ultrasound in abdominal malignancy. South Med J 1972;65:1331.
9. Holm HH, Rasmussen SN, Kristensen JK. Errors and pitfalls in ultrasonic scanning of the abdomen. Br J Radiol 1972;45:835.
10. Pond GD, Haber K. Echography: a new approach to the diagnosis of adrenal hemorrhage of the newborn. J Can Assoc Radiol 1976;27:40–44.
11. Yeh HC. Sonography of the adrenal glands: normal glands and small masses. AJR 1989;135: 1167–1177.
12. Sample WF. A new technique for the evaluation of the adrenal gland with gray scale ultrasonography. Radiology 1977;124:463–469.
13. Marchal G, Glin J, Verbeken E, et al. High resolution real-time sonography of adrenal glands: a routine examination? J Ultrasound Med 1986; 5:65–68.
14. Zapposodi F, Derchi LE, Rizzatto G. Ultrasonography of the normal adrenal glands: a study using linear array real time equipment. Br J Radiol 1986;59:759–764.
15. Oppenheimer DA, Carroll BA, Yousem S. Sonography of the normal neonatal adrenal gland. Radiology 1983;146:157–160.
16. Kangarloo H, Diament MS, Gold RH, et al. Sonography of adrenal glands in neonates and children: changes in appearance with age. J Clin Ultrasound 1986;14:43–47.
17. Mitty HA, Yeh HC. Radiology of the adrenals with sonography and CT. Philadelphia: WB Saunders, 1982.
18. Brownlie K, Kreel L. Computer assisted tomography of normal suprarenal glands. J Comput Assist Tomogr 1978;1:1–10.
19. Karstaedt H, Segel SS, Stanley RJ, Melson GL, Levitt RG. Computed tomography of adrenal gland. Radiology 1978;129:723–730.
20. Davies DV. Gray's anatomy, 34th ed. London: Longmans, Green, 1967:1601–1605.
21. Netter FH. Endocrine system and selected metabolic diseases (the CIBA collection of medical illustrations, Vol 4). Summit, NJ: CIBA Pharmaceutical Company, 1965:78–79.
22. Yamakita N, Yasuda K, Miura K. Delineation of adrenal in controls and non-tumors adrenal disorders by real-time ultrasonic scanner. Ultrasound Med Biol 1986;12:107–114.
23. McGraham JP, Myracle MR. Adrenal hypertrophy possible pitfall in the sonographic diagnosis of renal agenesis. J Ultrasound Med 1986; 5:265–268.
24. Yeh HC. Adrenal gland and nonrenal retroperitoneum. Urol Radiol 1987;9:127–140.
25. Yeh HC, Mitty HA, Rose J, Wolf BS, Gabrilove JL. Ultrasonography of adrenal masses: usual features. Radiology 1987;127:467.
26. Schaner EG, Dunnick NR, Doppman JL, et al. Adrenal cortical tumors with low attenuation coefficients: a pitfall in computed tomography diagnosis. J Comput Assist Tomogr 1978;2:11.
27. Bowerman RA, Silver TM, Jaffe MH, et al. Sonography of adrenal pheochromocytomas. AJR 1981;137:1227–1231.
28. Yeh HC, Pertsemildis D, Mitty HA. Pheochromocytoma: role of ultrasonography and CT. Presented at the 70th Annual Meeting of the Radiologic Society of North America, Washington, DC, November 1984.
29. Chang A, Glazer HS, Lee JKT, Ling D. Adrenal gland: MR imaging. Radiology 1987;163: 123–128.
30. Bernardino ME. Management of the asymptomatic patient with a unilateral adrenal mass. Radiology 1988;166:121–123.
31. Doppman JL, Miller DL, Dwyer AJ, et al. Macronodular adrenal hyperplasia in Cushing disease. Radiology 1988;166:347–352.
32. Glazer HS, Weyman PJ, Sagel SS, Levitt RG, McClennan BL. Nonfunctioning adrenal masses: incidental discovery on computed tomography. AJR 1982;139:81–85.
33. Soffer LJ, Iannaccone A, Gabrilove JL. Cushing's syndrome—a study of fifty patients. Am J Med 1961;30:129–146.
34. Copeland PM. The incidentally discovered adrenal mass. Ann Intern Med 1983;98:940–945.
35. Yeh HC, Mitty HA, Rose J, Wolf BS, Gabrilove JL. Ultrasonography of adrenal masses: unusual manifestations. Radiology 1978;127:475–483.
36. Yeh HC. Ultrasonography of the adrenals. Semin Roentgenol 1988;23:250–258.
37. Dunnick NR, Heaston D, Halvorsan R, Moore AV, Korobkin M. CT appearance of adrenocortical carcinoma. J Comput Assist Tomogr 1982;6:978–982.

38. Davies RP, Lam AH. Adrenocortical neoplasm in children: ultrasound appearance. J Ultrasound Med 1987;6:325–328.
39. Pagani JJ. Normal adrenal glands in small cell lung carcinoma: CT guided biopsy. Am J Roentgenol 1983;140:949–945.
40. Weber CL, Murphy ML. Adrenal hypofunction secondary to adrenocortical destruction by metastatic carcinoma of the lung. J Arkansas Med Soc 1971;68:181.
41. Forsythe JR, Gosink BB, Leopold GR. Ultrasound in the evaluation of adrenal metastases. J Clin Ultrasound 1977;5:31–34.
42. Robbins SL. Pathology, 3rd ed. Philadelphia: WB Saunders, 1967;1219–1240.
43. McLelland R, Landes RR, Ransom CL. Retroperitoneal pneumography a safe method using carbon dioxide. Radiol Clin North Am 1965;3:113–128.
44. Sample WF. Adrenal ultrasonograpy. Radiology 1978;127:461.
45. McLachalan MSF, Robert EE.Demonstration of normal adrenal gland by venography and gas insufflation. Br J Radiol 1971;44:664–671.
46. Vicks BS, Perusek M, Johnson J, Trio F. Primary adrenal lymphoma: CT and sonographic appearance. J Clin Ultrasound 1987;15:135–139.
47. Feldberg MAM, Hendriks MJ, Klinkhamer AC. Massive bilateral non-Hodgkin's lymphomas of the adrenals. Urol Radiol 1986;8:85–88.
48. Wilson DA, Nguyan DL, Tytle TL, Swaney CM, Muchmore HG. Sonography of the adrenal glands in chronic disseminated histoplasmosis. J Ultrasound Med 1986;5:69–73.
49. Wilms GE, Baert AL, Kint EJ, et al. Computed tomographic findings in bilateral adrenal tuberculosis. Radiology 1983;146:729–730.
50. Wilson DA, Muchmore HG, Tisdal RG, et al. Histoplasmosis of the adrenal glands studied by CT. Radiology 1984;150:779–783.
51. Paling MR, Williamson BRJ. Adrenal involvement in non-Hodgkin's lymphoma. AJR 1983; 141:303–305.
52. White SJ, Stuck KJ, Blane CE, Silver TM. Sonography of neuroblastoma. Am J Roentgenol 1983;141:465–468.
53. Pery M, Kaftori JK, Bar-Maor JA. Sonography for diagnosis and follow-up of neonatal adrenal hemorrhage. J Clin Ultrasound 1981;9:397–401.
54. Mittlestaedt CA, Volberg FM, Merten DR, et al. The sonographic diagnosis of neonatal adrenal hemorrhage. Radiology 1979;131:453–457.
55. Mineau DE, Koehler PR. Ultrasound diagnosis of neonatal adrenal hemorrhage. AJR 1979;132: 443–444.
56. Sarnaik AP, Sanfilippo DJ, Slovis TL. Ultrasound diagnosis of adrenal hemorrhage in meningococcemia. Pediatr Radiol 1988;18:427–428.
57. Foster DG. Adrenal cysts: review of literature and report of case. Arch Surg 1986;92:131–143.
58. Behan M, Martin EC, Muecke EC, et al. Myelolipoma of the adrenal: two cases with ultrasound and CT findings. AJR 1977;129:993–996.
59. Yeh HC. Adrenal sonography. In: Leopold GR, ed. Ultrasound in breast and endocrine disease. Clin Diagn Ultrasound 1984;12:101–130.
60. Kenny PJ, Stanley RJ. Calcified adrenal masses. Urol Radiol 1987;9:9–15.
61. Morrison SC, Comisky E, Fletcher BD. Calcification in the adrenal glands associated with disseminated herpes simplex infection. Pediatr Radiol 1988;18:240–241.
62. Subramanyam BR, Balthazar EJ, Horii SC. Sonography of accessory spleen. AJR 1984;143: 47–49.
63. Thrall JH, Freitas JE, Beierwaltes WH. Adrenal scintigraphy. Semin Nucl Med 1978;8:23.
64. Gross MD, Valk TW, Swanson DP, Thrall JH, Grekin RJ, Beierwaltes WH. The role of pharmacologic manipulation in adrenal cortical scintigraphy. Semin Nucl Med 1981;11:128–148.
65. Francis IR, Smid A, Gross MD, Shapiro B, Naylor B, Glazer GM. Adrenal masses in oncologic patients: functional and morphologic evaluation. Radiology 1988;166:353–356.
66. Mitty HA, Nicolis GL, Gabrilove JL. Adrenal venography: clinical radiographic correlation in 80 patients. AJR 1973;119:564–575.

CHAPTER 4

Ultrasonography of the Normal Kidney and Diffuse Renal Disease

NEIL T. WOLFMAN, M.D.
ROBERT E. BECHTOLD, M.D.
NAT E. WATSON, M.D.

Present-day ultrasound scanning of the kidney is performed almost exclusively with real-time systems. The kidney can be found quickly, its axis determined, and motion assessed.

Renal ultrasound is best performed in the coronal plane through the flanks with the patient in a supine or decubitus position (1–6). The right kidney is most often scanned along the anterior axillary line using the liver as an acoustic window. The left kidney is optimally scanned along the posterior axillary line using the spleen as the acoustic window for the upper pole (2, 7) (Fig. 4.1). Rosenberg and associates (8) have also used a fluid-filled stomach as an acoustic window for the left kidney.

Coronal scanning gives optimal delineation of the medial and lateral borders of the kidney and the encompassing perirenal and pararenal spaces (Fig. 4.2). This view also displays the collecting system in continuity from the calices to the ureteropelvic junction and proximal ureter and helps in the evaluation of hydronephrosis and parapelvic processes (3, 9) (Fig. 4.3). Vessels, particularly on the right, may be scanned in their longitudinal axis to evaluate such abnormalities as intravascular thrombus. In addition, the coronal plane correlates anatomically with other examinations such as the intravenous pyelogram (IVP).

Routine examination of the kidney includes coronal scanning along both the longitudinal and the transverse axes. The kidneys are usually imaged during deep inspiration so that the organ is in its most caudal position, out from beneath the overlying ribs, to allow easier scanning. Placing a rolled pillow or other bolster under the dependent flank in the decubitus position increases the space between the lower margin of the rib cage and the iliac crest, improving access for renal imaging.

Scanning in the prone position is possible but produces suboptimal images resulting from significant sound beam attenuation by the paravertebral muscles and interference of the ribs. Therefore, this position should be considered only as a last resort (1, 2, 4, 5). If the prone position must be used, placing a pillow under the patient's abdomen will help position the kidneys for better imaging.

NORMAL ANATOMY

Kidney

The kidneys are paired retroperitoneal organs located on either side of the vertebral column at the upper to midlumbar level. The left kidney is often more cephalad than the right (1). The renal axis is oblique, with the upper pole medial and posterior to the lower pole. The anterior position of the lower pole in reference to the upper pole is accentuated in the decubitus position. The ultrasonographer should be aware of the renal axis to obtain true longitudinal and transverse views.

The renal border is usually smooth but may be lobular because of persistent fetal lobation (Figs. 4.4 and 4.26). The renal parenchyma is composed of a variable number of lobes, each consisting of a central medullary pyramid enveloped by cortex; contrilobar cortex covers the pyramid base, and the septal cortex or column of Bertin is insinuated between the pyramids.

Marchal et al. (10) correlated the histologic structure of the kidney with its sonographic appearance. On ultrasound the adult cortex appears homogeneous, with low-level echoes less or equal in echogenicity to liver when measured at the same depth from the transducer (1, 2, 5, 11–13) (Fig. 4.4). Cortical echogenicity is a function of the complex histologic architec-

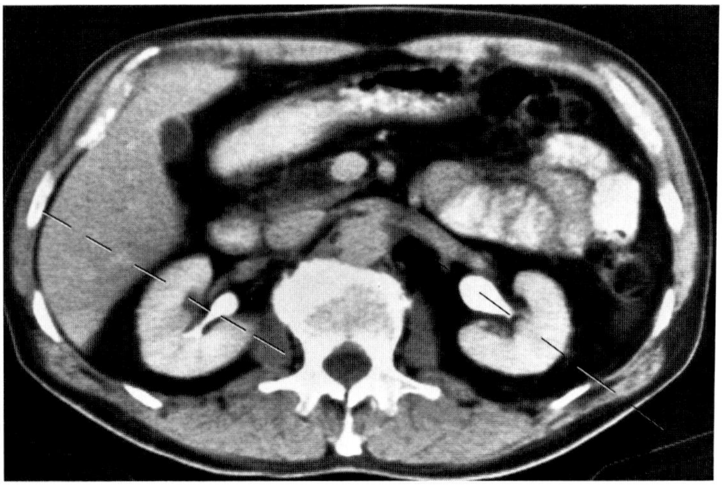

Figure 4.1. CT scan at the level of the midpole of both kidneys. The *dotted lines* represent the approximate planes for coronal imaging of the right and left kidneys.

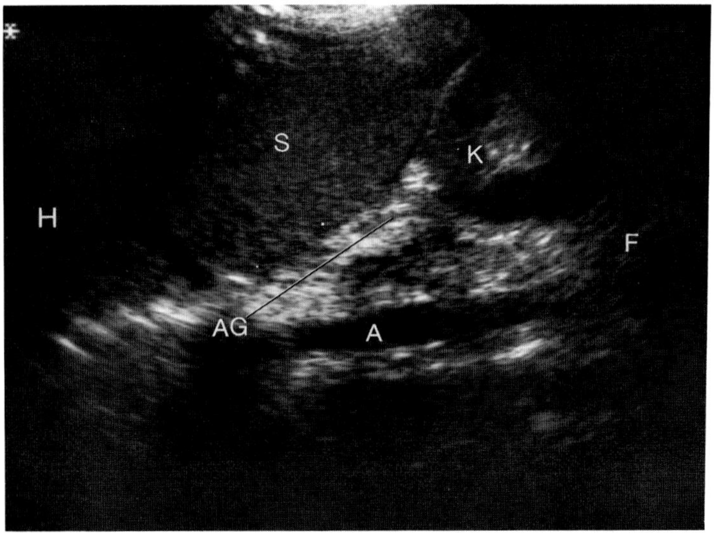

Figure 4.2. Longitudinal scan in the coronal plane along the left posterior axillary line demonstrates the upper pole of the left kidney (*K*) and surrounding structures, including the spleen (*S*), the aorta (*A*), and a portion of the left adrenal gland (*AG*). *H,* toward head of patient; *F,* toward feet of patient.

ture of the cortex, which contains a myriad of nephrons and vessels and therefore abundant acoustic interfaces. The medullary pyramids composed of the urine-filled collecting tubules and the loops of Henle are hypoechoic or anechoic (Fig. 4.4). They are easily differentiated from the cortex in the majority of patients. This differentiation is more difficult to see in obese patients (1, 4). Sonographic detection and appearance of the pyramids also varies with the patient's state of hydration; they are more readily seen with increased diuresis (14). The medullary pyramids are 1.2 to 1.5 cm thick (5). Aging causes progressive medullary fibrosis, and corticomedullary differentiation tends to fade (10). Progressive parenchymal atrophy is also noted with age and is associated with increasing sinus fibrolipomatosis and hilar enlargement.

In the majority of kidneys there is partial or complete fusion of some lobes. This usually occurs at the polar regions but can also be seen in the middle zone (1, 10, 15). Jones et al. (16) state that 70% of kidneys have at least one such compound pyramid. They appear as large, irregular, hypoechoic areas and should not be confused with local caliectasis, cysts, or a mass (Fig. 4.5). Compound pyramids are easier to see in children, who are often thin and in whom high-frequency transducers can be used.

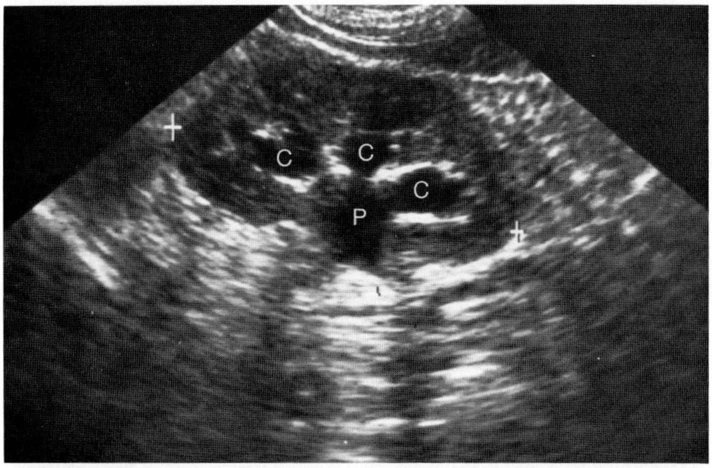

Figure 4.3. Longitudinal view in the coronal plane of the left kidney with hydronephrosis. The entire collecting system is imaged in this plane, which coincides with the axis of the collecting system. The dilated calices (*C*) can be followed into the pelvis (*P*).

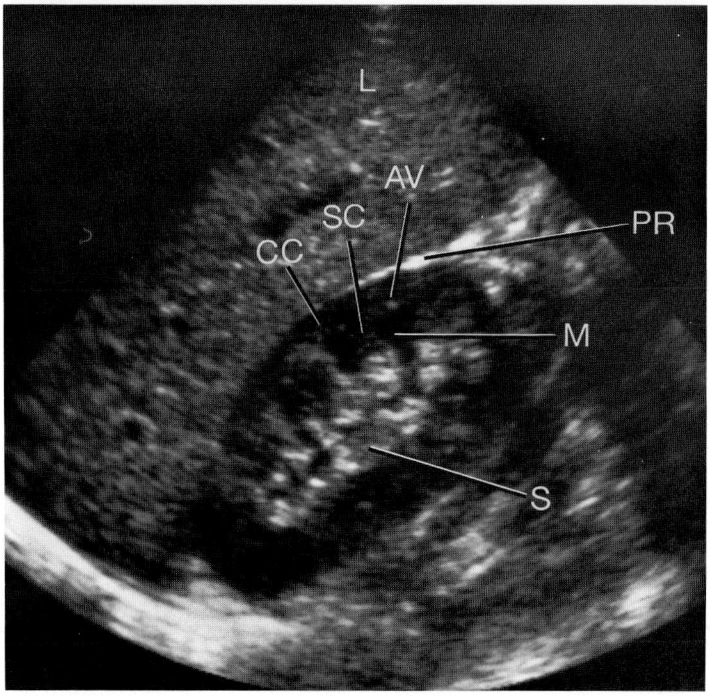

Figure 4.4. Longitudinal image of the right kidney demonstrating the renal anatomy and perirenal area. The renal parenchyma is less echogenic than that of the adjacent liver, a normal ultrasonic relationship. *CC,* centrilobar cortex; *SC,* septal cortex or column of Bertin; *M,* medulla; *AV,* arcuate vessels; *S,* renal sinus; *L,* liver.

The arcuate vessels reportedly visualized in 25% of cases (1, 12) and more frequently seen with real-time equipment, appear as discrete, echogenic, highly reflective punctate echoes at the corticomedullary junction and can be used to evaluate cortical thickness (5) (Fig. 4.4). Subsidiary interlobar arteries course in the corticomedullary junction in fused areas (12, 15). They are farther from the renal capsule and larger than arcuate arteries, but the two cannot be differentiated on ultrasound (Fig. 4.5). While lobar fusion can be seen, it is easily missed. The variable course of the different vessels could conceivably result in overestimation of cortical thickness.

The renal sinus contains the collecting system, vessels, lymphatics, and fatty and fibrous tissue. It appears on ultrasound in the longitudinal axis as an intensely echogenic, irregularly marginated oval in the midportion of the kidney (Figs. 4.4 and 4.6). Fat is primarily responsible for sinus echogenicity, although

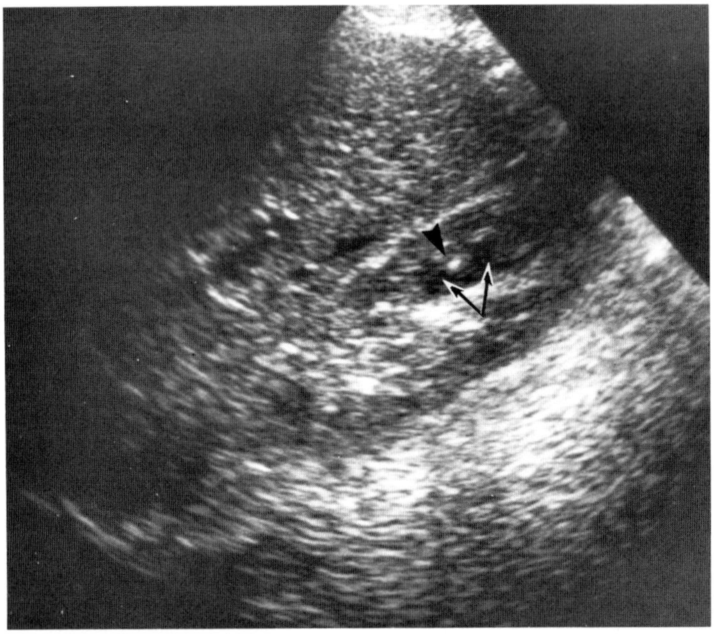

Figure 4.5. Longitudinal examination of the right kidney. Partial fusion of two lobes (*arrows*). The septal cortex is seen insinuating between a portion of the fused medullary pyramids. Note the punctate echogenic focus (*arrowhead*), which in this case represents a subsidiary interlobar vessel.

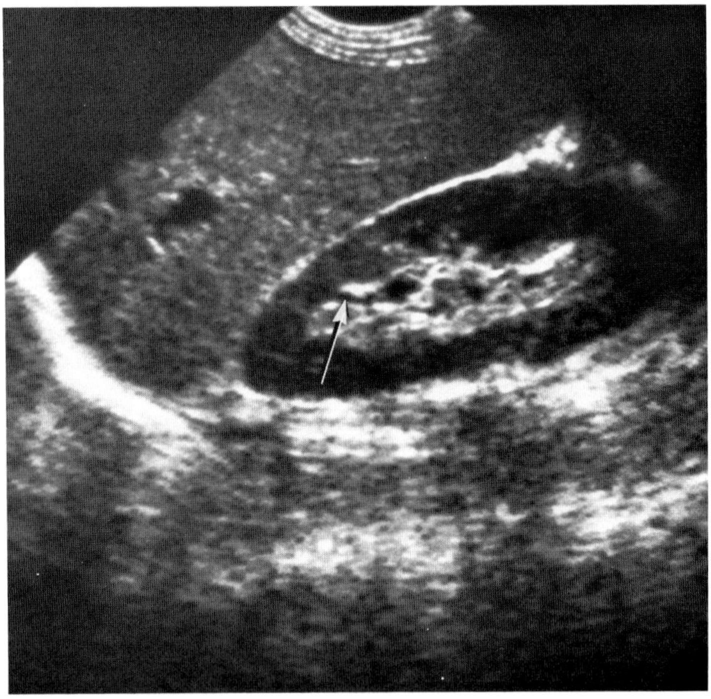

Figure 4.6. Longitudinal image of the right kidney demonstrating the central echogenic sinus region. Multiple anechoic areas within the sinus region represent portions of the collecting system and vascular structures. One calix and its infundibulum (*arrow*) are seen coursing from the tip of the medullary pyramid to the pelvis.

other structures are contributing factors (2). Portions of the collecting system may be imaged as anechoic structures within the echogenic sinus, depending on the state of hydration. In the well-hydrated patient, particularly one with a full bladder, both kidneys may appear minimally hydronephrotic. In the normal patient the collecting system should appear less distended after voiding. Vessels may also be seen coursing through the sinus, and Doppler techniques can be employed if necessary to differentiate them from collecting system components. An extrarenal pelvis when present may appear as a round or oval anechoic cystic structure just medial to the renal hilum (Fig. 4.7). It should not be confused with hydronephrosis.

Brandt et al. (17), scanning patients in the prone position, have reported normal renal dimensions: right kidney length 10.7 cm (SD 1.35), width 5 cm (SD 0.76), and anteroposterior dimension 3.95 cm (SD 0.15); left kidney length 11.1 cm (SD 1.15), width 5.3 cm (SD 0.8), and anteroposterior dimension 4.14 cm (SD 0.84). Size will vary with patient height, age, body habitus, and state of hydration. In many laboratories, for practical reasons, renal length is the single most common measurement recorded, but it is important to note that volume measurements are more sensitive than any one linear value.

Renal volume calculations are based on the formula for a prolate ellipsoid:

$$V = L \times W \times T \times 0.52$$

where L denotes the renal length, W the renal width, and T the anteroposterior dimension (1, 18–20). A corrected formula,

$$V = L \times W \times T \times 0.49$$

has also been used (21).

Vasculature

Real-time ultrasound has enhanced visualization of the renal vessels. Scanning is performed transversely to coincide with the vessel axis. The arteries are posterior to the veins at the level of the hilum.

The right renal artery arises from the anterolateral margin of the aorta. From its origin the artery courses anteriorly to the right diaphragmatic crus, behind the inferior vena cava and posteriorly to the renal hilum. At the origin it is best imaged by scanning from an anterior approach (Fig. 4.8), and a left lateral decubitus position can help in visualization of both the right and left arteries in some circumstances (22). The more distal portions of the artery are best imaged with transverse scanning in the coronal plane (Fig. 4.9). With longitudinal scanning the renal artery may be seen crossing posteriorly to the cava and may indent the caval wall (Fig. 4.10). On transverse scans, the crus of the diaphragm can simulate the renal artery, and care should be taken not to confuse the two structures (1) (Fig. 4.8).

The left renal artery originates from the posterolateral wall of the aorta and courses posterolaterally to the renal hilum. In our experience the left renal artery is the most difficult renal vessel to image in its entirety. Its origin, like that of the right artery, it best imaged from an anterior approach with the patient in supine or left lateral decubitus position (Figs. 4.8 and 4.11). Coronal imaging best demonstrates the distal portion.

Multiple renal arteries are present in approximately 25% of the population (2). Although such arteries may be imaged on ultrasound, particularly on the right side posterior to the inferior vena cava, they are often missed (1).

The right renal vein exits from the hilum and courses anteriorly and medially to enter the posterolateral aspect of the inferior cava (Figs. 4.9 and 4.12). This vein can be large enough to simulate an anechoic mass. It may also enlarge in patients with congestive heart failure (Fig.

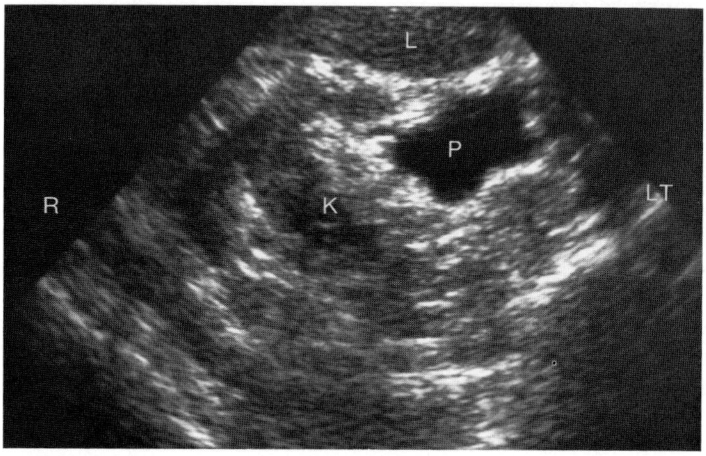

Figure 4.7. Transverse examination of the midpole of the right kidney (*K*) demonstrates an extrarenal pelvis (*P*). A small portion of the liver (*L*) anterior to the kidney is also seen on the image. *R*, right side of patient; *LT*, left side of patient.

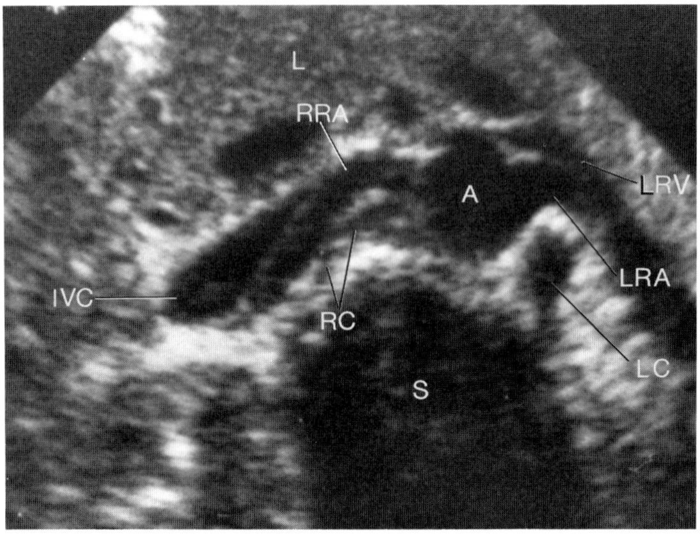

Figure 4.8. Transverse image, anterior approach of the aorta (*A*) at the level of the renal arteries. The proximal portion of the right renal artery (*RRA*) is well displayed as it exits from the aorta and proceeds to course behind the inferior vena cava (*IVC*). The origin of the left renal artery (*LRA*) is also imaged. Note the position of both the right crus and left crus (*RC, LC*) posterior to the arteries. In particular, the right crus can mimic the course of the renal artery and should not be confused with it. *LRV*, left renal vein; *S*, spine; *L*, liver.

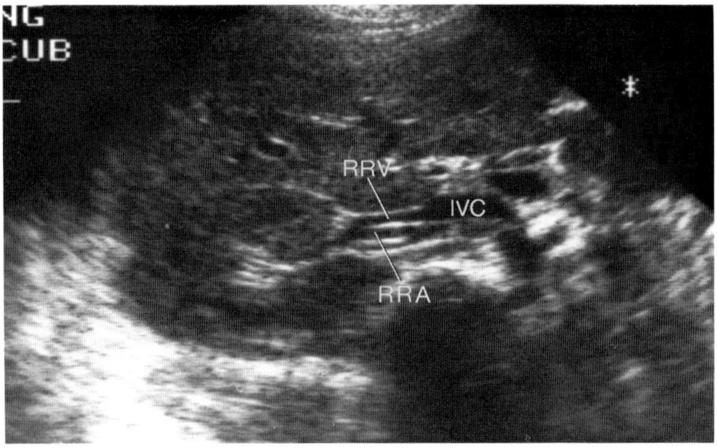

Figure 4.9. Transverse scan of the right kidney. The distal part of the right renal artery (*RRA*) is seen in its normal position coursing behind the right renal vein (*RRV*). It can be seen in this image entering into the kidney. In this image also note that the right renal vein can be seen in its entire course from the kidney to the inferior vena cava (*IVC*).

4.13). It is usually imaged in its entirety with transverse scanning in the coronal or modified coronal plane (23).

The left renal vein has a long course beginning anteromedially from the hilum, anterior to the renal artery. It then traverses the notch between the aorta and the superior mesenteric artery (SMA), either above or at the level of the transverse duodenum; it then continues toward the right and joins the inferior vena cava. The most proximal portion is imaged coronally (Fig. 4.14), and the remainder is best imaged transversely through the anterior abdominal wall (Fig. 4.15). The proximal left renal vein prior to its entry between the aorta and the SMA often appears focally distended (Figs. 4.16 and 4.11). This finding is thought to result from compression of the vein by the SMA and aorta. The transverse duodenum, which also crosses the midline between these two arteries, may contribute to this compression of the vein (24, 25). Care should be taken not to confuse this venous distention with a renal artery aneurysm (25), and with real-time ultrasound the distinction should not be a problem. Doppler analysis can easily differentiate between venous and arterial flow. Retroaortic and circumaortic renal veins are infrequent anomalies that are potentially visible on ultrasound (1, 26, 27) (Fig. 4.17). Their identification may be useful in planning for surgery.

Low-amplitude punctate echoes within the inferior vena cava and renal vein that move in the direction of blood flow have been described.

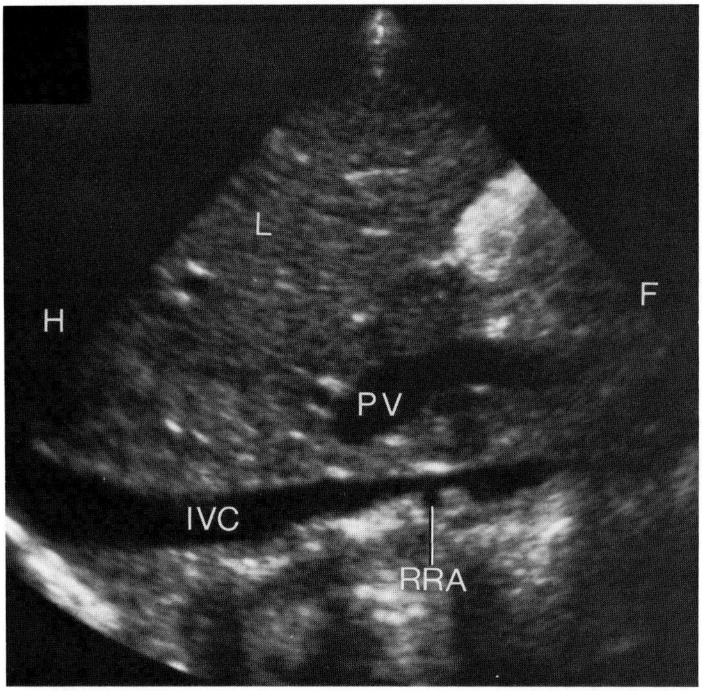

Figure 4.10. Longitudinal examination from anterior approach over the inferior vena cava (*IVC*). The right renal artery (*RRA*) is seen in cross section as it courses posterior to the vena cava. *L,* liver; *PV,* portal vein; *H,* toward head of patient; *F,* toward feet of patient.

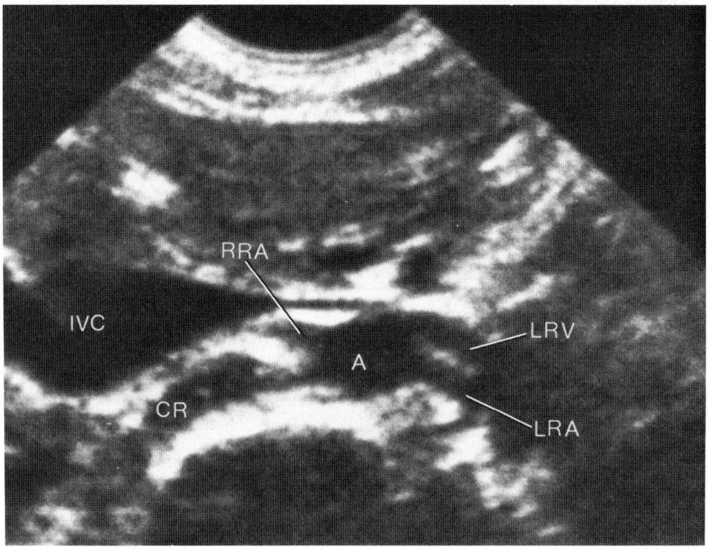

Figure 4.11. Transverse scan of the aorta at the level of the renal arteries. Note the origin of the left renal artery (*LRA*) from the posterolateral wall of the aorta (*A*). *RRA,* right renal artery; *LRV,* left renal vein; *IVC,* inferior vena cava; *CR,* right crus of the diaphragm.

These echoes, best seen in thin patients, are thought to result from the scattering of the sound beam by red blood cells (28).

In addition to its use in imaging the renal vasculature, Doppler ultrasound allows evaluation of flow characteristics (29–31). The renal artery shows a high systolic frequency shift, which then decreases gradually but continues throughout diastole, reflecting the low resistance of the system in the normal patient (Fig. 4.18). In the proximal portion of the artery a "window" under the spectral tracing is present because of almost uniform velocity shifts (32). Although the waveform remains similar throughout, gradual reduction in peak frequency and some spectral broadening are noted as tracings are taken more distally in the renal artery. The intrarenal vessels cannot be indi-

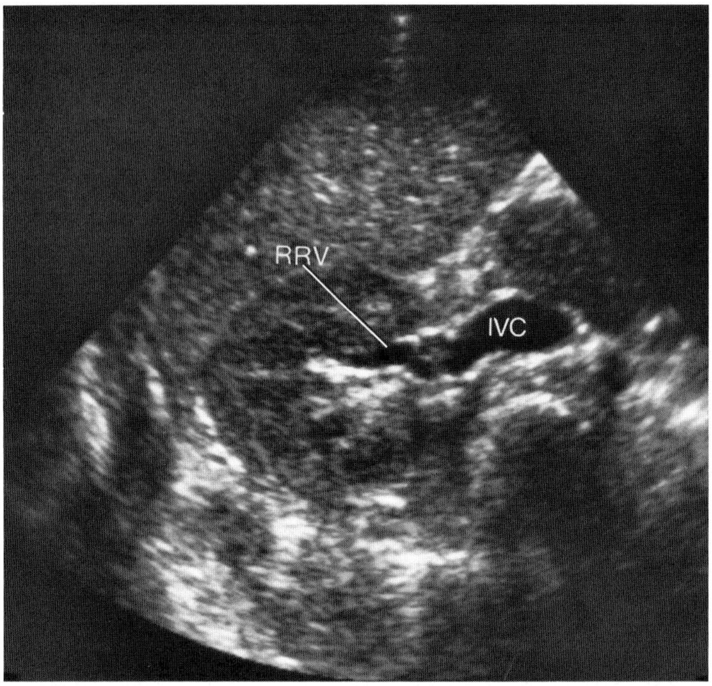

Figure 4.12. Transverse image of the right kidney demonstrating the entire course of the right renal vein (*RRV*) from the renal hilum to the inferior vena cava (*IVC*).

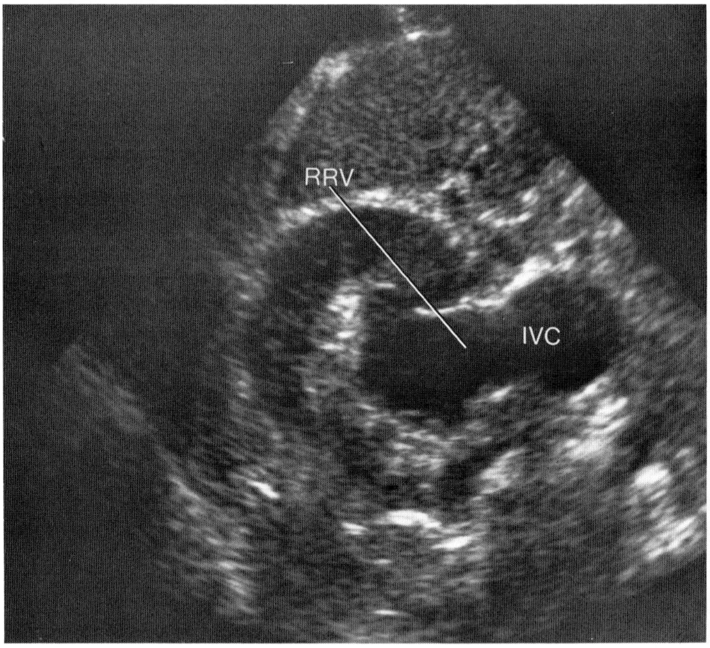

Figure 4.13. Transverse scan of the right kidney at the level of the hilum. The right renal vein (*RRV*) is grossly dilated in its entire course in this patient with congestive heart failure. *IVC*, inferior vena cava.

vidually imaged; however, placement of the Doppler gate in the expected area of the segmental, interlobar, and arcuate vessels will often give excellent arterial signals (Fig. 4.19). The spectral tracings are similar in form to those of the main renal artery (32, 33).

Normal extrarenal and intrarenal venous flow is characteristically continuous with echoes of multiple frequencies and slight variation due to respiratory and cardiac motion (29, 30) (Fig. 4.20). Mild fluctuations in renal vein size, seen particularly on the right, are due to

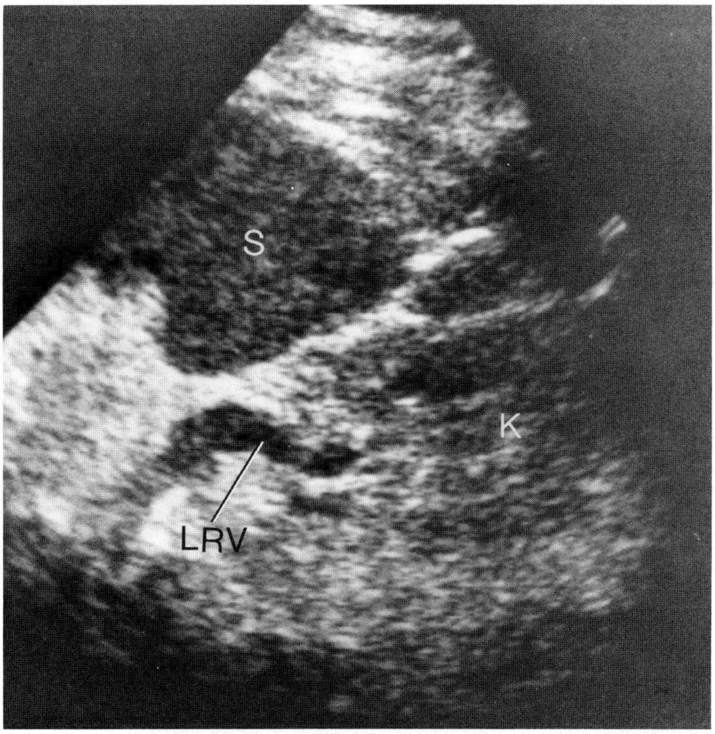

Figure 4.14. Transverse scan of the left kidney in coronal plane at the level of the renal hilum. The proximal portion of the left renal vein (*LRV*) can be seen exiting from the kidney (*K*). A portion of the spleen (*S*) adjacent to the kidney is also imaged.

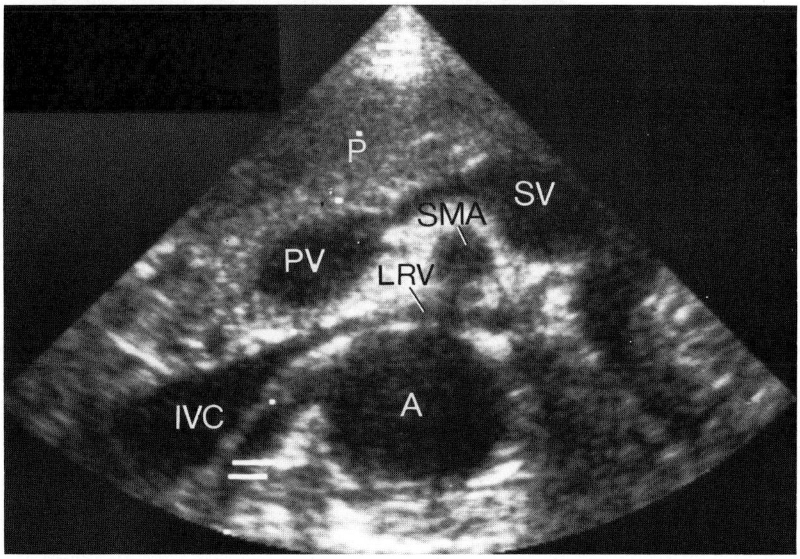

Figure 4.15. Transverse scan over the aorta (*A*) and inferior vena cava (*IVC*) at the level of the renal vessels. Note the left renal vein (*LRV*) as it courses between the superior mesenteric artery (*SMA*) and the aorta (*A*) and enters into the inferior vena cava. A Doppler cursor (*parallel white lines*) is positioned over the right renal artery. *SV,* splenic vein; *PV,* portal vein; *P,* pancreas.

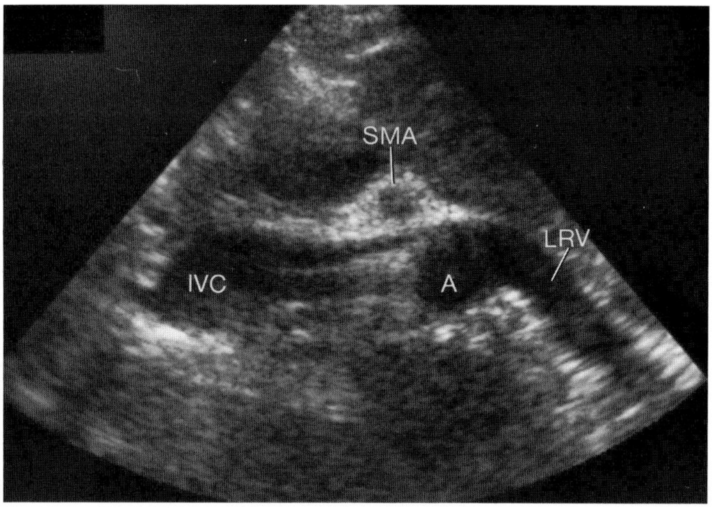

Figure 4.16. Transverse view over the aorta. There is focal distention of the left renal vein (*LRV*) prior to its entrance between the aorta (*A*) and the superior mesenteric artery (*SMA*). It then decreases in caliber and continues to the inferior vena cava (*IVC*).

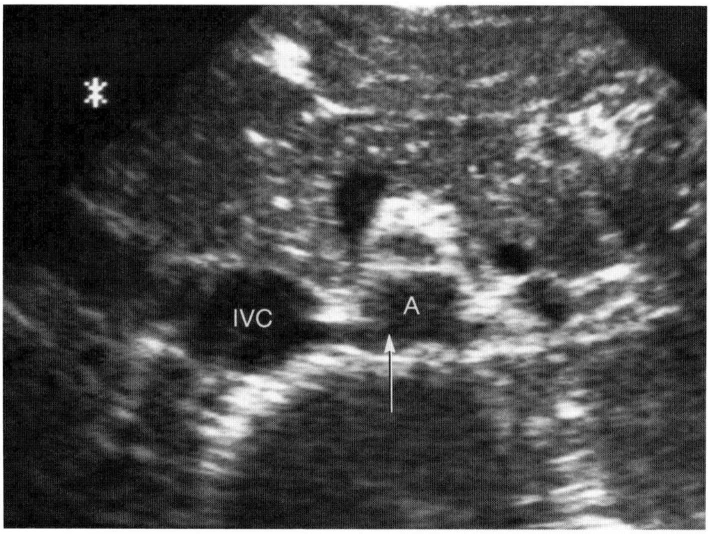

Figure 4.17. Transverse image of the aorta at the level of the renal vein. The retroaortic left renal vein (*arrow*) courses behind the aorta (*A*) and then enters into the inferior vena cava (*IVC*).

respiration and transmitted pulsations from the inferior vena cava (1, 2). The absence of pulsations may indicate renal vein thrombosis; this diagnosis can be confirmed by Doppler interrogation.

Retroperitoneal Spaces

The kidneys are located in the retroperitoneum, which is divided into three compartments: the anterior pararenal space, the posterior pararenal space, and, between these two, the perirenal space. A brief description of this region follows; more detailed descriptions can be found in the literature (34, 35).

The anterior pararenal space contains the aorta and inferior vena cava, their major branches, and the pancreas, all easily seen on ultrasound (Fig. 4.21). Portions of the duodenum, ascending colon, and descending colon are also located in this space.

The boundaries of the perirenal space are the anterior and posterior leaves of Gerota's fascia. Within the fascia lie the kidney and adrenal gland surrounded by the intensely echogenic perirenal fat (see Figs. 4.2, 4.4, and 4.9). The adrenal gland, especially when enlarged, can be seen on sonography, and techniques for its visualization are described (36–38) (Fig. 4.22). In most institutions, however, CT is the primary modality of imaging the adrenal glands.

The posterior pararenal space is composed primarily of fat that, like perirenal fat, is

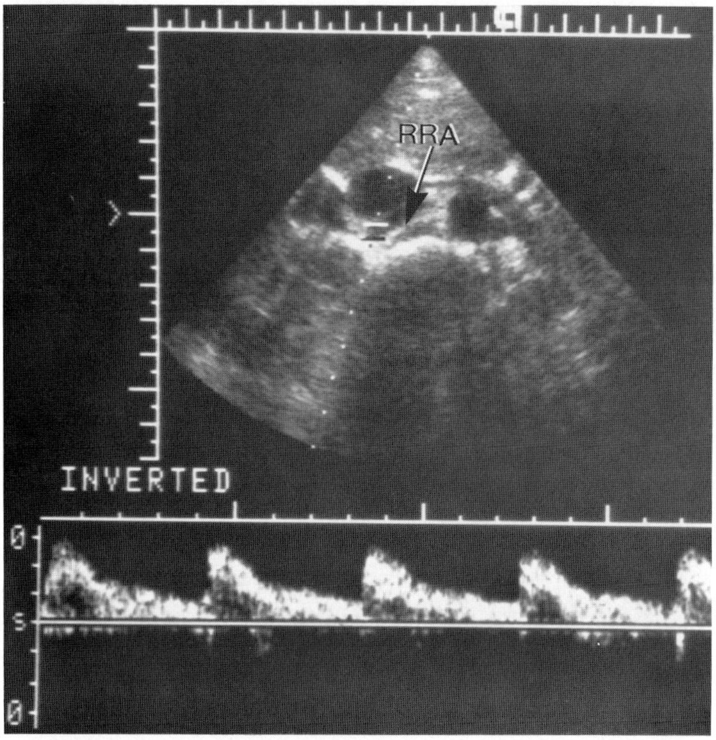

Figure 4.18. Transverse duplex Doppler examination of the proximal portion of the right renal artery (*RRA*). The Doppler gate is placed over the right renal artery. The spectral tracing seen below the image shows the characteristic waveform associated with the renal artery, consisting of a high systolic frequency shift that gradually decreases but is continuous throughout diastole. The *arrow* indicates the "window" in the spectral tracing (see text).

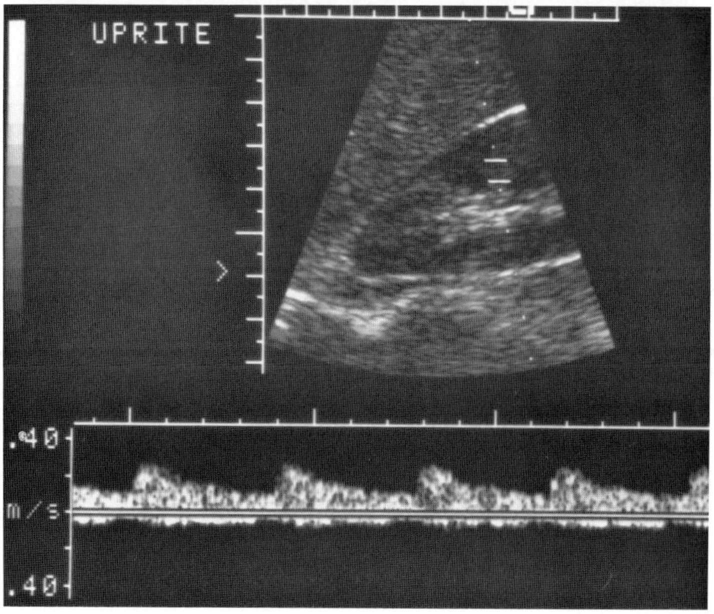

Figure 4.19. Duplex Doppler examination of the right kidney. The upper pole is visualized. The Doppler gate is over the region of the interlobar artery. Below the image is a normal spectral tracing seen in the intrarenal arteries demonstrating a systolic peak velocity with decreasing but continuous flow throughout diastole (see text).

highly echogenic. No organs reside in this space.

In the normal patient the fascia forming the boundaries of the retroperitoneal spaces in general is not defined on ultrasound, although it may be seen in some patients (Fig. 4.23).

The psoas muscles, located medially to each kidney adjacent to the vertebral column, are seen when scanning the kidneys in the coronal plane (Fig. 4.24). The quadratus lumborum muscles, positioned posteriorly to the kidneys, can also be seen depending on the plane of im-

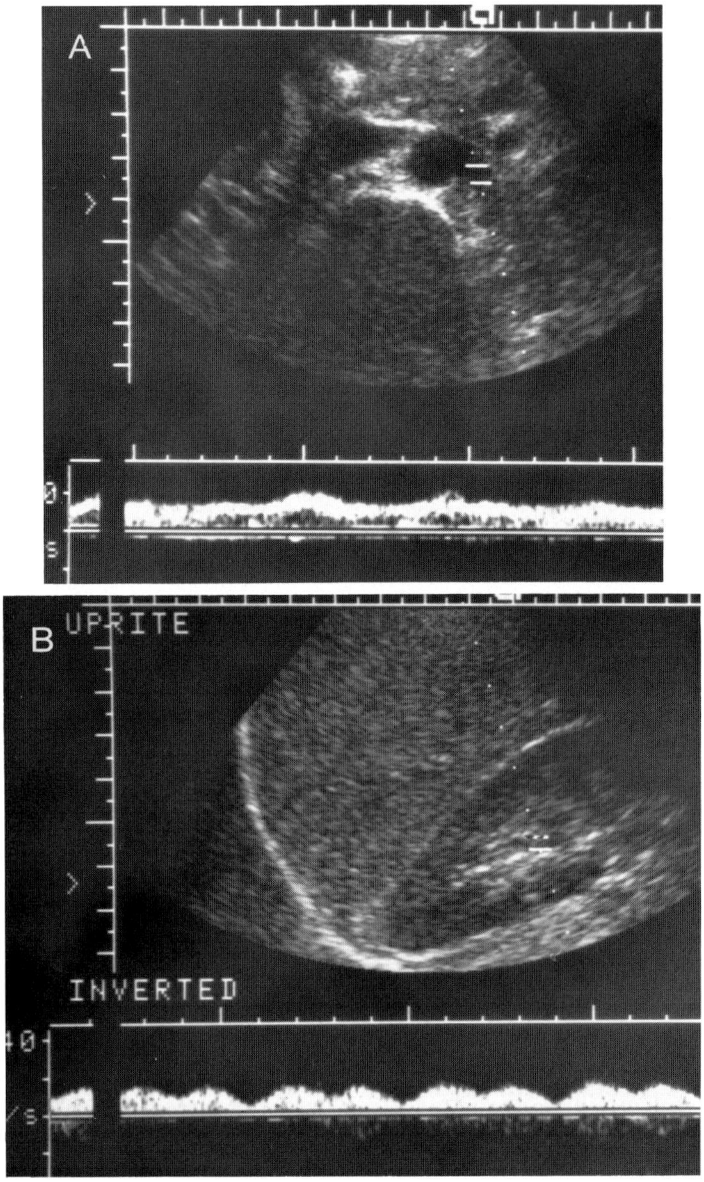

Figure 4.20. **A,** Duplex Doppler examination of the main left renal vein with the Doppler cursor over the vein. **B,** Duplex Doppler examination of the right kidney with a Doppler gate over an intrarenal vein in the sinus region. Both spectral tracings demonstrate the characteristic continuous flow pattern with multiple frequencies. Note the variation in the spectral tracing secondary to respiratory and cardiac motion.

aging. On real-time examination one can appreciate the mobility of the kidney and the encompassing perirenal area as they slide superiorly and inferiorly along the psoas muscles during respiration.

ANOMALIES

To this point the discussion has been limited to the anatomy and ultrasound appearance of the typical kidney. One should also be cognizant of common congenital anomalies that may be found incidentally during routine scanning. It is estimated that urinary tract abnormalities are present in approximately 10% of newborns (2). Failure to recognize these entities could result in a false diagnosis of a renal mass or other abnormality and lead to unnecessary workup and expense for the patient.

The hypertrophied column or septa of Bertin is one of the most common anomalies (39–41). It is thought to represent the fusion of the septal cortices of two adjacent lobes (39). It appears on ultrasound as a "mass" of isoechoic cortex that invaginates deeply into the parenchyma and indents the renal sinus, and is located most often at the junction of the upper and middle

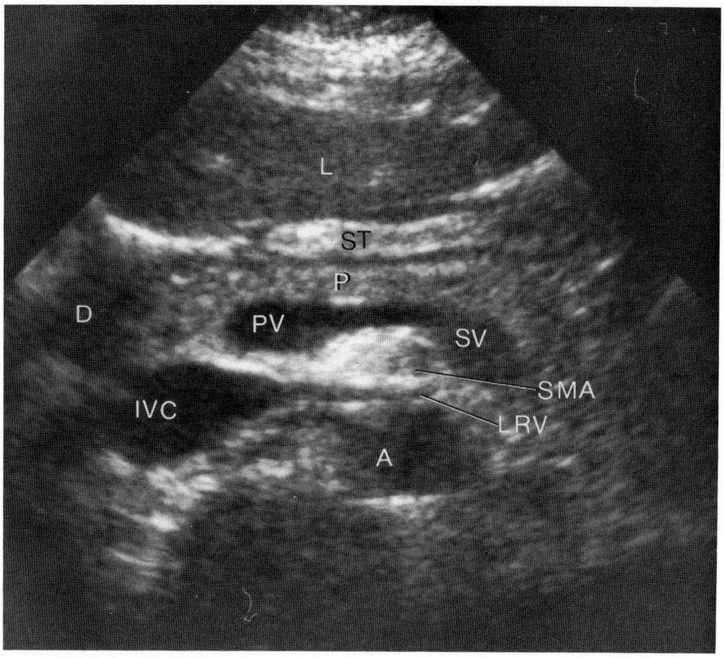

Figure 4.21. Transverse image of the upper abdomen demonstrating many of the structures seen in the anterior pararenal space, including the pancreas (*P*), the duodenum (*D*), the aorta (*A*), and the inferior vena cava (*IVC*). The stomach (*ST*) is seen directly anterior to the pancreas, and the left lobe of the liver (*L*) is seen anterior to the stomach. *LRV,* left renal vein; *SMA,* superior mesenteric artery; *SV,* splenic vein; *PV,* portal vein.

thirds of the kidney (39–41) (Fig. 4.25). In one large series a hypertrophied column of Bertin was noted in approximately 50% of kidneys, twice as often on the left (39). With this prevalence it is important not to misdiagnose the hypertrophied column as a neoplastic mass. As Lafortune et al. pointed out (39), needless nephrectomies were performed prior to the general awareness of this entity.

Fetal lobation, manifested as small indentations along the renal border, can persist in the adult kidney (Fig. 4.26). It is best appreciated on longitudinal sonograms. Anatomically, the indentations occur between the renal lobes and calices and not opposite a calix, as is the case when they are secondary to renal scarring (23).

Frequently the spleen will compress and flatten the upper lateral border of the left kidney. Just inferior to this compression the border is bulged, forming the "dromedary hump" (23) (Fig. 4.27). This pseudomass is recognizable on ultrasound because the parenchyma and its relation to the sinus region appear normal. On those occasions when a neoplastic lesion is still a diagnostic consideration, radionuclide imaging or contrast-enhanced computed tomography (CT) will help differentiate between the two.

Duplication of the renal collecting system is another common anomaly, with an estimated incidence of 0.25 to 10% (42). On ultrasound a cleft of normal renal parenchyma is visible, dividing two zones of the highly echogenic sinus (42) (Fig. 4.28). The level of duplication is usually not apparent on ultrasound.

The junctional parenchymal defect was first described by Fine and Keen (43). It represents an extension of the renal sinus to the renal surface and occurs when there is incomplete fusion of the embryonic superior and inferior parenchymatous masses (renunculi). It is most often found in the upper pole of the right kidney anteriorly and extending to the sinus, but it has been seen posteriorly in the lower pole as well (44). Hoffer et al. (44), in a prospective study of 100 pediatric sonograms, identified a junctional parenchymal defect in 46% of right kidneys and 19% of left kidneys. On ultrasound the defect appears as a triangular or round highly echogenic area that is continuous with the sinus and with the perirenal fat (44, 45) (Fig. 4.29). The defect, like the sinus, contains fat, which accounts for the similar echogenicity (45). The continuity from surface to sinus can be demonstrated by varying the axis of the transducer to coincide with that of the defect. This anomaly could be mistaken for renal scarring or a renal mass, but awareness of the entity and careful scanning should avoid confusion.

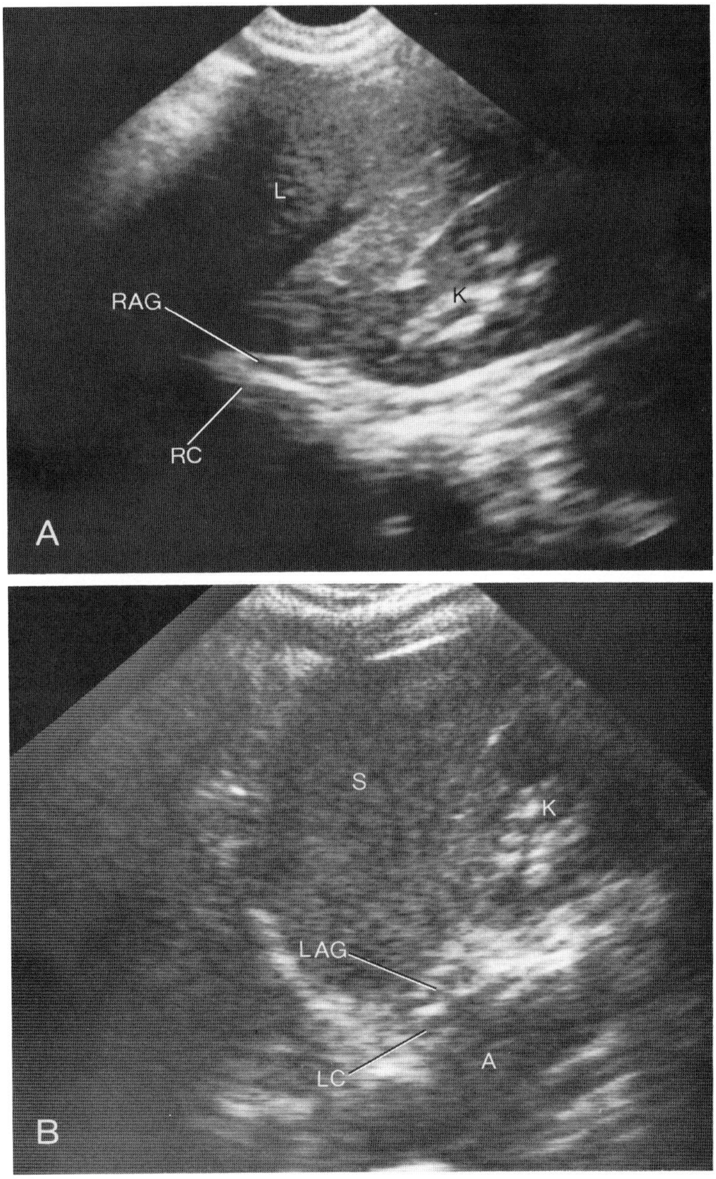

Figure 4.22. Longitudinal scans in the coronal plane of the right and left adrenal glands. **A,** The right adrenal gland (*RAG*) is seen in its relation to the upper pole of the kidney (*K*), the liver (*L*), and the right crus of the diaphragm (*RC*). The body of the adrenal gland and a portion of the limbs are visualized. **B,** Note the left adrenal gland (*LAG*) and its relationship to the upper pole of the left kidney (*K*), the spleen (*S*), and the left crus of the diaphragm (*LC*).

While a number of rare fusion anomalies have been described (46–48), horseshoe kidney is the most common fusion anomaly seen on ultrasound and occurs in 0.28% of the population (49, 50). It is the result of fusion of the metanephric blastema, which occurs in the fourth to eighth weeks of fetal development (49, 50). The kidneys are low in position with an abnormal axis, resulting from fusion of the lower poles across the midline by an isthmus (23, 49, 50). The isthmus is usually composed of functioning renal tissue but may rarely be fibrotic. The sinus regions are more ventrally positioned than normal, owing to incomplete rotation resulting from fusion. The horseshoe kidney is almost always supplied by aberrant arteries.

Horseshoe kidneys will be encountered during routine ultrasound examinations (Fig. 4.30). In the past, with static scanning units, this anomaly has been misdiagnosed as retroperitoneal adenopathy (50) and even pancreatitis (49). However, with real-time ultrasound the examiner can easily follow the renal axis,

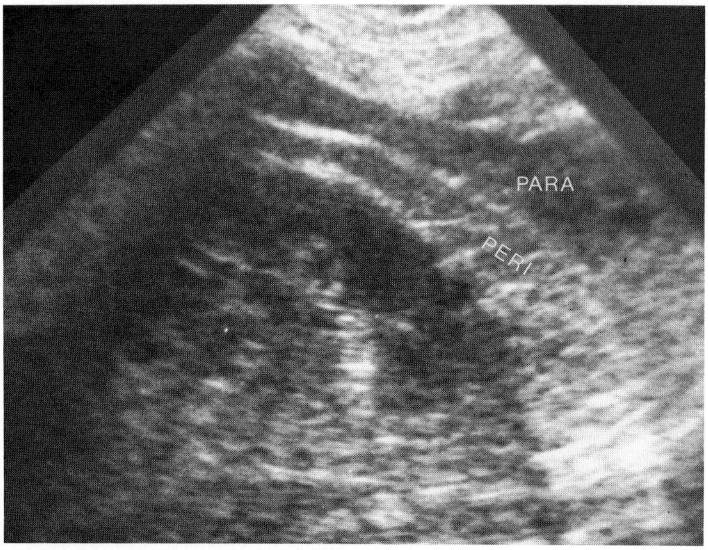

Figure 4.23. Longitudinal scan of the left kidney. The lower portion of the kidney is visualized. In this obese patient the perirenal space (*PERI*) can be differentiated from the pararenal space (*PARA*). During the real-time examination the kidney and perirenal fat moved with respiration, unlike the pararenal space, which remained immobile.

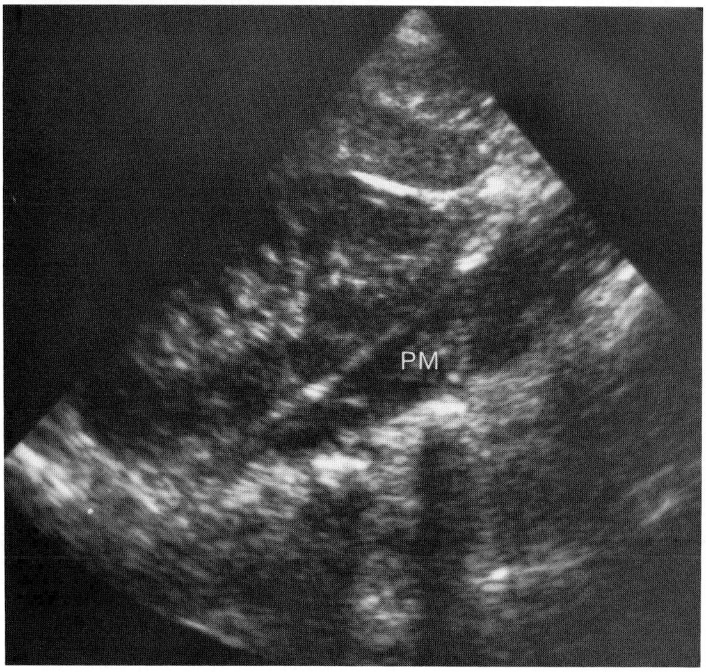

Figure 4.24. Longitudinal examination of the right kidney in the coronal plane. The psoas muscle (*PM*) is seen medial to the kidney and adjacent to the vertebral column. On real-time examination during respiration the kidney is mobile and "slides" along the psoas muscle.

and this fact, along with the general awareness of the possibility of horseshoe kidney, makes misdiagnosis unlikely.

Positional anomalies are also encountered, with the ptotic and ectopic kidney being the most common (23). The ectopic kidney is usually more caudad than normal, and the occurrence of an empty renal fossa should prompt a search inferiorly in the lower abdomen and the pelvis in an attempt to locate the affected kidney. Bowel often fills the empty renal fossa. Rarely the ectopic kidney is located in the thoracic cavity (51). Differential diagnosis includes a solitary kidney, renal agenesis, or dysgenesis. Particularly helpful is the fact that in cases of ectopia the normally positioned kidney is of normal size, whereas in the other conditions it usually undergoes compensatory hyper-

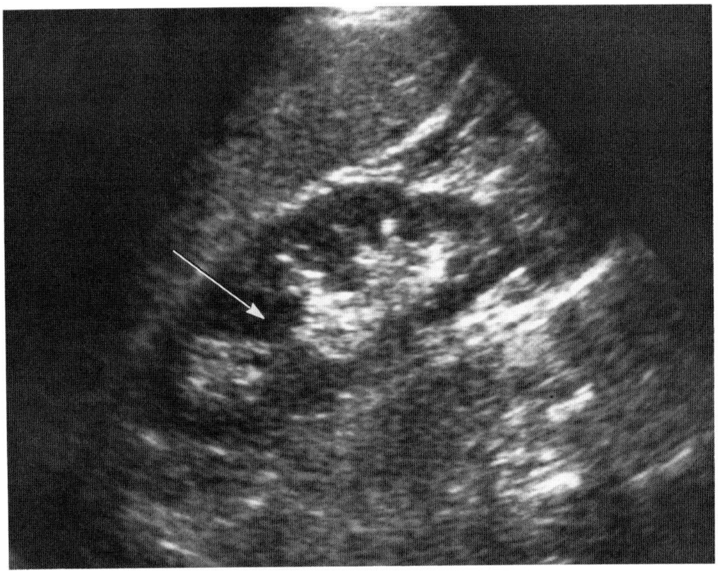

Figure 4.25. Hypertrophied column of Bertin. This longitudinal image of the right kidney demonstrates a hypertrophied column of Bertin (*arrow*) indenting the renal sinus located in its most typical position at the junction of the upper and middle thirds of the kidney. The parenchymal pattern and echogenicity of the hypertrophied column are identical to those of the remaining renal parenchyma in this kidney.

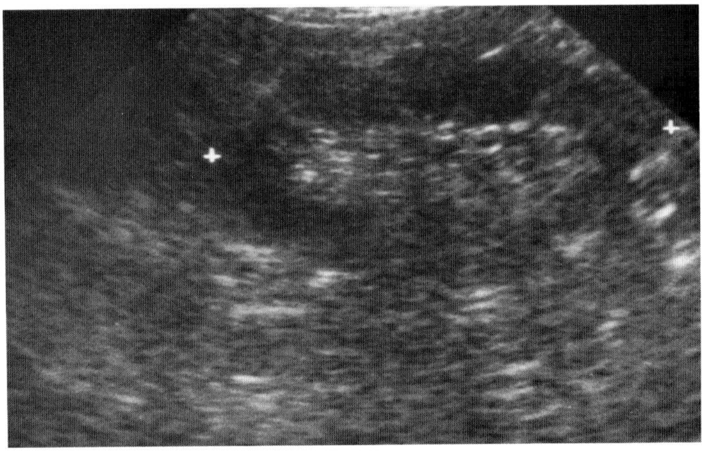

Figure 4.26. Fetal lobation. A longitudinal coronal scan of the left kidney. Fetal lobation is well demonstrated and seen as indentations along the renal border.

trophy. Ectopic kidney is often associated with other anomalies (48, 52, 53).

DIFFUSE DISEASE

The difficulties in interpreting the findings on ultrasonographic examination of the kidneys in diffuse renal disease are many and are discussed at some length in this chapter. Because of these difficulties, a systematic approach is desirable. There are two well-recognized and complementary approaches to renal parenchymal disease, which if integrated provide a reasonable basis for discussion. The first is the systematic approach to the radiologic diagnosis of parenchymal disease of the kidney as outlined by Davidson (54). This approach uses (*a*) primary uroradiologic elements of size, contour, and laterality and (*b*) secondary uroradiologic elements that describe the papillae, pelvoinfundibulo-caliceal system, parenchymal thickness, nephrogram, calcification, attenuation value, miscellaneous factors, and echogenicity. This last element, echogenicity, is the basis for the second approach, popularized by Rosenfield (12), which has been emphasized in the ultrasound literature. Before considering echogenicity in more detail, it may be of value to discuss the problems with and value of the elements of Davidson's approach that are applicable to sonography.

Size is one primary consideration in detecting and classifying renal parenchymal disease. Sizing kidneys accurately can be quite difficult. Volumetric analysis is too laborious for routine

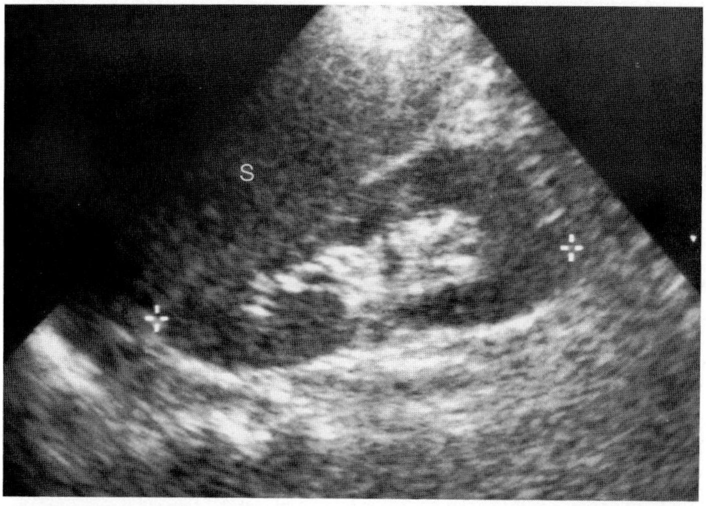

Figure 4.27. Dromedary hump. Longitudinal examination of the left kidney. The spleen (*S*) compresses the upper portion of the left kidney, and the inferior border has a bulged appearance representing the dromedary hump.

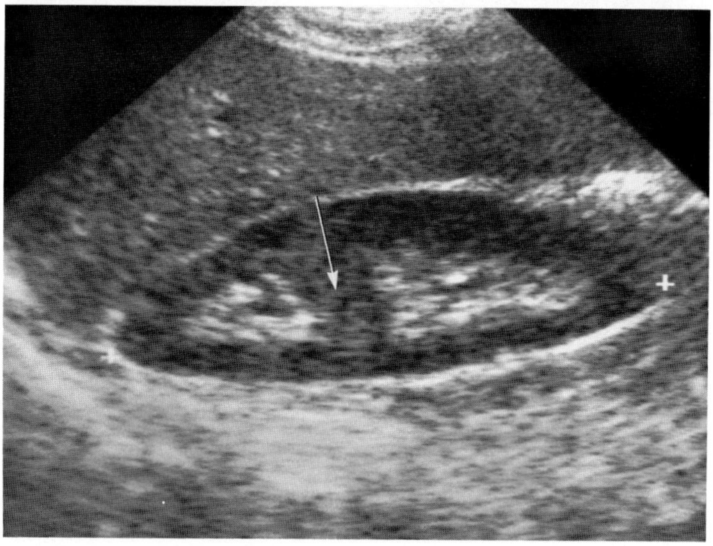

Figure 4.28. Duplicated renal collecting system. Longitudinal examination of the right kidney. A cleft of normal renal parenchyma (*arrow*) divides two zones of echogenic sinus, indicative of a duplicated collecting system.

clinical use, and, as mentioned earlier, the single measurement of renal length is generally used. Even this measurement can be problematic because of anatomic and technical considerations that may make even single measurements difficult in some patients. This difficulty leads to problems of reproducibility, which greatly affect the accuracy of studies designed to follow the course of disease with renal length as a criterion. One needs also to remember that there is no magnification in the ultrasonographic measurement as there is in uroradiography. Another consideration is that the size of the kidney may change in different stages of the same disease. For instance, the kidney involved with amyloidosis may be large, small, or normal in size. Despite these limitations, size considerations are frequently helpful from a practical clinical standpoint (Tables 4.1 and 4.2). It is quite helpful to demonstrate small hyperechoic kidneys in a patient who presents with renal failure. Although the etiology of the renal failure cannot be determined on the basis of this ultrasonographic picture, management decisions can be made. On the other end of the spectrum, it is also very helpful to demonstrate bilaterally enlarged kidneys. Although the diagnostic set is quite large for this finding, in clinical practice the majority of these cases will be associated with diabetes mellitus.

Two secondary uroradiologic elements are especially helpful ultrasonographically. They are

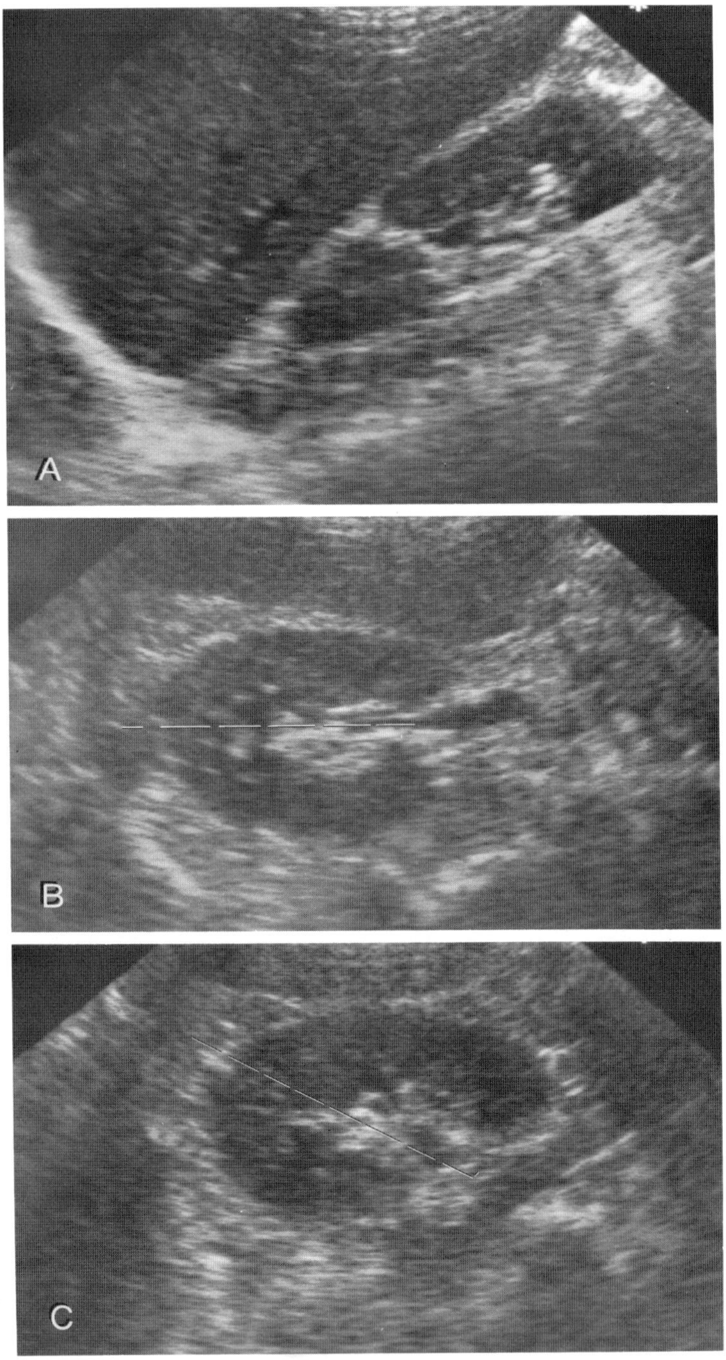

Figure 4.29. A, Junctional parenchymal defect. Longitudinal examination of the right kidney. Note the highly echogenic fat in this defect coursing from the sinus to the perirenal fat, at which point it has a more triangular appearance. **B** and **C,** Transverse scans through the upper portion (**B**) and the lower portion (**C**) of the kidney. Because of incomplete fusion of the superior and inferior renunculi, the axes of the superior and inferior portions of the kidney are different. This change in axis can be noted in transverse scanning, as is demonstrated by the *dashed lines* representing the axis of the kidney in its superior (**B**) and inferior (**C**) portions.

the degree of renal echogenicity and the distinction between changes involving the cortex and those primarily involving the medulla.

The distinctive secondary uroradiologic element demonstrated ultrasonographically in diffuse renal parenchymal disease is the degree of echogenicity (Tables 4.1 and 4.2). Rosenfield divided changes seen ultrasonographically into those producing a diffuse increase in cortical echoes ("Type I changes") and those causing focal distortion of parenchymal anatomy ("Type II changes") (12). Type I changes are associated with numerous diffuse renal parenchymal diseases, and the list has subsequently grown (Table 4.1). Grading of diffusely increased cortical echoes is generally done by comparing the

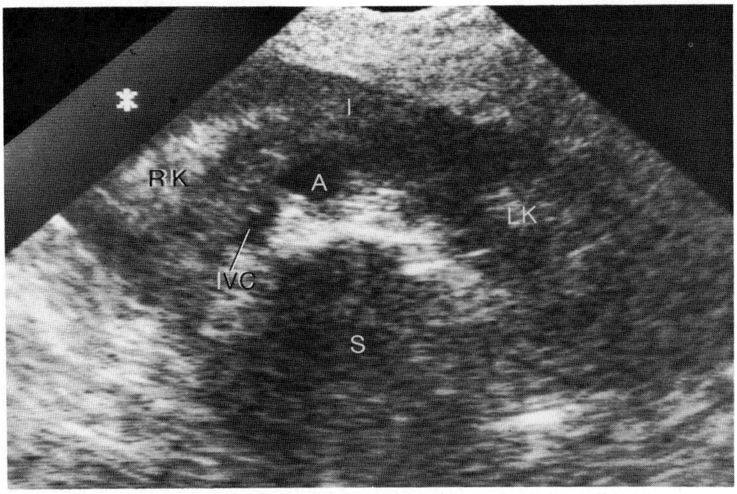

Figure 4.30. Horseshoe kidney. Transverse examination taken from the anterior abdominal wall. The right kidney (*RK*) and the left kidney (*LK*) and the connecting isthmus (*I*) are seen in this example. *S*, spine; *A*, aorta; *IVC*, inferior vena cava.

Table 4.1.
Diffuse Medical Renal Disease Causing Increased Cortical Echogenicity

Small Kidney	Normal or Enlarged Kidney
Nephrotic syndrome	Acute glomerulonephritides
Glomerulonephritis—chronic	Goodpasture's syndrome
Arteriolarnephrosclerosis	Systemic lupus erythematosus
Diabetes mellitus (late)	Diabetes mellitus
Medullary cystic disease	AIDS nephropathy
Amyloidosis (late)	
Papillary necrosis	Interstitial disease
Chronic pyelonephritis[a]	
Acquired cystic disease[a]	1. Inflammation
	a) Infections—acute pyelonephritis
	b) Immunologic
	2. Infiltrative disease
	a) Amyloidosis
	b) Leukemia (rare)
	c) Lymphoma (rare)
	d) POEMS syndrome
	Renal tubular diseases
	1. Acute tubular necrosis
	a) Ischemic
	b) Toxic
	1) Drug induced
	2) Ethylene glycol
	3) Myoglobinuria
	2. Tubular deposition disease
	a) Oxalosis
	b) Gout
	Adult polycystic disease[a]

[a] Irregular borders.

Table 4.2.
Diffuse Renal Disease Causing Decreased Cortical Echogenicity

Normal or Enlarged Kidney	
Uniform	Multifocal
Lymphoma (uncommon)	Lymphoma
Leukemia	
Acute pyelonephritis	Acute pyelonephritis
XGP[a]—diffuse	XGP[a]—segmental

[a] XGP, xanthogranulomatous pyelonephritis.

echogenicity of the renal parenchyma with that of the adjacent liver or spleen or with that of the renal sinus. Renal cortical echogenicity equal to or greater than that of the liver is generally considered abnormal. However, this finding is observed most often in patients with known or suspected renal disease, in whom increased echogenicity is found in 35 to 65% of cases. A more recent report indicates that in nonselected cases, many patients with normal renal function have renal cortical echoes equal to those of liver. This lax criterion of renal cortex echogenicity equal to or greater than liver is neither very sensitive (62%) nor very specific (58%) when applied to all patients referred for ultrasonographic evaluation. A stricter criterion, renal cortex echogenicity greater than liver, is much more specific (96%), but the sensitivity drops considerably (20%) (55).

Some technical considerations that may affect the echo return from the renal cortex and liver should be kept in mind. Because of the nonlinear compression of high- and low-level echoes, small differences in liver and renal parenchymal echoes may not be appreciated at high output settings. Lowering the output settings maximizes the difference in echogenicity (56). For greatest accuracy, the renal parenchyma should be compared to liver at an equal distance from the transducer. This ensures not only that the echoes are subject to the same gain compensation but also that they are in the same focal zone. The latter condition is important because the echo amplitude is greatest in the focal zone of the transducer and diminishes in the near and far fields (13, 56). Another pitfall to avoid is comparing echogenicity of structures that are examined through different acoustic windows. Because of the diminished sound attenuation of fluid, kidneys seen on the other side of ascites or fluid-filled structures such as the gallbladder or large cysts appear to have increased cortical echoes (57). It is also apparent that for a valid comparison, the echo texture of the liver must be normal (58). With all of these factors in mind, there is one group of patients in whom true increased cortical echogenicity does not represent disease: infants, whose renal cortical echogenicity is normally greater than that of the liver (13, 19, 59, 60). For more discussion, see Chapter 13.

Pathologic correlates of increased echogenicity were originally ascribed to increased amounts of collagen and calcium in the renal parenchyma. It was observed that the bulk modulus of supporting tissues, which contains more collagen, is 10,000 times that of the parenchyma of solid organs (56), and this collagen deposition may be the common pathologic finding in the many diseases that cause increased cortical echogenicity. Calcium causes increased echogenicity when seen not only in stones and vascular walls, but also in diseases of the medulla or cortex that are associated with calcium deposition.

Early reports correlating increased renal cortical echogenicity with the extent of cellular and sclerotic changes in the glomeruli have some validity. A more consistent correlation, however, has been found between increased renal echogenicity and interstitial infiltration, tubular pathology, or both (61–64). No patterns of increased echogenicity have been found to help in the differential diagnosis of diffuse medical renal diseases (Table 4.1) (58). This fact is not surprising, as the range of pathologic response in different diseases is quite limited. Tubular and interstitial changes usually follow glomerular changes and vice versa, so that all three components of the renal parenchyma are involved in most pathologic processes. Precise diagnosis usually depends on a combination of clinical history, urinary sediment evaluation, blood tests, and possibly biopsy. In some cases, even a combination of all of these does not provide an etiologic diagnosis, especially in end-stage renal disease (ESRD).

The ultrasonographic picture of ESRD is quite specific, as described below, but other stages of renal disease (acute, subacute, or chronic) cannot be determined from the echogenicity (64, 65).

The ultrasonographic appearance of most diffuse medical renal diseases is very similar (Tables 4.1 and 4.2). In mild cases, there may be no discernible changes from the normal (Fig. 4.31**A**). In more severe disease, either the cor-

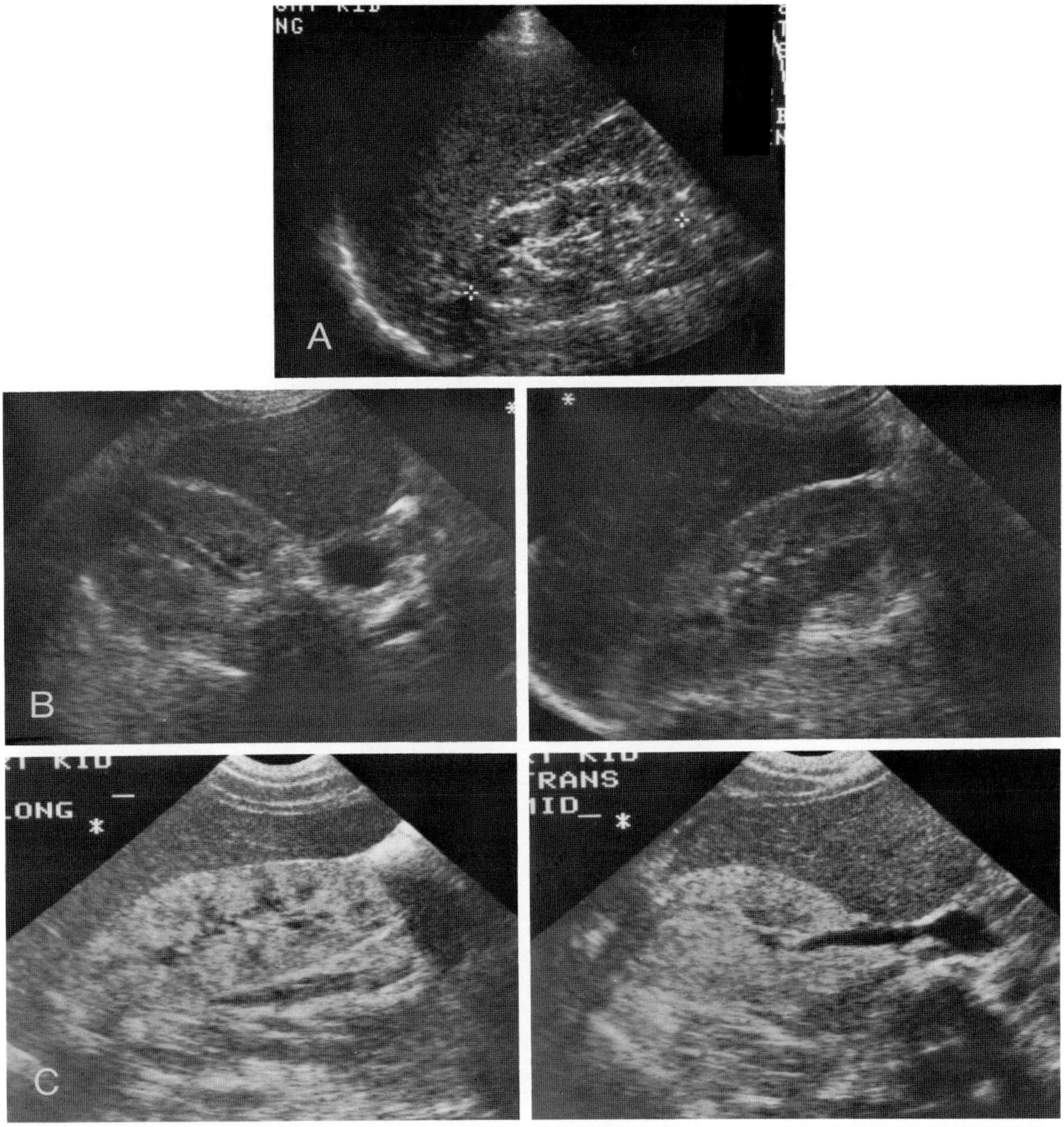

Figure 4.31. Cortical echogenicity compared to echogenicity of adjacent liver or spleen and renal sinus echoes. **A,** Chronic glomerulonephritis (longitudinal image). Serum creatinine 4.0. Renal length 9.4 cm. Renal cortical echogenicity equal to that of liver. **B,** Diabetes mellitus (longitudinal and transverse images). Serum creatinine 3.0. Renal length 14.5 cm. Cortical echogenicity greater than liver. **C,** Hypertension and end-stage renal disease (longitudinal and transverse images). Serum creatinine 11.0. Renal length 11 cm. Cortical echogenicity equal to that of renal sinus.

tex or the medulla may be more echogenic than the liver, and the corticomedullary differentiation may be quite pronounced (Fig. 4.31**B**). If the pathologic process resolves, the ultrasonographic picture may return to normal. If the disease progresses, several changes occur that reflect fibrosis of different areas of the kidney: (*a*) the cortex becomes progressively hyperechoic, (*b*) the corticomedullary differentiation becomes less pronounced as the medullary pyramids become more fibrotic, and (*c*) the renal sinus becomes less distinct (less echogenic) as fibrous tissue replaces highly reflective renal sinus fat (Fig. 4.31**C**). Overall, this fibrosis leads to progressive shrinkage of the kidney (5), producing the typical appearance of the small echogenic kidney of ESRD (Fig. 4.32**A**), which can be difficult to distinguish from the similarly echogenic perirenal fat (Fig. 4.32**B**). The degree of increased echogenicity does give an idea of the extent of the disease at the time of the examination but is not helpful in determining prognosis.

Ultrasound, in addition to depicting the small echogenic kidney with renal medical disease, is highly accurate and sensitive in diagnosing hydronephrosis (66–68). Therefore, azotemic patients are often referred to ultrasound to rule out hydronephrosis, a potentially curable cause of azotemia, and to assess renal size (69–71). The percentage of azotemic patients examined sonographically that will have hydronephrosis as the cause is directly related to the probability of the patient's having hydronephrosis, as assessed by history and clinical examination (70, 71).

Besides the majority of diffuse renal diseases resulting in increased parenchymal echogenicity, there is also a group of inflammatory and infiltrative diseases that on ultrasound produce a hypoechoic parenchyma (Table 4.2). The pathologic correlates of this appearance vary with the disease process. Therefore, although they share many ultrasonographic features, the more frequently encountered diffuse renal diseases excluding the end-stage kidney

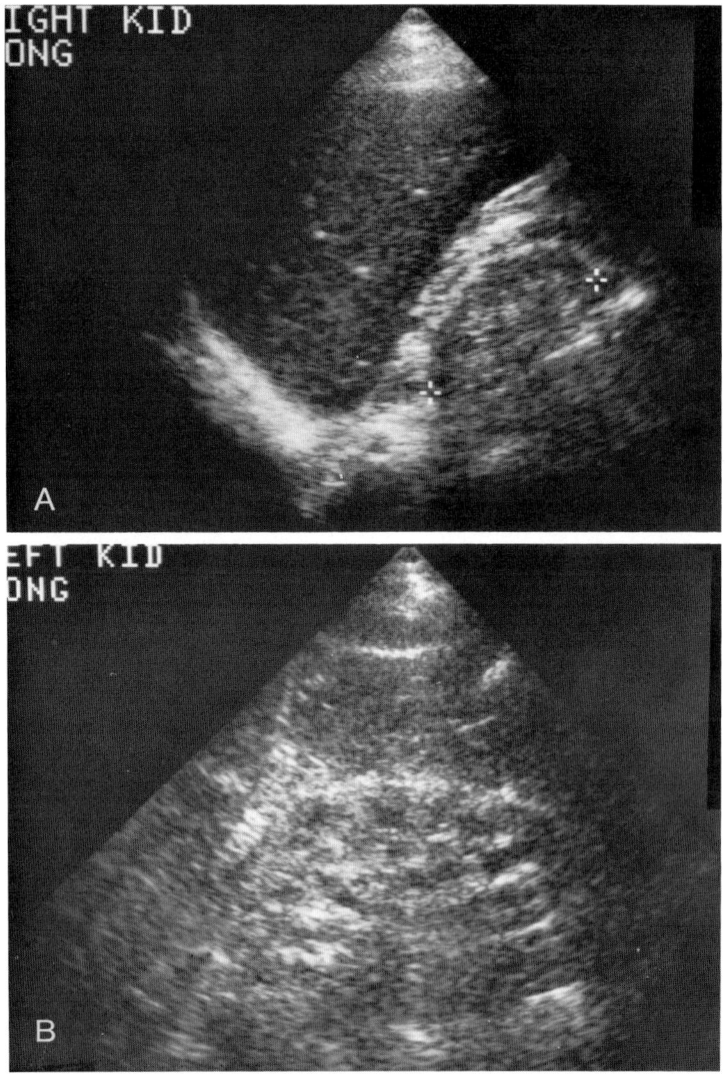

Figure 4.32. End-stage renal disease (ESRD). The typical picture is a small hyperechoic kidney. **A,** Hypertension and ESRD. Serum creatinine 14.7. Renal length 6.0 cm. Right kidney with increased cortical echogenicity. Pyramids are no longer discernible. **B,** Chronic glomerulonephritis. Serum creatinine 4.0. Renal length 9.0. Left kidney, note the difficulty in distinguishing the kidney from surrounding retroperitoneal structures when the spleen does not provide an acoustic window.

already described above are probably best considered individually, with particular attention to changes in size and echogenicity.

Glomerular Diseases

GLOMERULONEPHRITIS

Diseases involving primarily the glomeruli usually result from immunologic reactions involving the capillaries of the glomeruli. The glomerulonephritides fall into this category. The kidney can make only a limited number of responses to this injury. They include (*a*) cellular proliferation (endothelial, epithelial, and mesangial), (*b*) leukocytic infiltration, (*c*) thickening of the glomerular basement membrane, and (*d*) hyalinization and sclerosis. Damage to the glomeruli results secondarily in changes to other parts of the kidney, including the tubules, interstitium, and blood vessels (72). Clinically, patients with acute glomerulonephritis present with hematuria, hypertension, azotemia, and red cell casts in the urine (73). Nephrotic syndrome is often present.

Sonographically, acute glomerulonephritis is reported to show (*a*) normal to increased renal size, (*b*) marked increase in cortical echogenicity, and (*c*) prominent, sonolucent pyramids. As the disease process abates, these changes revert to normal (65, 73). The frequency with which increased cortical echogenicity is seen depends on the severity of the disease in the group studied rather than whether it is acute or chronic. A histologic correlate to account for increased echogenicity has not been found (73). Thinning of the parenchyma is only occasionally seen, and then usually in chronic disease (65).

SYSTEMIC LUPUS ERYTHEMATOSUS

In systemic lupus erythematosus (SLE), an autoimmune disorder involving multiple organs including the kidney in over half the patients, changes similar to those associated with glomerulonephritis have been described. Pathologically, SLE renal lesions include mesangial nephritis and focal proliferative, diffuse proliferative, and membranous glomerulonephritis. In addition to those glomerular lesions, vasculitis characterized by edema and perivascular infiltrate may be present. Tubulointerstitial lesions may also be present, especially in cases with diffuse proliferative glomerulonephritis. In a few cases, the tubulointerstitial lesion may predominate (72). Clinically, lupus nephritis varies from a mild proteinuria to a fulminant acute progressive glomerulonephritis, and prognosis usually correlates with the type and extent of renal involvement (74).

Sonographically, abnormalities in size and cortical echogenicity may be found. The size is most often normal even when there is significant renal impairment or proteinuria. If, however, the kidneys are enlarged or small, renal functional impairment is usually more severe. Changes in cortical echogenicity may include diffusely increased echogenicity or multiple focal areas of cortical hypoechogenicity (Fig. 4.33). In one study, patients with SLE who were referred for sonography had cortical echogenicity equal to (48%) or greater than (26%) that of the liver. In this study, a positive correlation was found between the degree of increased cortical echogenicity and the degree of renal impairment. Unfortunately, it provided no additional information not readily appreciated from laboratory studies routinely obtained in these patients (74). Areas of cortical hypoechogenicity have been suggested as a rather specific sign of SLE (75), though this observation has not been corroborated by others.

AIDS NEPHROPATHY

Ultrasonographic changes have been reported in some patients with nephropathy associated with AIDS. The pathologic change first emphasized in AIDS nephropathy was focal segmental glomerulosclerosis, a rather nonspecific pathologic finding (76). Global glomerulosclerosis has also been described. More recently, tubular changes ranging from mild dilatation to markedly dilated, irregular, and infolded tubules, with intratubular deposits of proteinaceous material and occasionally cyst-like structures of the cortex and medulla have been thought to better explain the changes seen at ultrasonography (77).

Clinically, renal abnormalities in AIDS patients range from proteinuria to renal insufficiency of varying severity. Renal involvement, seen in about one-third of patients, is an important cause of morbidity and mortality (77).

Ultrasonographically, kidneys involved with AIDS nephropathy have been normal in size to enlarged (Fig. 4.34). Cortical echogenicity is normal in about 35 to 40% of reported cases, with varying degrees of diffusely increased cortical echogenicity in the majority. The changes

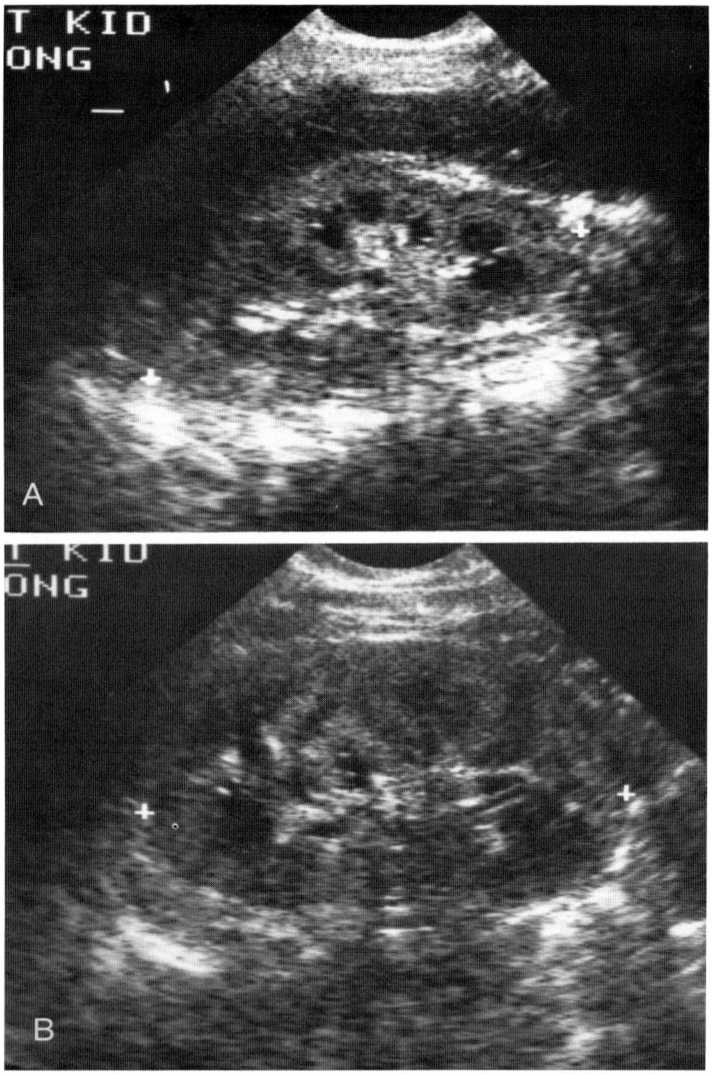

Figure 4.33. Systemic lupus erythematosus (SLE). **A,** Right kidney of patient with membranous SLE. Serum creatinine 4.2. Note the increased cortical echogenicity and prominent corticomedullary differentiation. **B,** Left kidney, same patient. In addition to increased cortical echogenicity, there are irregular areas of decreased echogenicity.

in echogenicity seen on ultrasound correlate pathologically with glomerular changes and to a greater degree with the tubular changes (76). Similar findings are present in patients with AIDS nephropathy, whether or not they use heroin (76, 77).

MISCELLANEOUS GLOMERULAR DISEASES

Many other diseases that pathologically affect primarily the glomerulus have been reported to cause diffusely increased echogenicity. They include some of the most common diseases affecting the kidney, such as arteriolarnephrosclerosis and diabetes mellitus (Fig. 4.35), as well as the less frequent Alport's disease and adult hemolytic uremic syndrome. The frequency of sonographic changes and their pathologic correlates have not been well documented at this time.

Tubular Diseases

ACUTE TUBULAR NECROSIS

Some changes seen ultrasonographically in diseases involving primarily the renal tubules are indistinguishable from those seen in diseases involving primarily the glomeruli. Acute tubular necrosis (ATN) is the most common cause of acute renal failure and is usually reversible. Tubular damage seen in ATN occurs in two relatively common conditions: ischemic

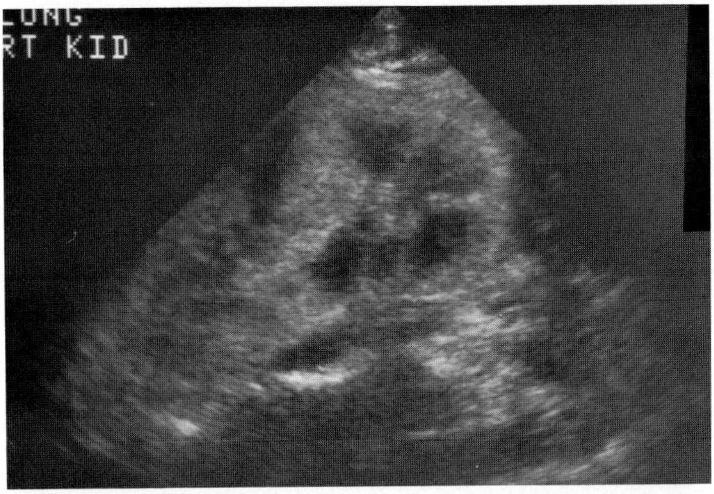

Figure 4.34. Nephropathy associated with intravenous cocaine abuse and AIDS. Serum creatinine 9.5. Note the marked increase in cortical echogenicity and large, relatively hypoechoic pyramids.

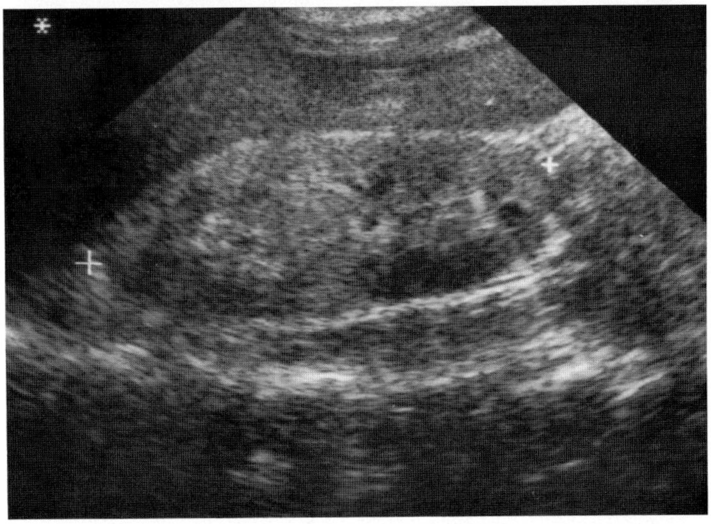

Figure 4.35. Diabetes mellitus. Serum creatinine 7.1. Note the large size (13.9 cm) and increased cortical echogenicity. Diabetes mellitus is the most common cause of renal enlargement with increased cortical echogenicity.

injury and damage due to a nephrotoxin (78). Pathologically, tubular damage resulting from ischemia is characterized by morphologic changes that are quite mild and may be difficult to see on routine histologic sections. Relatively small lengths of tubules show evidence of necrosis with rupture of the basement membranes and occlusion of the lumen by casts. There may be some interstitial edema and accumulation of leukocytes in the vasa recta. In toxic ATN, there is extensive necrosis of the proximal tubular segment, as well as casts in distal convoluted tubules and proximal collecting ducts. In toxic ATN, there is more severe tubular necrosis and swelling (72).

The clinical picture begins with the onset of oliguria or anuria lasting 10 to 20 days and often requiring dialysis. A diuretic phase follows, signaling the beginning of recovery (79). Eventually normal tubular function is restored.

Ultrasound is usually performed to rule out obstruction as a cause of the patient's oliguria. The difference in the extent and degree of tubular damage in ATN may explain the variable ultrasound appearance. There is general agreement that in renal transplants, ischemic ATN does not lead to change in size or increase in cortical echogenicity. This may also be true for ischemic ATN in native kidneys. Some have described occasional increase in echogenicity of the cortex (73).

ATN caused by toxins such as gentamicin (78), ethylene glycol (80), and myoglobinuria

(81), on the other hand, is reported to have increased cortical echogenicity with occasional enlargement of the kidneys globally or prominence of the renal pyramids.

A third form of ATN results from the intratubular block secondary to Tamm-Horsfall protein and gives the ultrasonographic picture of hyperechoic renal pyramids rather than cortex (78). Although Tamm-Horsfall proteins are seen in adult ATN, this clinical entity and its ultrasonographic picture have been reported only in newborns (5).

ACUTE CORTICAL NECROSIS

Acute cortical necrosis (ACN) is a rare cause of acute renal failure involving the cortex and sparing the medulla (79). It is usually associated in the adult with shock, sepsis, myocardial infarction, burns, toxemia of pregnancy, abruptio placenta, and postpartum hemorrhage, and is sometimes a complication of abdominal aortic surgery (73, 79, 82).

The exact mechanism causing ACN is unknown, but it is likely due to ischemia. Histologically there is necrosis of the tubular cells and leukocyte infiltration into the interstitium (73, 82). Calcification is often present at the boundary of the necrotic and viable tissue or throughout the cortex 24 hr or more after the initial insult (82).

Clinically ACN begins with anuria, mild fever, leukocytosis, and little in the way of physical findings (79). If only a portion of the cortex is involved, the patient usually survives. If, on the other hand, the entire cortex is involved, uremia usually develops, leading to death unless the patient receives dialysis or transplantation.

On ultrasound in ACN the cortex may initially be hypoechoic but most commonly the cortex is hyperechoic, because of calcium and collagen deposition (73). Other causes of cortical calcium deposition include oxalosis (83) and hypercalcemia from tumors (84). An interesting though rarely seen finding in cortical necrosis is an apparent hypoechoic rim around the periphery, perhaps representing the subcapsular cortex, which has been spared by capsular collaterals (82).

Interstitial Diseases

Diseases that affect primarily the renal interstitium may also be associated with ultrasonographic changes. The interstitial diseases can be divided into inflammatory and infiltrative types.

INFLAMMATORY DISEASES

Acute Pyelonephritis

Bacterial inflammatory disease of the kidney occurs along a spectrum of anatomic distribution and severity. Acute pyelonephritis, most commonly with *Escherichia coli* as the causative organism (85), is the most common inflammatory disease encountered. Most infections develop by ascending from the bladder along the subepithelial lymphatics of the collecting system (85, 86) to involve the lining membranes of the renal pelvis (acute pyelitis). Subsequently, spread occurs into the interstitium from the renal pyramids to focal areas in the cortex, which becomes swollen and edematous. The inflammatory reaction may remain focal, may become diffuse, may coalesce into an inflammatory mass without drainable pus (acute focal bacterial nephritis or acute lobar nephronia), or may progress to suppuration, forming microabscesses (87). These microabscesses may further coalesce into a carbuncle, or abscess (88). This is particularly likely when the host is immunocompromised, the organism is virulent, or the treatment is inadequate.

Extension outside the renal capsule or Gerota's fascia can occur, particularly when the renal infection is associated with obstruction, prior trauma, or intravenous drug abuse (85, 89).

Uncomplicated pyelonephritis is most common in the 15- to 35-year-old female, and is characterized by chills, fever, dysuria, flank pain, hematuria, pyuria, and bacteriuria. Morbidity is low and mortality vanishingly rare. Typical cases are recognized by symptoms alone, and uncomplicated cases are adequately treated with antibiotics. Imaging procedures are not usually necessary. Investigation into the origin of the infection is required only to exclude abscess or obstruction in female patients with recurrent urinary tract infections (UTIs), healthy male patients with UTI, or patients with severe symptoms not responding to treatment.

The ultrasound features of acute pyelonephritis parallel the spectrum of the pathologic findings and may demonstrate focal or diffuse renal disease. In uncomplicated cases the involved kidney may appear normal. The classic *acute focal bacterial pyelonephritis* (lobar nephronia) on ultrasound is a solid, poorly marginated, possibly wedge-shaped mass in a lobar distribution, without posterior acoustic enhancement. It contains low-level echoes that disrupt the corticomedullary junction (85, 87, 90). Uncommonly the lesion may be isoechoic (91) and rarely hyperechoic, particularly when complicated by hemorrhage (85).

An *abscess* appears sonographically as a poorly marginated, thick-walled cystic mass (86, 92), which may distort the renal contour. It exhibits a wide range of echogenicity, from nearly anechoic to highly echogenic, as a result of coagulative necrosis and microbubble formation (88). Posterior acoustic enhancement is usually present, denoting the fluid component of the lesion. It has been noted that small renal abscesses may resemble focal pyelonephritis (86).

In *diffuse* (Fig. 4.36) or *multifocal* (Fig. 4.37) acute pyelonephritis, the kidney is enlarged and hypoechoic (85, 86). The corticomedullary junction is obscured and the parenchymal echogenicity is reduced, accentuating the distinction between the parenchyma and renal sinus (85). Conversely, if the renal sinus is infiltrated with pus, the distinction between the parenchyma and renal sinus is reduced (85). Infrequently, diffuse pyelonephritis may produce diffusely increased cortical echogenicity (63) (Fig. 4.38). With extension, an anechoic zone around the kidney defined by Gerota's fascia can be seen (88).

Chronic Atrophic Pyelonephritis

Chronic atrophic pyelonephritis represents an old, healed lesion of focal pyelonephritis that has formed a cortical scar adjacent to a blunted calix. On ultrasound chronic pyelonephritis appears as a focal loss of parenchyma with increased echoes in the cortex and medulla (Fig. 4.39). A retracted calix adjacent to a cortical scar can be recognized as an echogenic zone if not distended with urine, or an anechoic zone if

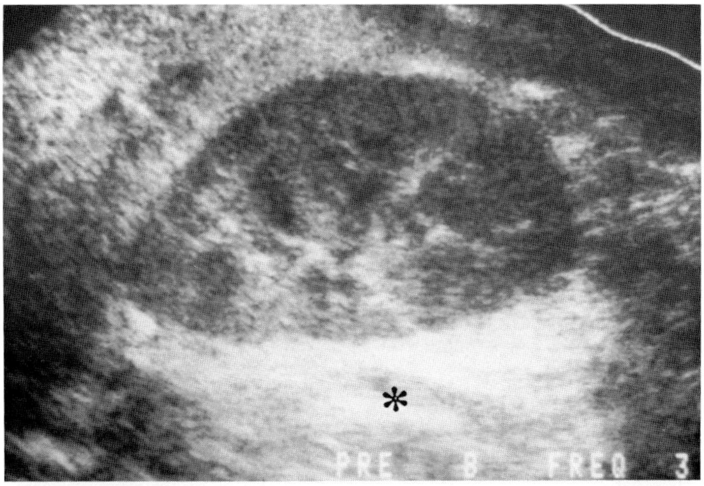

Figure 4.36. Acute diffuse pyelonephritis. Enlarged, rounded, smooth, uniformly hypoechoic kidney with preserved reniform shape. Note marked posterior acoustic enhancement, reflecting fluid component of interstitial inflammatory infiltrate (*asterisk*).

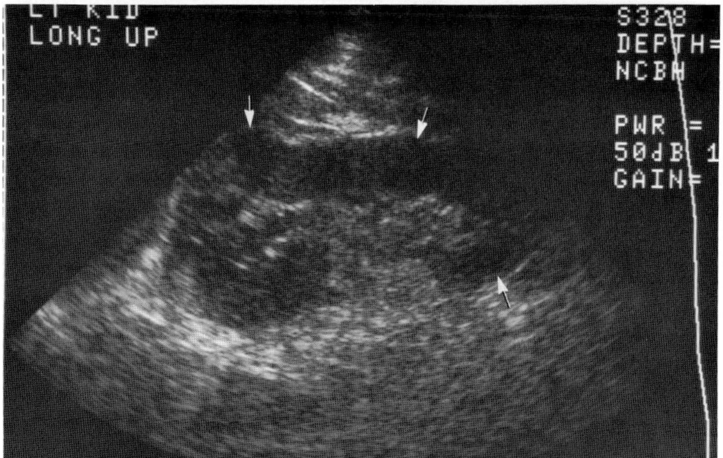

Figure 4.37. Acute multifocal pyelonephritis. Enlarged kidney with multiple hypoechoic regions in parenchyma, each reflecting a focal region of pyelonephritis (*arrows*).

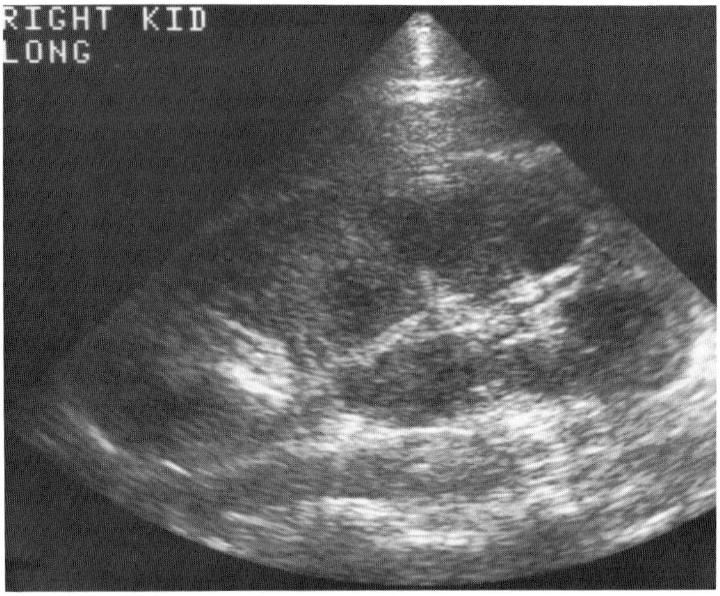

Figure 4.38. Acute pyelonephritis with increased cortical echogenicity. Enlarged kidney with increased distinction of medulla and cortex, and pronounced cortical echogenicity.

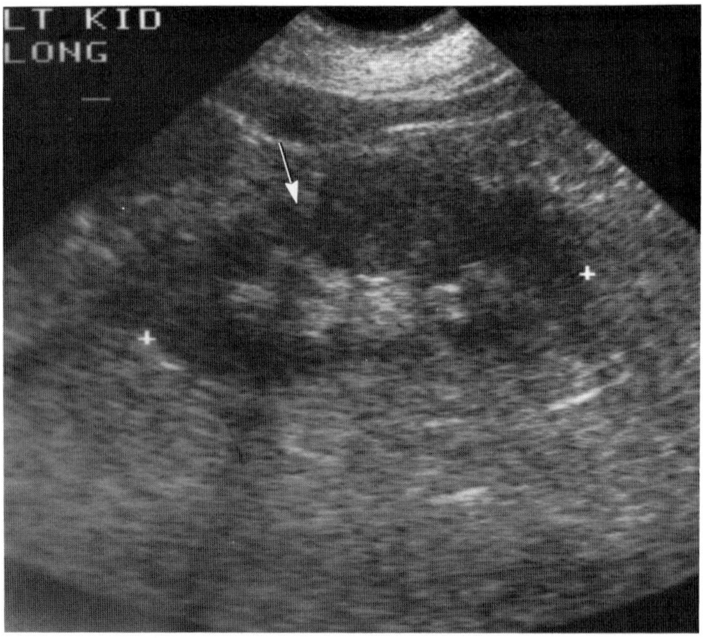

Figure 4.39. Chronic pyelonephritis. Small, scarred kidney with multiple contour indentations, some adjacent to extensions of renal sinus (*arrow*).

distended (93). This feature may be helpful in distinguishing between pyelonephritis and segmental ischemia, as the latter does not distort the collecting system. If the inflammatory process is diffuse, it will be repeated throughout the parenchyma to produce a small, scarred kidney.

Emphysematous Pyelonephritis

Other renal inflammatory conditions beyond the spectrum of acute to chronic pyelonephritis can develop and be seen on ultrasound. Emphysematous pyelonephritis is histologically considered to be a type of pyelonephritis rather than a separate entity (94). It is a fulminant, necrotizing process usually found in diabetics and most often caused by *E. coli* or *Proteus mirabilis*. In immunocompromised patients, especially renal transplant patients, it may result from *Staphylococcus aureus* (95). Approximately one-third of these cases begin with a urinary tract infection (85). Extreme renal ischemia caused by the inflammation induces the organism to ferment glucose to lactic acid and carbon dioxide, producing gas (85). In diabetics mortality is reported to be 90% without surgery and 36 to 50% with surgery (96).

The sonographic features of emphysematous pyelonephritis include renal enlargement and decreased echogenicity. Gas may be seen in the parenchyma, renal sinus, or perirenal space (97). The gas appears as hyperechoic structures with "dirty shadowing" (indistinct posterior acoustic shadowing) or "ring-down" artifacts (a repeating band of echoes within a posterior acoustic shadow) behind them.

Xanthogranulomatous Pyelonephritis

Xanthogranulomatous pyelonephritis (XGP) is the consequence of renal infection of some duration, often several months. There is usually associated pelvic obstruction from staghorn or other large calculi. Two forms exist, a diffuse form and a focal or tumefactive form. In the more common diffuse form, the inflammatory process begins in the pelvocalyceal system with the development of pyonephrosis as a result of infection behind the obstructing calculus. The renal parenchyma is then progressively destroyed and replaced with sheets of lipid-laden histiocytes called "foam" or "xanthoma" cells (85, 98). Extrarenal extension to the perirenal and pararenal spaces is common, and extension to the skin, the subphrenic and pleural spaces, and the back and psoas muscles has been reported (99). The less common focal or tumefactive form is a limited process resulting from obstruction by stone or stricture of an isolated portion of the collecting system.

XGP occurs more commonly in women, in patients with diabetes mellitus, and in middle age (fourth and fifth decades), although it has been described in all age groups (98, 100). Clinical signs are nonspecific and include pain, mass, weight loss, fever, and general malaise (98). A UTI is often present, most commonly associated with *P. mirabilis* and *E. coli,* and many have a history of chronic UTIs.

On sonographic examination, the kidney involved with diffuse XGP is globally enlarged with multiple hypoechoic or anechoic areas (Fig. 4.40). This is the result of replacement of the normal renal architecture by multiple fluid-filled masses corresponding to parenchymal necrosis, hemorrhage, and abscess formation (98). The reniform shape is preserved. The central echo complex is highly reflective (85, 97), and calculi with posterior shadowing may be seen. However, shadowing may be inapparent when extensive fibrosis is present (85). In some reports there is often marked hydronephrosis (98), whereas others report absence of caliceal dilatation (85). Occasionally no normal renal structures are present, and the renal fossa is occupied by multiple large inflammatory masses with irregular walls.

In *segmental XGP* there are focal areas of renal enlargement containing one or more hypoechoic or anechoic masses. The renal margin may be smooth or lobulated, and calculi and extrarenal extension may be evident (85).

Fungal Infection

Renal fungal infection arises through an ascending route in the majority of cases (85) and is usually caused by *Candida albicans* (101), although other less common fungal species such as *Aspergillus* and *Cryptococcus* may be the cause. Saprophytic fungal infection can be seen in immunocompromised patients, diabetics, those with underlying renal disease, or those undergoing therapy for genitourinary tract infection (85). With prolonged colonization of the urinary tract, a "fungus ball," consisting of fungal hyphae, may form in a portion of the renal collecting system.

Sonographically there is diffuse parenchymal swelling, which may progress to pyonephrosis, intra- and extrarenal abscesses, and most characteristically, the fungus ball, seen as one or more nonshadowing solid masses in the collecting system, more echogenic than the surrounding parenchyma (102).

Renal Tuberculosis

Renal tuberculosis, a less common infection, but one having a resurgence secondary to AIDS, usually arises from hematogenous spread from other foci, most frequently the lungs (85). Multiple abscesses form throughout the cortices of both kidneys (103) and give rise to a chronic granulomatous inflammatory process. Caseation necrosis, fibrosis, calcium deposition, and cortical destruction are also seen. The process may extend to the medullary pyramids and communicate with the collecting system, leading to granuloma formation, edema, fibrosis, and stricture formation (73). Macroscopic abnormalities are almost always unilateral; if the other kidney is affected, it is usually the result of ureteral reflux or obstruction from bladder changes, rather than progression of the primary hematogenous infection (103).

Tuberculosis may produce a normal sono-

Figure 4.40. Xanthogranulomatous pyelonephritis. **A,** Longitudinal image. **B,** Transverse image. Markedly enlarged, hypoechoic kidney with a large central calculus with posterior shadowing (*arrowhead*), and replacement of parenchyma by multiple hypoechoic regions, representing abscesses (*arrows*).

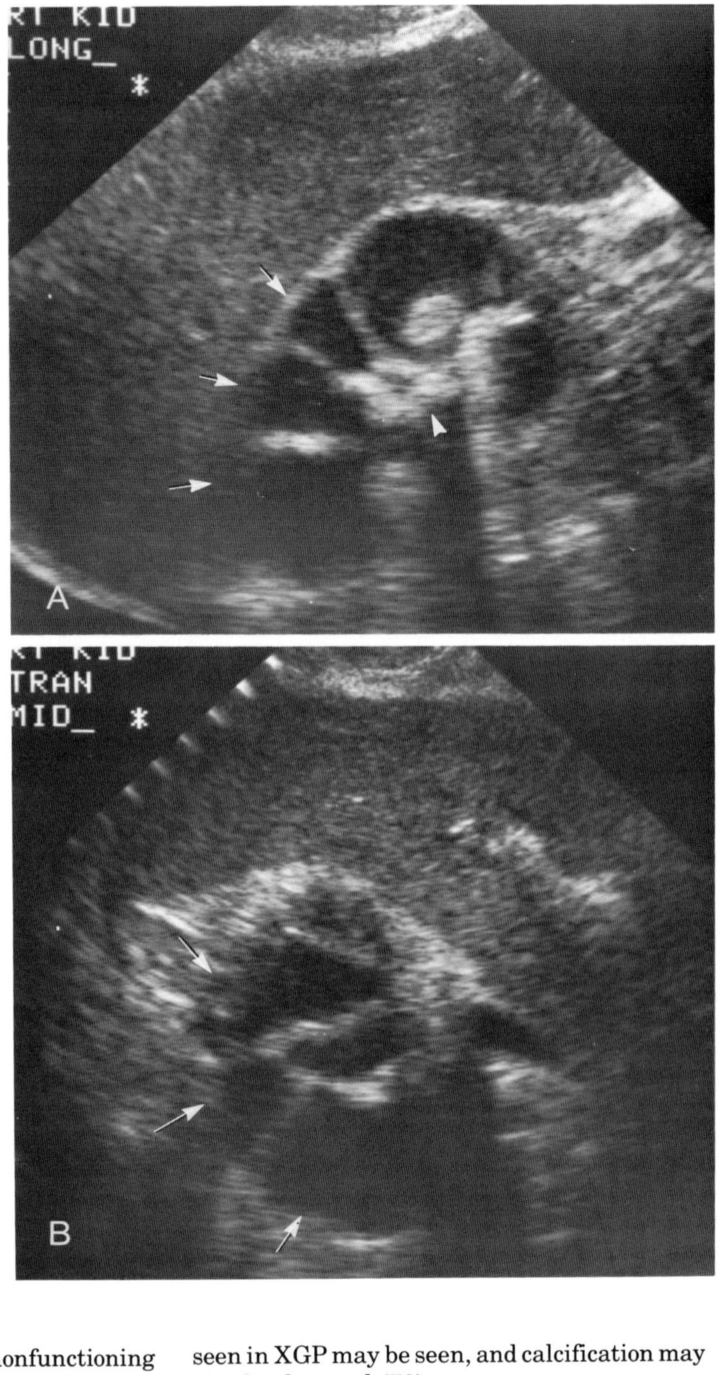

gram, even in the presence of a nonfunctioning kidney or excretory urography (104). There may be loss of the corticomedullary junction. More marked abnormalities include hydronephrosis with debris (85). Tuberculous strictures lead to dilatation and infection of portions of the collecting system, and appear as a focal dilated collecting system containing debris (105). Inflammatory masses similar to those seen in XGP may be seen, and calcification may also be detected (73).

Interstitial Nephritis

Interstitial nephritis not related to infection is thought to be the result of immunologic mechanisms. Pathologically, the kidneys may be slightly enlarged with edema of the interstitium and a mononuclear cell infiltration. In some cases, large numbers of eosinophils and neutrophils may be present. On occasion, giant-cell granulomas are seen. Variable degrees of tubular necrosis may be present (72). Although ultrasonic findings in specific interstitial disease entities have not been reported extensively, pathologic correlations have demonstrated increased cortical echogenicity in cases of interstitial abnormalities, particularly in active interstitial disease processes (13, 62).

INFILTRATIVE PROCESSES

Amyloidosis

Noninflammatory infiltration of the kidney occurs occasionally with amyloidosis, leukemia, and lymphoma. Renal involvement with amyloidosis is the major cause of death from this disease. Amyloidosis can be seen in primary form or secondarily associated with chronic inflammatory and infective processes, including rheumatoid arthritis, juvenile rheumatoid arthritis, familial Mediterranean fever, tuberculosis, ulcerative colitis, and osteomyelitis (73, 79). This reactive systemic amyloidosis has also been seen in patients with ankylosing spondylitis, Reiter's syndrome, scleroderma, dermatomyositis, systemic lupus erythematosis, Waldenström's macroglobulinemia, and multiple myeloma (73) (Fig. 4.41). Neoplastic diseases such as renal cell carcinoma and Hodgkin's disease have also been associated with amyloidosis.

The size of the kidney may be normal or enlarged initially. Later, the kidney contracts, possibly because of vascular compromise resulting from amyloid deposits. The glomerulus is the primary site of amyloid deposition, though interstitial peritubular tissues and vessels are also involved (72).

Ultrasonographically, amyloid renal disease is characterized by a size dependent on the stage of disease, and increased cortical echogenicity with preservation of corticomedullary differentiation (106) (Fig. 4.41). The cortical echogenicity is thought to be due to the amyloid deposition (106). Although the ultrasound findings are common to many diffuse processes, in the proper clinical settings their presence should suggest the possibility of renal involvement with amyloidosis.

Renal Leukemia

Renal leukemic infiltration is a common entity in childhood leukemia, found in up to 63% of patients dying from systemic leukemia (107, 108). It also has been reported to be present in adults (109), and in both groups it is more frequently seen in lymphocytic forms. Histologically, leukemic cells infiltrate the interstitium, crowding and replacing the tubules and to a lesser extent the glomeruli, resulting in renal enlargement (79). This infiltration and resultant renomegaly are usually diffuse and bilateral but can be focal and nodular (73). In approximately 15% of patients renal enlargement is present without evidence of leukemic infiltration. The etiology is unknown (109). Chemotherapy can cause tumor cytolysis and uric acid liberation, leading to obstructive nephropathy by urate crystal deposition (110).

Renal leukemia is often clinically silent, with other systemic dysfunctions predominating. However, hypertension and renal failure may be observed (111). While the renal failure seen in renal leukemia may be due to the leukemia itself, it often results from uric acid nephropathy and can be caused by hyperuricemia, septicemia, and hemorrhage (109, 112).

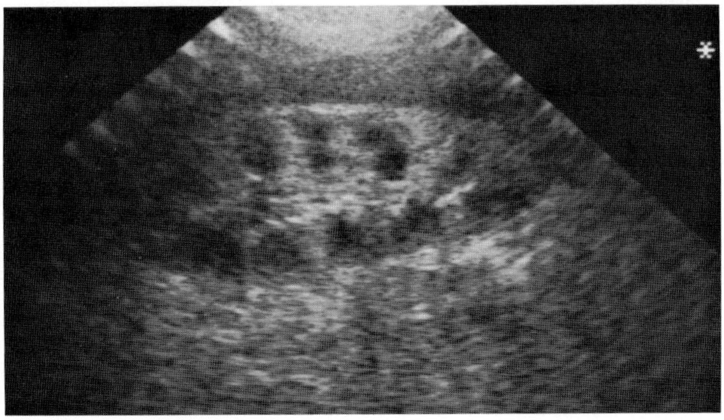

Figure 4.41. Multiple myeloma and renal failure. Serum creatinine 6.2. Renal length 12.2 cm. Note the increased cortical echogenicity and prominent corticomedullary differentiation.

Renal leukemic involvement results in the ultrasound appearance of renal enlargement with either normal or decreased echogenicity with a smooth contour (Fig. 4.42) (110). The hypoechoic appearance of the kidney is often nonuniformly distributed, so that multiple nodular areas of low-level echoes are seen in the parenchyma (112). If urate obstructive nephropathy is present, the renomegaly is accentuated by hydronephrosis. In either case the kidney will revert to normal with remission, and abnormal findings will recur during relapse (112). Diffuse coarse cortical echoes in involved kidneys have also been described (109).

Ultrasound has proved to be a useful clinical tool in monitoring patients with potential renal leukemia. It is more sensitive than urography in identifying parenchymal involvement (109), with the added advantages of no contrast requirement, independence of renal function, and use for serial examinations without radiation exposure. It is more useful in (*a*) demonstrating occult leukemia, (*b*) following response to therapy, (*c*) monitoring complications of chemotherapy and the disease itself such as bleeding and infection, and (*d*) assessing the kidney for hydronephrosis.

Renal Lymphoma

Renal lymphoma occurs in both primary and secondary forms and is much more common in non-Hodgkin's lymphoma than in Hodgkin's disease (113). Since the kidney does not contain lymphoid tissue, primary renal lymphoma is very rare (114–116). Most frequently the kidney is a secondary site of involvement from either hematogenous invasion or direct extension. Between 33 and 50% of patients dying with lymphoma have renal involvement at autopsy (113, 114). In fact, after the hematopoietic and reticuloendothelial systems, the urinary tract is the most common site of lymphomatous involvement (113). The incidence of renal involvement in highly aggressive AID-related lymphoma is approximately 11% (117).

Initially lymphomatous tumor proliferation occurs in the interstitium around nephrons, collecting ducts, and blood vessels (118) with preservation of lobular architecture and function (119). Progression leads to compression and obliteration of the tubules with less severe effects on the glomeruli (120). With continued growth the tumor destroys parenchymal support, and then growth becomes expansile (119).

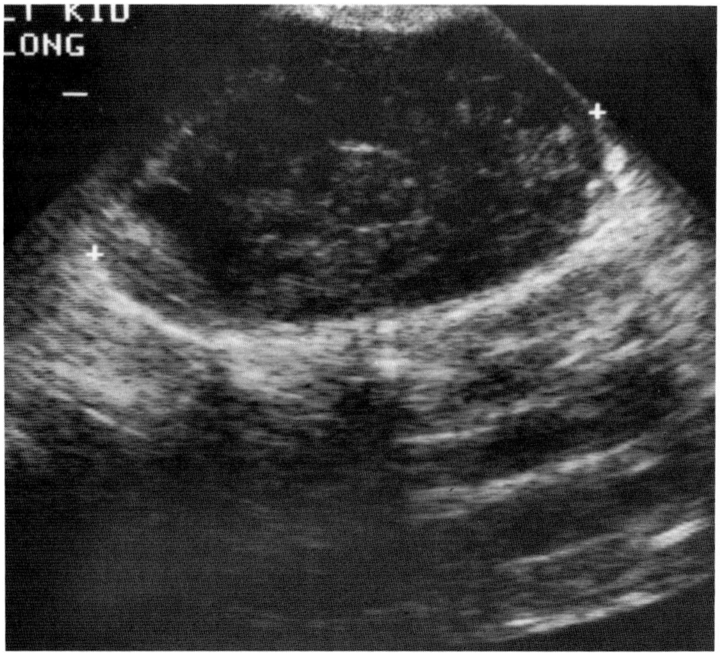

Figure 4.42. Renal leukemia. Large, inhomogeneous, hypoechoic kidney with smooth borders and with loss of renal sinus architecture.

If tumor growth is slow and reniform, reinform shape is preserved; if growth is rapid or nonuniform, contour is distorted (119).

Renal involvement is most often multinodular and bilateral. In a study by Richmond et al. (113), 74% of cases were bilateral and 61% had multiple nodules. Other patterns of involvement included invasion from retroperitoneal lymph nodes (11%), small solitary parenchymal nodules (7%), bulky single tumors (6%), diffuse infiltration (6%), and microscopic disease only (7%) (113).

Renal involvement with lymphoma is usually clinically silent. Occasionally abdominal pain, palpable mass, hypertension, oliguria, and macroscopic hematuria may be present, but renal failure secondary to lymphoma is rare (113, 121).

Ultrasound or computed tomography shows renal involvement in approximately 5% of patients who have lymphoma (119). The variable microscopic distribution of lymphoma in the kidney means that the sonographic appearance will also vary. The most common sonographic appearance is that of a normal-sized or enlarged kidney with multiple homogeneous hypoechoic or anechoic masses without sharply defined walls and with little or no posterior acoustic enhancement (122, 123) (Fig. 4.43). Occasionally, however, posterior acoustic enhancement is present (124), and the tumor masses may appear remarkably similar to cysts. Although the posterior wall may be slightly irregular and posterior acoustic enhancement slightly reduced (125) (Fig. 4.44), differentiation from a cyst in these cases is most difficult (115). In approximately 5% of the cases the organ is diffusely enlarged and hypoechoic without focal lesions (126–128). Rarely, renal sinus echoes are lost secondary to lymphomatous involvement (129). Lymphoma in retroperitoneal nodes may directly invade the kidney and distort the renal architecture (119, 128) or may extend along the ureter to invade the renal sinus (115). Lymphoma arising in the perirenal space (Fig. 4.45) presents as a hypoechoic mass that may infiltrate the renal sinus and may simulate hematoma or inflammatory tissue (130). Following chemotherapy the renal lymphomatous masses may become echogenic or may remain hypoechoic (124).

POEMS

Other infiltrative diseases such as POEMS (131) syndrome, a multisystemic plasma cell disorder consisting of polyneuropathy, organomegaly, endocrinopathy, m-protein increases, and skin changes may affect the kidneys. Ul-

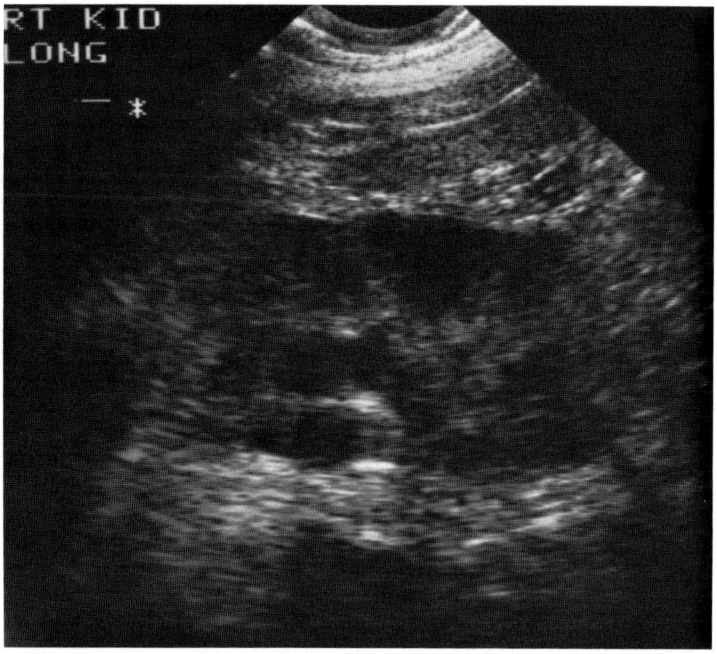

Figure 4.43. Renal lymphoma. Normal-sized kidney with irregular contour and multiple focal hypoechoic masses producing nonuniform appearance of parenchyma.

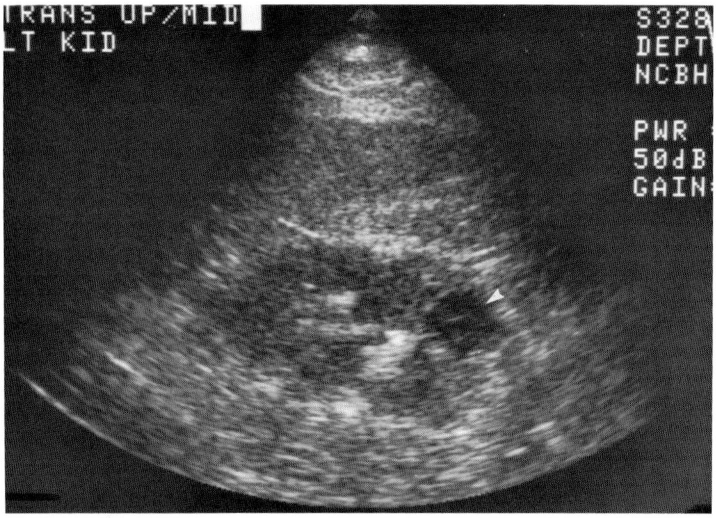

Figure 4.44. Renal lymphoma. Normal-sized kidney with single irregular hypoechoic mass (*arrowhead*).

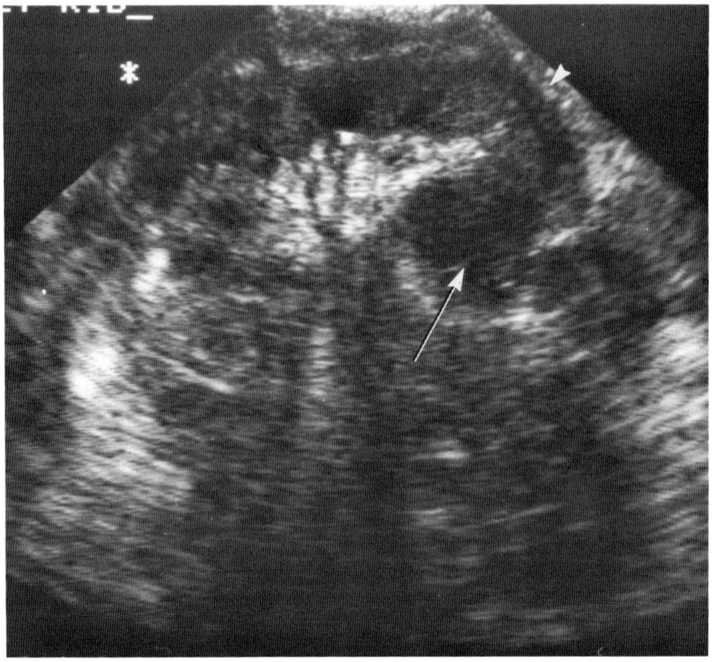

Figure 4.45. Perirenal lymphoma. Diffuse peripheral lymphoma appearing as a peripheral rim around the cortical margin (*arrowhead*). Intrarenal hypoechoic lymphomatous masses were also seen (*arrow*).

trasonographically there is renal enlargement, markedly increased cortical echogenicity, and decreased sinus echogenicity.

Nephrocalcinosis

Diffuse renal disease manifested by increased echogenicity primarily of the renal medulla is caused most commonly by nephrocalcinosis. Nephrocalcinosis occurs in many different clinical settings in which there is hypercalcemia. High calcium levels cause cellular damage followed by calcium deposition in tubular cells.

Usually, these renal calcium deposits are seen at the corticomedullary junction, but they may occur elsewhere. In medullary nephrocalcinosis, the normally sonolucent pyramids become densely echogenic, sometimes causing posterior acoustic shadowing (73) (Fig. 4.46). In the adult, hyperechoic pyramids are almost pathognomonic of medullary nephrocalcinosis from hypercalcemia (73, 132). In infancy, however, other conditions—including Tamm-Horsfall protein deposition (78), medullary sponge kidney (56), nephrophthisis (73), Cushing's syndrome (133), use of furosemide (134),

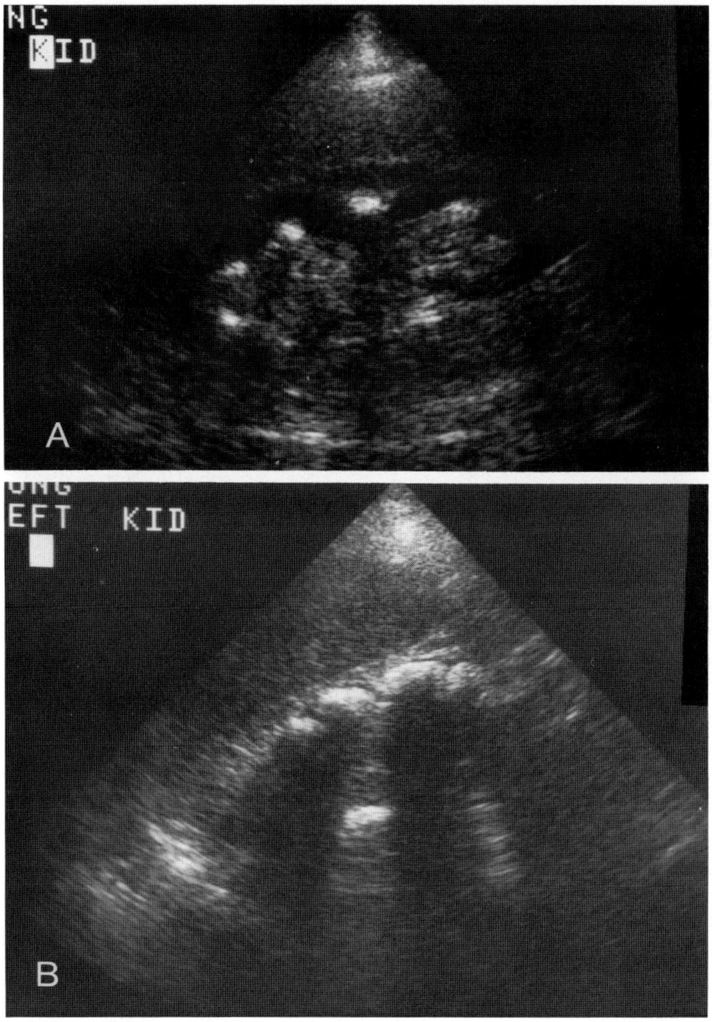

Figure 4.46. **A,** Medullary sponge kidney and nephrocalcinosis. Serum creatinine 1.0. Note hyperechoic renal pyramids with distal shadowing behind one. **B,** Medullary nephrocalcinosis secondary to Type I renal tubular acidosis. Note densely echogenic renal pyramids with posterior acoustic shadowing.

and Williams' syndrome (56)—may give a similar ultrasonographic picture.

Adult Polycystic Kidney Disease

Finally, two diffuse renal diseases causing predominantly cystic changes should be considered. Adult polycystic kidney disease (PCKD) is an autosomal dominant disorder with high penetrance but variable expressivity (135, 136). Although typically presenting in middle age, this disorder has been identified in some infants and children (73, 137).

In adult PCKD the kidneys are enlarged and contain a variety of cortical and medullary cysts, lined by epithelium, which have been regarded as distended nephrons (138). These occur most often in Bowman's capsule, the loop of Henle, and the proximal convoluted tubule (139). Some residual foci of normal renal parenchyma usually persist (135). These changes are classically bilateral but asymmetric (140). Other more limited forms of presentation, however, have been described, including unilateral PCKD (138) and segmental PCKD (141).

The majority of patients are adults when symptoms first arise, usually by the fourth or fifth decade. Symptoms include flank pain or mass, hypertension, hematuria, and chronic renal failure (136, 142). The rate of progression is variable and empirically, the larger the cysts, the more likely the patient will develop symptoms (136). Associated abnormalities are cysts in other organs, including the liver, spleen, pancreas, lung, ovaries, uterus, thyroid, seminal vesicles, and epididymis (136, 137, 139, 143). Though the liver is the most common nonrenal organ involved and may be enlarged, liver function tests remain normal (143, 144) unless portal venous hypertension ensues (145). Approximately 20% of patients have associated intracranial aneurysms, particularly of the basilar artery (135). Nephrolithiasis is also frequently associated with PCKD (146).

Sonographically the involved kidneys are enlarged and lobular, with multiple cysts of varying sizes (144, 147) (Fig. 4.47). The cysts may distort the central caliceal echoes (144) and expand the architecture of the kidney to the extent that its shape may be unrecognizable. Occasionally, calcium may be detected in the cyst walls (143). Small cysts may not be distinguished sonographically, making the diagnosis difficult. In these cases sonographically there are focally strong echoes within the cortex representing reflections from the cyst wall (144). Common cyst complications include hemorrhage and infection, both of which change cyst appearance from simple to complex with internal echoes (Fig. 4.48), which may cause difficulty in differentiating individual cysts. PCKD is easily identified with ultrasound, which unlike excretory urography is not dependent on

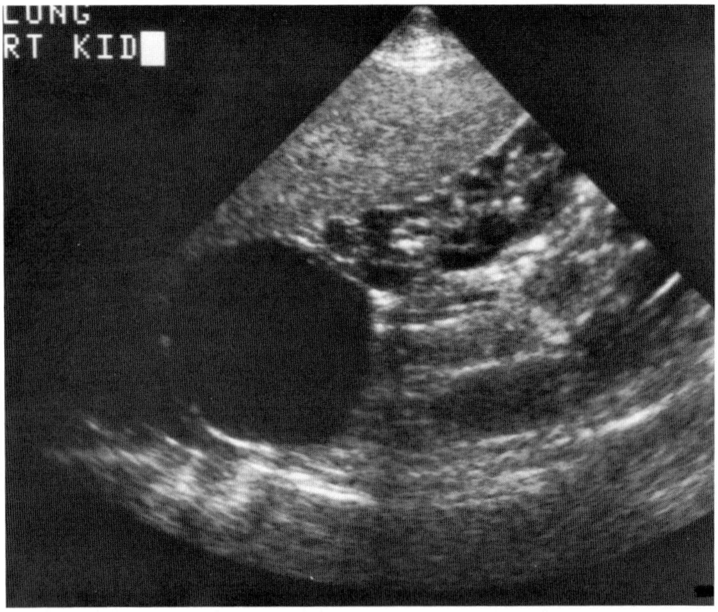

Figure 4.47. Polycystic kidney disease. Enormous kidney with multiple variably sized cysts which distort the renal parenchymal and sinus architecture.

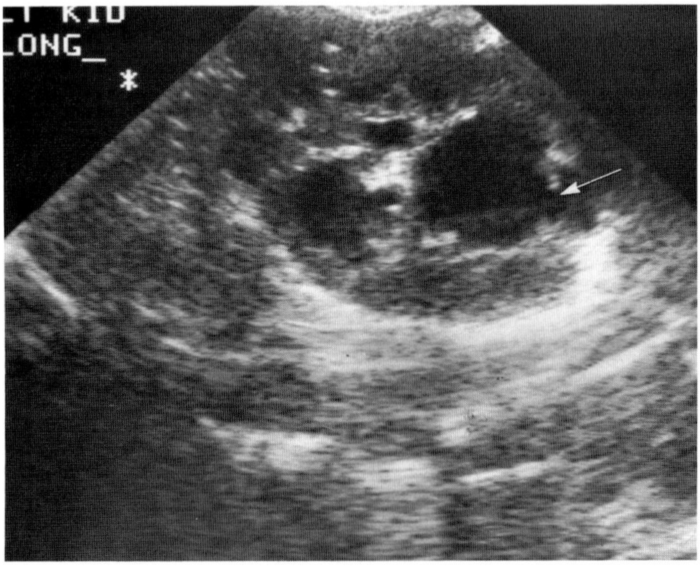

Figure 4.48. Complicated cyst in polycystic kidney disease. Fluid-debris level (*arrow*) in one of many cysts in affected kidney. The fluid-debris level moved with changes in patient position, and the debris always remained on the dependent aspect of the cyst.

renal function. Reports indicate that ultrasound is an effective screening study, and sonography has been determined to be the best available modality for presymptomatic evaluation of relatives of patients with PCKD (136, 148). Lawson et al. have suggested that ultrasound should be the procedure of choice for diagnosis, screening, and followup of PCKD (144).

Acquired Renal Cystic Disease

Acquired renal cystic disease (ARCD), the development of renal cysts and solid tumors in the native kidneys of patients undergoing long-term hemodialysis or peritoneal dialysis, was first described by Dunnill et al. in 1977 (149). ARCD is considered to be present when 40% or more of renal parenchyma is replaced by multiple cysts in chronically diseased kidneys (150–152). The formation of cysts is related to duration of disease (153, 154) and/or dialysis (155) and begins to accelerate after approximately 3 yr from the onset of the disease (156).

Although the pathogenesis of ARCD is uncertain, several theories have been advanced. It may represent an exaggeration of the normal process of retention cyst formation in the tubules of the kidney (157), or cysts in tubules may form because of interstitial fibrosis or obstruction by oxalate crystals (158). Other theories include vascular insufficiency (159) or cystogenic nephrotoxin caused by uremia, since ARCD may regress after transplantation, and since experimentally, agents such as diphenylalamine and dephenylthiazole have been shown to cause renal changes similar to ARCD (160–162). Controversy exists as to whether ARCD may be due to the longer survival of patients with end-stage renal disease who are undergoing dialysis, or to dialysis itself (163). The severity of ARCD has clearly been correlated with duration of time on hemodialysis, and patients dialyzed more than 3 yr have an 80% risk of contracting ARCD (159).

Pathologically the appearance of the kidney is variable. Kidneys may be small and contracted with multiple small cysts, or huge with multiple larger cysts (164). Cysts are filled with clear or bloody fluid. Histologically, the cyst lining is flattened cuboidal epithelium. With time, progressive hyperplasia of the cyst wall occurs, leading to dysplasia and formation of papillary tufts (153).

Complications include hemorrhage, stone formation, and, most worrisome, tumor formation. Reported solid tumors include papillary adenomas, tubular adenomas, and renal cell carcinoma (155, 165). The incidence of malig-

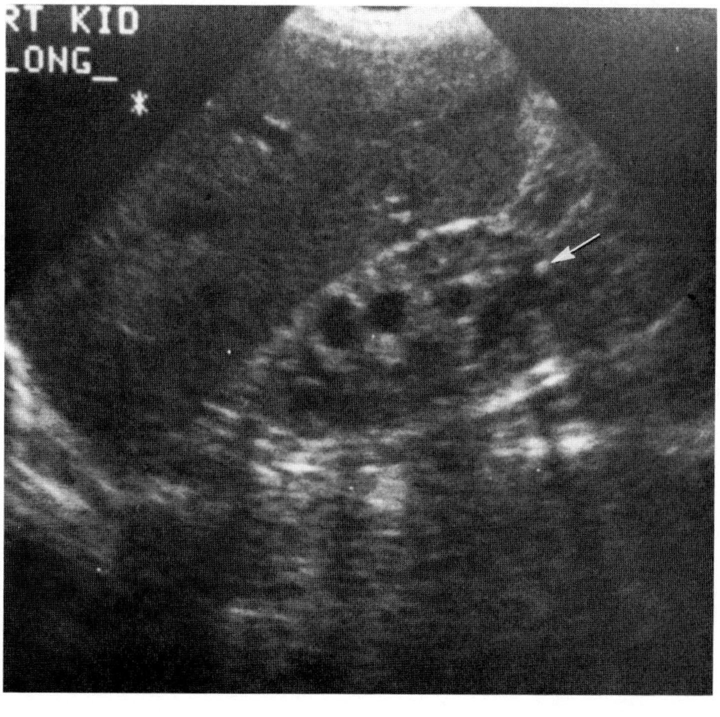

Figure 4.49. Acquired renal cystic disease. Small, smooth, hyperechoic kidney typical of chronic medical renal disease, with multiple cysts and a calculus (*arrow*).

nancy in ARCD is approximately 2500 times that of the normal population (153), and solid neoplasms are seen in 10 to 40% of patients with ARCD. Because the cytological appearance of the adenocarcinoma can be uniform, with little to suggest malignancy, all solid masses should be regarded as potentially malignant. Tumor pathogenesis is probably related to chronic uremia and immunosuppression (166) and to the dysplasia of the cyst wall seen histologically. The solid neoplasms usually develop after cyst formation but have been seen in patients who do not yet have ARCD (167).

Apart from experiencing the clinical features pertaining to chronic renal failure, patients with ARCD are usually asymptomatic. Acute pain and gross or microscopic hematuria may accompany either cyst hemorrhage or calculi formation. These episodes should be aggressively investigated to rule out accompanying malignancy.

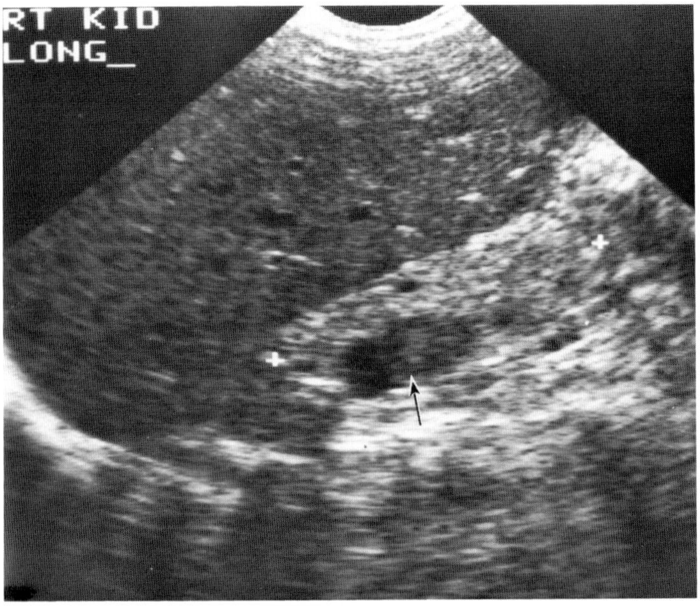

Figure 4.50. Malignant neoplasm in acquired renal cystic disease. Solid mass (*arrow*) in hyperechoic kidney adjacent to a cyst.

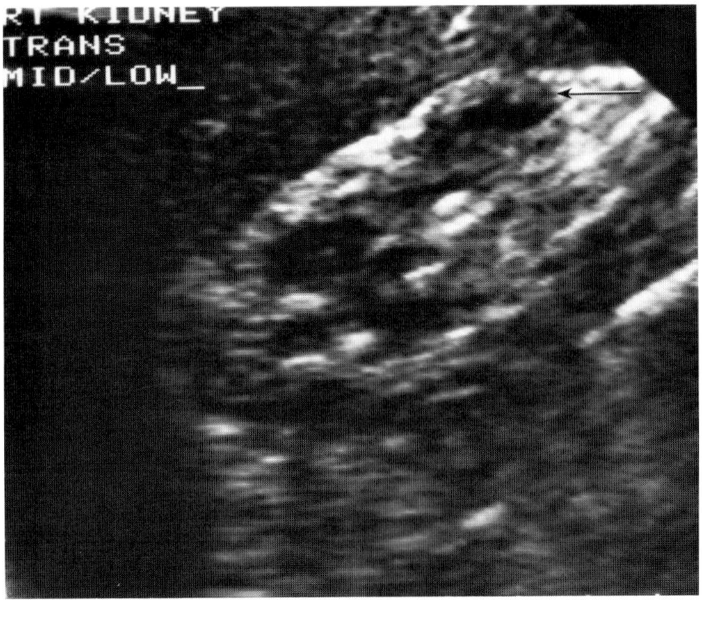

Figure 4.51. Complicated cyst in acquired renal cystic disease. Thick-walled cystic mass in anterior aspect of middle to lower pole (*arrow*) of hyperechoic kidney. This could exactly mimic a cystic malignancy, but had completely disappeared on a 4-month follow-up examination.

The sonographic findings center on the appearance of the cyst formation in chronically diseased kidneys. Initially, the cysts are not visualized and kidneys involved with ARCD are small (156) with a slight increase in echogenicity and no distinct corticomedullary junction (164) as seen in any chronically diseased kidney without ARCD. When cysts become visible they are diffusely distributed within the renal cortex (Fig. 4.49) and medulla and range in size from less than 1 cm to more than 2 cm (164, 168), creating a lobular contour. The cysts usually appear simple, unless marked by previous hemorrhage or infection, either of which creates complex features such as irregular and poorly marginated walls and internal echoes.

With time, the kidneys may enlarge and become more echogenic. As cysts increase in number, renal enlargement occurs despite progressive renal parenchymal atrophy (155, 156). Some authors advise yearly screening examinations in patients on dialysis to monitor for development of ARCD and to look for solid neoplasms (141) (Fig. 4.50). Nevertheless, the identification and characterization of solid masses and their distinction from cysts (Fig. 4.51) may be difficult (169).

Acknowledgments

We thank Raymond B. Dyer, M.D. for this careful review and suggestions regarding this manuscript, and Donna S. Garrison, Ph.D, for editorial assistance.

References

1. Wolfman NT, Karstaedt N. Ultrasound anatomy of the kidney. In: Resnick MI, Parker MD, eds. Surgical anatomy of the kidney. Mount Kisco, NY: Futura, 1982:109–141.
2. Hricak H. Renal ultrasound. In: Sarti DA. Diagnostic ultrasound text and cases. Chicago: Year Book, 1987:350–435.
3. Cubberley DA, Gosink BB, Forsythe J. Coronal sonography: a review of abdominal applications. J Ultrasound Med 1985;4:35–46.
4. Fleischer AC. Renal and urological sonography. In: Fleischer AC, James AE. Diagnostic sonography: principles and clinical applications. Philadelphia: WB Saunders, 1989:433–460.
5. Mittelstaedt CA. The urinary tract. In: abdominal ultrasound. New York: Churchill Livingstone, 1987:221–230.
6. Hicken P, Sauerbrei EE, Cooperberg PL. Ultrasonic coronal scanning of left upper quadrant. J Can Assoc Radiol 1981;32:107–110.
7. Finberg H. Renal ultrasound: anatomy and technique. Semin Ultrasound 1981;2:7–19.
8. Rosenberg ER, Clair MR, Bowie JD. The fluid-filled stomach as an acoustic window to the left kidney. AJR 1982;138:175–176.
9. Thompson IM, Kovac A, Geshner J. Coronal renal ultrasound: II. Urology 1981;17:210–213.
10. Marchal G, Verbeken E, Oyen R, Moerman F, Baert AL, Lauweryns J. Ultrasound of the normal kidney: a sonographic, anatomic and histologic correlation. Ultrasound Med Biol 1986; 12:999–1009.
11. Cook JH III, Rosenfield AT, Taylor KJW. Ultrasonic demonstration of intrarenal anatomy. AJR 1977;129:831–835.
12. Rosenfield AT, Taylor KJW, Crade M, DeGraaf CS. Anatomy and pathology of the kidney by gray scale ultrasound. Radiology 1978;128: 737–744.
13. Rosenfield AT, Siegel NJ. Renal parenchymal disease: histopathologic-sonographic correlation. AJR 1981;137:793–798.
14. Hricak H, Cruz C, Eyler WR, Madrazo BL, Romanski R, Sandler MA. Acute post-transplantation renal failure: differential diagnosis by ultrasound. Radiology 1981;139:441–449.
15. Hodson CJ. The renal parenchyma and its blood supply. Curr Probl Diagn Radiol 1978;7:1–32.
16. Jones BE, Hoffer FA, Teele RL, Lebowitz RL. The compound renal pyramid: a normal hypoechoic region on the pediatric sonogram. J Ultrasound Med 1987;6:515–518.
17. Brandt TD, Neiman HL, Dragowski MJ, Bulawa W, Claykamp G. Ultrasound assessment of normal renal dimensions. J Ultrasound Med 1982;1:49–52.
18. Jones TB, Riddick LR, Harpen MD, Dubuisson RL, Samuels D. Ultrasonographic determination of renal mass and renal volume. J Ultrasound Med 1983;2:151–154.
19. Han BK, Babcock DS. Sonographic measurements and appearance of normal kidneys in children. AJR 1985;145:611–616.
20. Moskowitz PS, Carroll BA, McCoy JM. Ultrasonic renal volumetry in children: accuracy and simplicity of the method. Radiology 1980; 134:61–64.
21. Hricak H, Lieto RP. Sonographic determination of renal volume. Radiology 1983;148:311–312.
22. Isikoff MB, Hill MC. Sonography of the renal arteries: left lateral decubitus position. AJR 1980;134:1177–1179.
23. Davidson AJ. Radiologic anatomy of the kidney. In: Radiology of the kidney. Philadelphia: WB Saunders, 1985:71–110.
24. Buschi AJ, Harrison RB, Brenbridge ANAG, Williamson BRJ, Gentry RR, Cole R. Distended left renal vein: CT/sonographic normal variant. AJR 1980;135:339–342.
25. Kurtz AB, Dubbins PA, Zegel HG, Cole-Beuglet C, Goldberg BB. Normal left renal vein mimicking left renal artery aneurysm. J Clin Ultrasound 1981;9:105–108.
26. Kinard RE, Orrison WW. Ultrasound demonstration of the retroaortic left renal vein. J Clin Ultrasound 1986;14:151–152.
27. Leekam RN, Gray RR, Matzinger MA, Grosman H. Ultrasound demonstration of a circumaortic left renal vein. J Clin Ultrasound 1985;13:366–368.
28. Wolverson MK, Nouri S, Joist JH, Sundaram M, Heiberg E. The direct visualization of blood

flow by real-time ultrasound: clinical observations and underlying mechanisms. Radiology 1981;140:443–448.
29. Taylor KJW, Burns PN, Woodcock JP, Wells PNT. Blood flow in deep abdominal and pelvic vessels: ultrasonic pulsed-Doppler analysis. Radiology 1985;154:487–493.
30. Rifkin MD, Pasto ME, Goldberg BB. Duplex Doppler examination in renal disease: evaluation of vascular involvement. Ultrasound Med Biol 1985;11:341–346.
31. Taylor DC, Kettler MD, Moneta GL, et al. Duplex ultrasound scanning in the diagnosis of renal artery stenosis: a prospective evaluation. J Vasc Surg 1988;7:363–369.
32. Rigsby CM, Burns PN, Taylor KJW. Renal duplex sonography. In: Taylor KJW, Burns PN, Wells PNT, eds. Clinical applications of Doppler ultrasound. New York: Raven Press, 1988: 201–245.
33. Hricak H, Taylor KJW, Marich K, Lue TF, Burns P. Doppler in urology. In: Hricak H, ed. Genitourinary ultrasound. New York: Churchill Livingstone, 1986:241–270.
34. Love L, Meyers MA, Churchill RJ, Reynes CJ, Moncada R, Gibson D. Computed tomography of extraperitoneal spaces. AJR 1981;136:781–789.
35. Meyers MA. Dynamic radiology of the abdomen. Normal and pathologic anatomy. 2nd ed. New York: Springer-Verlag, 1982:105–185.
36. Sample WF. Adrenal ultrasonography. Radiology 1978;127:461–466.
37. Günther RW, Kelbel C, Lenner V. Real-time ultrasound of normal adrenal glands and small tumors. J Clin Ultrasound 1984;12:211–217.
38. Marchal G, Gelin J, Verbeken E, Baert A, Lauwerijns J. High-resolution real-time sonography of the adrenal glands: a routine examination? J Ultrasound Med 1986;5:65–68.
39. Lafortune M, Constantin A, Breton G, Vallee C. Sonography of the hypertrophied column of Bertin. AJR 1986;146:53–56.
40. Mahony BS, Jeffrey RB, Laing FC. Septa of Bertin: a sonographic pseudotumor. J Clin Ultrasound 1983;11:317–319.
41. Leekam RN, Matzinger MA, Brunelle M, Gray RR, Grosman H. The sonography of renal columnar hypertrophy. J Clin Ultrasound 1983; 11:491–494.
42. Schaffer RM, Shih YH, Becker JA. Sonographic identification of collecting system duplications. J Clin Ultrasound 1983;11:309–312.
43. Fine H, Keen EN. The arteries of the human kidney. J Anat 1966;100:881–894.
44. Hoffer FA, Hanabergh AM, Teele RL. The interrenicular junction: a mimic of renal scarring on normal pediatric sonograms. AJR 1985;145: 1075–1078.
45. Carter AR, Horgan JG, Jennings TA, Rosenfield AT. The junctional parenchymal defect: a sonographic variant of renal anatomy. Radiology 1985;154:499–502.
46. Obley DL, Slasky BS, Bron KM. Right-sided splenorenal fusion with arteriographic, ultrasonic, and computerized tomographic correlation. Urol Radiol 1982;4:221–225.
47. Aragona F, Serretta V, Fiorentini L, Marconi A, Spinelli C. Combined renal and pyelic fusion with crossed ectopia of single ureter. Urology 1986;28:339–341.
48. McCarthy S, Rosenfield AT. Ultrasonography in crossed renal ectopia. J Ultrasound Med 1984;3:107–112.
49. Mindell HJ, Kupic EA. Horseshoe kidney: ultrasonic demonstration. AJR 1977;129:526–527.
50. Mendelson DS, Mitty HA, Janus C, Cohen BA. Horseshoe kidney mimicking adenopathy. Urol Radiol 1983;5:121–122.
51. Morcos SK. Intrathoracic kidney with a simple cyst in its upper pole diagnosed by ultrasound. J Clin Ultrasound 1985;13:127–129.
52. Ward JN, Nathanson B, Draper JW. The pelvic kidney. J Urol 1965;94:36–39.
53. Dretler SP, Olsson C, Pfister RC. The anatomic, radiologic and clinical characteristics of the pelvic kidney: an analysis of 86 cases. J Urol 1961;105:623–627.
54. Davidson AJ. A systematic approach to the radiologic diagnosis of parenchymal disease of the kidney. In: Radiology of the kidney. Philadelphia: WB Saunders, 1985:113–123.
55. Platt JF, Rubin JM, Bowerman RA, Marn CS. The inability to detect kidney disease on the basis of echogenicity. AJR 1988;151:317–319.
56. Rosenfield AT, Taylor KJW, Jaffe CC. Clinical applications of ultrasound tissue characterization. Radiol Clin North Am 1980;18:31–58.
57. Fontaine S, Lafortune M, Breton G, Vallée C. Ascites as a cause of hyperechogenic kidneys. J Clin Ultrasound 1985;13:633–636.
58. Hayden CK, Santa-Cruz FR, Amparo EG, Brouhard B, Swischuck LE, Ahrendt DK. Ultrasonographic evaluation of the renal parenchyma in infancy and childhood. Radiology 1984;152:413–417.
59. Haller JO, Berdon WE, Friedman AP. Increased renal cortical echogenicity: a normal finding in neonates and infants. Radiology 1982;142: 173–174.
60. Vade A, Lau P, Smick J, Harris V, Ryva J. Sonographic renal parameters as related to age. Pediatr Radiol 1987;17:212–215.
61. Hricak H, Cruz C, Romanski R, et al. Renal parenchymal disease: sonographic-histologic correlation. Radiology 1982;144:141–147.
62. Brenbridge AN, Chevalier RL, Kaiser DL. Increased renal cortical echogenicity in pediatric renal disease: histopathologic correlations. J Clin Ultrasound 1986;14:595–600.
63. Rosenfield AT. Ultrasound evaluation of renal parenchymal disease and hydronephrosis. Urol Radiol 1982;4:125–133.
64. Krensky AM, Reddish JM, Teele RL. Causes of increased renal echogenicity in pediatric patients. Pediatrics 1983;72:840–846.
65. Päivänsalo M, Huttunen K, Suramo I. Ultrasonographic findings in renal parenchymal diseases. Scand J Urol Nephrol 1985;19:119–123.
66. Ellenbogen PH, Scheible FW, Talner LB, Leopold GR. Sensitivity of gray scale ultrasound in detecting urinary tract obstruction. AJR 1978;130:731–733.

67. Talner LB, Scheible W, Ellenbogen PH, Beck CH Jr, Gosink BB. How accurate is ultrasonography in detecting hydronephrosis in azotemic patients? Urol Radiol 1981;3:1–6.
68. Lee JKT, Baron RL, Melson GL, McClennan BL, Weyman PJ. Can real-time ultrasonography replace static B-scanning in the diagnosis of renal obstruction? Radiology 1981;139: 161–165.
69. McClennan BL. Current approaches to the azotemic patient. Radiol Clin North Am 1979;17:197–211.
70. Ritchie WW, Vick CW, Glocheski SK, Cook DE. Evaluation of azotemic patients: diagnostic yield of initial US examination. Radiology 1988;167:245–247.
71. Stuck KJ, White GM, Granke DS, Ellis JH, Weissfeld JL. Urinary obstruction in azotemic patients: detection by sonography. AJR 1987; 149:1191–1193.
72. Nomura G, Kinoshita E, Yamagata Y, Koga N. Usefulness of renal ultrasonography for assessment of severity and course of acute tubular necrosis. J Clin Ultrasound 1984;12:135–139.
73. Green D, Carroll BA. Ultrasound of renal failure. In: Hricak H, ed. Genitourinary ultrasound. New York: Churchill Livingstone, 1986:55–88.
74. Stanley JH, Cornella R, Loevinger E, Schabel SI, Curry NS. Sonography of systemic lupus nephritis. AJR 1984;142:1165–1168.
75. Longmaid HE III, Rider E, Tymkiw J. Lupus nephritis: new sonographic findings. J Ultrasound Med 1987;6:75–79.
76. Schaffer RM, Schwartz GE, Becker JA, Rao TKS, Shih YH. Renal ultrasound in acquired immune deficiency syndrome. Radiology 1984; 153:511–513.
77. Hamper UM, Goldblum LE, Hutchins GM, et al. Renal involvement in AIDS: sonographic-pathologic correlation. AJR 1988;150:1321–1325.
78. Rosenfield AT, Zeman RK, Cicchetti DV, Siegel NJ. Experimental acute tubular necrosis: US appearance. Radiology 1985;157:771–774.
79. Davidson AJ. Diagnostic set: large, smooth, bilateral. In: Radiology of the kidney. Philadelphia: WB Saunders, 1985:221–254.
80. Walker JT, Keller MS, Katz SM. Computed tomographic and sonographic findings in acute ethylene glycol poisoning. J Ultrasound Med 1983;2:429–431.
81. Pardes JG, Auh YH, Kazam E. Sonographic findings in myoglobinuric renal failure and their clinical implications. J Ultrasound Med 1983;2:391–394.
82. Sefczek RJ, Beckman I, Lupetin AR, Dash N. Sonography of acute renal cortical necrosis. AJR 1984;142:553–554.
83. Wilson DA, Wenzl JE, Altshuler GP. Ultrasound demonstration of diffuse cortical nephrocalcinosis in a case of primary hyperoxaluria. AJR 1979;132:659–661.
84. Shuman WP, Mack LA, Rogers JV. Diffuse nephrocalcinosis: hyperechoic sonographic appearance. AJR 1981;136:830–832.
85. Piccirillo M, Rigsby CM, Rosenfield AT. Sonography of renal inflammatory disease. Urol Radiol 1987;9:66–78.
86. Morehouse HT, Weiner SN, Hoffman-Tretin JC. Inflammatory disease of the kidney. Semin Ultrasound CT MR 1986;7:246–258.
87. Zaontz MR, Pahira JJ, Wolfman M, Gargurevich AJ, Zeman RK. Acute focal bacterial nephritis: a systematic approach to diagnosis and treatment. J Urol 1985;133:752–757.
88. Kuligowska E, Newman B, White SJ, Caldarone A. Interventional ultrasound in detection and treatment of renal inflammatory disease. Radiology 1983;147:521–526.
89. Wicks JD, Thornbury JR. Acute renal infections in adults. Radiol Clin North Am 1979;17:245–260.
90. Rosenfield AT, Glickman MG, Taylor KJW, Crade M, Hodson J. Acute focal bacterial nephritis (acute lobar nephronia). Radiology 1979;132:553–561.
91. McCoy R, Kurtz AB, Rifkin MD, Kodroff MB, Bidula MM. Ultrasound detection of focal bacterial nephritis (lobar nephronia) and its evolution into renal abscess. Urol Radiol 1985;7: 109–111.
92. Funston MR, Fisher KS, van Blerk JP, Bortz JH. Acute focal bacterial nephritis or renal abscess? A sonographic diagnosis. Br J Urol 1982;54:461–466.
93. Kay CJ, Rosenfield AT, Taylor KJW, Rosenberg MA. Ultrasonic characteristics of chronic atrophic pyelonephritis. AJR 1979;132:47–49.
94. Lautin EM, Gordon PM, Friedman AC, Dourmashkin L, Fromowitz F. Emphysematous pyelonephritis: optimal diagnosis and treatment. Urol Radiol 1979;1:93–96.
95. de Wardener HE. The kidney: an outline of normal and abnormal function. 4th ed. Edinburgh: Churchill Livingstone, 1978.
96. Olazabal A, Velasco M, Martinez A, Villaricencio H, Codina M. Emphysematous pyelonephritis. Urology 1987;29:95–98.
97. Allen HA III, Walsh JW, Brewer WH, Vick CW, Haynes JW. Sonography of emphysematous pyelonephritis. J Ultrasound Med 1984;3:533–537.
98. Hartman DS, Davis CJ Jr, Goldman SM, Isbister SS, Sanders RC. Xanthogranulomatous pyelonephritis: sonographic-pathologic correlation of 16 cases. J Ultrasound Med 1984;3:481–488.
99. Goldman SM, Hartman DS, Fishman EK, Finizio JP, Gatewood OMB, Siegelman SS. CT of xanthogranulomatous pyelonephritis: radiologic-pathologic correlation. AJR 1984;142: 963–969.
100. Van Kirk OC, Go RT, Wedel VJ. Sonographic features of xanthogranulomatous pyelonephritis. AJR 1980;134:1035–1039.
101. Michigan S. Genitourinary fungal infections. J Urol 1976;116:390–397.
102. Stuck KJ, Silver TM, Jaffee MH, Bowerman RA. Sonographic demonstration of renal fungus balls. Radiology 1981;142:473–474.
103. Premkumar A, Lattimar J, Newhouse JH. CT and sonography of advanced urinary tract tuberculosis. AJR 1987;148:65–69.

104. Schaffer R, Becker JA, Goodman J. Sonography of tuberculous kidney. Urology 1983;22: 209–211.
105. Rosenfield AT, Taylor KJW, Dembner AG, Jacobson P. Ultrasound of renal sinus: new observations. AJR 1979;133:441–448.
106. Subramanyam BR. Renal amyloidosis in juvenile rheumatoid arthritis: sonographic features. AJR 1981;136:411–412.
107. Nies BA, Bodey GP, Thomas LB, Brecher G, Freireich EJ. The persistence of extramedullary leukemic infiltrates during bone marrow remission of acute leukemia. Blood 1965;26: 133–141.
108. Kirshbaum JD, Preuss FS. Leukemia: a clinical and pathologic study of one hundred and twenty-three fatal cases in a series of 14,400 necropsies. Arch Intern Med 1943;71:777–794.
109. Kumari-Subaiya S, Lee WJ, Festa R, Phillips G, Pochaczevsky R. Sonographic findings in leukemic renal disease. J Clin Ultrasound 1984; 12:465–472.
110. Gore RM, Shkolnik A. Abdominal manifestations of pediatric leukemias: sonographic assessment. Radiology 1982;143:207–210.
111. Viadana E, Bross IDJ, Pickren JW. An autopsy study of the metastatic patterns of human leukemias. Oncology 1978;35:87–96.
112. Goh TS, LeQuesne GW, Wong KW. Severe infiltration of the kidneys with ultrasonic abnormalities in acute lymphoblastic leukemia. Am J Dis Child 1978;132:1204–1205.
113. Richmond J, Sherman RS, Diamond HD, Craver LF. Renal lesions associated with malignant lymphomas. Am J Med 1962;32:184–207.
114. Lalli AF. Lymphoma and the urinary tract. Radiology 1969;93:1051–1054.
115. Hartman DS, Davis CJ Jr, Goldman SM, Friedman AC, Fritzche P. Renal lymphoma: radiologic-pathologic correlation of 21 cases. Radiology 1982;144:759–766.
116. Freeman C, Berg JW, Cutler SJ. Occurrence of prognosis of extranodal lymphomas. Cancer 1972;29:252–260.
117. Nyberg DA, Jeffrey RB Jr, Federle MP, Bottles K, Abrams DI. AIDS-related lymphomas: evaluation by abdominal CT. Radiology 1986; 159:59–63.
118. Hartman DS, Davidson AJ, Davis CJ Jr, Goldman SM. Infiltrative renal lesions: CT-sonographic-pathologic correlation. AJR 1988; 150:1061–1064.
119. Heiken JP, McClennan BL, Gold RP. Renal lymphoma. Semin Ultrasound CT MR 1986;7:58–66.
120. Petersen RO. Urologic pathology. Philadelphia: JB Lippincott, 1986:128–130.
121. Glicklich D, Sung MW, Frey M. Renal failure due to lymphomatous infiltration of the kidneys: report of three new cases and review of the literature. Cancer 1986;58:748–753.
122. Horii SC, Bosniak MA, Megibow AJ, Raghavendra BN, Subramanyam BR, Rothberg M. Correlation of CT and ultrasound in the evaluation of renal lymphoma. Urol Radiol 1983;5: 69–76.
123. Carroll BA, Ta HN. The ultrasonic appearance of extranodal abdominal lymphoma. Radiology 1980;136:419–425.
124. Kaude JV, Lacy GD. Ultrasonography in renal lymphoma. JCU 1978;6:321–323.
125. Heelan RT, Filippa DA. Lymphoma of kidney mimicking simple renal cyst on ultrasound. Clin Bull 1981;11:139–141.
126. Carroll BA. Ultrasound of lymphoma. Semin Ultrasound 1982;3:114–122.
127. Falappa P, Trodella L, Maresca G. Lymphomatous involvement of the kidneys: computed tomography and ultrasound demonstration. Diag Imaging 1980;49:266–268.
128. Heiken JP, Gold RP, Schnur MJ, King DL, Bashist B, Glazer HS. Computed tomography of renal lymphoma with ultrasound correlation. J Comput Assist Tomogr 1983;7:245–250.
129. Gregory A, Behan M. Lymphoma of the kidneys: unusual ultrasound appearance due to infiltration of the renal sinus. J Clin Ultrasound 1981;9:343–345.
130. Lindgren PG, Magnusson A, Hagberg H, Paulsen K. Perirenal lymphoma: report of a case. Acta Radiol Diagn 1986;27:433–435.
131. Arenson AM, Rubenstein JD, McKee JD. Renal ultrasound in POEMS syndrome. J Clin Ultrasound 1985;13:208–209.
132. Glazer GM, Callen PW, Filly RA. Medullary nephrocalcinosis: sonographic evaluation. AJR 1982;138:55–57.
133. Foley LC, Luisiri A, Graviss ER, Campbell JB. Nephrocalcinosis: sonographic detection in Cushing's syndrome. AJR 1982;139:610–612.
134. Cacciarelli AA, Young N, Levine AJ. Grayscale ultrasonic demonstration of nephrocalcinosis. Radiology 1978;128:459–460.
135. Grantham JJ. Polycystic renal disease. In: Earley LE, Gottschalk CW, eds. Strauss and Welt's diseases of the kidney. 3rd ed. Boston: Little, Brown, 1979:1123–1146.
136. Rosenfield AT, Lipson MH, Wolf B, Taylor KJW, Rosenfield NS, Hendler E. Ultrasonography and nephrotomography in the presymptomatic diagnosis of dominantly inherited (adult-onset) polycystic kidney disease. Radiology 1980;135: 423–427.
137. Bosniak MA, Ambos MA. Polycystic kidney disease. Semin Roentgenol 1975;10:133–143.
138. Hantman SS. Unilateral adult polycystic kidney. J Ultrasound Med 1982;1:371–374.
139. Davidson AJ. Diagnostic set: large, multifocal, bilateral. In: Radiology of the kidney. Philadelphia: WB Saunders, 1985:299–314.
140. Elkin M, Bernstein J. Cystic diseases of the kidney—radiological and pathological considerations. Clin Radiol 1969;20:65–82.
141. Kutcher R, Sprayregen S, Rosenblatt R, Goldman M. The sonographic appearance of segmental polycystic kidney. J Ultrasound Med 1983; 2:425–429.
142. Dalgaard OZ. Bilateral polycystic disease of the kidneys: a follow-up of two hundred and eighty-four patiets [sic] and their families. Acta Med Scand 1957;158 (suppl):328.
143. Kutcher R, Schneider M, Gordon DH. Calcification in polycystic disease. Radiology 1977;122: 77–80.

144. Lawson TL, McClennon BL, Shirkhoda A. Adult polycystic kidney disease: ultrasonographic and computed tomographic appearance. J Clin Ultrasound 1978;6:297–302.
145. DelGuercio E, Greco J, Kim KE, Chinitz J, Swartz C. Esophageal varices in adult patients with polycystic kidney and liver disease. N Engl J Med 1973;289:678–679.
146. Torres VE, Erickson SB, Smith LH, Wilson DM, Hattery RR, Segura JW. The association of nephrolithiasis and autosomal dominant polycystic kidney disease. Am J Kidney Dis 1988;11:318–325.
147. Kelsey JA, Bowie JD. Gray-scale ultrasonography in the diagnosis of polycystic kidney disease. Radiology 1977;122:791–795.
148. Sahney S, Sandler MA, Weiss L, Levin NW, Hricak H, Madrazo BL. Adult polycystic kidney disease: presymptomatic diagnosis for genetic counselling. Clin Nephrol 1983;20:89–93.
149. Dunnill MS, Millard PR, Oliver D. Acquired cystic disease of the kidneys: a hazard of long-term intermittent maintenance haemodialysis. J Clin Pathol 1977;30:868–877.
150. Feiner HD, Katz LA, Gallo GR. Acquired cystic disease of kidney in chronic dialysis patients. Urology 1981;17:260–264.
151. Smith JW, Sallman AL, Williamson MR, Lott CG. Acquired renal cystic disease: two cases of associated adenocarcinoma and a renal ultrasound survey of a peritoneal dialysis population. Am J Kidney Dis 1987;10:41–46.
152. Jabour BA, Ralls PW, Tang WW, Boswell WD Jr, Colletti PM, Feinstein EI, Massry SG. Acquired cystic disease of the kidneys: computed tomography and ultrasonography appraisal in patients on peritoneal and hemodialysis. Invest Radiol 1987;22:728–732.
153. Bretan PN Jr, Busch MP, Hricak H, Williams RD. Chronic renal failure: a significant risk factor in the development of acquired renal cysts and renal cell carcinoma. Case reports and review of the literature. Cancer 1986;57:1871–1879.
154. Bommer J, Waldherr R, van Kaick G, Ritz E. Acquired renal cysts in uremic patients—in vivo demonstration by computed tomography. Clin Nephrol 1980;14:299–303.
155. Thomson BJ, Jenkins DAS, Allan PL, Elton RA, Winney RJ. Acquired cystic disease of the kidney in patients with end-stage chronic renal failure: a study of prevalence and aetiology. Nephrol Dial Transplant 1986;1:38–43.
156. Takebayashi S. Sonographic evaluation of kidneys undergoing dialysis. Urol Radiol 1985;7:69–74.
157. Elliott HL, MacDougall AI, Buchanan WM. Acquired cystic disease of kidney [Letter]. Lancet 1977;2:1359.
158. Heptinstall RH. Chronic glomerulonephritis, end-stage kidney, and visceral changes in chronic renal failure. In: Pathology of the kidney. 3rd ed. Boston: Little, Brown, 1983;2:601–636.
159. Ishikawa I, Saito Y, Onouchi H, et al. Development of acquired cystic disease and adenocarcinoma of the kidney in glomerulonephritic chronic hemodialysis patients. Clin Nephrol 1980;14:1–6.
160. Carone FA, Rowland RG, Perlman SG, Ganote CE. The pathogenesis of drug-induced renal cystic disease. Kidney Int 1974;5:411–421.
161. Woodhouse MA, Offer J, Darmady EM. Diphenylamine induced polycystic kidneys compared with human polycystic kidneys: electron microscopical observations. Nephron 1965;2:253–254.
162. Darmady EM, Offer J, Woodhouse MA. Toxic metabolic defect in polycystic disease of kidney: evidence from microscope studies. Lancet 1970;1:547–550.
163. Budin RE, McDonnell PJ. Renal cell neoplasms: their relationship to arterionephrosclerosis. Arch Pathol Lab Med 1984;108:138–140.
164. Brendler CB, Albertsen PC, Goldman SM, Hill GS, Lowe FC, Millan JC. Acquired renal cystic disease in the end stage kidney: urological implications. J Urol 1984;132:548–552.
165. Scanlon MH, Karasick SR. Acquired renal cystic disease and neoplasia: complications of chronic hemodialysis. Radiology 1983;147:837–838.
166. Matas AJ, Simmons RL, Kjellstrand CM, Buselmeier TJ, Najarian JS. Increased incidence of malignancy during chronic renal failure. Lancet 1975;1:883.
167. Andersen BL, Curry NS, Gobien RP. Sonography of evolving renal cystic transformation associated with hemodialysis. AJR 1983;141:1003–1004.
168. McArdle CR, Grumbach K. Sonographic and computed tomographic appearances of acquired renal cystic disease. J Ultrasound Med 1983;2:519–520.
169. Coleman BG, Arger PH, Mulhern CB Jr, Pollack HM, Banner MP, Arenson RL. Gray-scale sonographic spectrum of hypernephromas. Radiology 1980;137:757–765.

CHAPTER 5

Ultrasonography of Renal Masses

JOSEPH R. DRAGO, M.D.
JEROME J. CUNNINGHAM, M.D.

Renal ultrasound is an important investigation of the kidney, especially in instances of suboptimal visualization or definition of the kidney with intravenous urography (IVU). Many lesions that cause urographic nonvisualization or poor visualization have typical diagnostic ultrasound appearances. In other instances, the combination of renal ultrasound and other noninvasive techniques may yield a specific diagnosis. Ultrasound is especially useful to establish the presence or absence of obstruction or to detect or characterize a renal mass.

Since the intravenous pyelogram is not a dynamic study but a static one, many limitations exist. Ultrasound, on the other hand, is a dynamic study with which the investigator can observe the kidney and juxtarenal structures throughout the examination. Other advantages of ultrasound are that it is safe, noninvasive, and inexpensive and can be done rapidly. This contrasts with IVU, which is time consuming, is associated with potentially serious (even fatal) reactions, and requires more direct surveillance by the radiologist to obtain a "tailored" radiological examination. On the other hand, since the ultrasonographer or physician is performing the sonogram, one can investigate many areas of concern at the initial examination as well as being able to obtain information regarding pararenal structures such as the liver, gallbladder, colon, spleen, ureters, and retroperitoneum. These are often not seen adequately on IVU. In many institutions ultrasound has largely replaced IVU, especially in the workup of patients with bladder outflow obstruction and also in any patient with elevation of BUN or creatinine. In the pediatric population, ultrasound has become the standard workup, in association with a voiding cystourethrogram, for children for urinary tract infections. The accuracy of ultrasound for detection of intrarenal or renal masses is approximately 95 to 96%. For equivalent-size masses, intravenous urography is often left behind with an accuracy of 70 to 75%, even when nephrotomography is carried out. Diagnosis of entities such as simple cortical cysts and columns of Bertin are rather routine with ultrasound but can be very difficult with IVU. Sonography can clearly demonstrate renal vein involvement with tumor and vena cava involvement with tumor, whereas IVU cannot. Ultrasound has become a standard "screening" test for patients with various urologic problems, including history of stones or prostate obstruction. Also, for drainage in certain cases it can be used as a therapeutic modality as an ultrasound guidance for percutaneous aspiration, percutaneous nephrostomy tube placement, or percutaneous biopsies without the need for contrast injection.

EXAMINATION TECHNIQUE

No patient preparation is needed or particularly helpful when sonographic examinations are done for evaluation of the kidneys for mass lesions. Prior to the study, the physician or technologist should review any urograms, CT scans, nuclear medicine examinations, or other pertinent radiological material that is available. The examiner should take advantage of the opportunity to read any medical records or laboratory reports that accompany the patient. If no clinical history has been provided, the patient should be interviewed and possibly examined for the presence of a palpable mass before the study begins. Most patients will have a pretty good idea as to the purpose of their visit to the ultrasound laboratory and they will often know a great deal of helpful information such as the location of a suspected lesion, or the fact that their urine contains blood, or that blood tests for renal function were abnormal.

As in any ultrasound study, the highest frequency transducer that will give diagnostic-quality images should be chosen. In adults, this will often prove to be a 3.5- to 5.0-MHz or equivalent crystal array. In a small person, a 5- to 6-MHz array might be practical; large persons may require a 2.25- to 3.5-MHz transducer. Real-time instrumentation will be employed most often. Linear array transducers are too bulky for successful renal scanning, so the study will almost always be done with a mechanical sector scanner, a computed sonography device, or a radial array unit.

The details of examination technique depend on the particular laboratory. We prefer to start with the patient completely supine and with both arms raised and folded above the head. Scanning of the right kidney through the right lower ribs using the liver as an acoustical "window" will be possible in the general area of the midaxillary line. Many longitudinal, transverse, and oblique sections should be performed and recorded. Next, we like to place the patient in left-side-down decubitus position and rescan the right renal area. This position often gives improved visualization, partly because the liver and kidney both tend to descend lower into the field of view, the hepatic flexure of the colon drops medially, and the rib interspaces tend to open up. The same examination sequence is repeated on the left side, although scanning usually has to be done more posteriorly and the decubitus position most often produces the better-quality images. Ideally, scans are done with suspended respiration or, even better, with the patient suspending respiration after deep inhalation.

On occasion, renal scanning for mass lesions may be optimized by putting the patient in unconventional positions. Upper-pole masses may sometimes be more visible with the patient sitting upright and the scan done from a posterior approach. Elevating the head of the bed may help with imaging of the right kidney. Rarely, one or the other kidney may be better seen with the patient prone.

It is always appropriate to examine both kidneys even if only one side was judged abnormal on a previous study. Imaging of the opposite kidney is obviously necessary when a lesion has been discovered that may require surgical intervention. The surgeon in this instance will be particularly anxious to know whether or not the kidney opposite the one he intends to remove or repair is healthy. Of course, if any tumor or potential tumor is discovered, a search for ascites, liver metastases, vascular involvement, adenopathy, or contralateral tumors is indicated.

RENAL CYSTS

Clinical Aspects of Renal Cystic Disease

Cysts are nonfunctioning parts of the kidney. Anatomic characteristics such as radiolucency and sharp margins are not necessarily identified on an excretory urogram. Renal sonography does not evaluate or require renal function, and therefore anatomic definition can be displayed even when renal failure exists or when urography is not possible. In this section, several specific cystic diseases are discussed and correlated with sonographic images. Characteristics of cysts have been outlined by many investigators; however, the work by Grossman et al. in 1983 (1) helped clarify the internal and external makeup of these cysts.

Clinical Correlations of Renal Cysts

Cystic disease of the kidney and simple renal cysts are common clinical conditions. While simple, uncomplicated cysts are relatively easy to diagnose and pose no health problem, complicated cystic lesions often create diagnostic dilemmas for the sonographer and the clinician. The many factors involved in clinical management of each have been the subject of many recent reviews (2–13).

The vast majority of patients with renal cysts are found when ultrasound imaging is performed to evaluate a patient with urinary tract or other abdominal or pelvic pathologic processes. If a renal mass is found, it is generally agreed that sonography should be the next study performed because of its noninvasive nature, information yield, and high degree of accuracy. However, if there are compelling clinical aspects that create the need for further assurance of the benignity of such a mass (e.g., unexplained hematuria or widespread metastatic disease), further confirmation is required. Further diagnostic pitfalls can be kept to a minimum with regard to the diagnosis of renal cysts if the following guidelines are observed:

1. All prior examinations (ultrasound, CT scans, or IVUs) should be available to the sonographer.
2. A clustering of several small cysts together may harbor a small incidental carcinoma that could be missed.
3. Vascular malformations or aneurysms can be mistaken for cystic disease.

4. Differential diagnosis of peripelvic cysts must be entertained.
5. Lesions that contain septations, or irregularities of the margin or calcium, should be considered suspicious and may be investigated further with CT scanning.

Ultrasonic Features of Renal Cysts

The great majority of persons seen in the ultrasound laboratory specifically for evaluation of renal cysts will fall into one of two major categories: the renal cyst was seen as an incidental finding during sonography for another reason such as suspected gallbladder disease, or a renal mass was seen or suspected on some radiological examination such as urography or CT scan and the referring physician wants characterization of the mass.

To meet strict criteria for diagnosis of a cyst, a renal mass lesion must satisfy the following tests: (*a*) geometric shape, either round or slightly oval; (*b*) internally echo free with no solid elements within the fluid-filled cavity; (*c*) a sharp and distinct interface between the cyst and adjacent renal tissue; (*d*) all borders distinctly defined, particularly posteriorly; and (*e*) little or no acoustical attenuation by the mass manifest by sound energy deposition distal to the lesion, a phenomenon commonly called "posterior enhancement," "good sound transmission," or "good through transmission." As deviations from these strict criteria increase, both qualitatively and quantitatively, the diagnosis of renal cyst becomes progressively more tenuous.

A very useful clinical classification for renal cysts has been proposed by Bosniak (2). Four categories are defined. Category I includes benign simple cysts that fulfill the strict criteria outlined above. Category II lesions are minimally complicated masses that show at least some deviation from the strict definition of a benign simple cyst. Category III lesions are complex masses that cannot be confidently diagnosed as benign or malignant based on radiological studies alone. Category IV masses are those that have malignant features.

Benign Cortical Cysts

The etiology of simple renal cysts remains uncertain. They generally are of no clinical significance and are very common in our population at large. Clinical significance depends on whether or not they cause distortion of the calices associated with local hydronephrosis, which could lead to obstruction, stasis, and increased instances of urinary tract infection. On the other hand, these simple cysts, if they are in a strategic position, may gain sufficient size, or by their location may be in a position to cause mechanically induced pain secondary to hydronephrosis. These cysts may lie anywhere along the cortex of the kidney, but if they are in the renal pelvis area they are called peripelvic cysts. Cysts generally contain yellow fluid and may become more common as patients age. Many varieties of cysts occur: simple cysts, multiloculaed cysts, hemorrhagic cysts, cysts with abscess in them, multiple simple cysts within the kidney, or the kidney may be replaced with cysts as in multicystic kidney disease. (2–16).

There are several conditions that on occasion may mimic the appearance of cysts and have similar characteristics on ultrasound (1, 2, 17, 18).

In occasional patients with large cysts, hydronephrosis may result or mechanical obstruction may occur, causing pain. These cysts may be merely aspirated and this may resolve the problem. On the other hand, if the cysts recur, surgical marsupialization of the cyst is necessary.

Most renal cysts arise from renal cortical tissue and thus these lie at the periphery of the kidney. Sizes are highly variable from a couple of millimeters to 20 or more centimeters. Figure 5.1 shows a typical category I cortical cyst. The lesion is round and echo free. All borders are sharp and clear and there is a distinct interface with normal renal parenchyma. Because the cyst is filled with clear fluid, acoustic energy passes unimpeded through the mass and this energy is deposited posteriorly as an explosion of reflections widely referred to as "posterior enhancement" or "good through transmission." In this situation, the diagnosis of benign cyst can be made with a confidence level approaching certainty. Figure 5.2 presents a similar case. The patient, an elderly man with renal artery stenosis, has marked atrophy of renal substance. An upper-pole mass with typical features of a category I cyst was an incidental finding in this instance. Again, the mass is slightly oval, the interface with normal kidney is sharp and abrupt, all borders are clearly defined, and posterior enhancement is conspicuous. Figure 5.3 also shows a typical benign cortical cyst. In this instance, the mass is completely surrounded by normal renal pa-

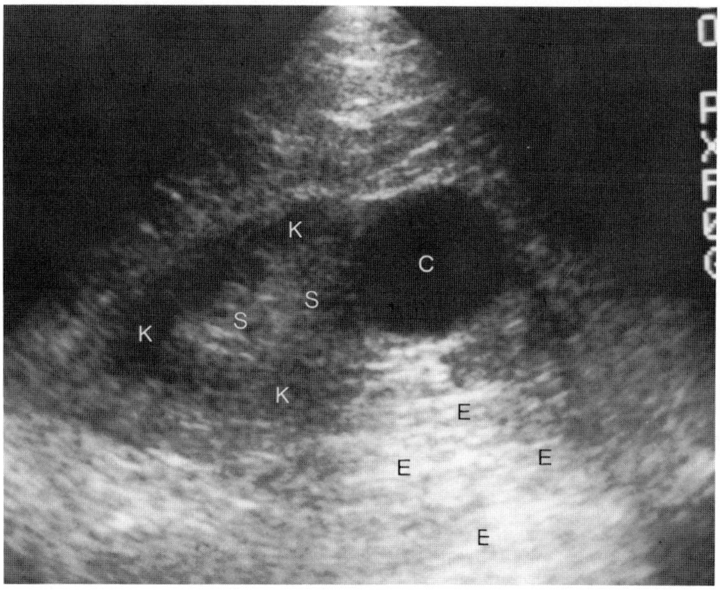

Figure 5.1. Benign cortical cyst. A rounded mass (*C*) is sharply delineated from adjacent normal kidney parenchyma (*K*) and renal sinus echoes (*S*). Acoustical enhancement (*E*) is conspicuous distal to the cyst.

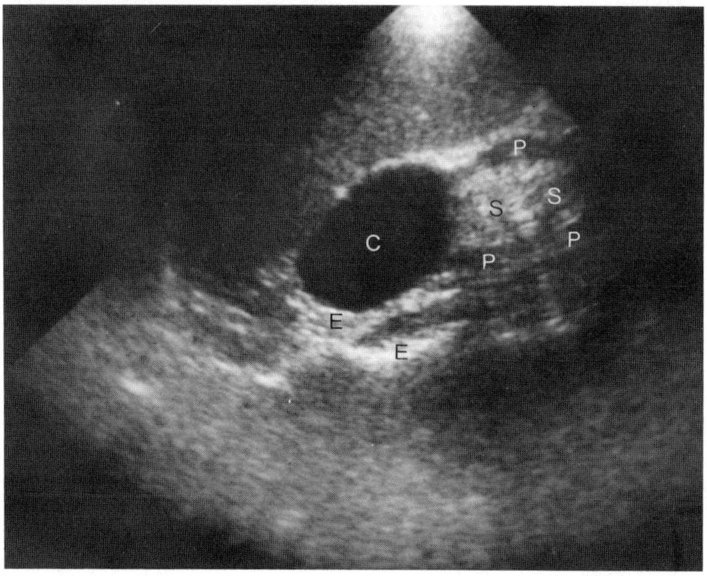

Figure 5.2. Benign cortical cyst in atrophic kidney. A typical cystic mass (*C*) arises from the upper pole of the left kidney. The parenchyma of the kidney (*P*) is globally thin and atrophic. The renal sinus echo complex (*S*) appears normal. There is acoustic enhancement (*E*) distal to the completely echo-free cyst.

renchyma and the renal border is not deformed. This is the usual sonographic finding when a patient is found to have a small low-attenuation renal lesion on a CT scan done for some unrelated reason. Often, it is not possible for the CT interpreter to distinguish between a solid mass and a small cyst, either because the patient cannot be given radiological contrast material or because CT volume averaging precludes accurate evaluation of these small structures.

Minimally Atypical Renal Cysts

A substantial percentage of renal cysts imaged in the ultrasound facility will have at least some minor deviation from the strict criteria necessary for the greatest degree of diagnostic confidence. In Bosniak's classification, these fall into category II (2). Examples of such cysts are those that contain septations, cysts that fulfill strict criteria except for a thin rim calcification, and cysts complicated by infection.

Category II cysts might also include lesions that appear hyperdense on CT scans, a finding attributed to hemorrhage (15).

Figure 5.4 shows a sharply demarcated sonolucent mass with very good posterior enhancement. Two minor atypical features are present. First, the cyst has a nongeometric, bilobed shape as a portion of the mass extends slightly beyond the renal outline and a larger portion extends into the parapelvic region. Next, the lesion is not completely free of internal echoes. There is a tiny, bright, linear "ping" just adjacent to the superior wall. These tiny wall reflections, which represent minor infoldings of the cyst wall or incomplete septations or synechiae, are seen commonly. Any time a wall irregularity is visible, the question of tumor within a cyst arises. But, put in perspective, minor wall irregularities are common, while tumor nodules within a benign cyst are increasingly rare. The image shown in Figure 5.5 also demonstrates a small wall irregularity. In addition, a multiband confluence of reverberation artifact can also be seen in the portion of the

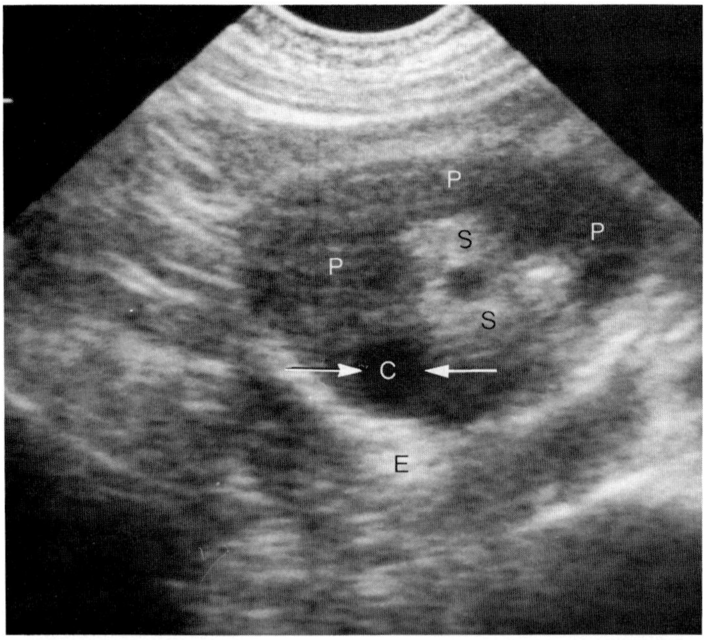

Figure 5.3. Small cortical cyst. A small sonolucent cystic mass (*C*) is completely surrounded by normal renal parenchyma (*P*). The central renal sinus echo complex (*S*) is normal. A small burst of acoustic enhancement (*E*) can be seen posterior to the cyst.

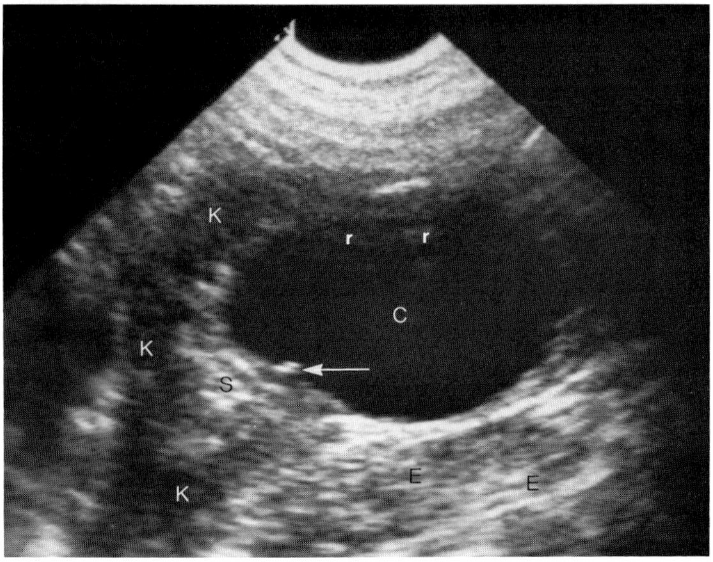

Figure 5.4. Large benign renal cyst. A large cystic mass (*C*) arises from the midportion of the adjacent kidney (*K*) and displaces the renal sinus echo complex (*S*) slightly. Reverberation echoes (*r*) are visible in the portion of the cyst nearest the transducer. A small infolding of tissue (*arrow*) produces a bright linear "ping" in the wall of the cyst.

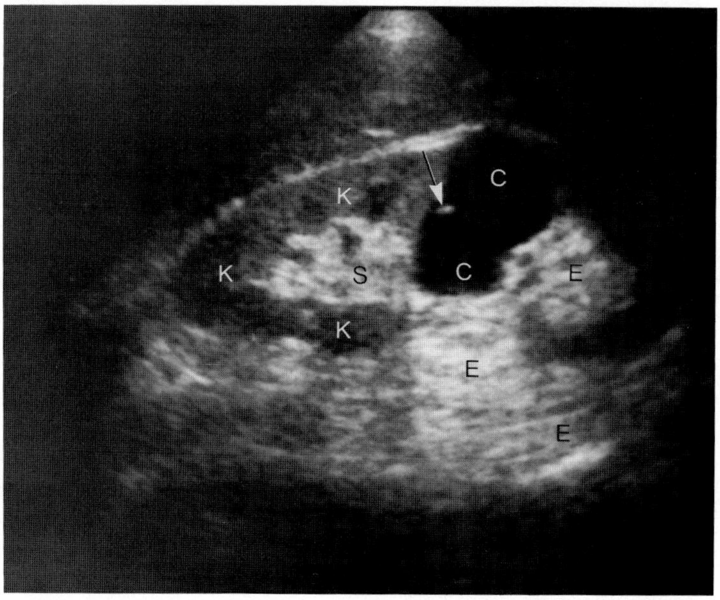

Figure 5.5. Benign cyst with atypical features. A lobulated cystic mass (*C*) arises from the lower pole of an otherwise normal kidney (*K*) and renal sinus echo complex (*S*). The cyst contains a bright echo (*arrow*) coming from a fragment of incomplete septation.

cyst that is nearest the transducer. Reverberations are exceedingly common in large fluid-filled structures, and experienced sonographers and physicians quickly learn to ignore them. Figure 5.6 is also an example of a category II, minimally atypical renal cortical cyst. This sharply defined, sonolucent mass has a lobulated shape. Posterior acoustic enhancement is excellent. There are two small wall irregularities and an incomplete septation. In spite of the deviations from strict criteria, the diagnosis of benign cyst can be made with confidence, and further evaluation with cyst puncture or CT needs to be done only if there is unexplained hematuria or clinical evidence that raises the possibility of a urinary malignancy.

The presence of thin septations inside a renal cyst is most often not a finding of clinical importance (14). There is general acceptance of the notion that one or two or three very thin, linear, complete or incomplete septations can be present inside an ordinary cyst and these should not create a diagnostic dilemma. Unfortunately, there is no general agreement on how many septations can be present before there are "too many," nor is there a consensus on how thick septations might be before they are "too thick."

Hemorrhagic and Infected Cysts

Benign cysts of the kidney may be altered by bleeding or infection to the point that they have to be classified in category III (that is, lesions that cannot be confidently diagnosed as benign or malignant with radiological study alone).

Patients with hemorrhagic cysts represent a serious problem for the clinician as well as the sonographer because it may be that these are indistinguishable from a clinical neoplasm that is cystic or a cyst that contains a neoplasm. Generally speaking, the clinical situation is one in which the patient presents with a mass or may present with a finding discovered by an abdominal imaging study such as a CT scan or ultrasound done for some unrelated reason. These lesions may also be associated with infection and may simulate a renal abscess. These lesions also, if they attain large size, may cause mechanical obstruction or urinary stasis and lead to infection or stones. In cases in which the cyst has become tremendously enlarged and hemorrhagic the patient may present with signs of shock clinically manifested by a drop in blood pressure and a rising pulse. This is a rare phenomenon, but it does occur (3, 19, 20).

The sonographic findings in hemorrhagic cysts cover a broad spectrum. Very frequently, no atypical findings are discovered at all. The lesion looks like a perfectly ordinary, simple, benign cyst. The presence of liquid blood or a combination of liquid blood and blood clots may form a fluid level or cause the entire cyst to become evenly echogenic and reduce the ability of the entire cyst to transmit the sound beam without significant attenuation. Blood clots may appear as solid masses with the cyst. An

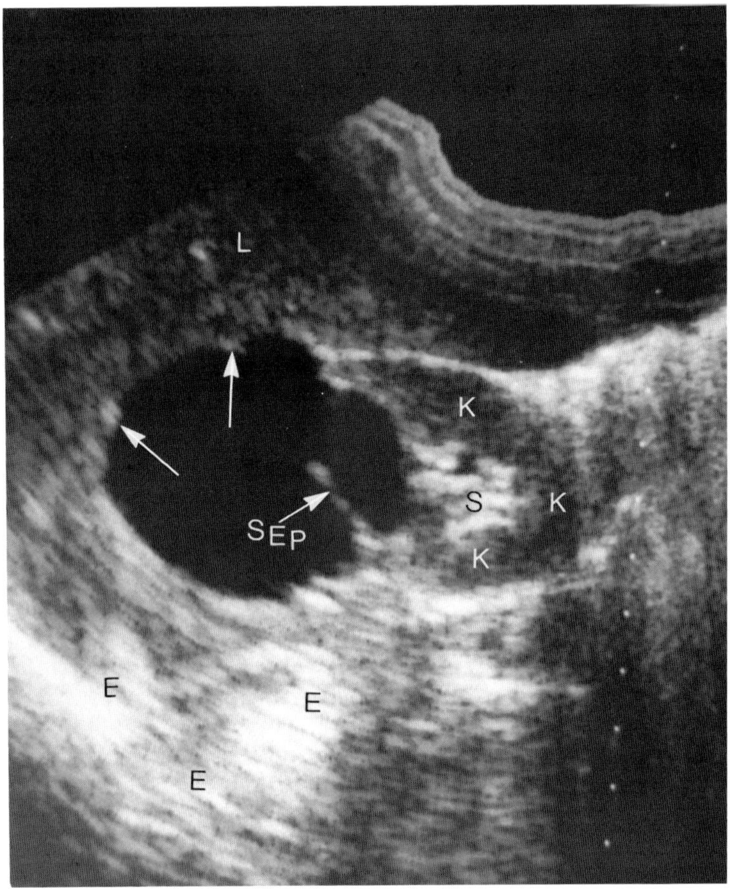

Figure 5.6. Septated cyst. A large, lobulated cystic mass containing an incomplete septum (*SEP*) arises from the upper pole of an otherwise normal kidney and central renal sinus echo complex (*S*). Two bright echoes (*arrows*) arise from small infoldings in the cyst wall. Acoustic enhancement (*E*) is conspicuous behind the cyst. *L,* liver.

example of this last presentation can be seen in Figure 5.7. This renal image was made when an elderly man experienced sudden flank pain and some minimal hematuria. Sonography shows a well-marginated renal mass with good posterior enhancement. A large, solid mass was visible within the cyst and this mass changed position as the patient assumed a variety of postures. Hemorrhage within a renal cyst was suspected. Because of medical problems unrelated to the urinary tract, CT and angiography done to evaluate the possibility of an occult malignancy causing hemorrhage were delayed for several weeks. Both of these studies were normal. The cyst fluid did not appear hyperdense on CT examination.

Just like hemorrhage, infection of a renal cyst produces a wide spectrum of sonographic findings. Even if the patient is very ill, no abnormality may be found aside from the usual findings for renal cyst. If thick pus has formed, a fluid level may be present. "Lumps" of infectious material will present as solid elements within the cyst. These lumps can obviously have an infinite variety of sizes and shapes. Images of an infected cyst are shown in Figure 5.8. The patient was a young man with a genetic neurovascular disease predisposing him to renal malignancy. A small renal mass was discovered by CT when evaluation for intraabdominal vascular malformation was done. The mass presented as a small, rounded lesion minimally deforming the renal outline. Acoustical transmission through the lesion was equal to solid renal tissue; there was no posterior enhancement. The lesion contained amorphous low-level echoes and several punctate calcifications. At surgery, excisional biopsy was done. The mass proved to be a simple cyst containing necrotic debris and bits of calcified material. The histologic diagnosis was a chronically infected medullary cyst.

Parapelvic Cysts

Renal parapelvic cysts originate in the renal hilum but do not communicate with the collect-

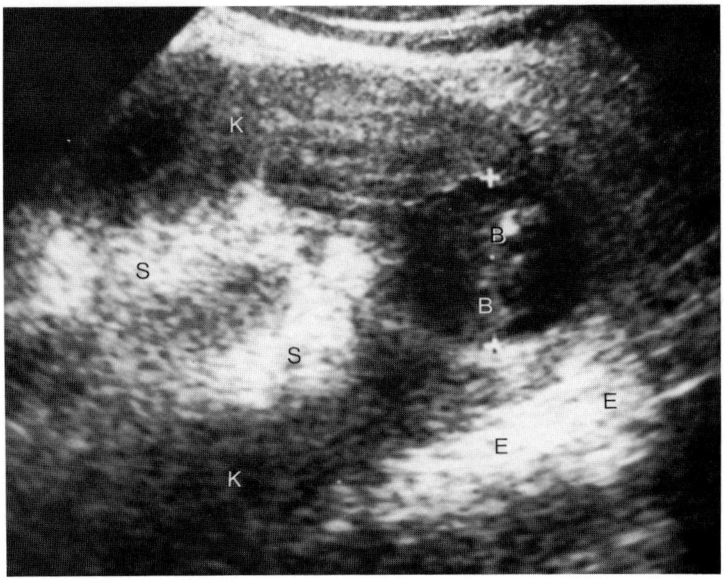

Figure 5.7. Hemorrhagic cyst. Magnification view of kidney (*K*) and central renal sinus (*S*) shows a cortical cyst (between *asterisks*). The cyst contains a solid irregular mass (*B*), which proved to be a blood clot. Acoustic enhancement (*E*) behind the mass is identified.

ing system. These cysts may mimic hydronephrosis on ultrasound examination. The origin of these parapelvic cysts generally is thought to be from the renal parenchyma in the vicinity of the renal hilus. The clinical significance and pathogenesis of such parapelvic cysts has been the subject of many discussions among urologists and radiologists for the past several years. Several theories have been developed to try to explain these cysts, including development from lymphatic channels or embryonic rests of renal tissues. Clinical manifestations are infrequent, but some complications attributable to parapelvic cysts include hydronephrosis secondary to mechanical obstruction, hypertension, infection secondary to mechanical obstruction and stasis, and hematuria. These cysts generally cause compression and may cause distortion of the renal collecting system, both the minor and major calices, and may result in obstruction that may result in calculus formation or pain. Large parapelvic cysts can cause venous or arterial compression and may also displace that kidney (17, 21).

Parapelvic cysts present echographically in one of two major forms (21). The more common presentation is multiple, noncommunicating, fluid-filled spaces filling the renal hilus. The cysts often have a variety of sizes and shapes. It is often difficult to completely clear reverberation and other artifactual echoes from the lesions, as the cystic spaces are intertwined among vessels, renal sinus fat, and elements of the collecting system (22). The second type of presentation takes the form of a single renal hilar cyst, often a very large one. In either instance, differentiation between parapelvic cysts and hydronephrosis is not always easy. In the case of multiple parapelvic masses, the sonographic appearance differs from hydronephrosis in that the cysts do not communicate with each other, there is no confluence toward a dilated ureter or tapered renal pelvis, and there is no characteristic appearance of dilated calices. In the instance of a single large parapelvic cyst, hydronephrosis may be excluded when the examiner sees the renal sinus echoes displaced away from the cyst and no dilated ureter or calices visible. In either instance, CT or urography may be necessary to establish the certain presence or absence of collecting system dilatation.

Figure 5.9 is an image of a patient with unilateral parapelvic cysts. There are multiple fluid-filled compartments with a variety of shapes and sizes. Many of the lesions return considerable echo reflections. Acoustic enhancement posterior to the affected kidney is conspicuous. Differentiation from hydronephrosis is difficult. Figure 5.10**A** and **B** show very similar findings in a patient with multiple parapelvic cysts. One of the cysts in the right kidney (Fig. 5.10**A**) has the deceptive appearance of a dilated renal pelvis. Excretory urography was necessary to show that the collecting system is not dilated (Fig. 5.10**C**). Rather, the

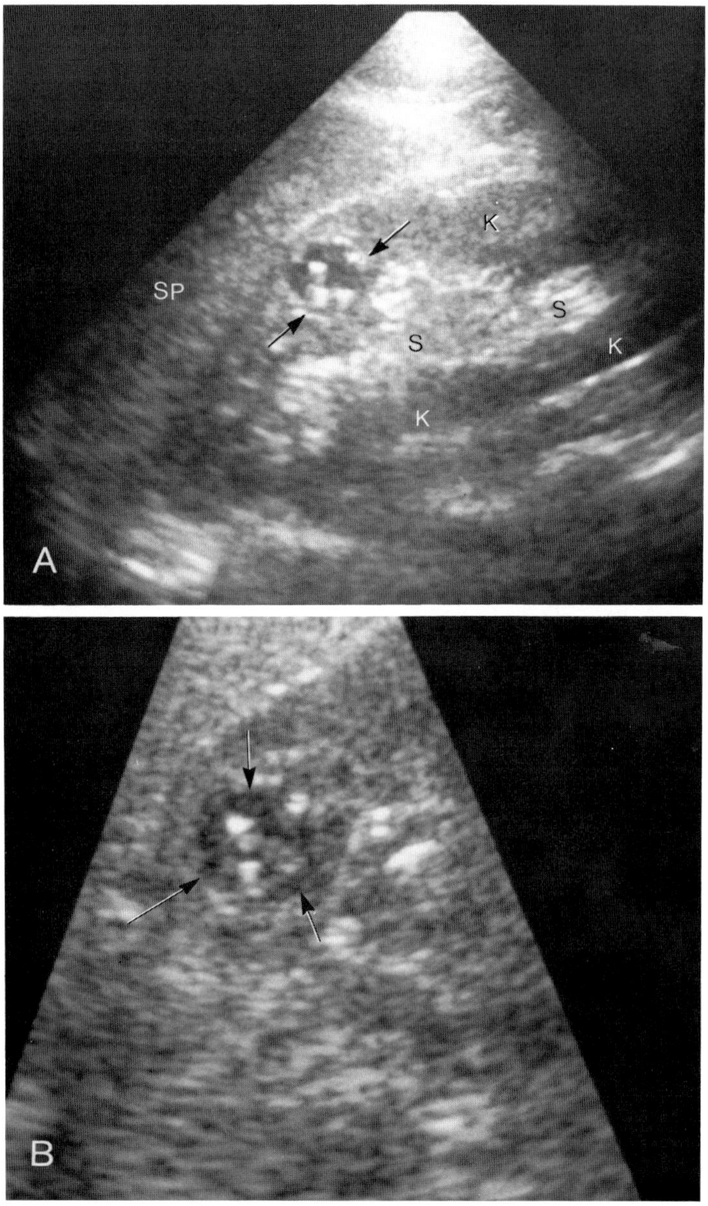

Figure 5.8. A, Infected cyst. A rounded cortical mass (*arrows*) contains several brightly reflective calcifications. The kidney parenchyma (*K*) and central sinus echoes (*S*) are otherwise normal. *SP,* spleen. **B,** Infected cyst. High-resolution view of infected cyst (*arrows*) shows poorly defined margins and a variety of internal echoes, including bright reflections from calcifications within necrotic debris. No acoustical enhancement is apparent distal to the cyst.

renal pelvis and infundibular structures are markedly stretched over the numerous cystic masses.

Figure 5.11 is a representative image from a patient with a single large parapelvic cyst. The fluid-filled mass fills the entire renal sinus and its slightly lobulated contour could readily be confused with a very dilated renal pelvis. This image can be usefully contrasted with the sonogram shown in Figure 5.12. In the latter case, the patient has a very dilated extrarenal pelvis. The characteristic ultrasonic findings of dilated calices communicating with an enlarged renal pelvis are shown. The renal pelvis converges toward the ureteropelvic junction in a characteristic tapered fashion.

Pyelogenic Cyst

Clinical features of a pyelogenic cyst or caliceal diverticulum have been debated by urologists for many years. The etiology and appropriate terminology for such a localized cystic swelling or dilatation of all or part of a calix is undetermined. It is not possible to distinguish

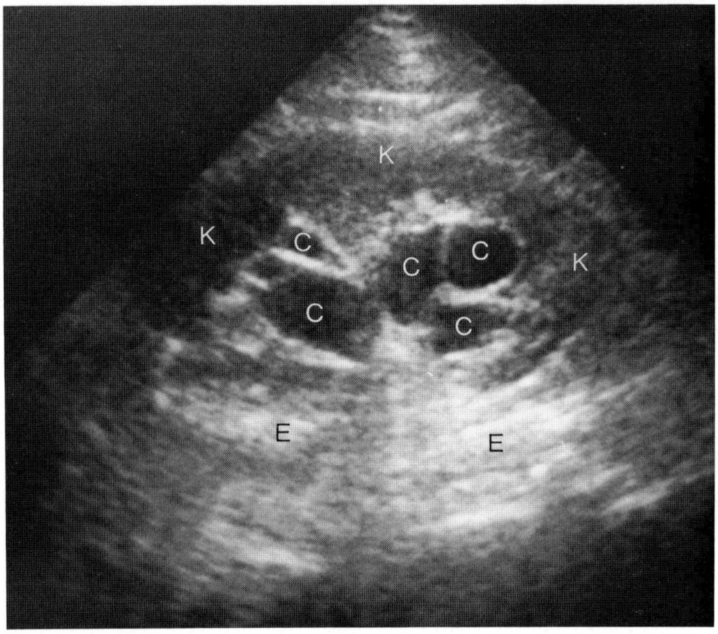

Figure 5.9. Unilateral parapelvic cysts. Multiple cystic spaces (*C*) lie in the hilum of the kidney (*K*). The cysts have a variety of sizes and shapes and many contain reverberation echoes. Acoustical enhancement (*E*) is visible posterior to the kidney.

these cysts from one another or even from a cortical cyst with ultrasound because they all appear as predominantly fluid-filled sacs and spaces within a kidney. A pyelogenic cyst or caliceal diverticulum is a cystic cavity in proximity to a normal calix. The diverticulum generally communicates with the calix or an infundibulum, but not with the renal pelvis, via a narrow channel. At times, this connection can be easily visualized with retrograde pyelography. The exact cause of the cystic areas can be congenital (such as Wolffian duct remnants) or inflammatory. Clinically speaking, these are silent unless stone formation occurs or debris within the cyst becomes infected. Then they may mimic intrarenal abscesses. On occasion, these infected patients may require percutaneous or operative drainage. In addition, pyelogenic cysts rarely achieve significant size to cause obstruction of other intrarenal structures, such as adjacent calices.

As would be predictable, the sonographic features of pyelogenic cyst are quite similar to those of a benign, simple cortical cyst. The examiner finds a rounded mass lesion in the renal parenchyma covered by a thin layer of cortex. The lesions may be single or multiple. The actual communication between a caliceal diverticulum and the caliceal fornix from which it is arising will not be visible, although this channel may be readily seen on urography or retrograde pyelograms. Figure 5.13 demonstrates a pyelogenic cyst complicated by stone formation. The lesion, as seen in Figure 5.13**A,** is a rounded, sonolucent mass with good margins and good posterior enhancement. The two small stones that have formed inside the diverticulum are readily visible in Figure 5.13. The larger of the two stones produced acoustical "shadowing" behind it.

Congenital Cystic Disorders

The great variety of complex cystic diseases that affect the kidney from birth onward are covered in Chapter 12. Two congenital cystic disorders are seen often enough in adults that a brief review is appropriate. These two disorders are polycystic kidney disease (PCKD) and multicystic dysplastic kidney disease (MCDK).

Polycystic Kidney Disease

Polycystic kidney disease of the adult is inherited as an autosomal dominant trait with a high penetrance. Most patients have the clinical components of their disease manifest by the fourth or fifth decade of life (17, 23, 24). There may be associated abdominal pathology such as pancreatic cysts and hepatic cysts. Members of a patient's family should be screened with ultrasound to see if they also have polycystic kidney disease. The main manifestations of adult polycystic kidney disease include pain, hypertension, and hematuria.

The disease is usually bilateral, but may be

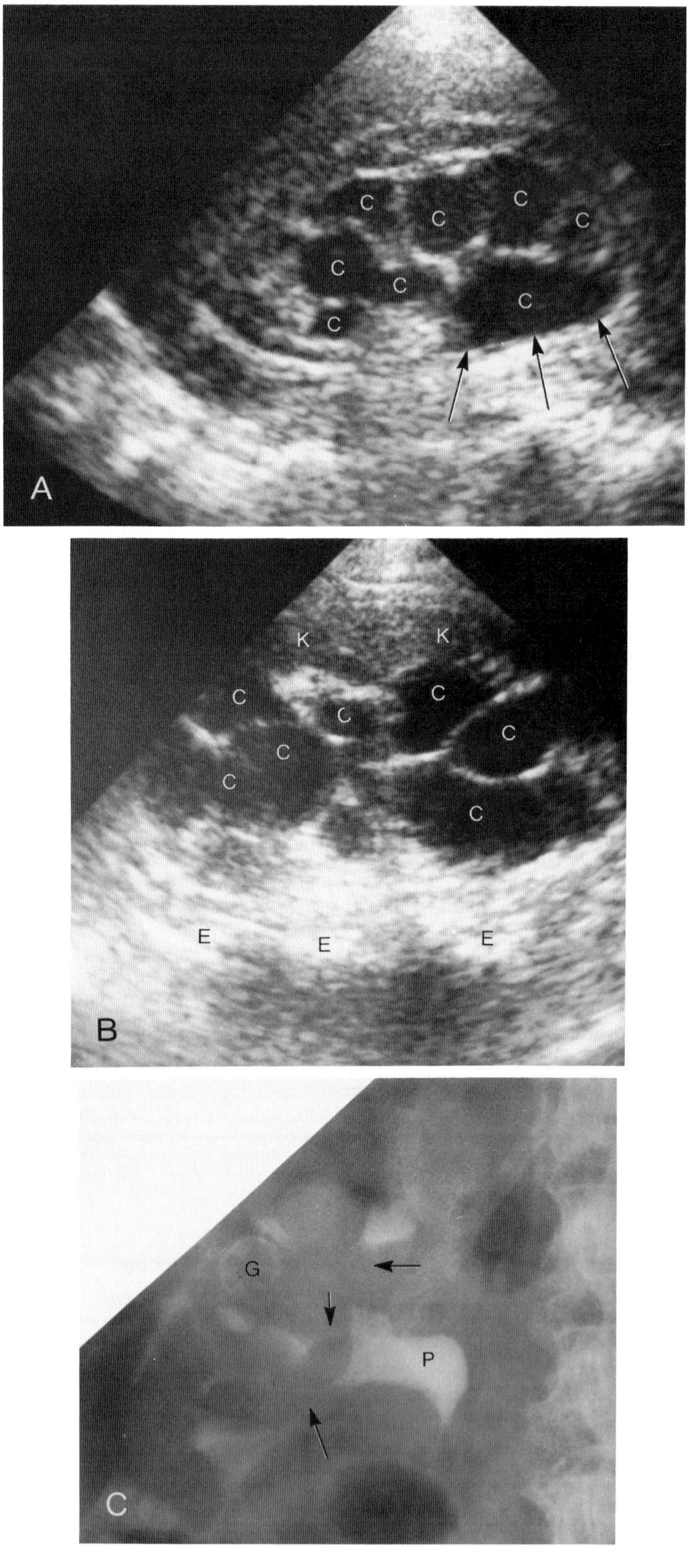

Figurc 5.10. A, Bilateral parapelvic cysts, right kidney. Numerous cysts fill the hilus of the kidney, simulating hydronephrosis. One of these cysts (*arrows*) is deceptively in the shape of the right renal pelvis. **B,** Bilateral parapelvic cysts, left kidney. A large number of cysts (*C*) literally fill the hilum of the left kidney (*K*). Coexisting hydronephrosis would be impossible to exclude. Acoustical enhancement (*E*) is conspicuous behind the kidney. **C,** Intravenous urogram of right kidney. The renal pelvis (*P*) and the infindibular structures (*arrows*) are stretched over some of the multiple parapelvic cysts. No hydronephrosis is present. An incidental gallstone (*G*) is visible.

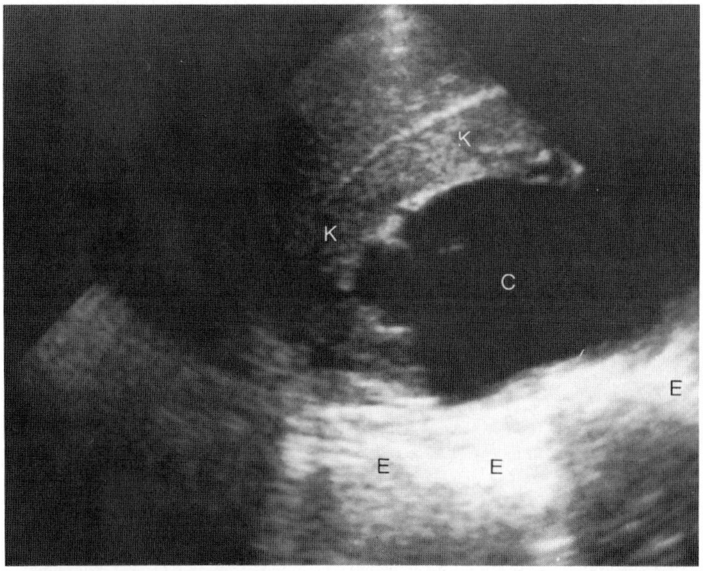

Figure 5.11. Parapelvic cyst. A very large, unilocular parapelvic cyst (*C*) fills the hilum of the kidney (*K*). The lesion closely simulates a very dilated renal pelvis. Much acoustic enhancement (*E*) occurs distal to the cyst.

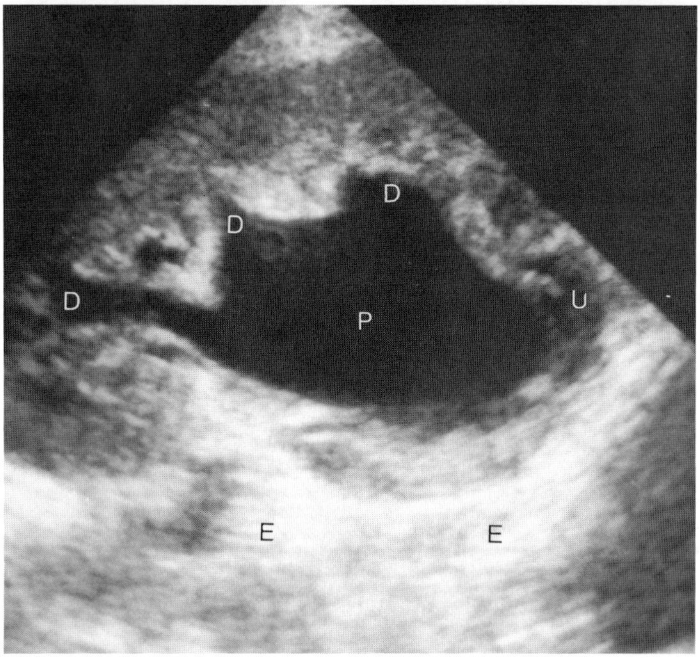

Figure 5.12. Dilated renal pelvis and calices. The image is shown in contrast to Figure 5.11. Dilated calices (*D*) communicate with an enlarged renal pelvis (*P*). The pelvis tapers toward a dilated ureter (*U*). Much acoustical enhancement (*E*) occurs distal to the large pelvis.

asymmetrical with innumerable cysts of different size arising from both the cortex and medulla. The end result is often progressive renal failure occurring approximately 10 to 15 years after the onset of symptoms or diagnosis. Many patients with this problem go on to renal transplantation. The main causes of death in this group of patients include uremia, cerebral hemorrhage, and cardiac disease. Associated clinical findings include one or more cerebral aneurysms (20%), cardiovascular abnormalities, neurofibromatosis, and renal carcinoma (23).

Multicystic Dysplastic Kidneys

In a pediatric age group, two of the most common causes for abdominal masses include hydronephrosis and multicystic dysplastic kidney (MCDK). It is critical to distinguish between the two, as their treatment differs markedly. Currently, if the patient has hydronephrosis, treatment should be aimed at relieving the

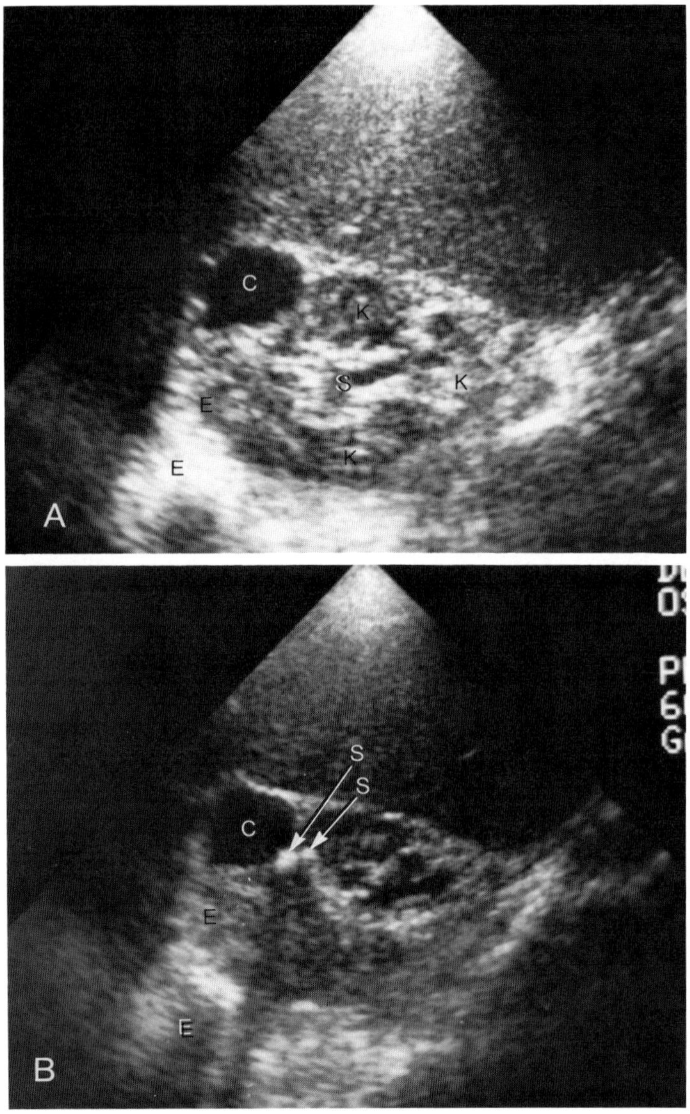

Figure 5.13. A, Pyelogenic cyst. A rounded, echo-free, cystic mass (*C*) with distal enhancement (*E*) sharply abuts the kidney (*K*) and normal renal sinus (*S*). **B,** Stones in pyelogenic cyst. Additional image of patient shown in **A** shows two stones (*arrows, S*) at the base of the pyelogenic cyst (*C*). Acoustic enhancement (*E*) is redemonstrated.

obstruction, either internally or percutaneously or by definitive surgical correction. Even kidneys with a thin parenchymal cortex may be salvaged. A classic multicystic kidney disease (Potter type II) results from complete ureteral obstruction, usually before the eighth to ninth fetal week. Because of interference with ureteral branching and budding, there is a decreased division of tubules in the collecting system and an inhibition in maturation of the nephrons. The terminal portions of these enlarged collecting tubules develop into cysts joined by massive sheets of small connective tissue fibers. When there is a case of incomplete or partial obstruction, renal development is complete but there is the occurrence of internal hydronephrosis with dilatation of the pelvic caliceal system and obstruction of this system. This is usually the case with developmental problems after the 36th week of gestation. In the second trimester, if incomplete obstruction occurs, results may be in the large range of the clinical pathologic spectrum mentioned above with varying degrees of cyst formation and caliceal dilatation, as well as changes that are dysplastic in the kidneys themselves. This combination of dysplasia with dilatation has been referred to by some as the hydronephrotic type of multicystic dysplastic kidneys (1, 25). If the diagnosis of multicystic kidney disease can be made with assurance with the aid of ultrasonography, surgical exploration is often delayed until 9 to 12 months of age. On the other hand, surgical therapy and excision may be permanently delayed if the family and patient are willing to undergo careful, close follow-up to determine any changes in the size of this mass.

A conventional example of multicystic kidney disease in a newborn is presented in Figure 5.14. Figure 5.14**A** shows a normal right kidney in a neonate. Little sinus fat is present. The renal pyramids are very large relative to renal parenchyma and the pyramids are conspicuously sonolucent, a fact that explains the frequent error made by inexperienced examiners when they confuse normal renal pyramids with multiple cysts or dilated calices of hydronephrosis. Figure 5.14**B** is an image of the left kidney in the same baby. On physical examination the child was found to have a left upper quadrant mass likely representing an enlarged spleen. The sonogram shows that the mass is a large kidney. The renal substance has been completely replaced by a confluent mass of in-

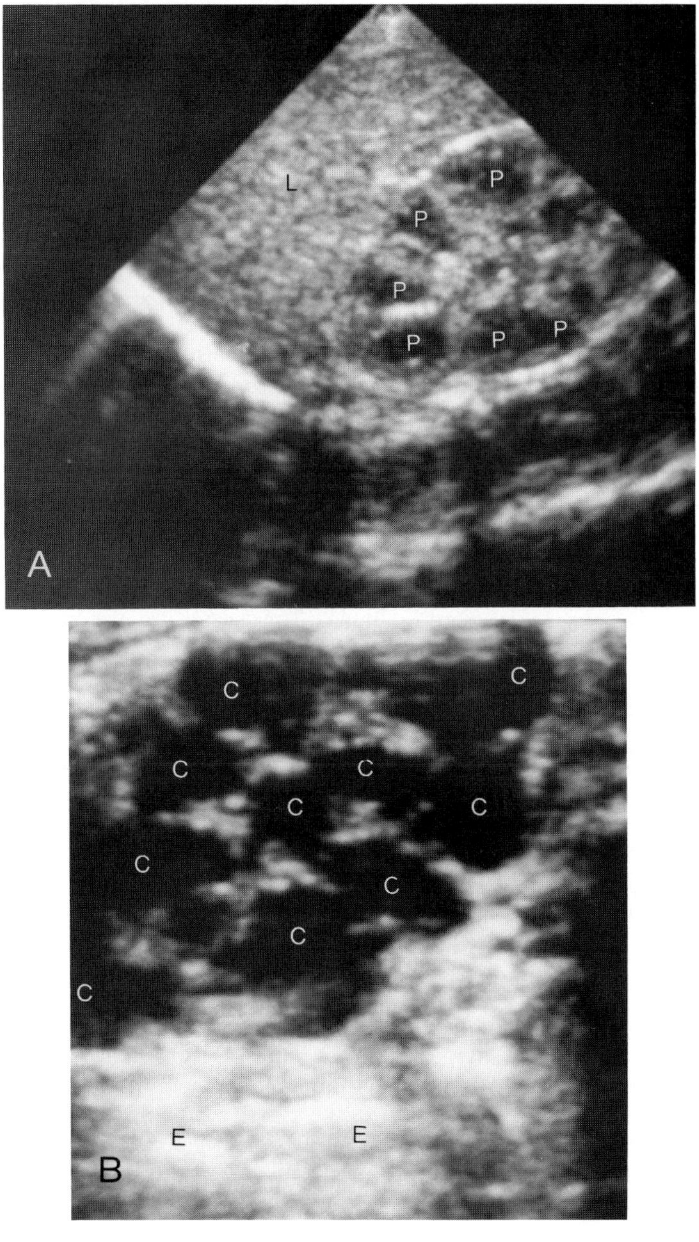

Figure 5.14. **A,** Normal right kidney. Images of the right renal fossa inferior to the right lobe of the liver (*L*) show a normal kidney. The normal sonolucent pyramids (*P*) can easily be mistaken for renal cysts. **B,** Multicystic left kidney. Images of the left renal fossa in the same patient as in **A** reveal a confluent mass of multiple cysts (*C*). No normal renal parenchyma is present. Distal enhancement (*E*) is demonstrated behind the cluster of cysts.

numerable cysts, the usual sonographic pattern in MCDK. The ureter and renal artery are absent in multicystic kidney, so these structures will not be visualized. Rarely, the multicystic kidney will not be seen as a bag of multiple cysts but, instead, the kidney will be gone and replaced by a simple single sac of fluid. If the multicystic kidney is not removed in early childhood, the edges of some or all of the cysts may calcify in an "eggshell" fashion.

Sonography is particularly useful in the setting of MCDK in two other respects. First, although MCDK is thought of as a unilateral disease, there is a high incidence of contralateral abnormalities, including ureteropelvic junction obstruction and contralateral cystic disorders (26). Thus ultrasound of the opposite kidney is particularly necessary when multicystic kidney is discovered on one side. Another important use for sonography in MCKD relates to the numerous documented cases that many multicystic kidneys, left untreated, simply shrivel up and literally disappear (27). Such patients are often diagnosed later in life as having unilateral renal agenesis. Thus, if the attending physician chooses, a child with MCKD may be observed with sonography to see if spontaneous regression occurs.

When sonography is done in the setting of PCKD, of course, bilateral abnormalities are expected. In general, the kidneys of such patients are enlarged if the disease is discovered in adulthood. The renal parenchyma will be barely recognizable if recognizable at all. Innumerable cysts of a great variety of sizes and shapes will be present. Often such patients are referred to exclude urinary obstruction because blood urea and creatinine are measured and found elevated. This would be a futile task for the examiner under most circumstances, because it will not usually be possible to distinguish dilated calices from the hundreds of cysts that might be present. If cysts become hemorrhagic or infected, it may be possible to visualize these with sonography. The clear fluid in such a cyst may be changed to reflective fluid, or fluid levels may be visible.

Figure 5.15**A** is an image of the left kidney of a young woman in the second trimester of pregnancy who presented with severe right flank pain, fever, and bloody, purulent urine. The left kidney is enlarged with many cysts and little recognizable renal parenchyma. The patient's right kidney is shown in Figure 5.15**B.** The kidney is huge, and many clear cysts are visible. Other cysts are filled with evenly echogenic material representing areas of both infected and uninfected hemorrhage. The patient required more than 1 month's treatment with intravenous antibiotics and bed rest before her symptoms subsided.

Figure 5.16 shows a somewhat atypical presentation for PCKD. Numerous cysts are visible, but overall the kidney is only slightly enlarged. The patient had presented with constitutional symptoms and was found to have renal failure.

Multilocular Renal Cysts

Multilocular renal cysts is a rare nonhereditary disease that is limited, generally speaking, to one area of one kidney. The involved cystic part of the kidney tends to be well encapsulated and consists of multiple noncommunicating cysts sharply separated from the surrounding normal tissues (16, 28). This entity does not have a defined etiology. Its behavior is generally benign. Several theories of pathogenesis have resulted in numerous names for these lesions: multilocular cyst, benign cystic nephroma, cystic Wilms' tumor, cystic hypertoma, cystic lymphangioma, and Perlmann's tumor (29–31). If nephroblastic elements occur in multilocular cysts, they are usually present in the childhood group.

Multilocular cysts have been described in all age groups, about evenly distributed between children and adults. The major complaint that causes the patient to seek medical care is an abdominal mass. These cysts are also interesting in that at least half of the cysts contain calcium deposits of different configurations. These configurations may be curvilinear, granular, or stellate. Peripheral calcifications have also been noted in some patients with multilocular cystic disease. If the cysts do not attain large size, they are not responsible for obstruction, stasis, and infection. Treatment may be conservative. However, there is often difficulty in distinguishing between these multilocular cysts and renal neoplasm (18). Care must be taken with regard to the ultrasound examination to help differentiate these from lesions in which there is a tumor growing in the cyst wall. In certain cases, however, it may be difficult to distinguish their appearance from that of a necrotic tumor or a tumor within a cyst. In those cases, additional studies such as CT scanning may be quite helpful, as may be surgical exploration.

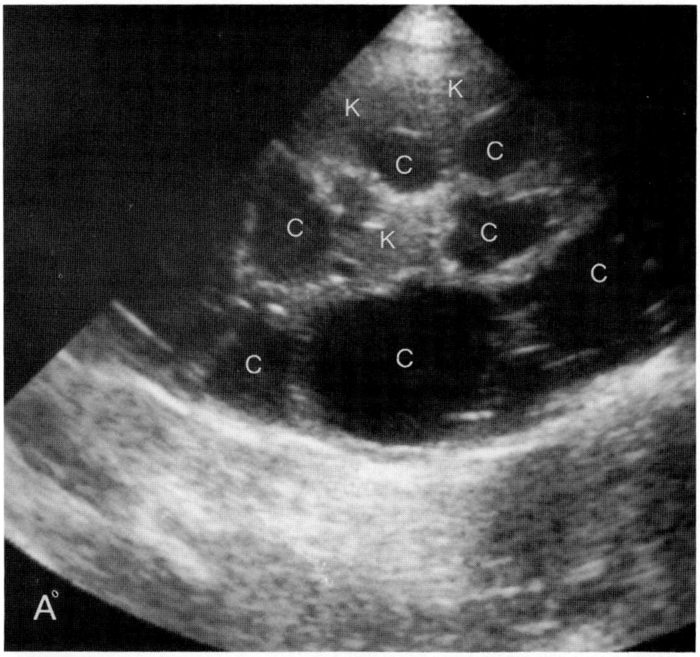

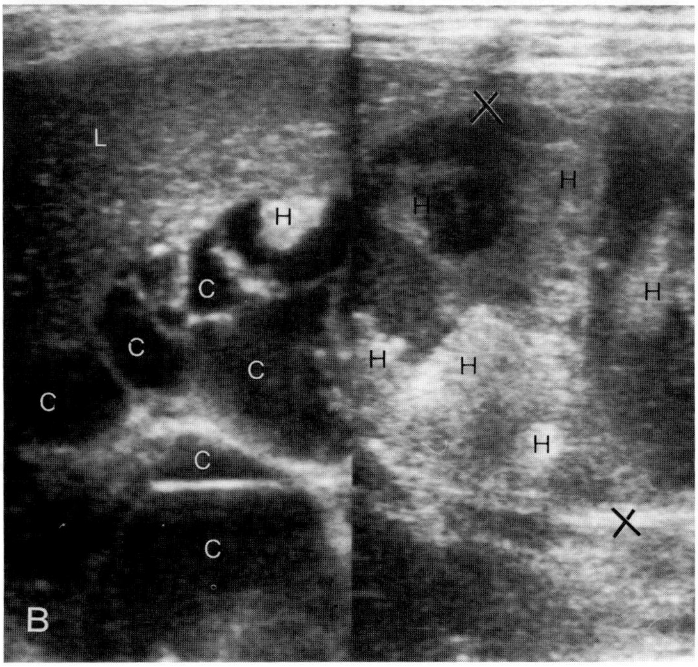

Figure 5.15. A, Polycystic kidney disease, left kidney. The kidney consists mostly of a number of variably sized cysts (*C*). A few scattered areas of unaffected kidney parenchyma (*K*) are visible. **B,** Polycystic kidney disease, right kidney. The right kidney is huge and a large number of cysts (*C*) are visible. A very large multiseptated cyst (between *X*'s) contains multiple areas of hemorrhage (*H*). The patient had gross hematuria, infected urine, and pain. *L,* edge of right lobe of liver.

Renal sonography demonstrates a large mass in the kidneys with multiple fluid masses separated by highly echogenic septations with normal renal tissue in the rest of the kidney. The excretory urogram, however, shows nonfunctioning of this mass, but in the rest of the kidney the caliceal system may appear normal, distorted, or have massive hydronephrosis, depending on the exact position, location, and extent of the mass. On IVP, the mass may not be distinguishable from Wilms' tumor; however, sonography easily distinguishes this (25, 32).

Sonographic findings in multilocular cystic masses are illustrated with the cases presented in Figures 5.17 and 5.18. Figure 5.17 is the image of a 44-year-old man with chronic lym-

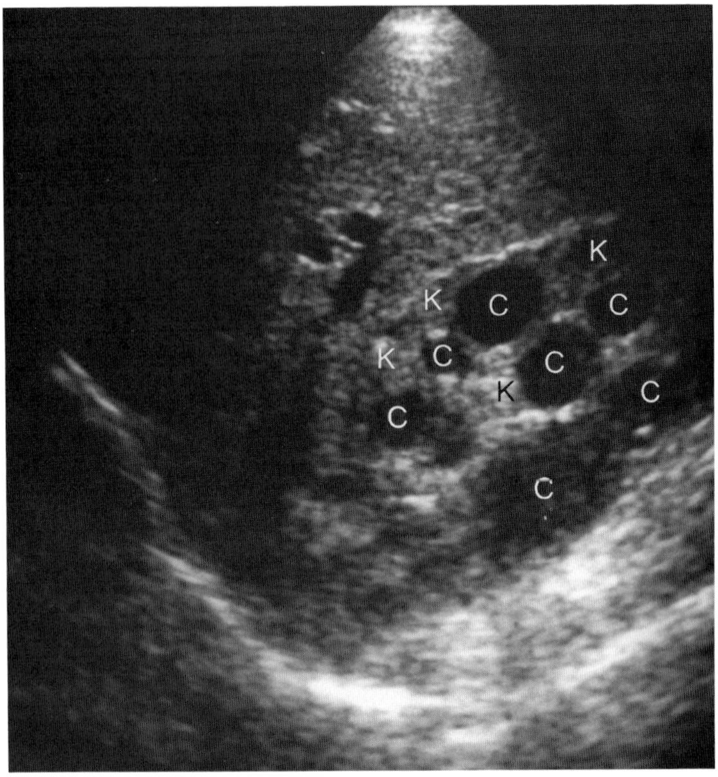

Figure 5.16. Polycystic kidney disease. The kidney is approximately normal in size. Many cysts (*C*) are visible. Bands and nodules of remaining normal renal parenchyma (*K*) can still be seen.

phocytic leukemia who had a large left upper abdominal mass presumed to be an enlarged spleen. After adequate chemotherapy, there was no change in the size of the mass. Sonography demonstrated that the lower half of the kidney was normal. The upper half was replaced by a very large mass consisting of a well-demarcated collection of cysts of various sizes and shapes, all of which appeared to contain clear fluid. Only a differential diagnosis can be offered in such an instance (19, 33). Multicystic carcinoma is unlikely, as the lesion is well demarcated from the kidney and none of the cysts contain hemorrhage or solid elements. Also, the septations separating the cysts are thin. The sonographic appearance is appropriate for multilocular cystic nephroma, although this particular clinical entity usually occurs more often in middle-aged women. A well-defined mass of variably sized cysts could represent the localized form of polycystic kidney disease, which can occur segmentally or unilaterally, or the segmental form of multicystic dysplastic kidney (34). The lesion appears to be a collection of separate cysts, so a multiseptated solitary cyst is unlikely. The mass of discrete cysts does not have the sonographic appearance of cystic degeneration in a preexisting solid mass such as a hematoma, abscess, or tumor. In that setting, altered fluid, thick septations, and solid mass admixed with the cysts would be expected. On occasion, a cluster of benign, simple cysts may fortuitously form a confluent multicystic mass. In this particular case, CT scans on two occasions and sonography on several occasions have shown no convincing solid elements or hemorrhage and no change over a 6-year observation period. The patient refuses surgical removal.

A typical multilocular cystic nephroma is shown in Figure 5.18. The patient was a middle-aged woman, as is usual. A renal mass was found at the time of urography for an uncomplicated urinary infection. Ultrasound showed a well-circumscribed mass that was clearly separated from normal kidney. The mass consisted of a collection of small but variably sized cysts, most of which are quite small. The larger cysts on the surface closest to the transducer could be shown to be free of internal echoes, but the smaller cysts located more deeply in the tumor were difficult to characterize, partly because of acoustic enhancement arising from the more anterior and larger cysts. Angiography showed

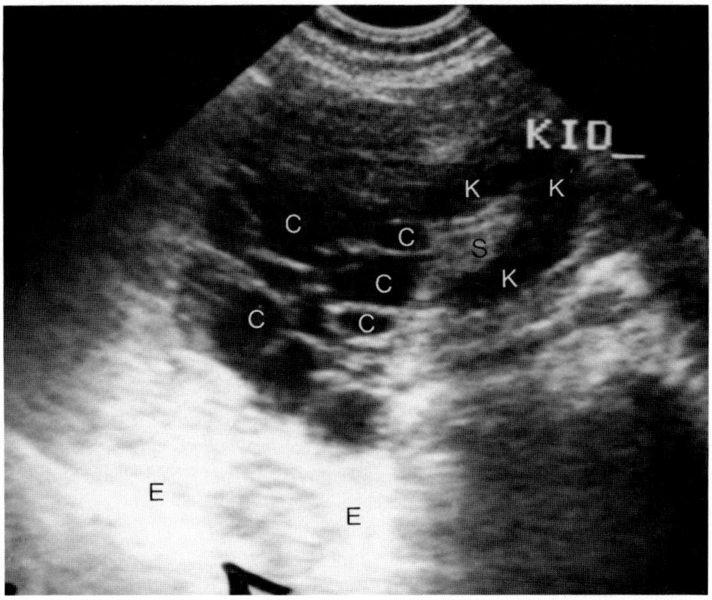

Figure 5.17. Multilocular cystic mass. The lower pole of the kidney, including renal parenchyma (*K*) and renal sinus structures (*S*) appears normal. There is a large multiseptated cystic mass replacing the upper pole. The lesion consists of many variably sized cysts (*C*) separated by thin, echogenic septations. Strong acoustical enhancement (*E*) can be seen from the lesion.

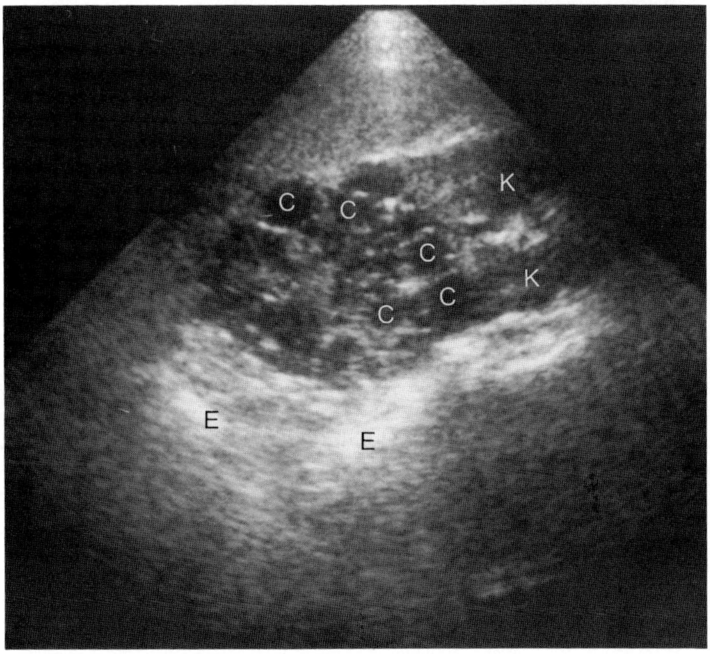

Figure 5.18. Multilocular cystic nephroma. The upper pole of the left kidney (*K*) has been replaced by a well-marginated cystic mass. The mass consists of many cysts (*C*). A number of the smaller cysts, particularly those located posteriorly, are not individually recognizable because of reverberation echoes and thick septations. Slight acoustic enhancement (*E*) lies distal to the nephroma.

an avascular mass. By CT and sonography, the lesion has to be classified in category III: whether it is malignant or benign is indeterminate by radiological study. Surgery and pathological examination revealed a well-encapsulated mass of many cysts containing a thick gelatinous fluid. Microscopic examination confirmed a multilocular cystic nephroma.

Cancer in a Cyst

Renal cysts must be carefully analyzed and evaluated with ultrasonography to be sure that there is a smooth fluid–cyst wall interface without internal projections. Cancer in a cyst has been reported to occur in approximately one in a thousand cases of renal cyst (7, 8). However, our personal experience is that it is even rarer than that. In terms of clinical presentation, if the patient has a large cyst, he or she will present with intraabdominal distress, obstruction, or mechanical symptoms of pain or may present with an abdominal mass observed by an examining physician or the patient himself or herself. In such cases, ultrasound examination is carried out as one of the first diagnostic tests. If it is not a clear cyst, then other investigations may be necessary, including cyst puncture and cystography. Generally speaking, there is no difference in terms of clinical presentation of a tumor within a cyst compared with any other abdominal or renal cystic mass. In occasional patients, a large renal tumor may become cystic secondary to necrosis in tumor. Whether this is the case of a "cyst that contains a tumor" or a "tumor that has become cystic" remains unclear. Suffice it to say that a renal cyst with a cancer in it is one that does not satisfy all the ultrasonic criteria of a simple cyst.

The sonographer doing ultrasound studies may discover links between renal cysts and renal cancer in one of four settings. First, renal cysts are so common that if a patient has a renal malignancy, he or she automatically has a 50% chance of having a coexisting renal cyst based purely on chance alone. Second, many renal cancers undergo cystic degeneration, as such tumors are very prone to necrosis and hemorrhage. Third, rare renal cancers, something less than 5%, are inherently cystic masses with malignant elements. Finally, there are extremely rare instances of cancer growing in an otherwise benign renal cyst.

An example of this last entity is shown in Figure 5.19. The echogram in this case was made when a 60-year-old woman presented with gross hematuria. A large circular mass was found arising from the lateral aspect of the lower pole of the right kidney. The mass was round and posterior enhancement was good. However, there was a soft-tissue nodule. Cyst puncture yielded bloody fluid. Partial nephrectomy was done because the mass appeared to be a benign cyst with hemorrhage at surgery. Histologic sections of the wall of the cyst, however, showed a poorly differentiated adenocarcinoma.

RENAL CELL CARCINOMA

Renal cell carcinoma is the most common primary malignancy of the kidney in the adult population. This tumor tends to have a slow doubling time, but despite this fact the prognosis tends to be poor with a survival rate of approximately 40 to 50% 10 years following radical nephrectomy (20). On the other hand, if the cancer is totally confined to the kidney, there is a 60 to 70% 5-year survival and a 40 to 50% 10-year survival. For this reason, early diagnosis of these lesions are quite important. For the clinician, renal cell carcinoma can pre-

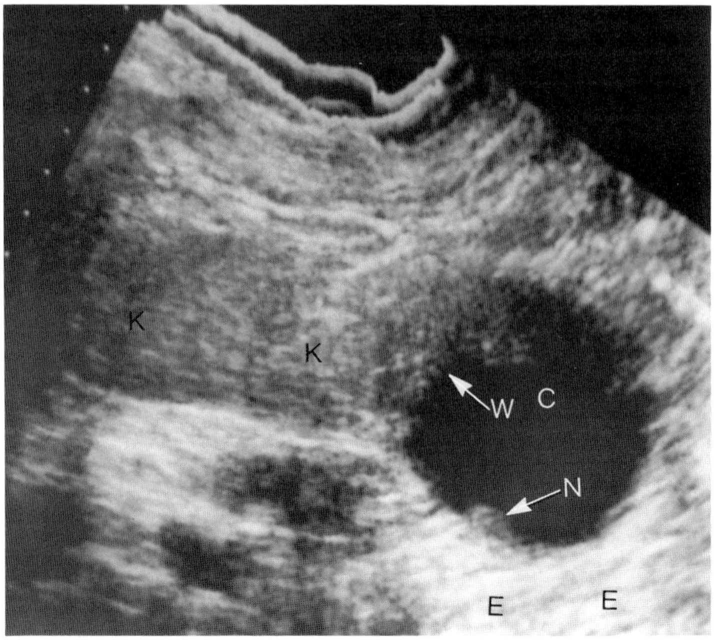

Figure 5.19. Adenocarcinoma within a cyst. A large cyst (*C*) arising from the lateral border of the kidney (*K*) contains an area of focal wall thickening (*arrow, W*) and a small nodule (*N*). Biopsy of these elements showed adenocarcinoma.

sent a variety of clinical signs and symptoms that make the diagnosis difficult. It is often called the great masquerader of abdominal masses. The tumor can present in a variety of growth patterns. Papillary adenocarcinomas are commonly avascular in contrast with the other patterns, which are generally vascularized (35). This may account for their slow and nonaggressive behavior compared to the vascularized tumors.

Over the past decade, computerized tomography and ultrasound have dramatically improved the detection of renal mass lesions. Simple cysts and angiomyolipomas have specific features on both diagnostic modalities that permit confident diagnosis. The remaining renal mass lesions are often not specifically characterized by these modalities. Renal arteriography has been used to aid the diagnosis of these renal masses. However, because of the invasive nature of angiography and somewhat nonspecific findings, especially in nonvascular renal tumors, more attention has been paid to CT scanning and ultrasound. When renal tumors have high arteriovenous shunts giving rise to high blood velocities due to pressure gradients, duplex Doppler scanning may be of benefit. Several investigators, including Ramos and others, have described their work with the Doppler ultrasound and this is helpful in discriminating between benign and malignant renal mass lesions (36–38).

Diagnosis of a renal malignancy sometimes cannot be made even with an intravenous pyelogram (IVP) of good quality, including tomography. Unless the clinician has a high index of suspicion, this may be inadequate in that there are several cases reported in which the IVP has been normal and either CT scanning or ultrasound has diagnosed a tumor on subsequent follow-up study (39). Renal tumors that cannot be diagnosed on IVP are those that, because of their size, location, or coexistent renal abnormalities, are not seen as a discrete mass lesion altering the contour of the kidney. The questions exist as to when and how aggressively to pursue the diagnosis of renal cell carcinoma. The answer is when a high clinical suspicion exists due to a variety of clinical and laboratory findings, further diagnostic evaluation other than intravenous urography must be carried out. It is well known that approximately two-thirds of all patients with renal cell carcinoma who have been diagnosed before death have either microscopic or commonly gross hematuria. About half of these patients may have abdominal pain and about 20% have palpable mass. A smaller but highly significant percentage of patients may have a toxic hepatic dysfunction as typified by abnormal liver function tests, or they may have fever, hypercalcemia, or hypertension. Many patients, however, are asymptomatic (40–43).

SONOGRAPHY OF HYPERNEPHROMAS

Hypernephromas are encountered in the ultrasound laboratory in a great variety of clinical settings. Many are incidental findings, an accidental discovery during sonography for gallbladder disease or other unrelated disorder. Some patients are referred for examination because they have a clinical complex that suggests renal cancer, unexplained hematuria for instance, and their attending physician recognizes the insensitivity of urography as a "screening" method for this disorder (39). Still others may have been examined with CT or urography and an indeterminate mass found. Some patients are sent for sonography in search of a primary tumor to explain a pathological fracture or positive lymph node biopsy for adenocarcinoma.

As would be entirely predictable, no pathognomonic sonographic pattern for hypernephroma exists. The tumors may be any size when discovered, ranging from a few millimeters to many centimeters. Variable amounts of hemorrhage and necrosis are common. No link has even been convincingly established between reflectivity and vascularity or histology, so renal cell carcinomas present seemingly randomly among lesions that are hyperechoic, hypoechoic, or isoechoic. No special characteristics of papillary versus nonpapillary tumors have been observed when these masses were studied with sonography (44). In the Mayo Clinic series of 102 renal cancers examined with echography, about one-third were less than 4 cm, about one-third were 4 to 8 cm, and about one-third were greater than 8 cm (45). The tumors were randomly distributed between the right and left sides and the upper, middle, and lower poles. Acoustic transmission distal to the lesion was equal to conventional renal tissue in the great majority of the 102 masses. Those with internal cystic components sometimes exhibited posterior enhancement, and 5% showed decreased through transmission with respect to normal kidney.

The basic presentation of the usual hypernephroma is that of a solid mass observed in any other organ system. Internal echoes are present. These may be low-level gray reflections or bright acoustic returns from calcifications. The mass has an indistinct interface with normal renal structures. Posterior enhancement is not often present in the absence of cystic change or a very homogeneous histology. The borders of the mass may well be quite irregular, and the shape of the lesion is most often nongeometric. There are no special, reliable, and consistent findings that help separate malignant solid renal masses from benign ones.

Small hypernephromas tend to be evenly echogenic; they have not had time to develop degeneration and hemorrhage. The lesions have not had time to grow into bulky masses, so these small tumors are often minimally border-deforming. The sonograms shown in Figure 5.20 were made when an asymptomatic elderly lady was found to have a large, palpable right upper quadrant mass. The mass was a large incidental hepatic cyst. This hepatic cyst served as a convenient acoustic window into the right renal bed. The upper posterior border of the right kidney was deformed slightly by an evenly echogenic mass. The mass slightly indented the renal sinus echoes. The borders of the mass had an indistinct interface with the rest of the kidney. Acoustic transmission behind the mass was unaffected compared to normal kidney. A localized hypernephroma was found at surgery. Figure 5.21**A** and **B** were obtained when a patient with highly vascular brain metastases was examined for a possible occult malignancy of the kidney. Sonography showed a poorly marginated, evenly reflective

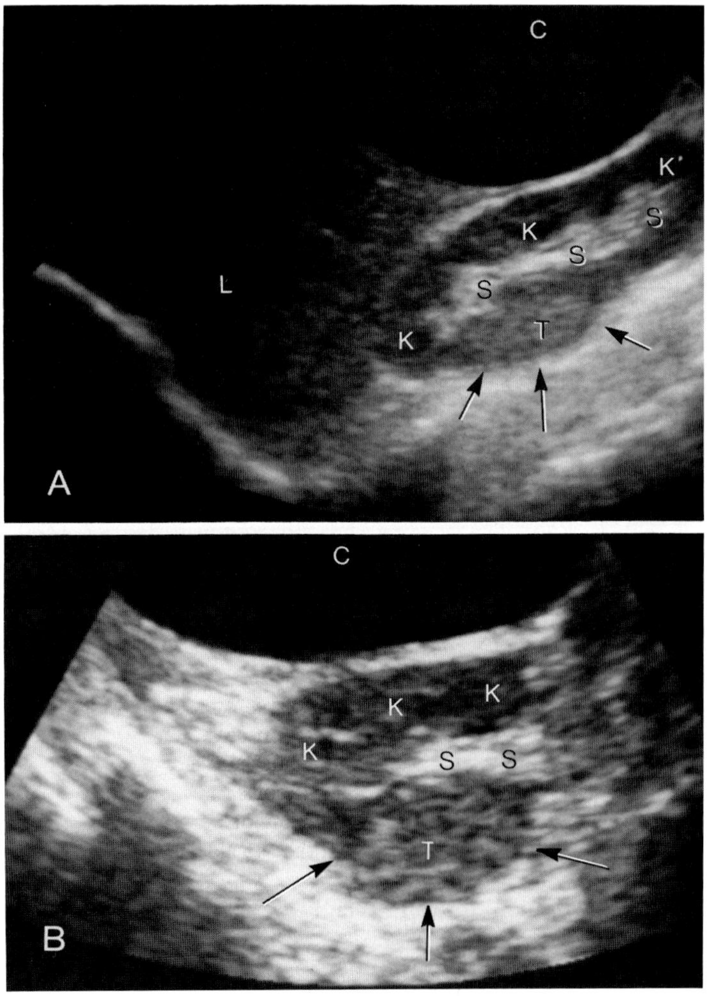

Figure 5.20. **A,** Small hypernephroma, longitudinal view. A small, evenly echogenic tumor mass (*T, arrows*) slightly indents the renal sinus (*S*) echo complex of the right kidney (*K*). The lesion is seen well because of an overlying large cyst (*C*) in the liver (*L*). Acoustic transmission through the mass is the same as through normal kidney. **B,** Small hypernephroma, transverse view. The large hepatic cyst (*C*) again overlies the right kidney (*K*), allowing redemonstration of the small, evenly echogenic tumor (*T, arrows*) indenting the renal sinus (*S*). The echo pattern of the tumor is better appreciated in this high-resolution view.

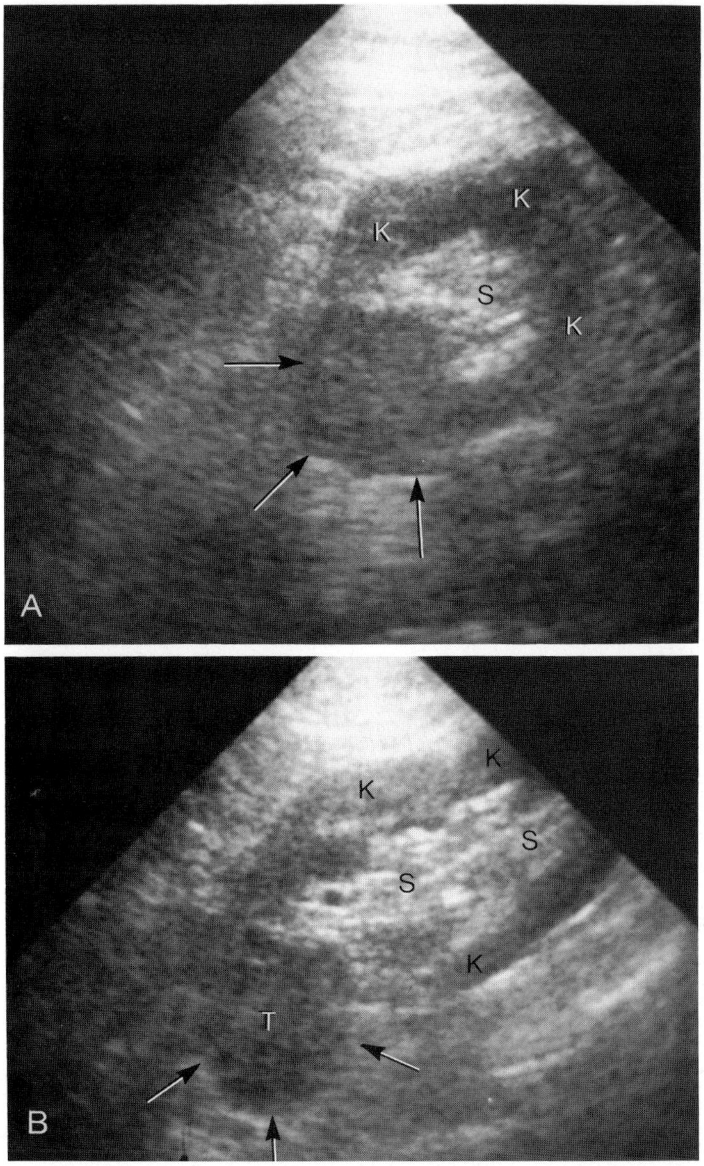

Figure 5.21. **A,** Small hypernephroma, transverse view. The renal contour is minimally deformed by this small, evenly echogenic mass (*arrows*) indenting the renal sinus echo complex (*S*) of the kidney (*K*). Acoustic transmission through the mass is not significantly enhanced. **B,** Small hypernephroma, longitudinal view. Border contour disruption by the tumor (*T*) is better appreciated on the longitudinal view. The renal sinus echo complex (*S*) of the kidney (*K*) is minimally indented by the tumor.

mass with global low-level reflections. Acoustical transmission was slightly enhanced distal to the lesion. The interface with normal renal parenchyma was indistinct. The findings are typical of a small solid renal lesion. In another patient the border of the right kidney was distinctly abnormal when a patient with bone metastases was examined with sonography (Fig. 5.22). There was a small, well-marginated mass, evenly echogenic except for a few tiny sonolucencies. Acoustic transmission through the small mass was the same as through normal kidney. Bone biopsy showed clear cell adenocarcinoma. In contrast, there is no deformity of the renal border shown in the hypernephroma demonstrated in Figure 5.23. This asymptomatic patient, who had numerous nodules demonstrated on a routine chest film, has a small, evenly echogenic mass that is not exophytic. Instead, the mass deforms and invades the renal sinus. Liver metastases are present.

Large bulky tumors are demonstrated in the examples that follow. Figure 5.24 shows a very large, bulky tumor arising from the superior pole of the right kidney. The intrinsic echo pattern is overall quite sonolucent with patchy clusters of low-amplitude reflections. Acoustic transmission through the mass is neither en-

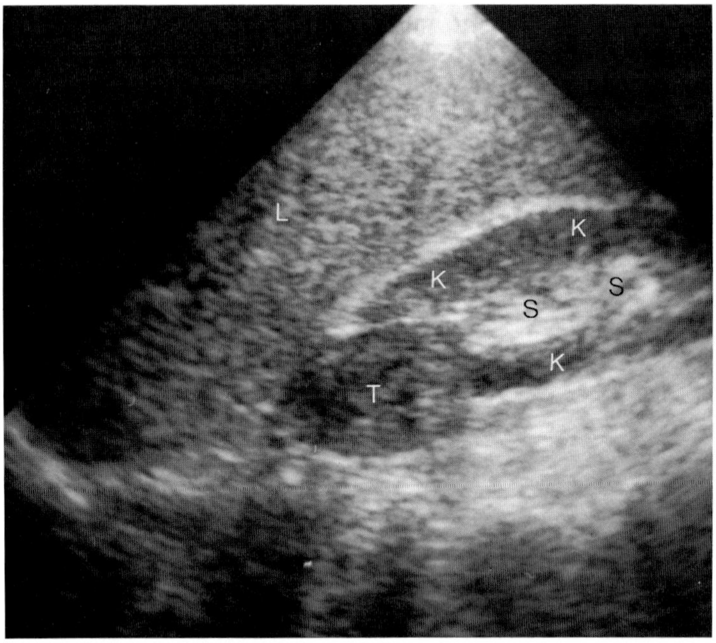

Figure 5.22. Small hypernephroma. An evenly echogenic tumor (*T*) containing only a few scattered sonolucent areas extends well beyond the border of the kidney (*K*). The renal sinus echo complex (*S*) is only slightly impinged upon. Sound transmission through the tumor is the same as for normal kidney.

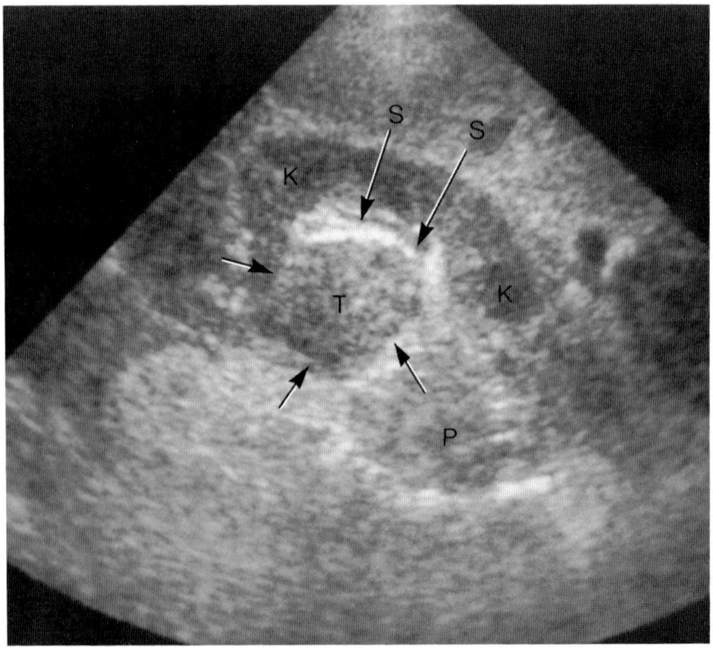

Figure 5.23. Small invasive hypernephroma, transverse view. A small, evenly echogenic tumor (*T*) does not distort the border contour of the kidney (*K*). The renal sinus echo complex (*S*) is thinned and stretched, suggesting collecting system invasion. *P*, psoas muscle.

hanced nor impeded through the lesion; transmission is the same as in the unaffected portions of the kidney. Figure 5.25 shows a very large, bulky, and nodular tumor with tumor nodules visible in renal parenchyma as well as the large exophytic mass. Very little uninvolved kidney remains. The mass is irregular and lobulated. Acoustic transmission through the lesion was the same as through normal kidney. The lesion was highly vascular at the time of arteriography. Interestingly, the same patient had a simultaneous oncocytoma of the opposite kidney and an invasive bladder cancer that eventually required radical cystectomy. A large, bulky hypernephroma with little surviving normal kidney tissue is shown in Figure

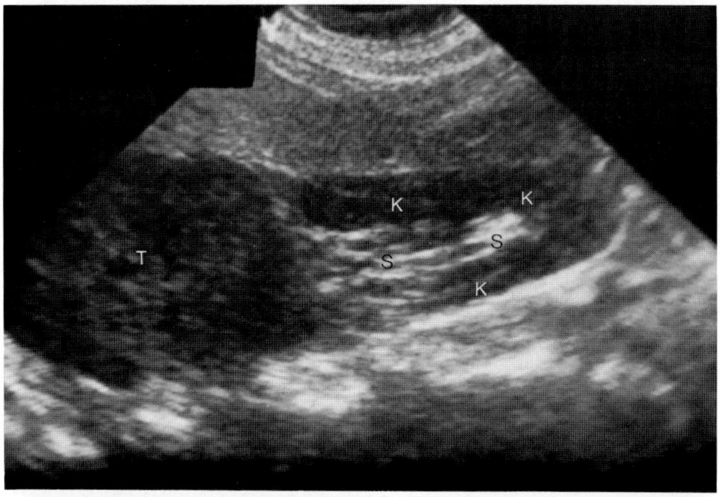

Figure 5.24. Large hypernephroma, longitudinal view. A large, bulky tumor (*T*) arises from the upper pole of the kidney (*K*) with slight displacement of the superior central renal sinus echo complex (*S*). Acoustical transmission through the tumor is the same as through normal kidney. Overall, the tumor is quite sonolucent with scattered patchy clusters of low-amplitude echoes.

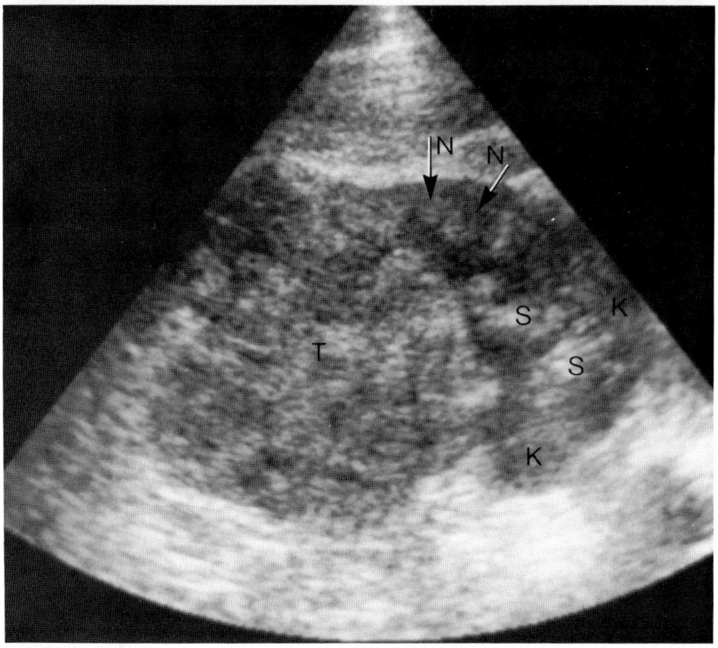

Figure 5.25. Bulky, nodular tumor. A large, irregular tumor (*T*) arises from barely recognizable residual renal tissue (*K*) and remaining central sinus echo complex (*S*) of the right kidney. The tumor consists of many reflective nodules of various sizes. Some of the nodules have been secondarily deposited in renal parenchymal tissue (*N*).

5.26. The mass has undergone extensive cystic degeneration and there are irregular fluid-filled spaces admixed with the solid elements of the tumor. In spite of the large area of cystic degeneration, there is no significant acoustic enhancement behind the lesion. Figure 5.27**A** and **B** were made when an elderly, previously healthy woman presented with gross painless hematuria which started suddenly. A very large, rounded, solid renal mass can be seen arising laterally from the right kidney. The tumor pattern shows low- and moderate-amplitude, patchy, nonhomogeneous reflections. The tumor mass is well demarcated from the normal kidney. Blood clots can be seen filling the renal pelvis on the right. Sonography of the left kidney (Fig. 5.27**B**) was positive. The renal sinus echo complex is depressed posteriorly by a very large nodular mass, a synchronous hypernephroma. Both lesions were studied with CT scanning and arteriography. Both were highly vascular. The right kidney had to be embolized to control hemorrhage. No further treatment has been given, and the patient is well and actively working in her business several months later. A somewhat similar situation is

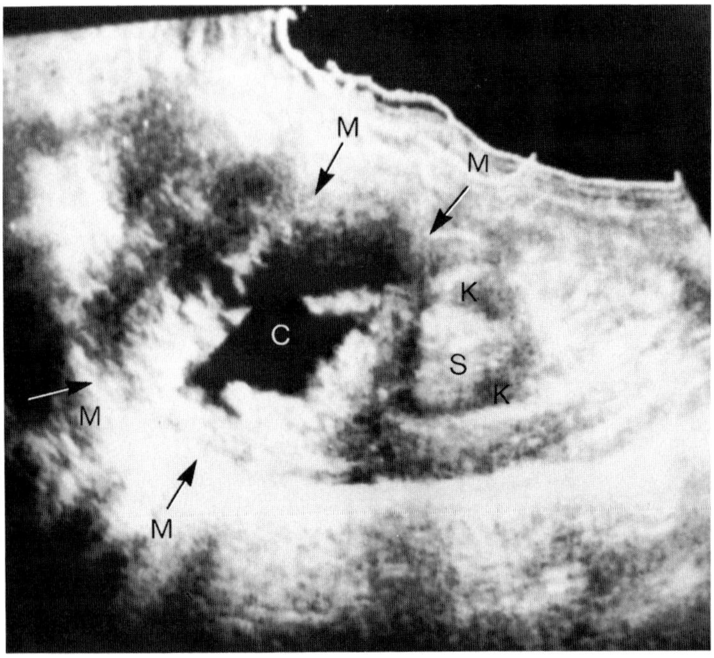

Figure 5.26. Bulky tumor with cystic degeneration. A small portion of residual renal tissue (*K*) and renal sinus echoes (*S*) are still visible in spite of a very large bulky mass (*M*) replacing much of the kidney. Internally, the mass shows large, irregular areas of cystic degeneration (*C*).

depicted in Figure 5.28. The patient had a nephrectomy 1 year earlier for apparently localized renal cell carcinoma. He presented with hematuria at the time of the sonogram shown in Figure 5.28. The echogram demonstrates a rounded, well-demarcated nodule arising from the posterior aspect of the midportion of the remaining right kidney. Homogeneous low-level reflections are recorded from the mass. The acoustical transmission is neither increased or decreased below the tumor. Wedge resection was performed to remove the metastatic (or synchronous) clear cell carcinoma.

The images shown in Figure 5.29**A** and **B** were made when an 85-year-old woman was referred for fever and right flank pain, which persisted following 6 weeks of treatment at a community hospital for a presumed infected renal hematoma. The patient had fallen and she began to have right flank pain, hematuria, and, later, fever. Urography and CT scans were interpreted as showing a renal hematoma. Sonography done on admission demonstrated a very large, quite reflective, minimally nodular solid tumor with evidence of collecting system invasion (Fig. 5.29**A**). Doppler study near the interface of the mass and adjacent normal-appearing kidney was positive for strong Doppler signals. Doppler shift exceeded 4 kHz. This finding has been reported to be a helpful adjunctive piece of evidence of separate benign renal lesions or avascular hypernephromas from vascular malignancies (46). The high Doppler signals may arise from large arterioveneous shunts. At surgery, a bulky adenocarcinoma of the kidney was found as suspected. Collecting system invasion was diagnosed grossly by the pathologist, but frank mucosal penetration was not confirmed on histological sections.

An avascular hypernephroma is shown in Figure 5.30. The kidney in this instance contains a large mass with just a very few scattered internal, low-level echoes. The mass is sharply demarcated from the remaining normal kidney. Acoustical transmission through the mass is poor and the lesion has a poor posterior border. Arteriography showed an avascular mass. At surgery a perfectly ordinary hypernephroma was found. There were no histological features present to explain the lack of internal echoes or the avascular appearance on arteriography.

If a renal tumor or suspected renal tumor is identified, it is fully appropriate to extend the echographic study to estimate clinical stage, even though CT is the most comprehensive modality for tumor staging (47). The liver should be examined, of course, for metastases. All quadrants of the abdomen should be searched for ascites. The opposite kidney should be examined with extra care to evaluate its intrinsic

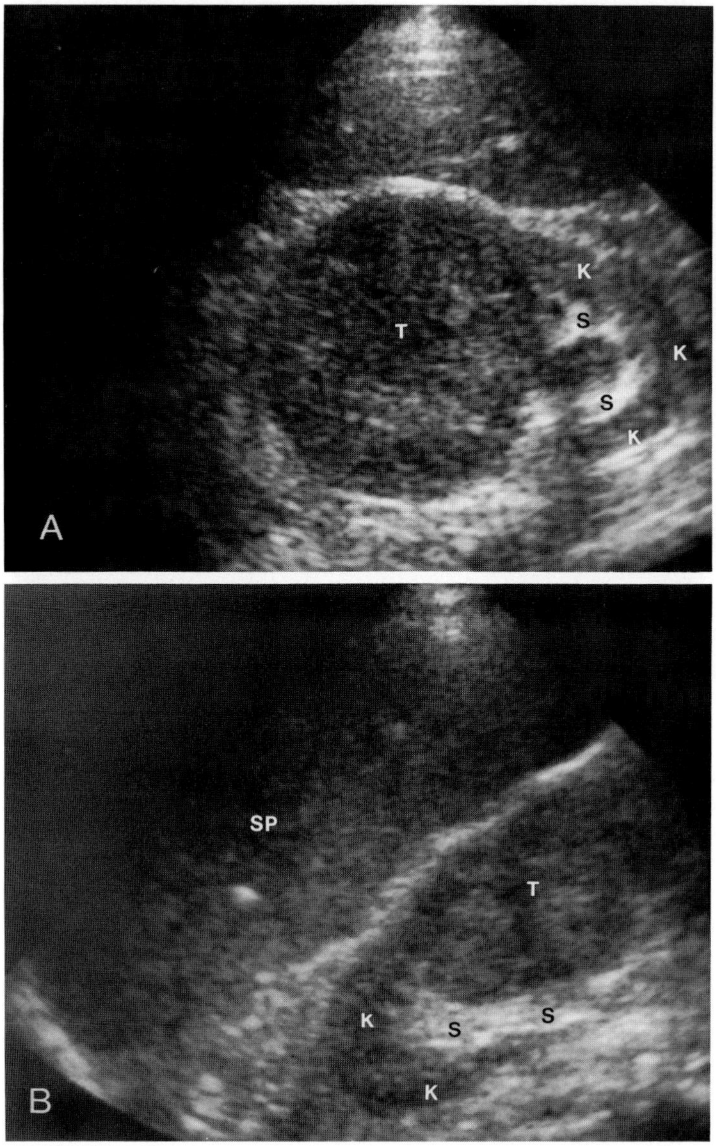

Figure 5.27. **A,** Bilateral hypernephromas, right kidney. A very large, rounded, nonhomogeneously echogenic tumor mass (*T*) arises from the lateral border of the right kidney (*K*). The central sinus echoes (*S*) are separated by a dilated renal pelvis containing echogenic blood clot. **B,** Bilateral hypernephromas, left kidney. A large, bulky, irregular tumor mass (*T*) greatly depresses the central sinus echo complex (*S*) of the left kidney (*K*). The tumor has a patchy and nodular echo pattern. *SP,* spleen.

status as well as to conduct a search for synchronous disease. The renal vein and inferior vena cava are of particular interest and should be carefully studied for tumor extention. Appropriate areas within the abdomen should be imaged for any evidence of enlarged lymph nodes.

The image shown in Figure 5.31 was made when a patient with previous nephrectomy for renal carcinoma on the left was examined for evidence of recurrent disease. Both a liver metastasis and a large nodule of tumor inside the inferior vena cava were visible on the first transverse scan taken of the upper abdomen.

METASTASES TO THE KIDNEY

The reported incidence of renal metastases at autopsy varies between 2 and 20% (48–50). Only relatively recently have the clinical and imaging characteristics of these lesions been recognized (51, 52). Radiologically and sonographically, metastatic lesions may appear similar to renal cell carcinoma. However, metastases are generally multiple and small and may be bilateral. However, 2 to 3% of renal cell carcinomas also exhibit this pattern (50). Several patterns of metastases to the kidney have been evaluated. Patients with gastrointestinal malignancy usually have larger, more exophyt-

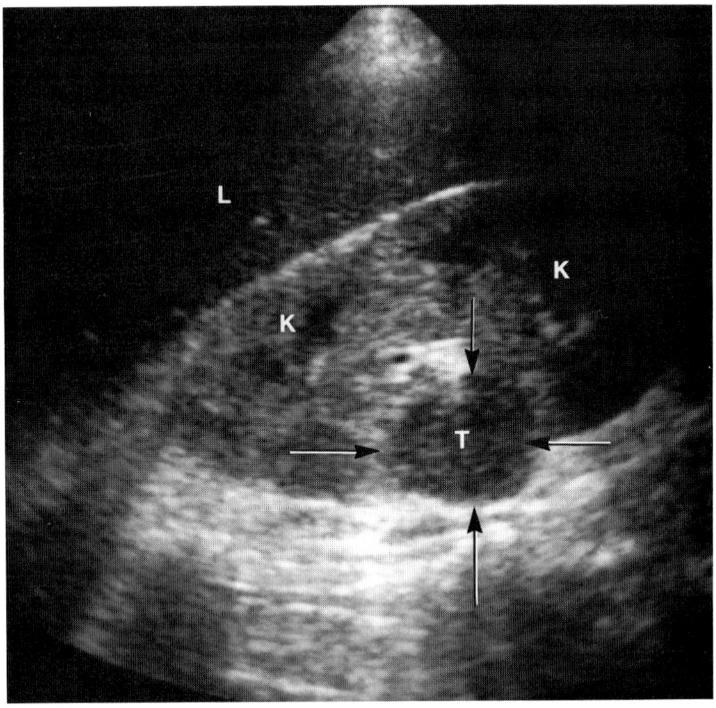

Figure 5.28. "Metastatic" hypernephroma. A conspicuous rounded nodule of evenly reflective tumor (*T*) arises from the posterior border of the right kidney (*K*). The patient had a left nephrectomy for hypernephroma 1 year earlier, at which time the right kidney appeared normal. *L*, liver.

ic renal masses than metastases from other causes. Melanoma and lung carcinoma involve the kidney and perinephric fat in a contiguous fashion. Metastases from breasts, lung, and head and neck primary tumors tend to be small and multiple in more than two-thirds of cases (53–55).

Metastatic tumor to the kidney is the most common renal malignancy. Even so, sonography of this lesion is not well studied or understood. Most patients with renal metastases have widespread disease, and deposits in the kidney are just another manifestation of generalized dissemination. Further, most such patients have no symptoms. Meticulous renal sonography for detection and characterization of often subtle renal masses is not often performed in this clinical setting. If urinary tract echography is done the examination is usually focused on the question of the presence or absence of obstruction.

The sonographic appearance of metastatic lesions as reported in the literature is nonspecific. Most often, multiple, poorly reflective, small, solid nodules are discovered (48, 56). But there is a very broad spectrum of ultrasonic presentations. Some metastatic lesions are highly avascular, others almost vascular. Some may contain areas of cystic degeneration or necrosis; others remain homogeneously solid. Hemorrhage may or may not be present.

The image shown in Figure 5.32 shows a small, poorly defined but highly reflective solid nodule in the upper pole of the right kidney. Acoustic transmission through the lesion is slightly enhanced compared to the normal kidney. The lesion was one of many metastatic deposits of choriocarcinoma present in this young woman. When a young man was found to have a mediastinal mass on a preemployment physical examination, an abdominal CT scan was done to evaluate the possibility of adenopathy. None was seen, but a small, low-attenuation lesion was found in the right kidney. This lesion appeared to be a cyst by CT criteria. Sonography, however, showed that the mass was solid (Fig. 5.33). The lesion was a sharply defined nodule minimally deforming the right lateral renal border. The mass was uniformly echogenic, returning medium-amplitude echoes; acoustic transmission through the mass was good. Small areas of cystic degeneration were present. Biopsy showed melanoma. Generally speaking, metastases to the kidney from melanoma are small and multiple. At least one patient with large cystic masses containing tumor nodules has been reported, however (57). The image shown in Figure 5.34 rep-

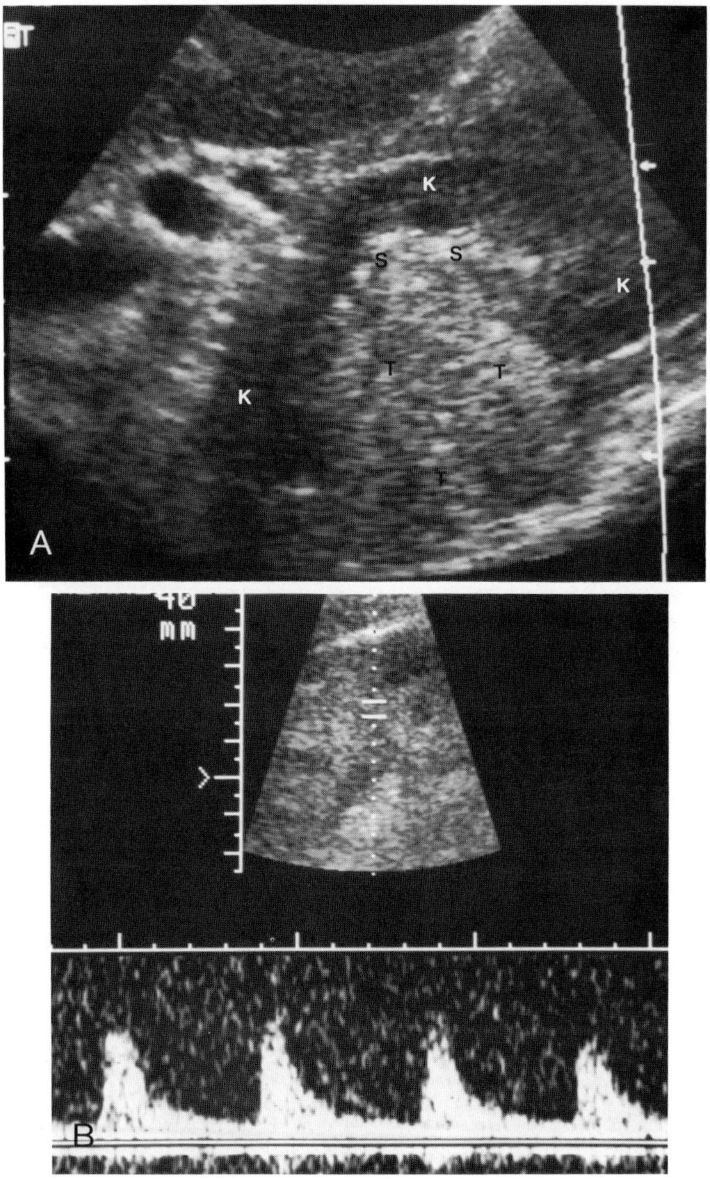

Figure 5.29. **A,** Hypervascular hypernephroma. A large, bulky tumor mass (*T*) extends into and appears to invade the sinus (*S*) echo complex of the right kidney (*K*). At surgery, invasion of the collecting system was present grossly but not confirmed with histological sections. **B,** Hypervascular hypernephroma. Doppler study of the tumor shown in **A** shows strong arterial signals arising near the junction of the tumor mass and right kidney. Presumably these strong Doppler signals arise from arteriovenous communications at the tumoral margin.

resents a selected view from a sonogram obtained after a woman with ovarian carcinoma had urography as a follow-up study for recurrent disease. A large right renal mass was found. The sonogram showed a very large tumor arising from the anterior aspect of the right kidney. The mass is evenly echogenic; calcifications are conspicuous inside the mass. The gallbladder is displaced. The right renal collecting system is not invaded or displaced. Surgical exploration and histologic sections confirmed the sonographic diagnosis of metastatic ovarian carcinoma to the right kidney.

TRANSITIONAL CELL CARCINOMA

Transitional cell carcinoma of the kidney is the third most common cancer in a renal unit after metastatic disease and hypernephroma. Clinically, the few signs of presentation could include microscopic or gross hematuria. In an occasional patient with a large intrarenal pelvic mass, hydronephrosis may occur. In addition, tumors of the upper ureter may also cause obstruction and dilatation of the renal collecting system. The use of urography, ultrasound, and urinary cytology have been helpful in the

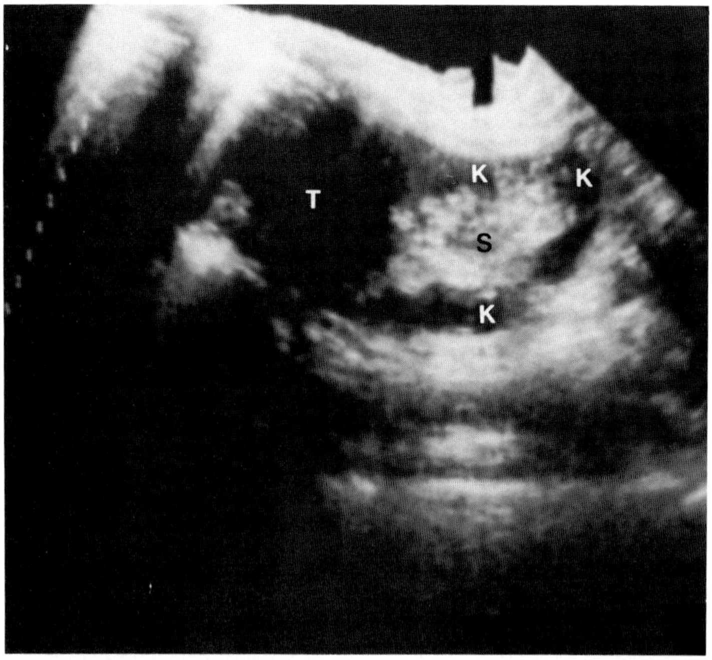

Figure 5.30. Hypovascular hypernephroma. A very weakly reflective solid mass (*T*) arises from the upper pole of the left kidney (*K*), slightly displacing the renal sinus echo complex (*S*). The mass was avascular at arteriography. At surgery, adenocarcinoma was found.

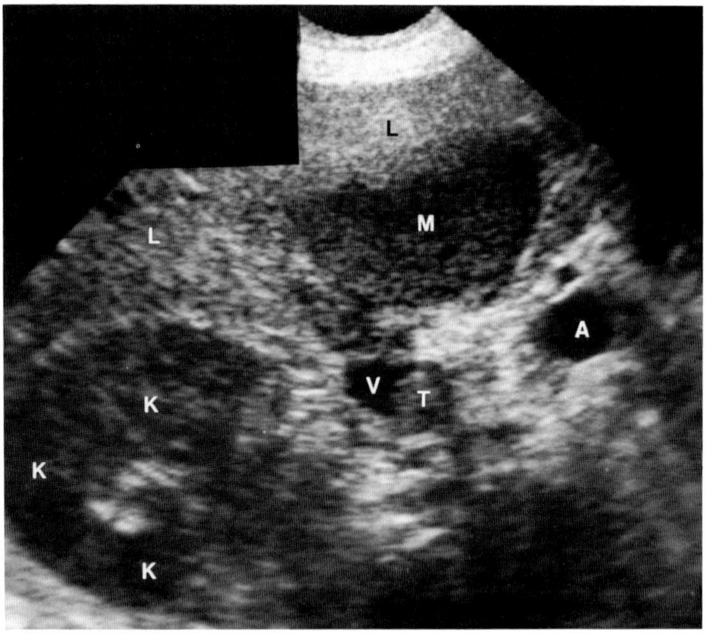

Figure 5.31. Metastatic hypernephroma. A nodule of tumor (*T*) is visible adherent to the left lateral wall of the inferior vena cana (*V*). There is a large metastatic tumor (*M*) in the left lobe of the liver (*L*). The aorta (*A*) and right kidney (*K*) are identified.

diagnosis. One of the problems with diagnosing transitional cell carcinoma is that small lesions may be missed by any modality, including ultrasound, IVP, arteriography, and CT scanning. Arteriography is notably poor for diagnosing transitional cell carcinoma of the renal pelvis, because most tumors are not vascular. Urinary cytology has been helpful, especially in high-grade tumors. Cytology is not of much benefit in patients with low-grade (grade 1 or 2) lesions. The reason for this is that the cells mimic normal cellular architecture and it is difficult for the cytopathologist to diagnose transitional cell tumors with certainty. Of late, our laboratory and others have used cell flow and DNA indices along with cytology in eval-

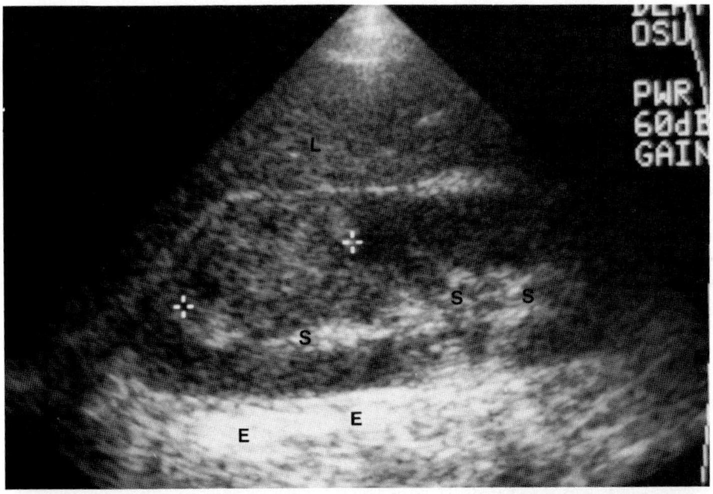

Figure 5.32. Metastatic choriocarcinoma. There is a focus of brightly reflective echoes in the anterior aspect of the upper pole of the right kidney (between *asterisks*). The renal sinus echoes (*S*) are thin in the region of the metastatic tumor. Acoustic transmission is slightly enhanced (*E*) distal to the tumor. *L,* liver.

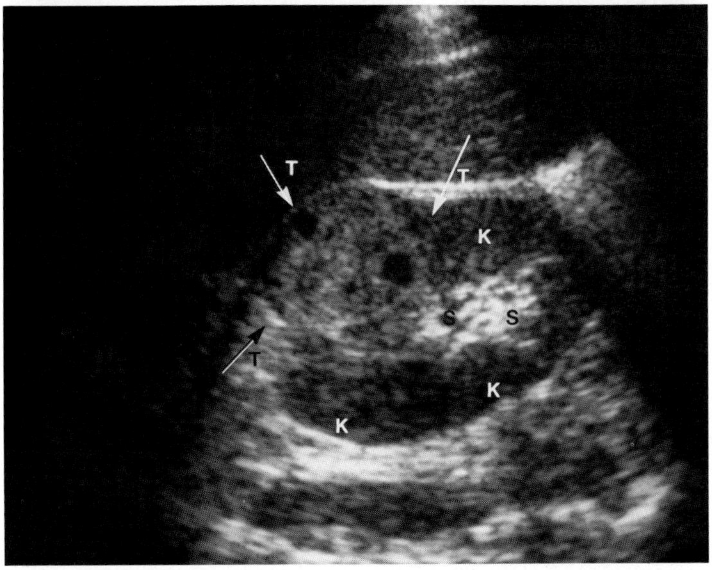

Figure 5.33. Melanoma metastatic to the kidney. A well-marginated, round tumor (*T, arrows*) with two areas of cystic degeneration inside arises from the lateral aspect of the kidney (*K*), slightly impinging upon the renal sinus (*S*) echo complex.

uating transitional cell carcinoma in patients. A high index of suspicion is necessary in patients with microscopic or gross hematuria, and these patients should be evaluated with an upper-tract as well as a lower-tract study.

The sonographer or physician performing echography of the kidney does not often detect transitional cell malignancy of the kidney because most such lesions are not bulky enough to form a grossly visible mass. The effect of transitional cell tumor on the collecting system will readily be found if an isolated hydrocalix or other segmental or global obstructive process has occurred. When bulky tumor is present in an adequate quantity to be detectable with echography, one of three patterns may be recognizable. The most frequent and "classic" presentation is that of a solid mass lying inside or splitting the central renal sinus echo complex (58). Other patterns include amputation of a portion of the renal sinus, invasion of the kidney and replacement of a renal parenchyma with a bulky sonolucent mass, or actual visualization of tumor within the ureter or renal pelvis.

The sonogram shown in Figure 5.35 was made when an elderly man with hematuria was found to have a renal pelvic filling defect on both intravenous urography and retrograde pyelography. The sonogram shows an irregular solid nodule in the collecting system without alteration of acoustical transmission. In particular, there is no acoustic "shadowing," as would be seen with a urinary calculus. Surgery con-

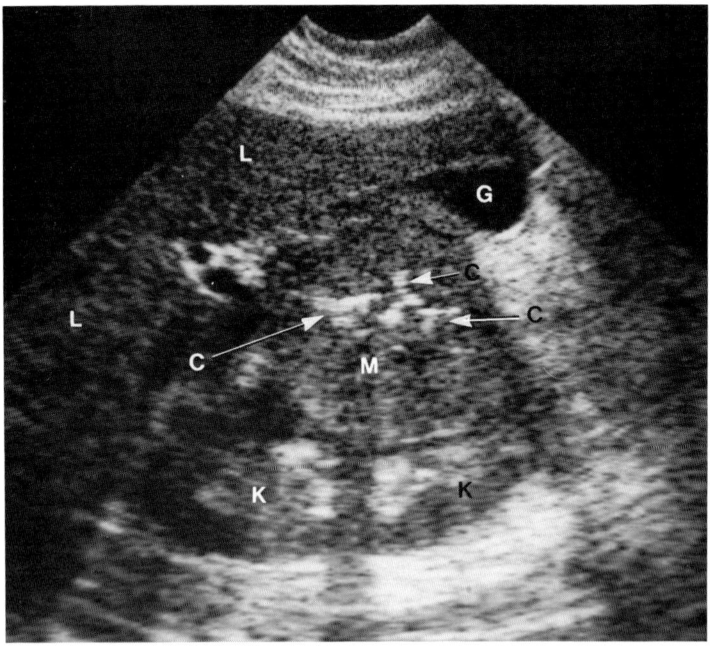

Figure 5.34. Cancer of the ovary metastatic to the kidney. The gallbladder (*G*), under the right lobe of the liver (*L*), is displaced forward by a bulky mass (*M*) arising from the anterior aspect of the right kidney (*K*). The mass contains several calcifications (*C*). Metastatic, calcified ovarian carcinoma was found at nephrectomy.

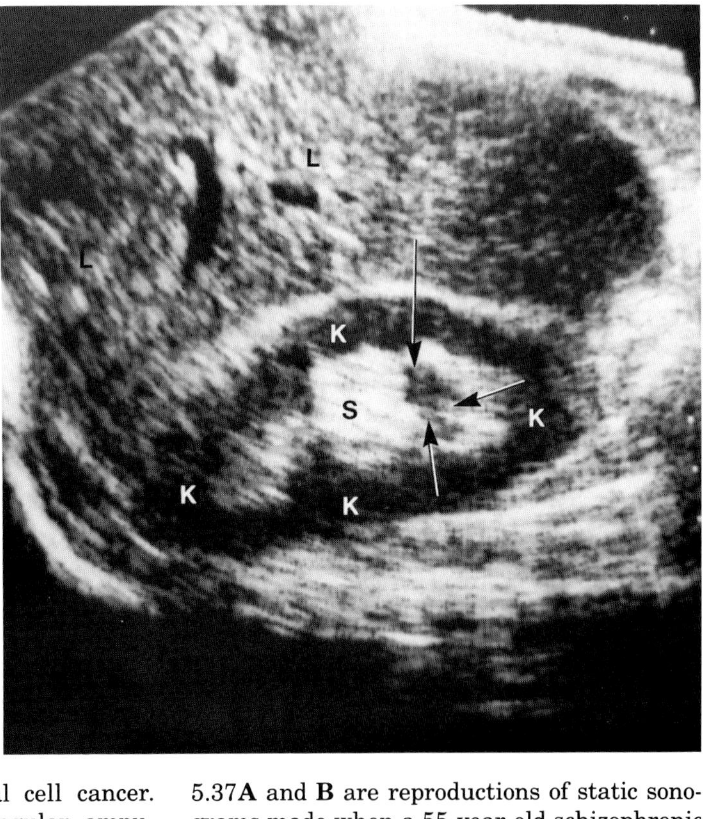

Figure 5.35. Transitional cell carcinoma. There is an irregular nodule of solid tissue (*arrows*) in the inferior portion of the renal sinus echo complex (*S*) of the right kidney (*K*). No acoustical shadowing is present below the lesion, indicating that it is not a stone. An adherent blood clot would have the same appearance. *L*, liver.

firmed a nodule of transitional cell cancer. Figure 5.36 shows partial, irregular amputation of the renal sinus echoes without any definite solid mass visible in the area of amputation. An infiltrating transitional cell malignancy was discovered at surgery. Figure 5.37**A** and **B** are reproductions of static sonograms made when a 55-year-old schizophrenic man was seen passing grossly bloody urine. The right kidney is normal. The left kidney has been nearly replaced by a very large, sonolucent tumor containing only a few scattered me-

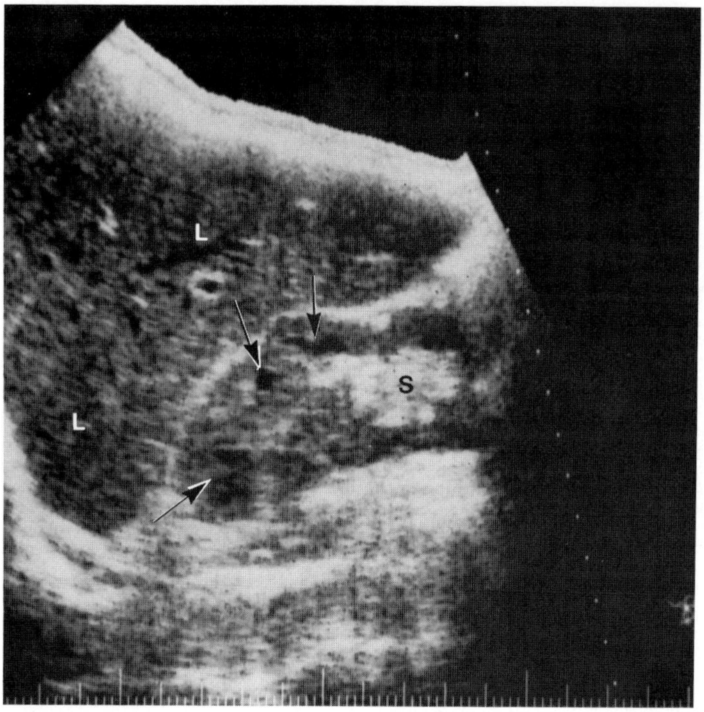

Figure 5.36. Transitional cell carcinoma. The central renal sinus echo complex (*S*) of the right kidney shows irregular amputation in the upper pole region. Sonolucent renal pyramids are preserved (*arrows*). *L*, liver. (Reprinted with permission from Cunningham JJ. Ultrasonic demonstration of renal collecting system invasion by transitional cell cancer. J Clin Ultrasound 1982;10:339–341.)

dium-amplitude reflections. A huge, bulky transitional cell malignancy was removed at the time of nephrectomy. The image shown in Figure 5.38 is a high-resolution view of the left renal pelvis of a 60-year-old man who had gross hematuria and left flank pain. Sonography showed that the renal pelvis was slightly dilated and there were papillary-appearing, irregular, solid masses adherent to the mucosal surface. The appearance would be typical for tumor nodules of transitional cell. The findings were falsely positive, however. Numerous biopsies and urine cytologies were negative. Follow-up sonography showed that the lesions had disappeared. Ultimately, the patient was found to have acute leukemia with low platelets. Presumably, the "classic" sonographic lesions and renal bleeding were caused by the bleeding diathesis of leukemia.

When sonography discloses a bulky mass suspected of being transitional cell tumor, careful examination of the renal vein and inferior vena cava is indicated. Detection of tumor extention into these structures is quite possible with ultrasound, and the clinical implications for such findings are profound (59).

RENAL LYMPHOMA

Lymphoma is common. Wentzell and Berkheiser reported on malignant lymphomas in the *Journal of Urology* 1955 (60). It is reported that 53% of patients with widespread lymphoma will have involvement in the kidney (61). Despite its widespread occurrence in patients with diffuse lymphoma, only about 10 or 15% of the patients will have symptoms that are clinically referable to the kidney. In less than 0.5% is renal lymphoma of an infiltrative type the sole cause of death. Clinically, four important characteristics and patterns have been described for renal lymphoma: solitary nodules, multiple nodules, infiltration (focal or diffuse), and engulfment by contiguous retroperitoneal structures. There is often concomitant thickening of peripelvic fascia and occasional hydronephrosis. In patients with clinically symptomatic renal lymphomas either hematuria or hydronephrosis with obstruction and pain are the main clinical features (62–65).

Many different types of clinical solid neoplasms may involve the kidney, including lymphoma and lymphosarcoma. Intravenous urography reveals generalized renal enlargement with stretching of the calices. Even with marked nodular involvement, the kidney retains its reniform shape (20). Considering lymphomatous disease as a diagnosis in renal masses one must be aware of the fact that metastases to the kidney are twice as common as primary tumors but are very rare.

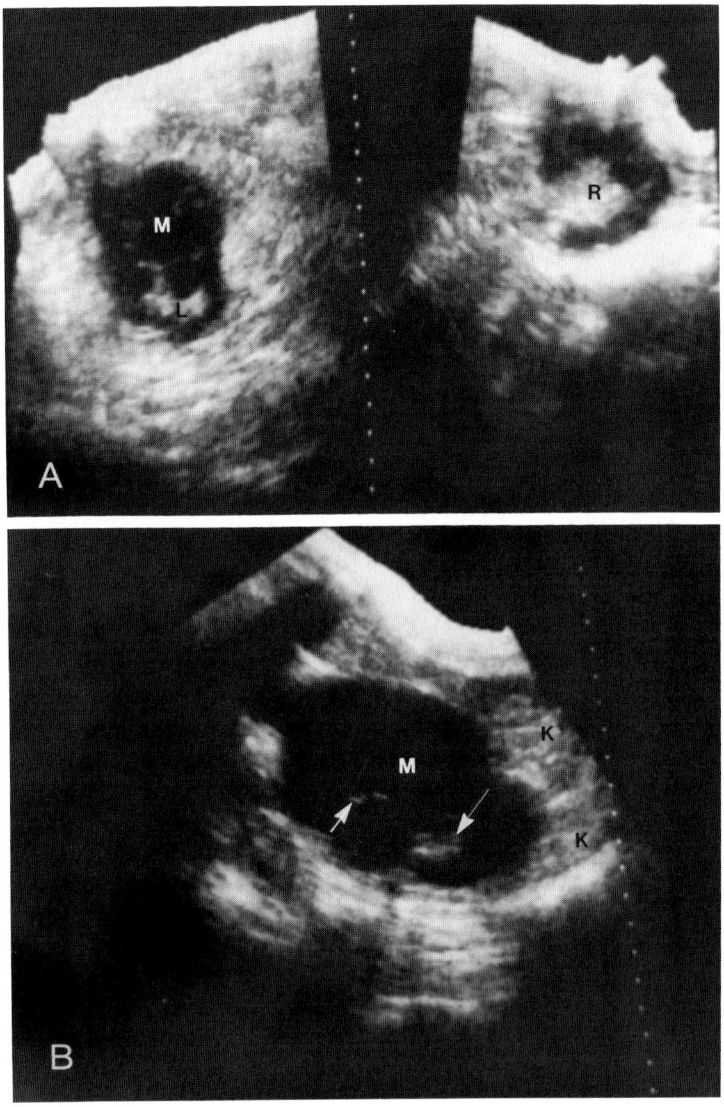

Figure 5.37. **A,** Bulky transitional cell carcinoma. Prone transverse sonogram shows a normal-appearing right kidney (*R*). There is a large, poorly reflective mass (*M*) replacing much of the left kidney (*L*). **B,** Bulky transitional cell carcinoma. Longitudinal view of the left kidney shown in **A** shows a very large sonolucent mass (*M*) arising from a small residual amount of unaffected kidney substance (*K*). The mass contains a few clusters of low-amplitude reflections.

Generally speaking, patients with lymphoma involving the intraabdominal organs are most often evaluated with CT scanning. Sonography can play a role in this disorder when CT findings need further clarification or if patients with lymphoma present with renal failure. In the setting of renal failure, sonography is a quick and efficient way to determine if the cause is ureteral obstruction (stones, lymphadenopathy, or ureteral invasion), replacement of renal substance by tumor nodules, or vascular compression (66).

Sonographic findings of renal lymphoma are classically those of a solid nodule or nodules of variable size that are poorly reflective, have ill-defined borders, no enhanced through transmission, and homogeneous low-amplitude internal echoes (66). The tumor masses may be single, multiple, or diffusely infiltrative (67).

Figure 5.39 shows a conventional example of renal involvement in a man with disseminated non-Hodgkin's lymphoma. A large, weakly reflective mass is visible in the posterior aspect of the upper pole of the kidney. Several smaller nodules are visible just anterior to the central sinus. The kidney is not obstructed.

COLUMN OF BERTIN

A prospective sonographic analysis of the kidneys in over 125 adults, recently reported by

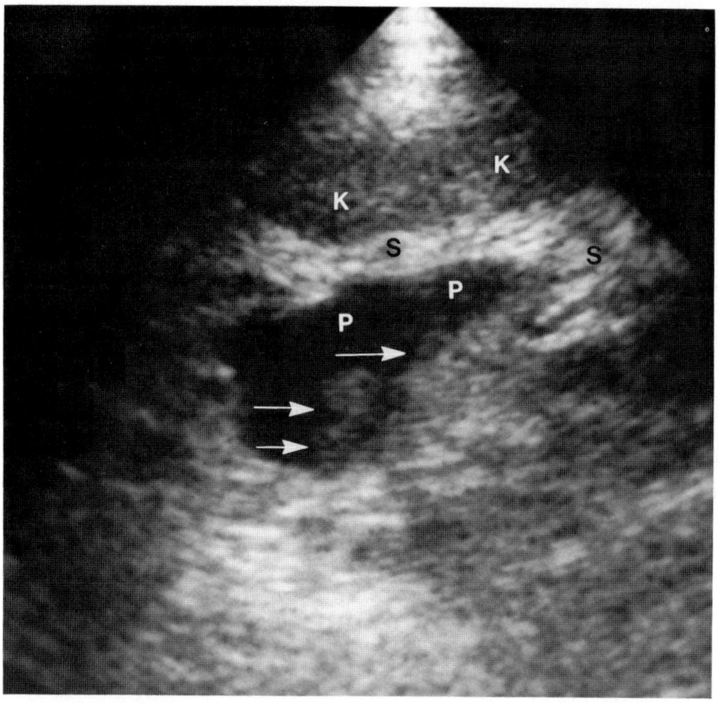

Figure 5.38. Adherent blood clot simulating papillary tumor. High-resolution sonogram of the left kidney in a man with hematuria shows clumps of irregular solid tissue (*arrows*) inside a mildly dilated renal pelvis (*P*) splitting the central sinus echo complex (*S*) of the left kidney (*K*). The lesions later proved to be adherent blood clots rather than papillary transitional cell tumor.

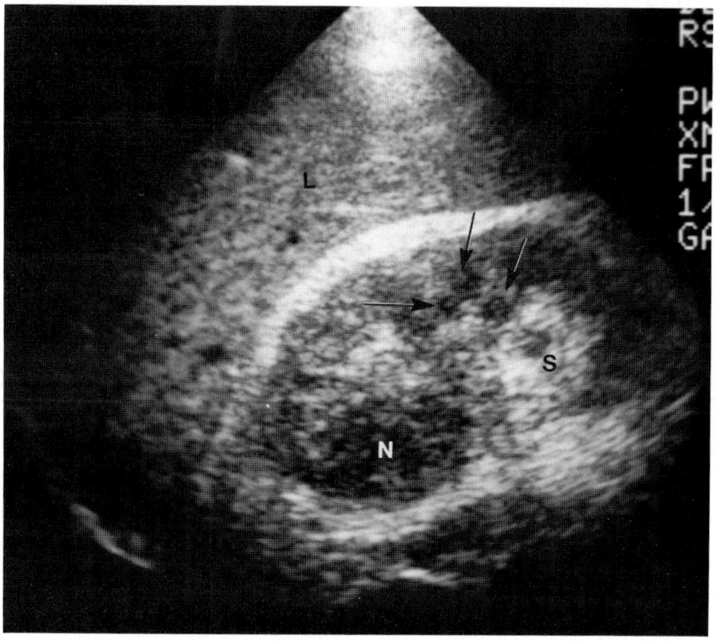

Figure 5.39. Lymphoma of the kidney. There are poorly marginated, sonolucent nodules (*arrows, N*) of a variety of sizes in the right kidney visible under the right lobe of the liver (*L*). A portion of the renal sinus echo complex (*S*) is visible on this coronal section.

Lafortune et al. (68), revealed clinical evidence of radiologic renal mass disease and a high percentage of patients with large columns of Bertin. This entity, however, is not new. It was initially described in 1744 by the French anatomist Joseph Bertin (69). While Bertin's original studies called attention to the concept that some columns are bigger than others and often protrude deeply into the renal medulla, it was not until the late 1960s that ultrasonographers became aware of their need for concern for the differentiation of this lesion from renal cell carcinoma (70–75). The ultrasonic characteristics of a hypertrophied column of Bertin have been defined as isoechoic cortical masses projecting into and indenting the hyperechogenic renal sinus. The in vivo incidence of this phenomenon occurs in almost 45 to 50% of people evaluated in that they have at least one mass. These masses or columns of Bertin can vary in extent and size but must be recognized as benign conditions. Approximately one in seven patients may have two areas of hypertrophied columns.

The hypertrophied column of Bertin has been a challenge, especially since the use of IVP with nephrotomography has become routine. Because it does simulate in many respects a renal mass, this entity may have been responsible for unnecessary nephrectomies prior to the days of angiography. Many synonyms exist for the term "column of Bertin," including renal pseudotumor, focal nodular hyperplasia, cortical invagination with prominent column of Bertin, lobar sysmorphism, benign cortical rest, cortical nodule, and recently, large cloisons (69–75).

The ultrasound characteristics of these hypertrophied columns are unique, and the only possible pitfall in differential diagnosis may be that of cancer. However, with careful analysis of the echogenicity of such a cyst and its acoustic enhancement, differentiation can be made from hypertrophied columns of Bertin. Of more than passing interest for the clinician is that the vast majority of these hypertrophied columns do not distort the renal architecture, in terms of the outer contour of the kidney, in any way. This is clearly not the case in the vast majority of renal cell carcinomas, and this is an important characteristic that helps distinguish this from a hypernephroma.

A large renal cortical column of Bertin is the most common benign mass encountered by the physician or technologist doing renal sonography. Most often the mass is found on the left at the junction of the upper and middle thirds. The mass consists of normal renal cortex intruding in a thumb-like fashion into the renal sinus, so its echographic appearance is entirely predictable. A typical examination is shown in Figure 5.40. A large, blunt nodule, isoechoic with normal renal substance, intrudes into and is enveloped by the renal sinus. No acoustical shadowing or enhancement is present. The renal border is not deformed. When all characteristic sonographic features of a large renal column are fulfilled, as in this instance, no further patient evaluation is needed (68).

A somewhat atypical instance of large column of Bertin that did require additional radiologic study is shown in Figure 5.41. The patient had left flank pain and inflammatory cells in the urine. Sonography shows a large focal mass in the anterior aspect of the left kidney. The mass is isoechoic with adjacent renal cortex which is being "looked at" with the most perpendicular portion of the sonic beam. The polar and posterior portions of the kidney are not as

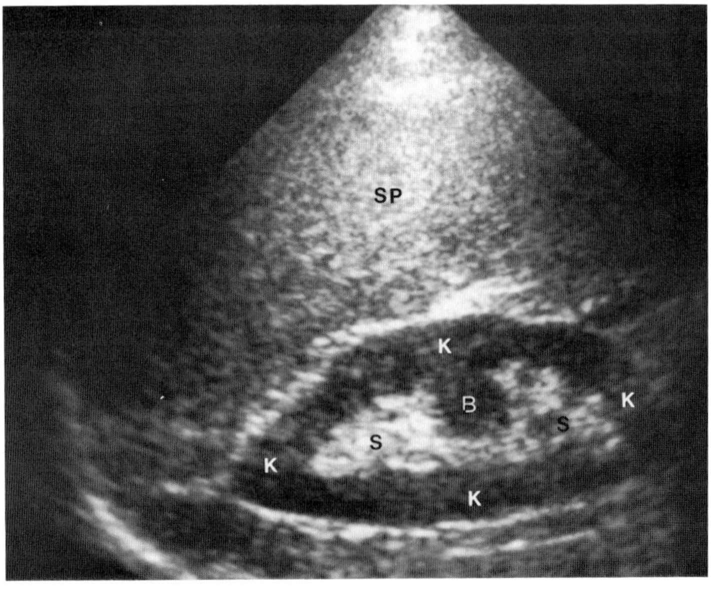

Figure 5.40. Column of Bertin. There is a large renal column of Bertin (*B*) intruding into the renal sinus echo complex (*S*) of the left kidney (*K*). The renal column has a thumb-like configuration, and the column is isoechoic with normal renal parenchyma. *SP,* spleen.

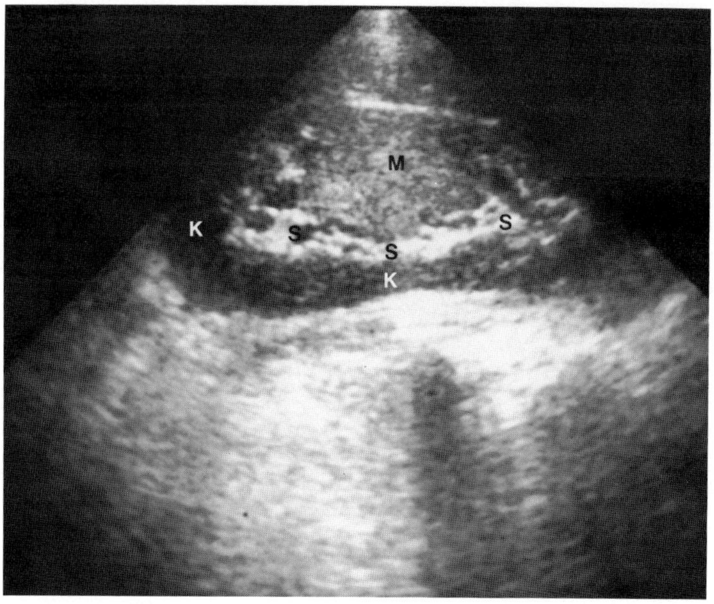

Figure 5.41. Atypical column of Bertin. A rather large reflective mass (*M*) indents the renal sinus echo complex (*S*). The mass is isoechoic with immediately adjacent renal parenchyma but it is less reflective than the kidney tissue at the extreme poles (*K*) of the kidney. The mass proved to be a large nodule of normal renal parenchyma.

reflective. In a setting similar to this, CT scans, nuclear renal scans, or arteriography may be required to exclude an abscess, tumor, or hematoma. The lesions shown in Figure 5.40 ultimately proved to be nothing more than a large renal column.

ANGIOMYOLIPOMA

Angiomyolipomas are generally benign tumors composed of fat, muscle, and blood vessels. A renal lesion corresponding to angiomyolipomas was first described by Morgan et al. in 1911 (76). The abundance of these three biologic elements is quite varied, and tumors may range predominantly from lipomatous to leiomyomatous. Angiomyolipomas are sharply demarcated from adjacent renal parenchyma, and local invasion is rare.

Fifty to eighty percent of renal angiomyolipomas are associated with tuberous sclerosis (77). Tuberous sclerosis is a syndrome transmitted by an autosomal dominant gene exhibiting incomplete penetrance. Characteristic findings of this include epilepsy, mental retardation, adenoma sebaceum, subungual fibromas, and cystic lesions of the lung.

The natural history of these tumors has not been well described and the stimulus for growth remains unknown. Many angiomyolipomas remain clinically occult. However, those that present symptomatically typically do so with hematuria, flank pain, or mass. We had a patient recently who presented with the clinical symptoms of shock (78).

The question clinically is what to do with these lesions and how to follow up on the patients. Patients whose tumors are less than 4 cm and who have not shown any sign of progression may be studied with periodic ultrasound or CT scans. For lesions that grow larger than 4 cm or lesions that initially present larger than this size with any suggestive history of intrarenal bleeding, these patients may be managed either with selective renal arterial embolization or, as in the case of several patients we have seen, with partial nephrectomy.

The majority of angiomyolipomas studied in the ultrasound laboratory are seen incidentally when renal sonography or sonography of some other organ in the abdomen, such as the gallbladder, is being imaged (79). Other times, the patient has some specific complaint, such as tuberous sclerosis or fat-containing mass seen at urography, which prompts a specific sonogram for angiomyolipoma.

The echographic features of these choristomas are entirely predictable. These masses contain variable amounts of fat, muscle, and vascular tissue and these elements cause a brightly reflective mass (80). Small angiomyolipomas found by accident while scanning for a nonurological complaint are shown in Figures 5.42 and 5.43. In each instance, a very strongly reflective, very bright small nodule is

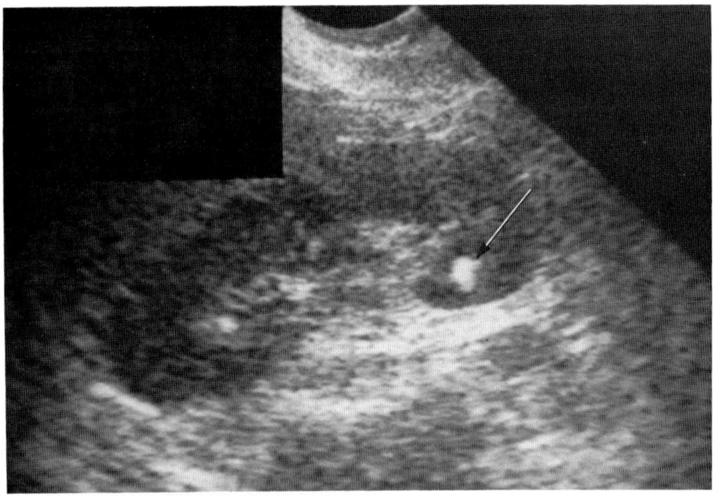

Figure 5.42. Small angiomyolipoma. A small incidental angiomyolipoma presents as a very focal, brightly echogenic mass (*arrow*) in the lower pole of the kidney.

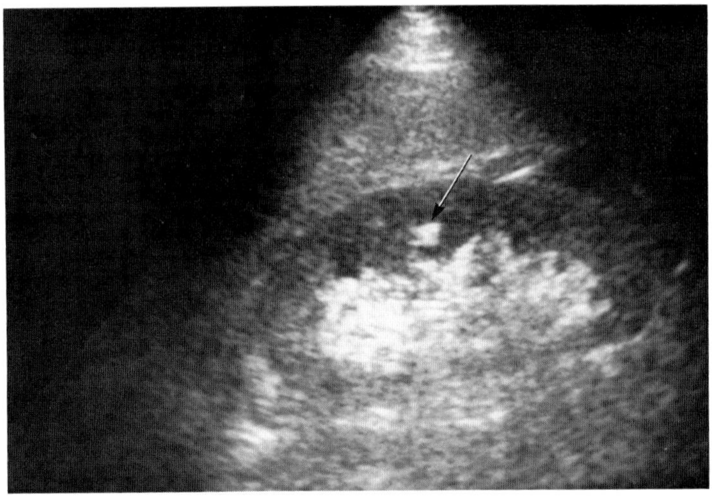

Figure 5.43. Small angiomyolipoma. A brightly echogenic angiomyolipoma (*arrow*) can be seen in the anterior midkidney.

visible against the more lucent renal parenchyma. Neither lesion shows acoustical shadowing or "ring down," but small angiomyolipomas can do either under the right technical circumstances, particularly when imaging a lesion close to the body surface with a high-frequency instrument. If there is any clinical evidence to suggest malignancy in a setting such as this and it is crucial to exclude hypernephroma, CT scanning for the presence of fat is indicated. Fat does not occur in hypernephromas, so the most strenuous effort must be made at the time of CT scanning to demonstrate this material (81). If fat is found, the confident diagnosis of angiomyolipoma has been established.

A larger angiomyolipoma can be seen in Figure 5.44. The images were made when a young physician collapsed during a cardiac catheterization procedure. Figure 5.44**A** shows that the patient has a huge angiomyolipoma arising from the lateral aspect of the right kidney. The lesion is so highly attenuating that only the more superficial portion is fully illuminated with the ultrasound beam. He also had smaller tumors in the parenchyma of both the right and left kidneys (Figure 5.44**A** and **B**). The treatment for him was a partial right nephrectomy. There were no clinical stigmata of tuberous sclerosis or similar disorder.

The kidney consists of several individual elements that fuse together, leaving the potential for small irregularities and spaces in the renal border. On occasion, these spaces may fill with extensions of renal sinus fat, a normal variant sometimes called the "junctional parenchymal

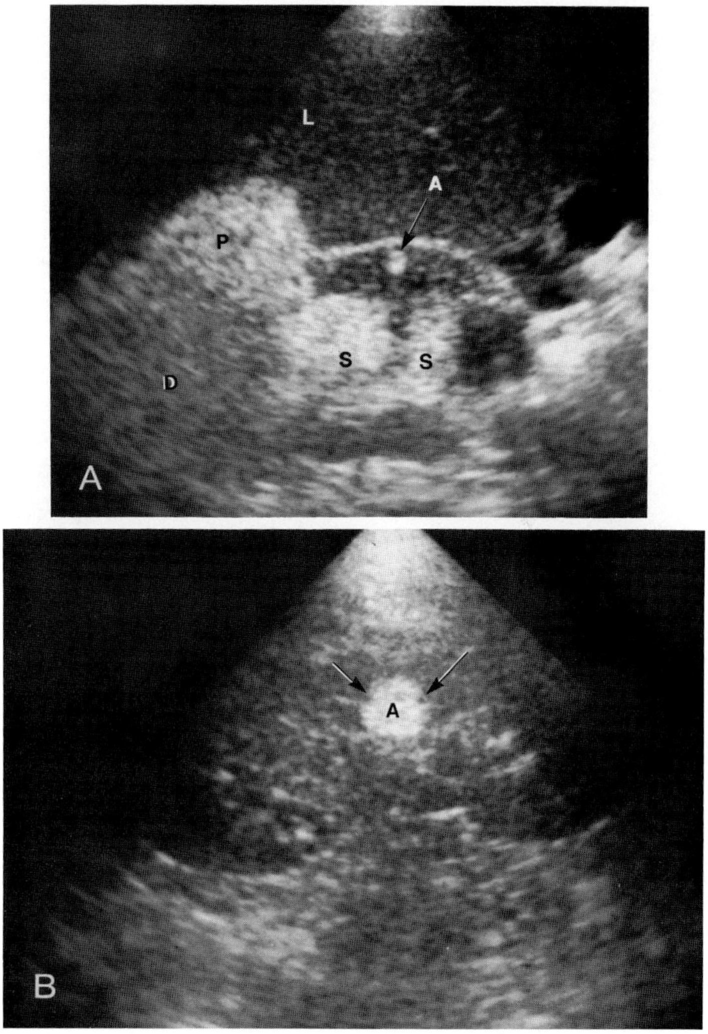

Figure 5.44. **A,** Large angiomyolipoma, right kidney. There is a very large, bulky angiomyolipoma arising from the lateral aspect of the right kidney. The portion proximal (*P*) to the transducer is brightly echogenic. Beam attenuation causes the more distal portion (*D*) to be less brightly illuminated. The reflectivity of the tumor is close to the reflectivity of the renal sinus echo complex (*S*). A small cortical angiomyolipoma is also visible (*arrow, A*). *L,* liver. **B,** Large angiomyolipoma. Sonogram of the left kidney made in the patient whose right kidney is shown in **A.** There is a small, rounded cortical angiomyolipoma (*arrows, A*) in the midportion of the kidney.

defect." A junctional parenchymal defect may easily be mistaken for a small angiomyolipoma, as shown in Figure 5.45. The finding is a small, brightly reflective, triangular collection of fat found most frequently in the anterior aspect of the upper pole of the right kidney (82).

RENAL ONCOCYTOMA

A preoperative diagnosis of renal oncocytomas has been difficult. Several investigators have attempted to classify and categorize the various ultrasonic considerations and the diagnosis (83). In a recent series of 15 histologically confirmed renal oncocytomas, lesions were evaluated for homogeneity, echogenicity, margination, venous invasion, and nodal enlargement. Sixty-six percent of the tumors were less than 5.5 cm in diameter, homogeneous, and well circumscribed. Three lesions were greater than 8 cm in diameter and contained areas of central necrosis or calcification. These three were nonspecific for renal oncocytoma. One lesion of the larger size, 12 cm, contained a central scar. These masses of the larger size tend to be inhomogeneous and, at best, moderately circumscribed. Since about 6 to 8% of renal cell carcinomas have this appearance, the homogeneous, well-marginated renal mass that is isoechoic with cortex and less than 5 cm in diameter is as likely to represent a renal cell carcinoma as it is an oncocytoma. This clinical entity of renal oncocytomas has only been recognized in the last 14 years with the work of Klein and others. Clinicians have become increasingly aware of this neoplasm as a distinct pathologic entity. Various descrip-

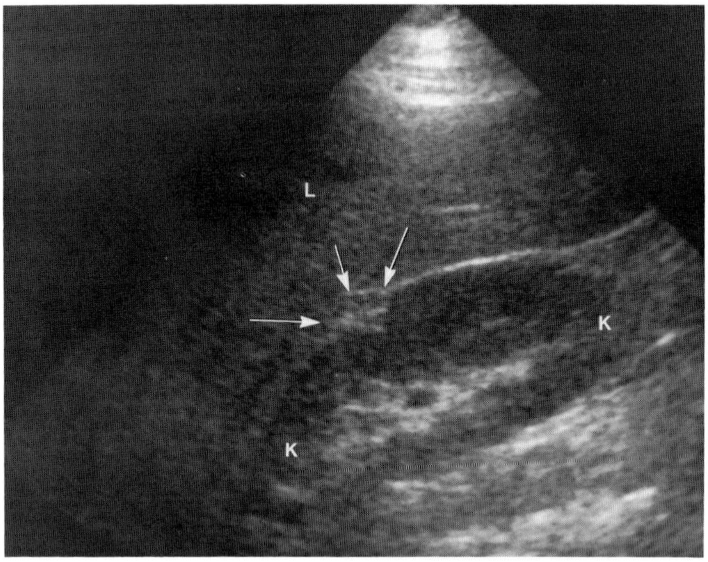

Figure 5.45. Junctional parenchymal defect. There is a small, triangular collection of fat (*arrows*) in a groove at the junction of the upper and middle thirds of the right kidney (*K*). This normal variant can easily be mistaken for an angiomyolipoma. *L*, liver.

tions of its angiographic and CT characteristics have been reported, and yet specific criteria for precise preoperative diagnosis have not been established (84–92).

Ultrasound has become the pivotal mechanism for distinguishing cystic from solid lesions and has proved helpful in several cases of oncocytoma diagnosis in our institution. The preoperative suggestion of an oncocytoma would offer the surgeon the choice of fine-needle aspiration biopsy for cytology prior to exploration. This has been used by several investigators (93, 94). As a standardized approach this may still be somewhat controversial. However, needle aspiration is particularly useful in selected patients who may be debilitated or in those with a solitary kidney. In these patients, preoperative distinction between malignant and benign tumors would influence the extent and type of surgery performed. If cytologic evaluation revealed a typical well-differentiated, large uniform cell with small, smooth nuclei and an eosinophilic cytoplasm (oncocytes), the surgeon may elect to perform less than radical surgery. Oncocytes, however, may be present in small numbers in renal cell carcinoma and that is why this criterion alone cannot be used for establishing the benign nature of lesions. Literature does suggest that if sonographic findings suggest a homogeneous lesion smaller than 5.5 cm that is isoechoic with renal parenchyma and well-demarcated margins, this should alert the physician to consider the possibility of an oncocytoma. However, small renal cell carcinomas less than 4 cm may be homogeneously solid with well-defined margins as well. These tumors account for about 5 to 6% of renal cell carcinomas (20). Finally, tumors larger than 6 cm with necrosis or calcification cannot be sonographically distinguished from renal cell carcinoma. Several investigators have reported isolated cases of renal oncocytoma with "spoke-wheel" appearance on sonographic evaluation similar to that seen in angiography, but this criterion cannot be taken as 100% diagnostic (95).

Renal oncocytomas represent approximately 6% of all renal tumors that were preoperatively considered to be carcinoma. Also, others would agree that since 1976 the incidence appears to be increasing (89). To cloud the issue further, the high survival rate in older studies of renal cell carcinoma patients, especially among those with low-grade, well-differentiated tumors, could be a result of misclassifications of oncocytomas as renal cell cancers. In general, the gross picture of an oncocytoma is that of a well-demarcated, partially encapsulated, rounded, solid mass. They characteristically have a tan brown color and they range in size from only tenths of centimeters to as large as 26 cm (84, 86, 95, 96). This is in distinction to the necrotic, yellow, often invasive characteristics of the typical renal cell tumor. Despite these obvious differences between the classic oncocytoma and a renal cell carcinoma, confusion still exists, and it is only with a high index of suspicion that the ultrasonographer can alert the clinician to the possibility of oncocytoma diagnosis and may thereby obtain cytologic fine-needle aspiration and help in certain cases of this difficult entity to diagnose.

The sonographic appearance of oncocytoma is more or less identical with that of a hypernephroma or any other solid mass except for two specific sets of circumstances. Small, well-defined renal masses less than 5.5 cm in diameter should prompt consideration of oncocytoma as a diagnostic possibility, even though small hypernephromas may have an identical presentation (83). If a homogeneously reflective renal mass is fairly large and it contains a stellate-central "scar" or lucent zone, oncocytoma should also be considered in the differential diagnosis (83, 97). It is worth emphasizing, however, that the absolute diagnosis of oncocytoma can be established only at surgery or needle biopsy.

Figure 5.46 was made when a patient with Goodpasture's syndrome had renal sonography because of rising creatinine. The kidneys were not obstructed, but a very small rounded mass was found arising from the anterior medial cortex. The mass was well demarcated and isoechogenic with normal renal substance. The preoperative sonographic diagnosis of oncocytomas was confirmed at later surgery. Figure 5.47 shows the left kidney of the patient whose right kidney, containing a hypernephroma, has been previously presented in Figure 5.24. Sonography of the left kidney as shown in this image shows a large, lobulated, highly reflective renal mass with good acoustic transmission. The interface between the mass and adjacent kidney is ill defined. The right kidney had to be removed because of an extensive infiltrating hypernephroma. The mass in the left kidney was removed with partial nephrectomy to spare renal tissue. It proved to be an oncocytoma.

Figure 5.48 shows a renal mass with classic features of oncocytoma. A large tumor is homogeneously echogenic and there is a large, central, stellate "scar." Nephrectomy, however, revealed a conventional renal adenocarcinoma.

INTRARENAL COMPENSATORY HYPERTROPHY

The condition of intrarenal compensatory hypertrophy may occur with varying frequency in patients who have suffered inflammatory renal diseases or subtotal renal infarcts. Essentially, the clinical problem is whether or not this is a mass that has the characteristics of being malignant and should be operated on. This is often seen in cases with pyelonephritic kidneys in which scarring occurs in the polar area of the kidney, and the middle portion of the kidney may hypertrophy and give rise to a pseudotumor effect on intravenous pyelography. Patients with such problems need to have ultrasound evaluation for definitive diagnosis.

The single confirmed case of this entity we have seen showed a predictable echographic pattern (Figure 5.49). There is a smooth bulge of tissue isoechoic with normal renal substance

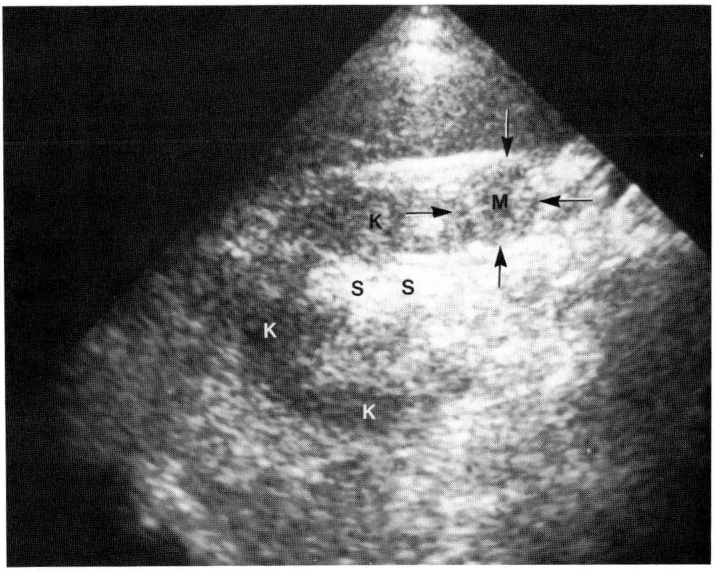

Figure 5.46. Small oncocytoma. A rounded mass (*arrows, M*) arises from the medial border of the kidney. The mass is isoechoic with normal kidney. The renal sinus echo complex (*S*) and kidney parenchyma (*K*) are normal.

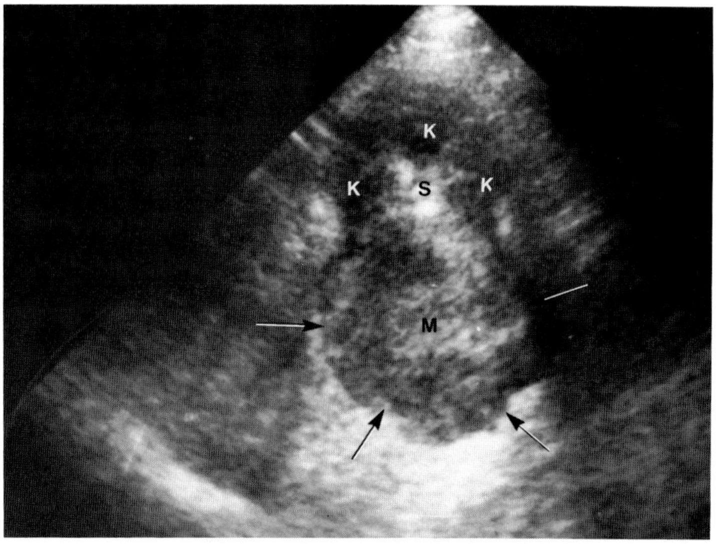

Figure 5.47. Large oncocytoma. A bulky, lobulated mass (*M, arrows*) blends imperceptibly with normal renal sinus echoes (*S*) and renal parenchyma (*K*). The mass, an oncocytoma, is indistinguishable from a hypernephroma.

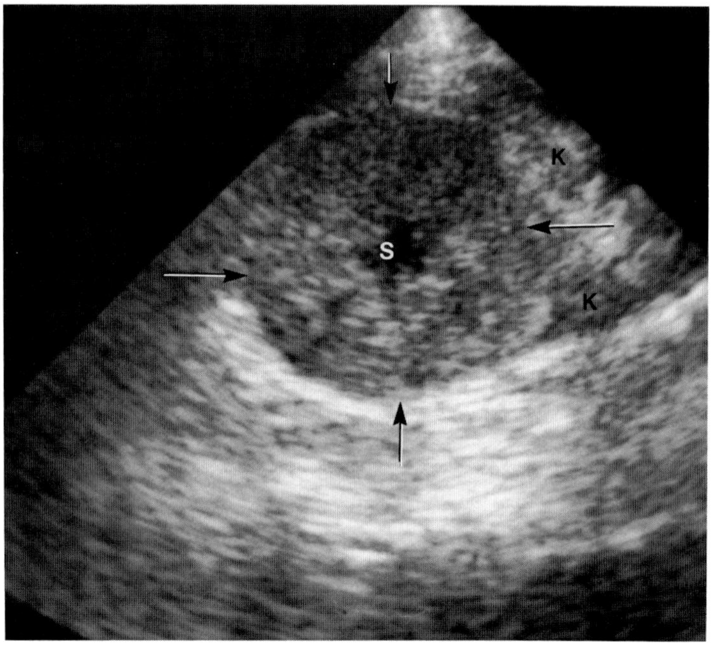

Figure 5.48. Hypernephroma simulating oncocytoma. A bulky mass (*arrows*) arises from adjacent kidney (*K*) tissue. The mass contains a stellate scar, a finding associated with oncocytomas. At surgery, a conventional hypernephroma was found.

in an otherwise severely atrophic kidney damaged by reflux nephropathy and chronic infection.

RENAL INFARCT

Renal infarct may be segmental or complete. In cases of complete renal infarction the entire kidney, over time, becomes small. Clinical symptoms of acute renal infarct simulate those of trauma: pain, decreased perfusion, and poor visualization on IVP. The injury responsible for this in the case of trauma is an intraarterial intimal tear which produces an intimal flap, leading to nonperfusion of the renal unit. In case of a partial infarct, hypertension may occur. Patients with incomplete infarction need routine follow-up to monitor for hypertension (98).

The clinical symptom complex associated with infarction is called the postinfarction syndrome. This is typified by flank pain, nausea and occasional fever. This has been associated

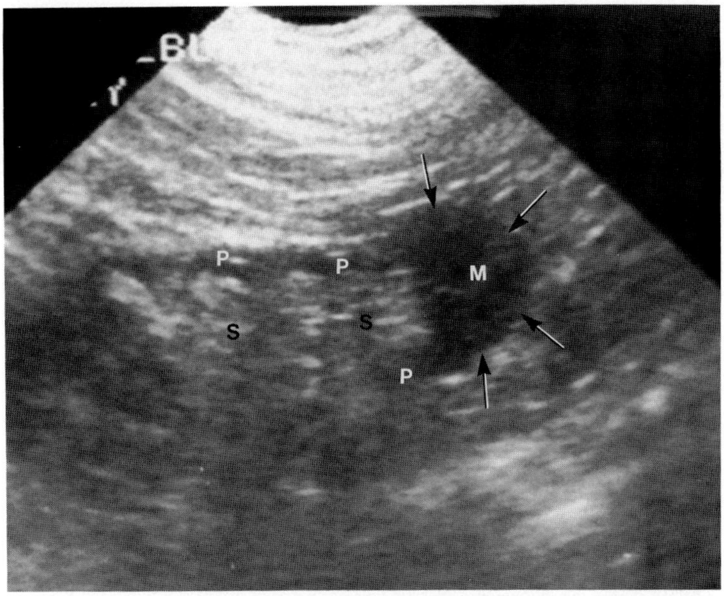

Figure 5.49. Intrarenal compensatory hypertrophy. There is an isoechoic, smooth mass (*arrows, M*) arising from the lower pole of the kidney. The kidney parenchyma (*P*) is very atrophic. Renal sinus echoes (*S*) are unremarkable.

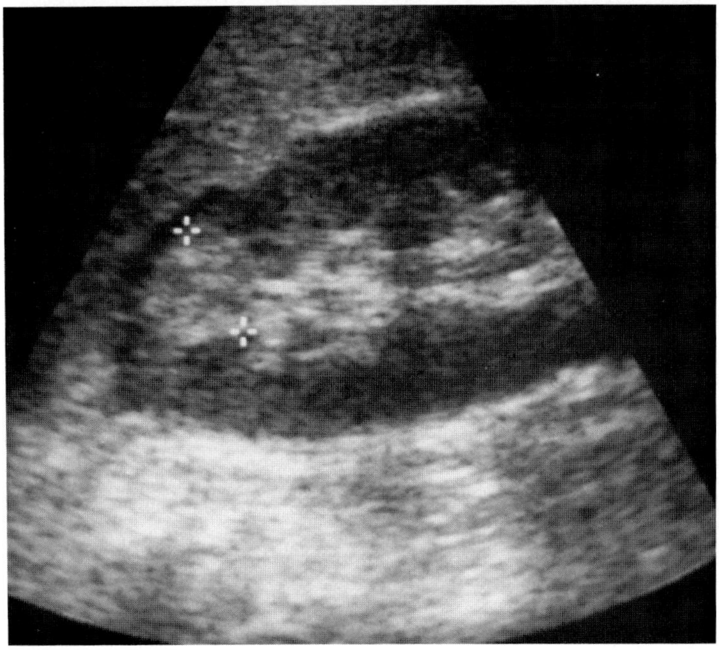

Figure 5.50. Recent infarct of the kidney. A brightly echogenic, rounded infarct can be seen between the asterisks. The lesion was not present on sonograms done 1 day earlier, prior to percutaneous transluminal angioplasty of the right renal artery.

with patients who have intentional renal infarction prenephrectomy as a planned part of a subsequent nephrectomy for renal cancer.

Most renal infarcts will involve compromise of the main renal artery, and the sonographic changes will mostly present as a diffuse decrease in the size of the kidney with global atrophy of the renal parenchyma. Focal infarcts caused by embolic disease can cause mass lesions as shown in Figures 5.50 and 5.51. Later, a deep focal cortical scar may form at the site of the infarct. The image shown in Figure 5.50 was made 1 day after transluminal angioplasty of the right renal artery. The patient began to have right flank pain and hematuria at the conclusion of the procedure. Sonography shows a rounded, brightly reflective zone in the upper pole of the right kidney. A hemorrhagic

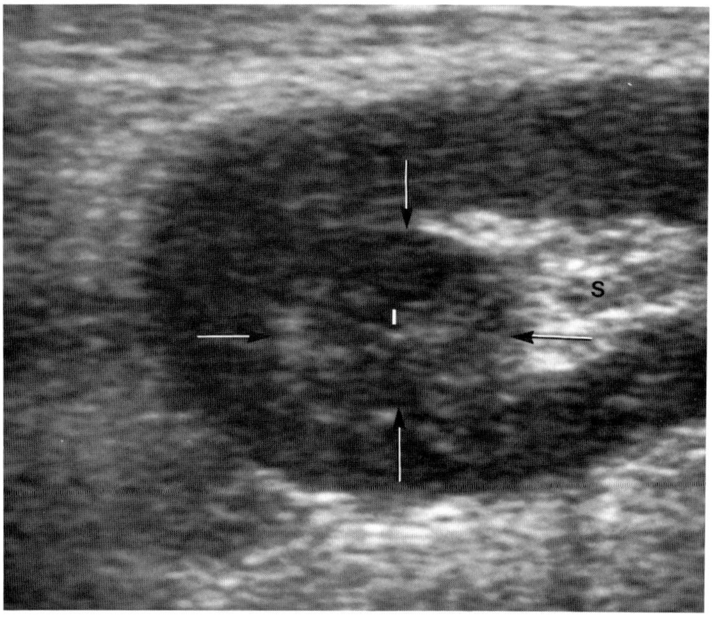

Figure 5.51. Remote infarct of the kidney. A rounded, poorly marginated mass (*arrows, I*) partly effaces the renal sinus echo complex (*S*). The mass contains scattered low-level linear reflections.

infarct caused by renal emboli was confirmed with repeat angiography. The remainder of the kidney was normal on both sonography and the repeat angiogram. A focal old infarct was found with needle biopsy of the kidney whose image is shown in Figure 5.51. The renal sinus is partly effaced by a rounded mass containing a few low-level reflections and exhibiting normal acoustic transmission compared to normal kidney. Necrotic renal tissue and chronic inflammatory cells were found, presumably caused by an embolus when the transplant had been done several weeks earlier.

The echographic appearance of a renal infarct cannot be described in terms of "typical changes." The appearance will vary depending on the age of the infarct, underlying renal disease, extent of the lesion, and influence of any treatment that might have been administered.

RENAL HEMATOMA

The most important clinical aspect of renal hematoma is the accurate demonstration of the structural and functional entity of the entire urinary tract because it is important to have this anatomical information in planning appropriate therapy, whether conservative nonoperative or surgical (operative) therapy. Renal trauma is often the cause of perirenal hematoma or renal hematoma. This may be associated with a motor vehicle accident or with percutaneous biopsy of the kidney. Patients suspected of having renal trauma are ordinarily evaluated initially by excretory urography or CT. Ultrasound has recently played a complementary role when the kidney cannot be visualized with intravenous urography or when the anatomic detail of the kidney requires better definition. Additionally, ultrasound is very useful in evaluating a perinephric fluid collection, which may occur with perirenal or renal hematomas. Ultrasound is useful in evaluating patients who are clinically stable, especially for type II trauma. Type I trauma is a renal contusion that may show little in the way of clinical signs and symptoms except for microscopic hematuria. A type III injury usually presents with shock and a shadow kidney and is often evaluated in the emergency room by emergency CT scanning or arteriography after the patient has been stabilized with large amounts of fluid replacement. The type II injury is a renal fracture that in most instances has a clinical picture of a patient who is stable, in whom microscopic or gross hematuria may occur, but who otherwise does not require any operative intervention. It is this patient who is at risk for developing a urinoma or a perirenal hematoma (99–101). In these instances ultrasound is very helpful in following a patient's progress longitudinally.

It is not possible to describe a "classic" sonographic appearance for hematomas related to the kidney and urinary tract. Much depends on the age of the lesion, the space in which the blood is located, the presence or absence of organization, fibrosis, or scar formation, and the speed of blood clot lysis relative to the time of sonography. Some common clinical examples follow.

Figure 5.52 is an image derived from a sonogram done 1 day after percutaneous renal biopsy. The patient had pain and hematuria beginning several hours after the procedure, which had apparently been uncomplicated. There were prebiopsy sonograms available to compare with those shown in Figure 5.52 to ascertain changes. The lateral border of the right kidney is swollen and there is a homogeneous increase in echoes at the site of the parenchymal biopsy, indicating increased reflectivity caused by tissue hemorrhage. Blood in the adjacent perinephric space appears quite different. The thin layer of extrarenal acute hemorrhage is echolucent and appears much like any other uncomplicated fluid that might appear in this body space.

Perinephric hematoma 3 days old had quite a different appearance in a patient whose kidney was perforated during the placement of a ureteral stent for retroperitoneal fibrosis (Figure 5.53). Blood entrapped in the space between the renal fascia and the renal capsule was moderately homogeneously reflective, more reflective than adjacent normal kidney. The renal border is deformed by the tense mass. Two bright echoes from portions of the ureteral stent are visible in the central sinus region.

A third example of acute hematoma can be seen in Figure 5.54. In this instance, an elderly lady with a vague history of falling 1 week earlier presented to her local hospital with right flank pain and hematuria. Urography showed a poorly functioning, displaced right kidney. CT scan was said to show a large necrotic right renal tumor invading the inferior vena cava, and the patient was referred for nephrectomy. Sonography demonstrated a markedly compressed but normal appearing right kidney. There was a huge, evenly echogenic, subcapsular mass present. The mass greatly displaced the inferior vena cava medially and anteriorly and greatly narrowed the inferior vena cava. CT scans and arteriograms confirmed the sonographic impression of subcapsular hematoma. There was no evidence of tumor. The age of the lesion was unknown, but the patient had complained of symptoms for about 1 week prior to sonography.

RENAL ABSCESS

Acute pyelonephritis in adult patients will resolve promptly after appropriate antibiotic

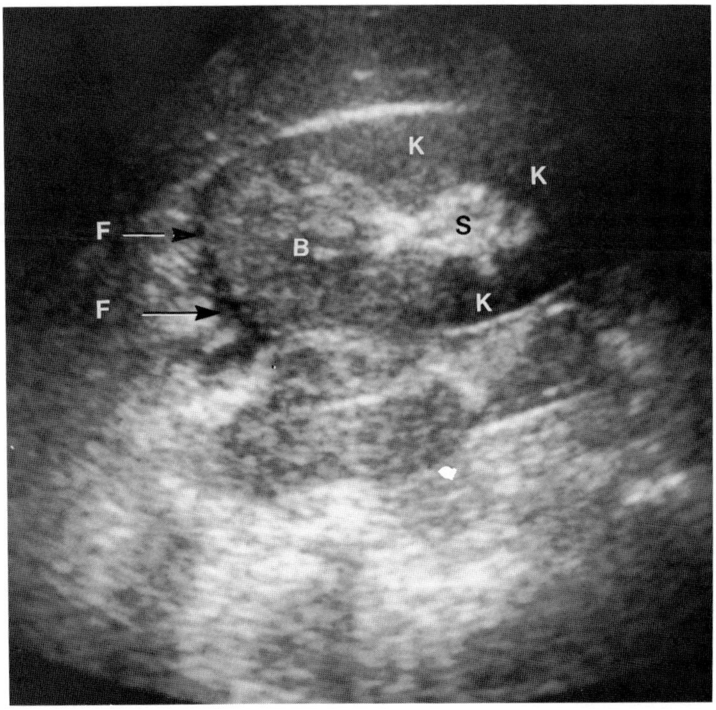

Figure 5.52. Postbiopsy hemorrhage. A poorly defined zone of increased reflectivity (*B*) can be seen at the biopsy site. There is a small collection of perinephric fluid (*F*), presumably blood. Renal sinus echoes (*S*) and kidney parenchyma (*K*) are otherwise normal.

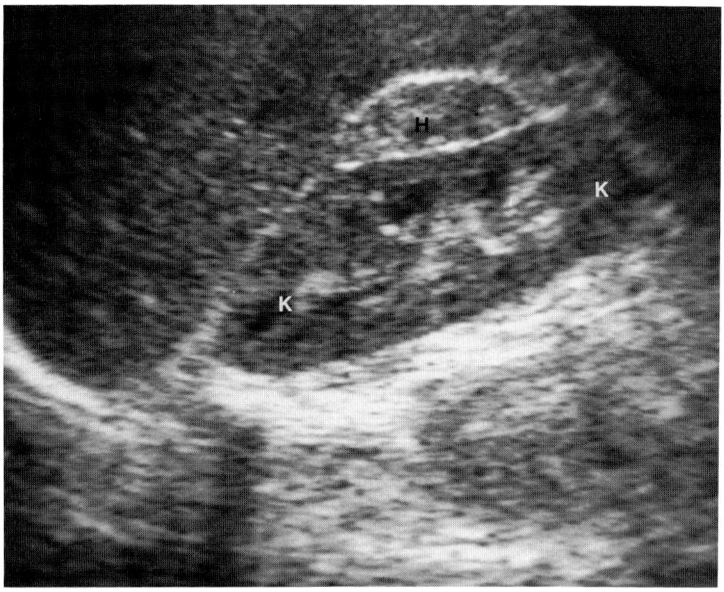

Figure 5.53. Perirenal hematoma. A moderately reflective, oval-shaped hematoma (*H*) lies between the renal fascia and the renal capsule at the site where the kidney was perforated with a ureteral catheter. The kidney (*K*) appears normal.

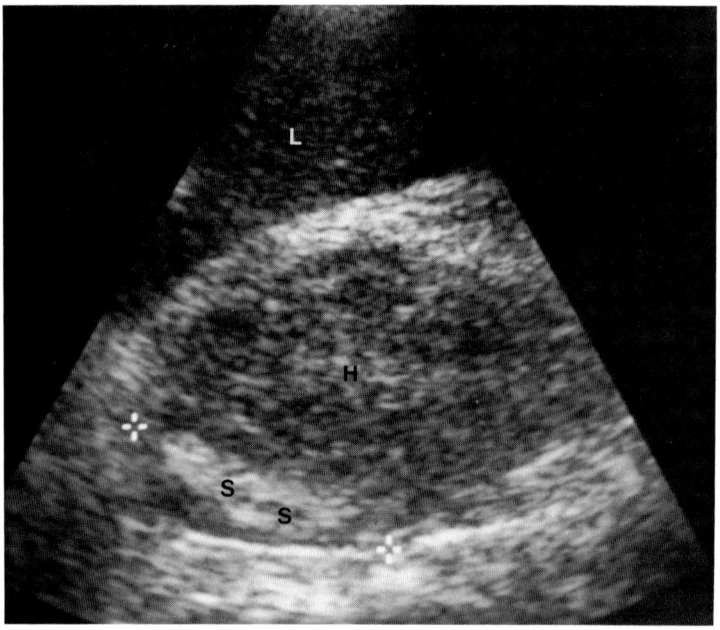

Figure 5.54. Large subcapsular hematoma. A normal kidney (between *asterisks*) with a normal renal sinus echo complex (*S*) is very compressed by a huge, diffusely reflective, subcapsular hematoma (*H*). *L*, liver.

therapy has been instituted, providing obstruction or congenital abnormalities leading to decreased antibiotic delivery to the tissue are not present. Recent radiological literature described characteristics of infection both on CT scanning and sonography (102). Patients who fail to respond to initial medical management require evaluation for obstruction or an abscess, and therefore radiologic investigation is necessary. Until recently, IVP and arteriography have been the primary methods used for evaluating patients with suspected renal abscesses. However, this has changed over the last several years with the advance of ultrasonography and CT, and these have largely replaced the aforementioned studies. Several reports have documented the use of both these modalities in the diagnosis (and in some cases the treatment) of perirenal and renal infections (102–109). Abscesses must be at least 2 to 3 cm

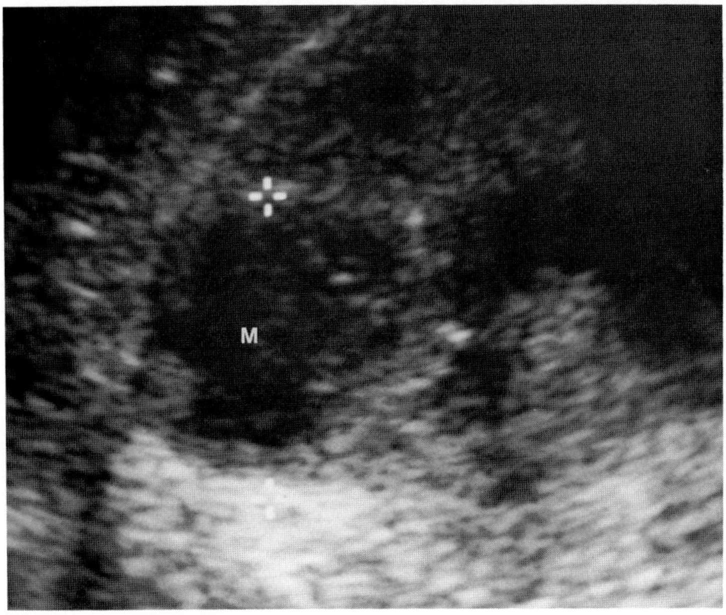

Figure 5.55. Focal nephronia. A large, weakly reflective mass (*M, asterisks*) with thin overlying cortex. Only a few scattered low-level echoes are visible within the localized inflammatory mass.

in diameter to be routinely detected sonographically. Abscesses smaller than 1 cm clearly have been missed by ultrasound. In addition to the size limitation, ultrasound cannot define gradual thickening or detect slight alterations in perinephric fat, as these alterations obviously occur in increments smaller than 1 cm. Ultrasound, however, is very useful in directing skinny-needle aspiration of suspected abscess masses and, in cases, may be the approach that leads to percutaneous drainage of these abscesses with antibiotic irrigation. Ultrasound may often underestimate the extent of involvement of renal masses that are inflammatory in nature because of its limitations in detecting small masses. Ultrasound can also be useful in the diagnosis of focal bacterial nephritis, because these appear as hypoechoic solid masses without definable walls.

Abscesses, however, appear as either a complex fluid collection or a hypoechoic mass with poor through transmission. Other characteristics may demonstrate a focal hypoechoic lesion with a solid mass in the entities called focal or multifocal bacterial nephritis.

CT examination is probably more useful than sonography when renal abscess is suspected for two major reasons. First, the sonographic features of renal abscess and other inflammatory diseases of the kidney are very nonspecific (110). Abscesses may be early, late, or chronic. These lesions contain variable mixtures of blood, infected debris, necrotic tissue, urine, pus, stones, gas, and a great variety of other tissue elements. Thus, their sonographic ap-

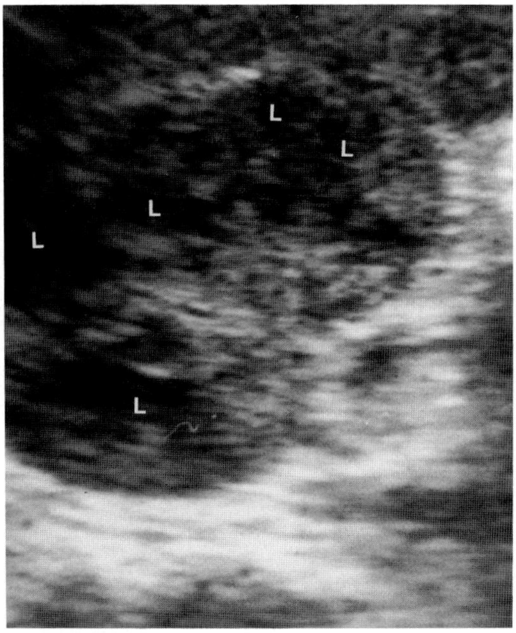

Figure 5.56. Multiple renal abscesses. Transverse sonogram shows a number of lucent, poorly defined zones within the kidney. Some of the larger areas of sonolucency (*L*) are identified.

pearances show infinite variety. A second reason to favor CT scanning over sonography is the disturbing number of false-negative examinations and the number of studies that underestimate the extent of the disease process (102).

Renal abscess formation often starts with a focus of "lobar nephronia," which may present as a poorly defined sonolucent area with low-level echoes. Alternatively, there may be a focus of highly reflective tissue, which is caused by both acutely inflamed tissue area and hemorrhage (111). Focal nephronia, an acutely inflamed area without drainable pus, is demonstrated in Figure 5.55. A reasonably well-defined mass is present in the upper pole of the right kidney. There are scattered low-level echoes. Sound transmission through the lesion is good. Figure 5.56 shows multiple renal abscesses in an acutely ill, immunocompromised young woman with leukemia. Multiple areas of poorly defined sonolucency are present throughout the kidney. Acoustic transmission through the renal unit is enhanced. Figure 5.57 was obtained when an elderly lady who was previously well presented with sepsis. Neither kidney was obstructed, but there were many

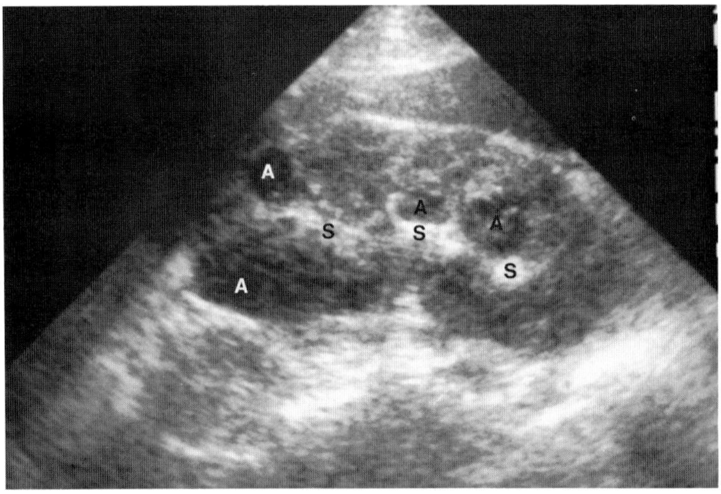

Figure 5.57. Multiple renal abscesses. Sonogram of this elderly lady with sepsis showed a number of nodular areas of poor reflectivity, which later proved to be renal abscesses. Some of the larger abscesses (*A*) are identified. The renal sinus echo complex (*S*) is thinned but no hydronephrosis is present. At autopsy, a great number of small microabscesses were also present.

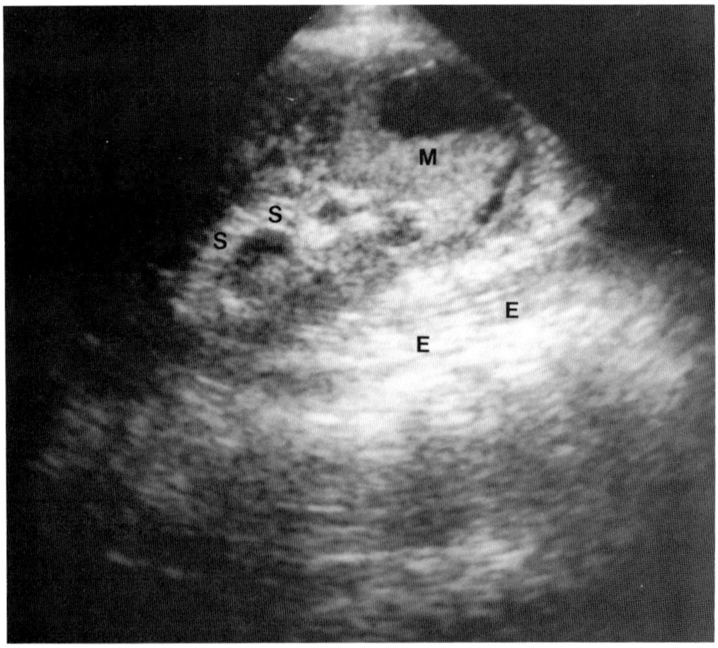

Figure 5.58. Large renal abscess. The lower pole of the kidney has been replaced by a circular mass (*M*) consisting of fluid and an irregular, echogenic mass of infectious debris and necrotic kidney tissue. The renal sinus echo complex is intact in the upper pole without hydronephrosis. There is acoustical enhancement (*E*) behind the abscess. The patient was a diabetic.

circular, poorly defined areas of decreased reflectivity and a generalized nonhomogeneous parenchymal pattern. Literally hundreds of abscesses of various sizes were found at autopsy.

Figure 5.58 displays a more advanced stage of abscess formation. There is a very large, thick-walled cystic mass in the lower pole of the kidney of this young diabetic woman with severe signs of acute renal infection. The cystic space is filled with a large clot of necrotic debris and pus. The upper pole of this same kidney was relatively unaffected, as seen by CT and sonography. A more chronic abscess forming a renal mass can be found in the images shown in

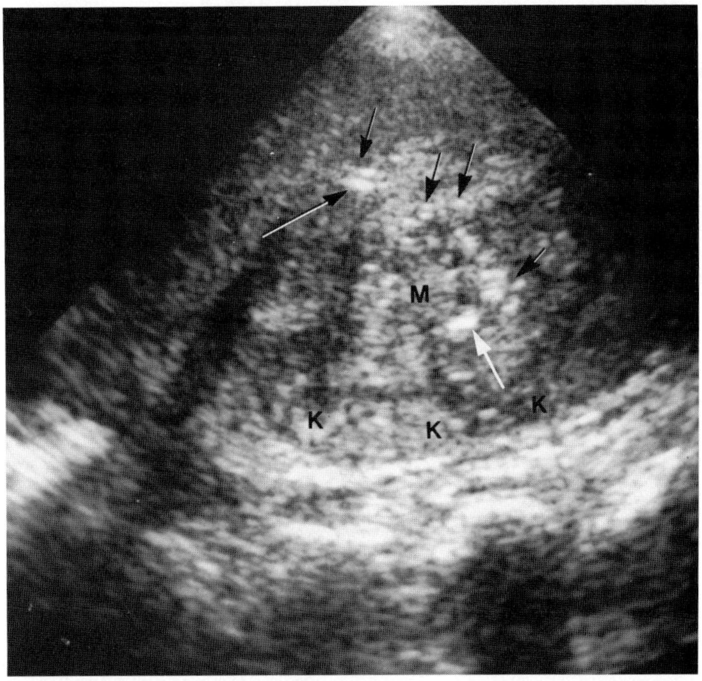

Figure 5.59. Large chronic renal abscess. A thin rim of highly echogenic kidney (*K*) is compressed by a huge reflective mass (*M*). Several bright echoes within the mass (*arrows*) arise from small calcifications and small collections of gas.

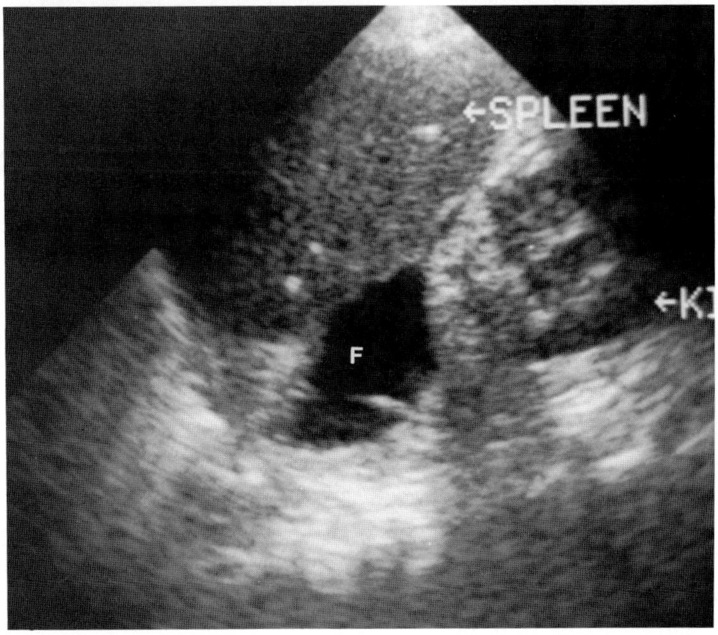

Figure 5.60. Perinephric infected fluid. A collection of sonolucent infected urine (*F*) can be seen between the spleen and the left kidney (*KI*). The upper-pole calices of the kidney are slightly dilated and filled with echogenic fluid from a pyonephrosis.

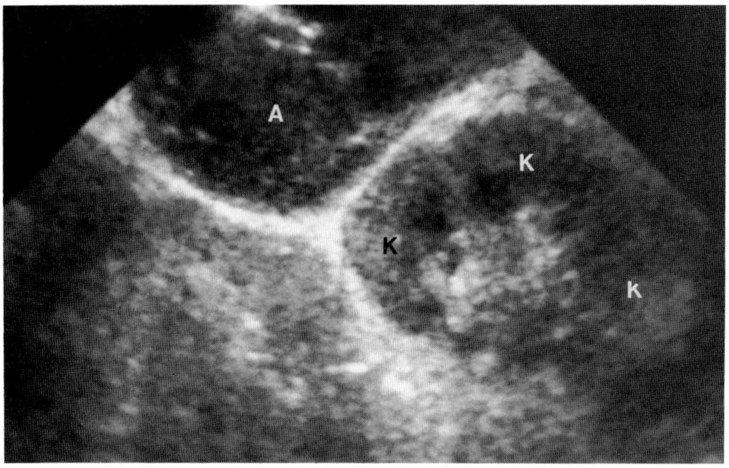

Figure 5.61. Large perirenal abscess. The kidney (*K*) appears normal. A well-circumscribed mass (*A*) lies adjacent to the kidney. The abscess contains mostly low-level echoes with an occasional bright reflection from gas bubbles. The air collections are not large enough to demonstrate traditional "ring down."

Figure 5.62. Perirenal pseudoabscess. An irregular collection of fluid (*F*) containing a few scattered linear echoes lies adjacent to a normal-appearing kidney (*K*). The patient had abdominal pain, marked tenderness, and fever in the area. At surgery, an incarcerated perirenal small bowel hernia was found.

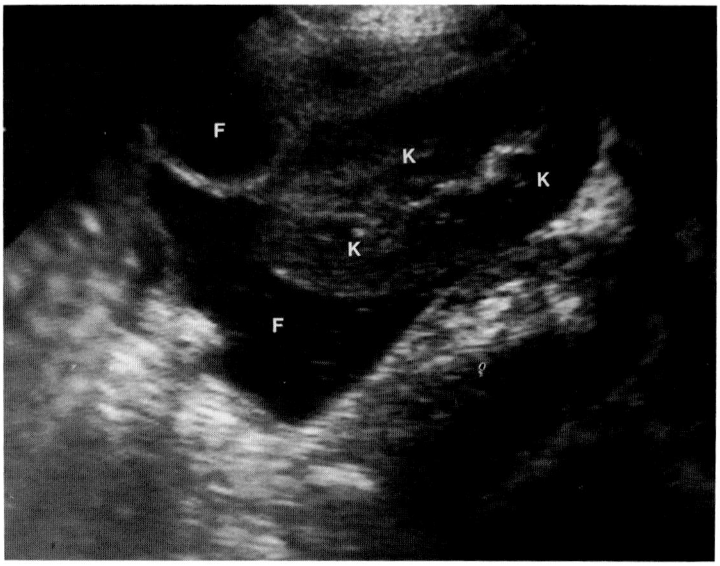

Figure 5.59. The kidney has been nearly replaced except for a thin echogenic rim. The abscess is a large, rounded, heterogeneous mass containing bright reflections. On the CT scan these reflections were seen to be both calcifications and microcollections of gas. The abscess had been present for several weeks. Nephrectomy was required.

Abscess collections are very frequently found adjacent to rather than in the kidney. Examples are shown in Figures 5.60 and 5.61. In Figure 5.60, infected urine has leaked out into the perinephric space between the upper pole of the left kidney and the spleen. The collecting system of the kidney is mildly dilated because of stone disease. Figure 5.61 shows a more organized process in the perinephric space. A well-marginated abscess contains low-level echoes and few microcollections of gas bubbles in this severely ill post–renal transplant patient. An interesting false-positive lesion in a renal transplant patient can be seen in Figure 5.62. The patient had bowel distention, severe tenderness in the region of the graft, fever, and increased white blood cell count. Sonography suggests a perirenal abscess with a few linear septations. The patient worsened on drug therapy, and surgery was performed. An incarcerated loop of bowel herniated through the peritoneum over the transplant was found. There was no renal abscess or perinephric fluid present.

References

1. Grossman H, Rosenberg ER, Bowie JD, Ram P, Merten DF. Sonographic diagnosis of renal diseases. AJR 1983;140:81–85.
2. Bosniak MA. The current radiological approach to renal cysts. Radiology 1986;158:1–10.
3. Pollack HM, Banner MP, Arger PH, Peters J, Mulhern CB Jr, Coleman BG. The accuracy of gray-scale renal ultrasonography in differentiating cystic neoplasms from benign cysts. Radiology 1982;143:741–745.
4. Jaffe CC, Rosenfield AT, Sommer FG, Taylor KJW. Technical factors influencing the imaging of small anechoic cysts by B-scan ultrasound. Radiology 1980;135:429–433.
5. Filly RA, Sommer FG, Minton MJ. Characterization of biological fluids by ultrasound and computed tomography. Radiology 1980;134:167–171.
6. Kissane JM. Congenital malformations. In: Heptinstall RH, ed. Pathology of the kidney. 3rd ed. Boston: Little, Brown, 1983:83–140.
7. McClennan BL, Stanley RJ, Melson GL, Levitt RG, Sagel SS. CT of the renal cyst: is cyst aspiration necessary? AJR 1979;133:671–675.
8. Emmet JL, Levine SR, Woolner LB. Coexistence of renal cyst and tumor. Incidence in 1007 cases. Br J Urol 1963;35:403–410.
9. Fishman MC, Pollack HM, Arger PH, Banner MP. High protein content: another cause of CT hyperdense benign renal cysts. J Comput Assist Tomogr 1983;7:1103–1106.
10. Zirinsky K, Auh YH, Rubenstein WA, Williams JJ, Pasmantier MW, Kazem E. CT of the hyperdense renal cyst: sonographic correlation. AJR 1984;143:151–156.
11. Balfe DM, McClennan BL, Stanley RJ, Weyman PJ, Sagel SS. Evaluation of renal masses considered indeterminate on computed tomography. Radiology 1982;142:421–428.
12. Kim WS, Goldman SM, Gatewood OMB, Marshall FF, Siegelman SS. Computed tomography in calcified renal masses. J Comput Assist Tomogr 1981;5:855–860.
13. Weyman PJ, McClennan BL, Lee JKT, Stanley RJ. CT of calcified renal masses. AJR 1982;138:1095–1099.
14. Rosenberg ER, Korobkin M, Foster W, Silberman PM, Bowie JD, Dunnick NR. The significance of septations in a renal cyst. AJR 1985;144:593–595.
15. Sussman S, Cochran ST, Pagani JJ, et al. Hyperdense renal masses: a CT manifestation of hemorrhagic renal cysts. Radiology 1984;150:207–211.
16. Grossman H, Winchester PH, Chisari FV. Roentgenographic classification of renal cystic disease. AJR 1968;104:319–331.
17. Witten DM, Myers GH Jr, Utz DC. Emmett's clinical urography. ed 4. Philadelphia: WB Saunders, 1977:974–986.
18. Feldberg MAM, Van Waes PFGH. Multilocular cystic renal cell carcinoma. AJR 1982;138:953.
19. Hartman DS, Davis CJ, Sanders RC, Johns TT, Smirniotopoulos J, Goldman SM. The multiloculated renal mass: considerations and differential features. Radiographics 1987;7:29–52.
20. Skinner DG, Lieskovsky G, eds. Diagnosis and management of genitourinary cancer. Philadelphia: WB Saunders, 1988:83–180.
21. Hidalgo H, Dunnick NR, Rosenberg ER, Ram PC, Korobkin M. Parapelvic cysts: appearance on CT and sonography. AJR 1982;138:667–671.
22. Baltarowich OH, Kurtz AB. Sonographic evaluation of renal masses. Urol Radiol 1987;9:79–87.
23. Kutcher R, Sprayregen S, Rosenblatt R, Goldman M. The sonographic appearance of segmental polycystic kidney. J Ultrasound Med 1983;2:425–429.
24. Lee JKT, McClennan BL, Kissane JM. Unilateral polycystic disease. AJR 1978;130:1165.
25. Grossman H. Integrated imaging for the evaluation of the urologic diseases of childhood. Urol Clin North Am 1980;7:177–199.
26. Kleiner B, Filly RA, Mack L, Callen PW. Multicystic dysplastic kidney: observations of contralateral disease in the fetal population. Radiology 1986;161:27–29.
27. Pedicelli G, Jequier S, Bowen A, Boisvert J. Multicystic dysplastic kidneys: spontaneous regression demonstrated with US. Radiology 1986;160:23–26.
28. Akhtar M, Qadeer A. Multilocular cyst of kidney with embryonic tissue. Uroradiology 1980;16:90–94.
29. Banner MP, Pollock HM, Chatten J, Whitzleben C. Multilocular renal cysts. AJR 1981;136:239–247.
30. Boggs LK, Kimmelstiel P. Benign multilocular cystic nephroma: report of two cases of so-called multilocular cyst of the kidney. J Urol 1956;76:530–541.
31. Joshi VV. Cystic, partially differentiated nephroblastoma: an entity in the spectrum of infantile renal neoplasia. Perspect Pediatr Pathol 1980;5:217–263.
32. Wood BP, Muurahainen N, Anderson VM, Ettinger LJ. Multicystic nephroblastoma: ultrasound diagnosis (with a pathologic-anatomic commentary). Pediatr Radiol 1982;12:43–47.
33. Wills JS. Cystic adenocarcinoma of the kidney mimicking multilocular renal cyst. Urol Radiol 1983;5:51–53.
34. Kutcher R, Sprayregen S, Rosenblatt R, Goldman M. The sonographic appearance of segmental polycystic kidney. J Ultrasound Med 1983;2:425–429.
35. Bard RH, Lord B, Fromowitz F. Papillary adenocarcinoma of kidney. II. Radiographic and biologic characteristics. Urology 1982;19:16–19.
36. Taylor KJW, Ramos I, Carter D, Morse SS,

Snower D, Fortune K. Correlation of Doppler US tumor signals with neovascular morphologic features. Radiology 1988;166:57–62.
37. Taylor KJW, Ramos I, Morse SS, Fortune KL, Hammers L, Taylor CR. Focal liver masses: differential diagnosis with pulsed Doppler US. Radiology 1987;164:643–647.
38. Ramos I, Fernandez LA, Morse SS, Fortune KL, Taylor KJW. Detection of neovascular signals in a 3 day Walker 256 rat carcinosarcoma by CW Doppler ultrasound. Ultrasound Med Biol 1988;14:123–126.
39. Kass DA, Hricak H, Davidson AJ. Renal malignancies with normal excretory urograms. AJR 1983;141:731–734.
40. Clayman RV, Williams RD, Fraley EE. The pursuit of the renal mass. N Engl J Med 1979; 300:72–74.
41. Prout GR Jr, Garnick MB. The kidney and ureter. In: Holland JF, Frei E III, eds. Cancer medicine. Philadelphia: Lea & Febiger, 1982:1880–1896.
42. Harvey HR, Thomas JL, Bernadino ME, Barnes TA, Lewis E. Pitfalls in diagnosis of exophytic renal tumors. Urology 1982;20:218–222.
43. Plaine LL, Hinman F Jr. Malignancy in asymptomatic renal masses. J Urol 1965;94:342–347.
44. Press GA, McClennan BL, Melson GL, Weyman PJ, Mauro MA, Lee JKT. Papillary renal cell carcinoma: CT and sonographic evaluation. AJR 1984;143:1005–1009.
45. Charboneau JW, Hattery RR, Ernst EC III, James EM, Williamson B, Hartman GW. Spectrum of sonographic findings in 125 renal masses other than benign simple cyst. AJR 1983;140:87–94.
46. Kuijpers D, Jaspers R. Renal masses: differential diagnosis with pulsed doppler US. Radiol 1989;170:59–60.
47. Johnson CD, Dunnick NR, Cohan RH, Illescas FF. Renal adenocarcinoma: CT staging of 100 tumors. AJR 1987;148:59–63.
48. Choyke PL, White EM, Zeman RK, Jaffe MH, Clark LR. Renal metastases: clinicopathologic and radiologic correlation. Radiology 1987; 162:359–363.
49. Pascal RR. Renal manifestations of extrarenal neoplasms. Hum Pathol 1980;11:7–17.
50. Abrams HL, Spiro R, Goldstein HM. Metastases in carcinoma: analysis of 1,000 autopsied cases. Cancer 1950;3:74–85.
51. Hietala SO, Wahlqvist L. Metastatic tumors to the kidney: a post mortem, radiologic and clinical investigation. Acta Radiol Diagn (Stockh) 1982;23:585–591.
52. Bhatt GH, Bernadino ME, Graham SD Jr. CT diagnosis of renal metastases. J Comput Assist Tomogr 1983;7:1032–1034.
53. Mitnick JS, Bosniak MA, Roghberg M, Megibow AJ, Raghavendra BN, Subramanyan BR. Metastatic neoplasm to the kidney studied by computed tomography and sonography. J Comput Assist Tomogr 1985;9:43–49.
54. Smith EB, Dunnick NR, Nelson P, Hammond CB. Renal metastases of malignant gestational trophoblastic disease: the use of intravenous urography in staging. Gynecol Oncol 1985;20: 317–324.
55. Walther PJ, Marks LS, Stern D, Smith RB. Renal metastasis of adenocarcinoma of the lung: massive hematuria managed by therapeutic embolization. J Urol 1979;122:398–400.
56. Pollack HM, Banner MP, Amendola MA. Other malignant neoplasms of the renal parenchyma. Semin Roentgenol 1987;22:260–274.
57. Tipton A, Goldman SM, Fishman EK, Arnold P. Cystic renal melanoma: CT/ultrasound correlation. Urol Radiol 1987;9:39–41.
58. Grant DC, DE GJ, Yoder IC, Newhouse JH. Sonography in transitional cell carcinoma of the renal pelvis. Urol Radiol 1986;8:1–5.
59. Hartman DS, Pyatt RS, Dailey E. Transitional cell carcinoma of the kidney with invasion into the renal vein. Urol Radiol 1983;5:83–87.
60. Wentzell RA, Berkheiser SW. Malignant lymphomatosis of the kidneys. J Urol 1955;74: 177–185.
61. Richmond J, Sherman RS, Diamond HD, Carver LF. Renal lesions associated with malignant lymphomas. Am J Med 1962;32:181–207.
62. Heiken PJ, Gold RP, Schnur RJ, King DL. Computerized tomography in renal lymphomas with ultrasound correlation. J Comput Assist Tomogr 1983;7:245–255.
63. Jafri SZH, Bree RL, Amendola MA, Glazer G, Schwab RE, Francis IR, Borlaz AG. CT of renal and perirenal non-Hodgkin lymphoma. AJR 1982;138:1101–1105.
64. Araki T. Leukemic involvement of the kidney in children. CT features: J Comput Assist Tomogr 1982;6:781–784.
65. Mettler FA. In: Crawford ED, Borden TA, eds. Genitourinary cancer surgery. Philadelphia: Lea & Febiger, 1982:436–437.
66. Horii SC, Bosniak MA, Megibow AJ, Raghavendra RN, Subramanyam BR, Rothberg M. Correlation of CT and ultrasound in the evaluation of renal lymphoma. Urol Radiol 1983;5: 69–76.
67. Hartman DS, Davis CJ, Goldman SM, Friedman AC, Fritzsche P. Renal lymphoma: radiologic-pathologic correlation of 21 cases. Radiology 1982;144:759–766.
68. Lafortune M, Constantin A, Breton G, Vallee C. Sonography of the hypertrophied column of Bertin. AJR 1986;146:53–56.
69. Bertin EJ. Memoire pour servir a l'histoire des reins. In: Histoire de l'Academie Royale des Sciences. Paris: Academie Royale des Sciences, 1744:77–111.
70. King MC, Friedenberg RM, Tena LB. Normal renal parenchyma simulating tumor. Radiology 1968;91:217–222.
71. Felson B, Moskowitz M. Renal pseudotumors: the regenerated nodule and other lumps, bumps, and dromedary humps. AJR 1969;107: 720–729.
72. Meaney TF. Errors in angiographic diagnosis of renal masses. Radiology 1969;93:361–366.
73. Popky GL, Bogash M, Pollack H, Longacre AM. Focal nodular hyperplasia. J Urol 1969;102: 657–660.

74. Lopez FA. Renal pseudotumors. AJR 1970;109: 172–184.
75. Charghi A, Dessureault P, Drouin G, et al. Malposition of a renal lobe (lobar dysmorphism): a condition simulating renal tumor. J Urol 1971;105:326–329.
76. Morgan GS, Staumfjord JV, Hall EJ. Angiomyolipoma of the kidney. J Urol 1951;65: 525–529.
77. Berg JW. Malignant hamartomatous angiomyolipomyoma in a case with solitary metastasis. From bronchogenic carcinoma. Cancer 1955;8:59–63.
78. Drago JR, Nesbitt JA, Leb R. Renal angiomyolipomas. J Surg Oncol 1988;38:64–67.
79. Raghavendra BN, Bosniak MA, Megibow AJ. Small angiomyolipoma of the kidney: sonographic-CT evaluation. AJR 1983;141: 575–578.
80. Bret PM, Bretagnolle M, Gaillard D, Plauchu H, Labadie M, Lapray JF, Roullaud Y, Cooperberg P. Small, asymptomatic angiomyolipomas of the kidney. Radiology 1985;154:7–10.
81. Bosniak MA, Megibow AJ, Hulnick DH, Horii JB, Raghavendra BN. CT diagnosis of renal angiomyolipoma: the importance of detecting small amounts of fat. AJR 1988;151:497–501.
82. Carter AR, Horgan JG, Jennings TA, Rosenfield AT. The junctional parenchymal defect: a sonographic variant of renal anatomy. Radiology 1985;154:499–502.
83. Goiney RC, Goldenberg L, Cooperberg PL, Charboneau JW, Rosenfield AT, Russin LD, McCarthy S, Zeman RK, Gordon PB, Rowley BA. Renal oncocytoma: sonographic analysis of 14 cases. AJR 1984;143:1001–1004.
84. Klein MJ, Valensi QJ. Proximal tubular adenomas of kidney with so-called oncocytic features: a clinicopathologic study of 13 cases of a rarely reported neoplasm. Cancer 1976;38: 906–914.
85. Yu GSM, Rendler S, Herskowitz A, Molnar JJ. Renal oncocytoma: report of five cases and review of literature. Cancer 1980;45:1010–1018.
86. Barth KH, Menon M. Renal oncocytoma: further diagnostic observations. Diagn Imaging 1980;49:259–265.
87. Johnson RJ, Thurman AE, Metter JB, Bannaya GA. Oncocytoma of kidney. Urology 1979; 14:181–185.
88. Weiner SN, Bernstein RG. Renal oncocytoma: angiographic features of two cases. Radiology 1977;125:633–635.
89. Merino MJ, Livolsi VA. Oncocytomas of the kidney. Cancer 1982;50:1852–1856.
90. Ambos MA, Bosniak MA, Valensi QJ, Maayag MA, Lefleur RS. Angiographic patterns in renal oncocytomas. Radiology 1978;129:615–622.
91. Levine E, Huntrakoon M. Computed tomography of renal oncocytoma. AJR 1983;141: 741–746.
92. Wasserman NF, Ewing SL. Calcified renal oncocytoma. AJR 1983;141:747–749.
93. Lafortune M, Breton G. Echographic demonstration of an oncocytoma. J Can Assoc Radiol 1983;34:144–146.
94. Rodriguez CA, Buskop A, Johnson J, Fromowitz F, Koss LG. Renal oncocytoma: preoperative diagnosis by aspiration biopsy. Acta Cytol 1980;24:355–359.
95. Lieber MM, Tomera KM, Farrow GM. Renal oncocytoma. J Urol 1981;125:481–485.
96. Ejeckam G, Tolnai G, Karkar K, McCaughey WTE. Renal oncocytoma: study of eight cases. Urology 1979;14:186–189.
97. Quinn MJ, Hartman DS, Friedman AC, Sherman JL, Lautin EM, Pyatt RS, Ho CK, Csere R, Fromowitz FB. Renal oncocytoma: new observations. Radiology 1984;153:49–53.
98. Reuter SR, Pomeroy PR, Chuang VP, et al. Embolic control of hypertension caused by segmental renal arterial stenosis. AJR 1976;127: 389–392.
99. Smith MJV, Seidel RF. Accidental trauma to the kidneys in children. J Urol 1966;96: 845–847.
100. Kauffman RA, Powbin R, Babcock BS. Upper abdominal trauma in children imaging evaluation. AJR 1984;142:449–469.
101. Saunders RC, Mennon S, Saunders AD. Complementary uses of nuclear medicine and ultrasound in the kidney. J Urol 1978;120:521–527.
102. Hoddick W, Jeffrey RB, Goldberg HI, Federle MP, Laing FC. CT and sonography of severe renal and perirenal infections. AJR 1983; 140:517–520.
103. Rauschbolb EN, Sandler CM, Sumant P, Childs TL. Computed tomography of renal inflammatory disease. J Comput Assist Tomogr 1982; 6:502–506.
104. Edell SL, Bonavita JA. The sonographic appearance of acute pyelonephritis. Radiology 1979;132:683–685.
105. Gelman ML, Stone LB. Renal caruncle: early diagnosis by retroperitoneal ultrasound. Urology 1979;6:103–107.
106. Schneider M, Becker JA, Striano S, Compos E. Sonographic-radiographic correlation of renal and perirenal infections. AJR 1976;127: 1007–1014.
107. Hoffman EP, Mindelzun RE, Anderson RU. CT in acute pyelonephritis associated with diabetes. Radiology 1980;135:691–695.
108. Lee KTL, McClennan BL, Melson GL, Stanley RJ. Acute focal bacterial nephritis: emphasis on grey scale sonography and computed tomography. AJR 1980;135:87–92.
109. Rosenfield AT, Glickman MG, Taylor KJW, Crade M, Hodson J. Acute focal bacterial nephritis (acute lobar nephronia). Radiology 1979;132:553–561.
110. Morehouse HT, Weiner SN, Hoffman JC. Imaging in inflammatory disease of the kidney. AJR 1984;143:135–141.
111. Rigsby CM, Rosenfield AT, Glickman MG, Hodson J. Hemorrhagic focal bacterial nephritis: findings on gray-scale sonography and CT. AJR 1986;146:1173–1177.

CHAPTER 6

Sonography of Acute and Chronic Renal Failure

BHASKARA K. RAO, M.D.
PATRICK J. BRYAN, M.D.

Renal failure is not a cascade of sharply defined stages but a continuum of progressive inability of the kidneys to maintain normal homeostatic functions. Mild "impairment" of renal function is detectable only by imposing unusual demands on kidneys, as during concentration and dilution tests. Renal "insufficiency" is a further reduction in homeostasis without a significant change in body fluid composition. Renal "failure" represents a stage of functional loss when kidneys are unable to maintain biochemical homeostasis, resulting in altered body fluid composition. "Uremia" is an end-stage clinical syndrome to which all progressive renal diseases ultimately converge.

Renal failure may be acute or chronic. Acute renal failure develops over a short span of time (hours to days) from renal or nonrenal (pre- and postrenal) causes and leads to rapid oliguria, anuria, and uremia if untreated. Chronic renal failure is due to progressive bilateral parenchymal disease occurring over a prolonged period (weeks to months). The rapidity of parenchymal destruction determines the extent of renal damage necessary before uremia ensues.

The causes of chronic and acute renal failure are numerous (Tables 6.1 and 6.2). Sonography plays an important role in the noninvasive diagnosis of renal failure and in guiding invasive procedures like biopsy and nephrostomy. In this chapter, discussion is confined to sonography of the important diseases of native kidneys that result in renal failure. Sonography of renal failure in transplants is discussed in Chapter 14.

NORMAL RENAL SONOGRAM

On high-resolution sonograms, the capsule is seen as a thin echogenic line confining the renal parenchyma. By convention, the renal cortex is considered less echogenic than the liver, and when renal echogenicity is equal to or greater than that of liver a renal abnormality is suspected (1, 2). Recent observations reveal that 72% of patients have normal renal function when their renal and hepatic echogenicities are equal. When the kidney is more echogenic than the liver, the specificity and positive predictive values for renal disease are 96% and 67%, respectively (3). The renal echogenicity depends on several intrinsic factors, such as the state of hydration and the severity of edema or fibrosis, and extrinsic factors such as the time : distance gain compensation curve setting, total gain, beam focal zone location, and presence of ascites (Fig. 6.1). The authors consider that decrease or loss of corticomedullary definition and renal echogenicity greater than that of the liver indicate parenchymal renal disease. In neonates and infants up to 6 months of age, the normal cortex is considerably echogenic and the renal pyramids are markedly hypoechoic (4). The renal pyramids appear as hypoechoic triangular areas with a lucent orifice at the papilla. The infundibular and caliceal wall is seen as a thin echogenic line surrounded by a variable amount of echogenic fat (central echo complex) (5). At the renal hilum, the arteries are seen as pulsatile echogenic tubes with thick walls. The veins are seen as thin-walled tubes that vary in size with respiration. In the renal parenchyma, interlobar and arcuate arteries are seen as echogenic and pulsatile lines around the renal pyramids.

ABNORMAL SONOGRAM IN RENAL FAILURE

Certain general principles are noteworthy in the sonographic investigation of renal failure. Sonography is insensitive for diagnosis of mild or early parenchymal disease, as subtle

Table 6.1.
Causes of Chronic Renal Failure

Primarily glomerular diseases
Chronic glomerulonephritis
Acute glomerulonephritis
Other glomerulonephritis
Primarily tubular diseases
Chronic hypercalcemic states
Aminoaciduria syndromes
Toxic nephropathy (drugs, chemicals, toxins, metals)
Radiation nephritis
Hyperoxaluria
Vascular diseases
Intrinsic renovascular disease
Hypertensive nephropathy
Hemolytic-uremic syndrome
Radiation nephritis
Polyarteritis nodosa
Diabetic nephropathy
Extrarenal renovascular disease
Bilateral renal artery stenosis
Bilateral fibromuscular hyperplasia
Bilateral renal artery thrombosis
Bilateral renal vein thrombosis
Collagen diseases
Diffuse systemic sclerosis
Disseminated lupus erythematosis
Polyarteritis nodosa
Metabolic renal diseases
Primary hyperparathyroidism
Primary hyperoxaluria
Hyperuricemia
Diabetic nephropathy
Analgesic nephropathy
Amyloidosis
Infections
Chronic pyelonephritis
Tuberculosis
Acquired immunodeficiency syndrome
Infiltrative processes
Lymphoma
Leukemia
Amyloidosis
Sarcoidosis
Glycogen storage diseases
Congenital anomalies
Polycystic disease
Medullary cystic disease
Hypoplastic kidneys
Horseshoe kidneys with obstruction
Chronic obstructive disease
Upper tract
Calculi
Neoplasm
Retroperitoneal fibrosis
Lower tract
Calculi
Prostatomegaly
Urethral valves

Table 6.2.
Causes of Acute Renal Failure

Prerenal
Hypovolemia
Hypotension
Salt depletion
Arterial occlusion
Parenchymal
Acute cortical necrosis
Acute glomerulonephritis
Acute pyelonephritis
Toxic nephropathy
Hemolytic-uremic syndrome
Acute tubular obstruction
Postrenal
Acute renal vein thrombosis
Acute urinary tract obstruction
Calculi
Trauma

changes in renal echogenicity are difficult to recognize. The primary role of sonography in renal failure is to differentiate obstructive from parenchymal causes so that the obstruction can be relieved by an appropriate invasive procedure. Further, sonography provides direct guidance for nephrostomy and biopsy procedures. In parenchymal disease, sonography may identify a specific pattern and direct investigative approach to a limited group of diseases from a large gamut (Tables 6.3 to 6.6). Doppler sonography is also useful in identifying vascular causes of renal failure.

In general, reduction in echogenicity is due to inflammation, edema, or cellular infiltration (e.g., pyelonephritis, acute renal vein thrombosis, lymphoma). An increase in renal echogenicity is due to glomerulosclerosis, tubular atrophy, interstitial cellular infiltration, or deposition of calcium, protein, glycogen, etc. In the late stage, several parenchymal diseases produce a sonographic picture of a small, shrunken, and diffusely hyperechoic kidney with thin cortex and indistinct corticomedullary definition (Fig. 6.2) (1, 2). In the sonographic evaluation of renal failure, an attempt is made to:

1. Identify the number, location, and size of the kidneys;
2. Assess their echogenicity;
3. Detect renal obstruction and estimate the severity of cortical loss;
4. Localize the site and determine the cause of obstruction;
5. Detect vascular occlusion; and

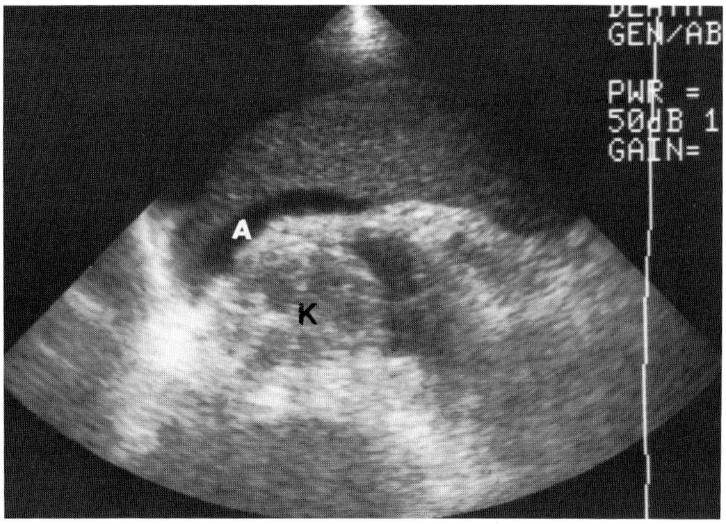

Figure 6.1. Transverse sonogram of the abdomen. Right kidney (*K*) appears highly echogenic due to excellent ultrasonic beam transmission through ascites (*A*), an artifact.

6. Provide follow-up information during and after therapy.

CHRONIC RENAL FAILURE

Progressive destruction of greater than 70% of total renal parenchyma can result in chronic renal failure. The numerous causes of chronic renal failure can be classified as (*a*) primarily glomerular diseases, (*b*) primarily tubular diseases, (*c*) vascular diseases, (*d*) collagen diseases, (*e*) metabolic renal diseases, (*f*) infections, (*g*) infiltrative processes, (*h*) congenital anomalies, and (*i*) chronic obstructive diseases. Due to the overlapping of underlying pathologic processes, some diseases can be classified into more than one group.

Table 6.3.
Hyperechoic Normal-Sized Kidneys

Newborn and infants
Dehydration
Hypovolemia
Myoglobinuria
Early parenchymal diseases
Early nephrocalcinosis
Early oxalosis
Leukemia
Glycogen storage disease

Table 6.4.
Hyperechoic Large Kidneys

Transient nephromegaly of newborn
Glomerulonephritis in infants
Acute infantile pyelonephritis
Radiocontrast nephropathy in infants
Early diabetic nephropathy
Autosomal recessive polycystic disease
Amyloidosis
Glycogen storage disease
Leukemia
Subacute renal vein thrombosis
Acute nephrotoxicity
Subacute cortical necrosis

Primarily Glomerular Diseases

CHRONIC GLOMERULONEPHRITIS

Chronic glomerulonephritis is one of the most common causes of chronic renal failure.

Table 6.5.
Hyperechoic Small Kidneys

Hypertension
Diabetes
Chronic glomerulonephritis
End-stage parenchymal diseases
Calcium nephropathy
Oxalosis
Hyperuricemia
Chronic renal vein thrombosis
Alport's syndrome
Chronic cortical necrosis

Table 6.6.
Hypoechoic Large Kidneys

Acute pyelonephritis
Acute renal vein thrombosis
Nephroblastomatosis
Bilateral Wilms' tumors
Lymphoma
Autosomal dominant polycystic disease
Multicystic dysplasia
Acute radiation nephritis

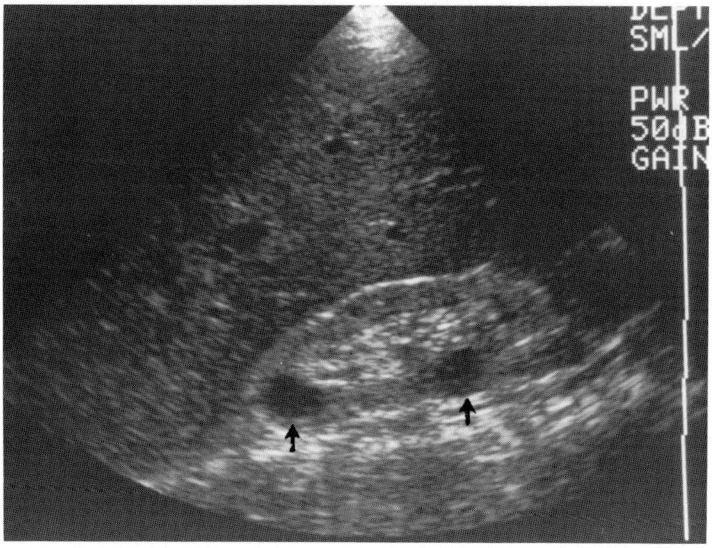

Figure 6.2. Longitudinal sonogram of right kidney. Small hyperechoic kidney with loss of corticomedullary differentiation, and cortical cysts (*arrows*) in chronic glomerulonephritis.

Pathologically, the disease is characterized by progressive inflammation of glomeruli, which become replaced by sclerosis and scarring. In the early stage, the kidneys may be enlarged, normal, or slightly reduced in size and show smooth contour. They appear pale yellow and have a fine granular texture. On sonograms, the kidneys vary in size and show smooth outlines. The cortical echogenicity is increased and the corticomedullary differentiation is accentuated. If pyramids are involved, they may be isoechoic with the cortex. In the late stage, the kidneys are small, contracted, pale, and coarsely granular with predominance of scarring and atrophy. On sonograms, the kidneys are small, irregular, and highly echogenic with poor corticomedullary distinction (1, 2, 6). In "end-stage" disease, focal cortical depressions due to scarring, small cysts, and calcifications may be seen (Fig. 6.3). When kidneys become isoechoic with the perinephric fat, they may be identified only by the presence of renal vessels at the hilum.

ACUTE GLOMERULONEPHRITIS

Progressive nonsuppurative inflammation of glomeruli in both kidneys can produce acute or chronic renal failure. A spectrum of entities (which include membranoproliferative glomerulonephritis, focal glomerulonephritis, antiglomerular basement membrane antibody disease, benign acute hemorrhagic nephritis, diffuse interstitial nephritis, and glomerulonephritis secondary to subacute bacterial endocarditis, systemic lupus erythematosus, and anaphylactoid purpura) produce diffuse or multifocal edematous swelling of kidneys with focal hemorrhages. On sonograms, the kidneys show mild to moderate enlargement, normal contour, diffuse cortical hyperechogenicity, enlarged pyramids, and absence of hydronephrosis (Fig. 6.4) (7, 8). Ultimately, recurrent episodes of acute glomerulonephritis may produce chronic renal failure and sonographic changes similar to those in chronic glomerulonephritis.

Primarily Tubular Diseases

Chronic tubular disease is due to sclerosis and atrophy or progressive intraluminal deposition of calcium salts or proteins.

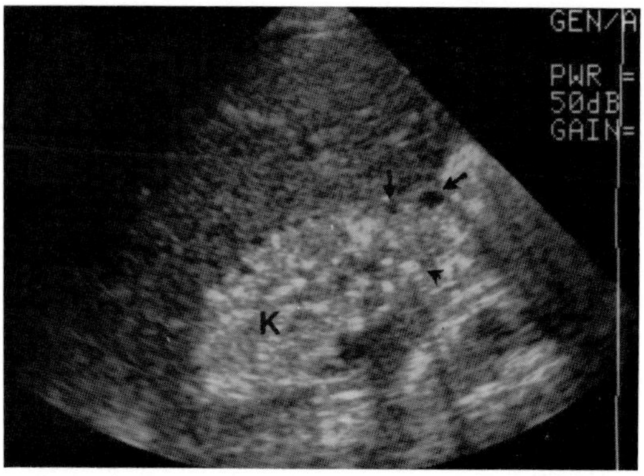

Figure 6.3. Longitudinal sonogram of right kidney. Small, intensely echogenic kidney (*K*) with loss of corticomedullary distinction, small peripheral cysts (*arrows*), and focal parenchymal calcifications (*arrowhead*) in end-stage renal disease due to chronic glomerulonephritis.

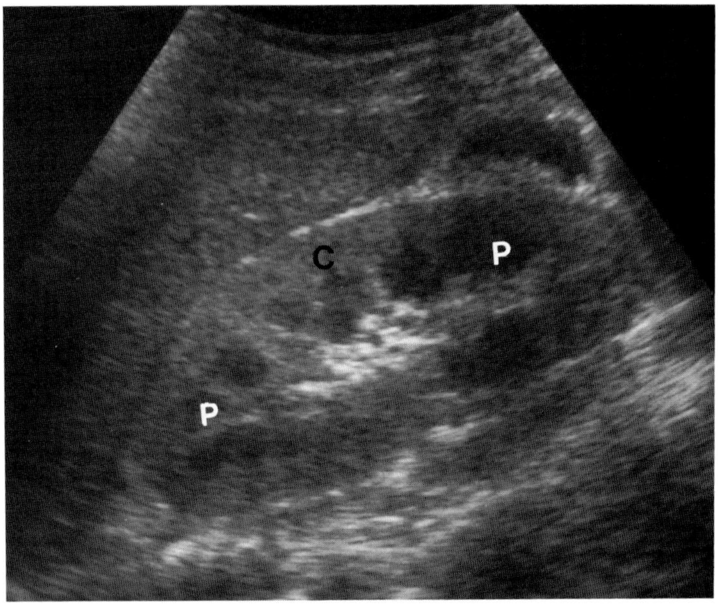

Figure 6.4. Longitudinal sonogram of right kidney. Enlarged kidney with hyperechoic cortex (*C*) and prominent hypoechoic pyramids (*P*) due to acute glomerulonephritis.

CALCIUM NEPHROPATHY

Several chronic hypercalcemic states such as hyperparathyroidism, diffuse metastatic bone disease, vitamin D intoxication, milk alkali syndrome, sarcoidosis, idiopathic hypercalcemia, infantile hypercalcemia, etc., and metabolic diseases such as De Toni-Fanconi syndrome, primary hyperoxaluria, hyperuricemia, cystinuria, tyrosinosis, etc., produce tubular deposition of calcium salts or amino acids, interstitial calcification, glomerular hyalinization, and intertubular and periglomerular fibrosis. Malignant neoplasm is the most common cause of hypercalcemia in the general population (9). The sonographic appearance of the kidneys depends on the site and severity of calcification. The calcinosis may be diffuse or focal and involve the cortex, medulla, or both (Fig. 6.5) (9, 10).

Cortical calcinosis is rare and occurs in primary hyperoxaluria, Fabry disease, the nail patella syndrome, sickle cell disease, chronic glomerulonephritis, renal cortical necrosis, Alport's syndrome (hereditary nephritis), and after methoxyflurane abuse or anesthesia (Figs. 6.6 and 6.7).

Medullary nephrocalcinosis is more common and is seen in dehydrated infants and in patients with renal tubular acidosis of any cause, oxalosis, hypercalcemic states, papillary necrosis, medullary sponge kidney, infantile and juvenile types of polycystic kidneys, Cushing's syndrome, enzyme disorders, vascular phenomena, and AIDS. Calcinosis in the cortex and medulla is seen in primary and secondary hyperoxaluria (10–12). On sonograms, the kidneys are often small or normal and rarely increased in size. Their echogenicity is increased at the sites of calcification, and acoustic shadowing may be present (Fig. 6.8) (13). Nephrocalcinosis and lithiasis are better seen

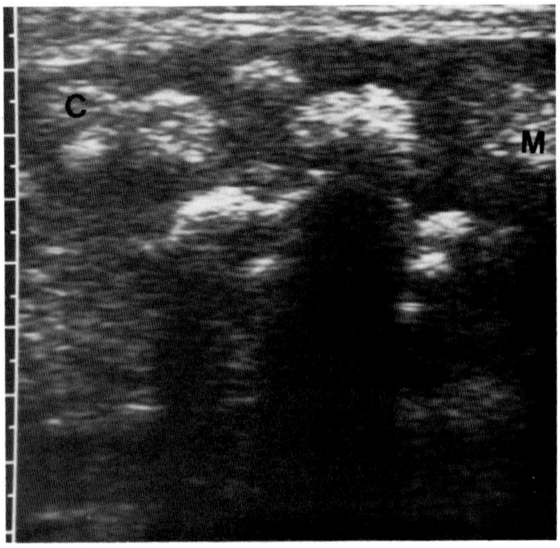

Figure 6.5. Longitudinal sonogram of left kidney. Large echogenic foci due to cortical (*C*) and medullary (*M*) calcifications in a patient with renal tubular acidosis.

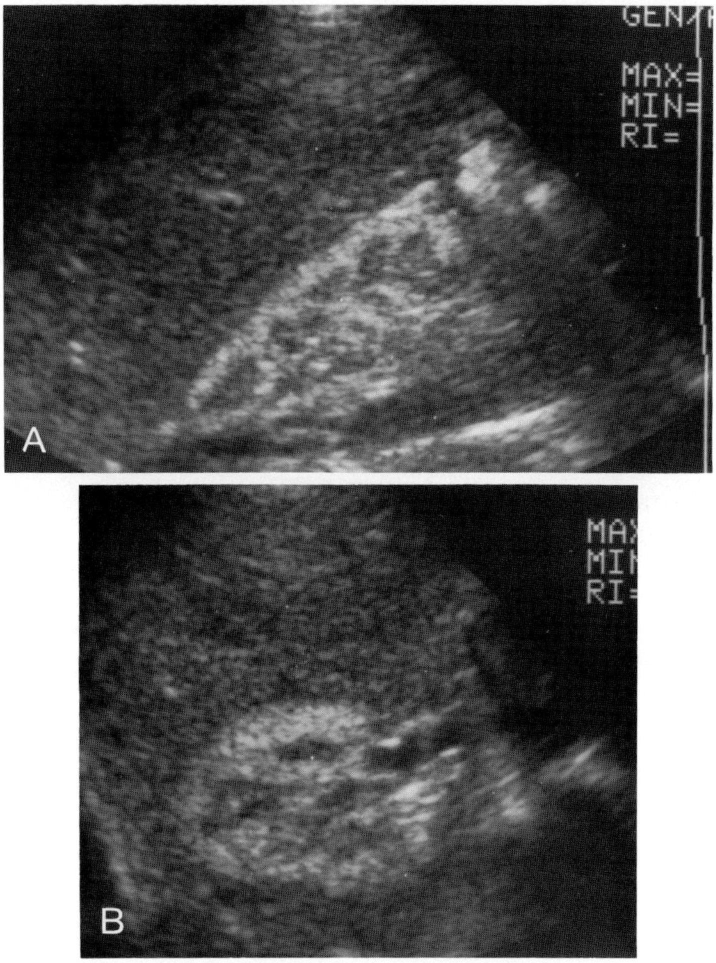

Figure 6.6. Longitudinal (*top*) and transverse (*bottom*) sonograms. Intensely echogenic cortex and slightly echogenic pyramids due to methoxyflurane-induced cortical calcinosis.

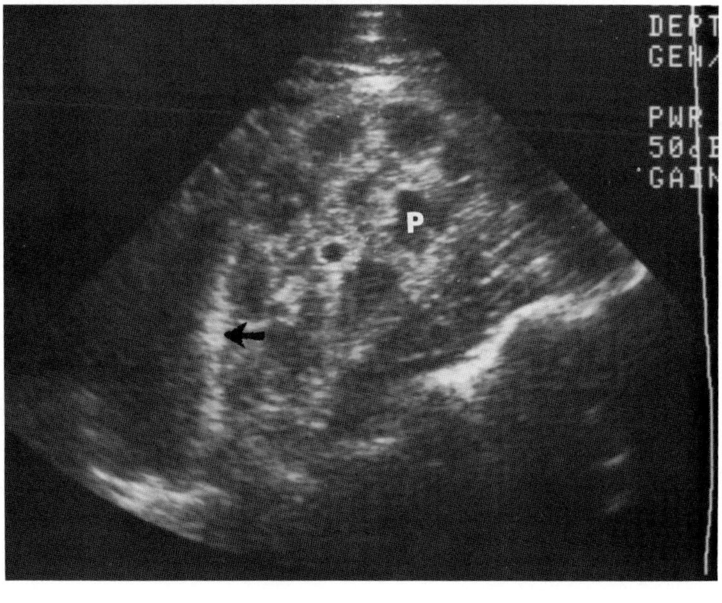

Figure 6.7. Longitudinal sonogram of right kidney. Highly echogenic cortex (*arrow*) due to cortical calcinosis with enlarged pyramids (*P*) in patient with Fabry disease.

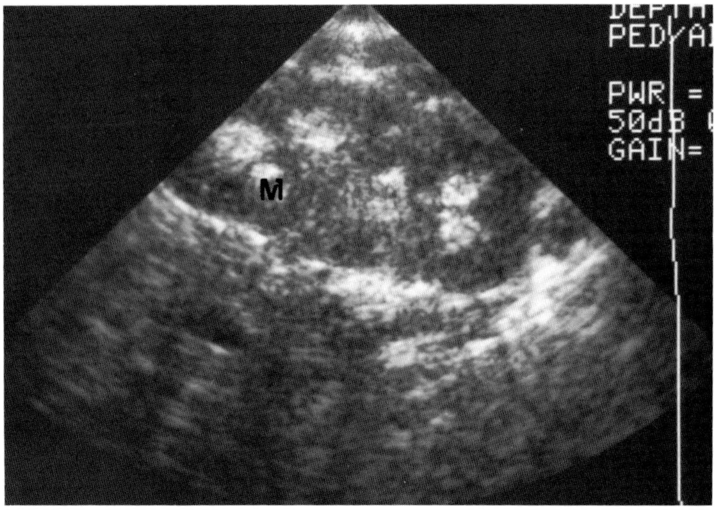

Figure 6.8. Longitudinal sonogram of right kidney. Highly echogenic pyramids due to extensive medullary calcinosis (*M*) in a hypercalcemic child.

on sonograms than on plain radiographs, tomograms, or urograms (14, 15). Computed tomography is highly sensitive for detection of early and small calcifications but is expensive for routine and serial imaging.

HEREDITARY AMINOACIDURIA SYNDROMES

Aminoaciduria syndromes such as cystinosis, tyrosinemia, and De Toni-Fanconi syndrome are characterized by proteinuria, crystalluria, renal tubular acidosis, and other clinical features. The pathologic changes include mesangial sclerosis and hypercellularity in glomeruli, glomerular hyalinization, interstitial infiltrates or fibrosis, and, in the late stage, tubular atrophy. On sonograms, the kidneys are small, smooth, and hyperechoic. The increase in echogenicity may be diffuse or limited to the cortex or medulla. Calculi may be present in the calices or pelvis (9, 10, 13). Calcification may be seen in the pyramids or cortex (Fig. 6.9).

TOXIC NEPHROPATHY

A variety of diagnostic contrast media, drugs (antibiotics, analgesics, antidiuretics, anticoagulants, anesthetics, anticancer drugs, antihypertensives, etc.), organic solvents, and chemicals produce acute or chronic renal failure, depending on their dose, length of exposure, and site of action. In general, acute toxic effect manifests as tubular necrosis, and chronic toxic effect as interstitial nephritis. Pathologic features of toxic nephropathy include acute cortical necrosis, nephrocalcinosis, nephrolithiasis, and interstitial nephritis. Nephrolithiasis and calcinosis from furosemide and papillary necrosis from phenacetin are the most common drug-induced changes observed by serial sonography (Fig. 6.10) (16, 17). Mercurial salts and lead produce tubular degeneration and cal-

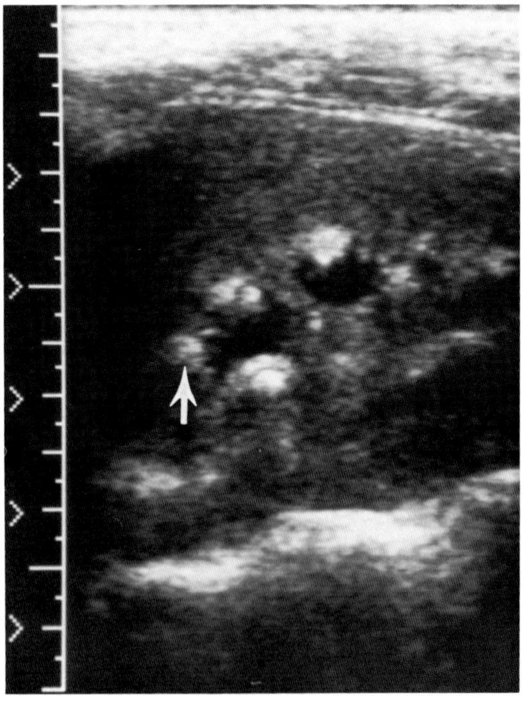

Figure 6.9. Longitudinal sonogram of right kidney. Intensely echogenic calcinosis in pyramids (*arrow*) and caliectasis in a child with De Toni-Fanconi syndrome.

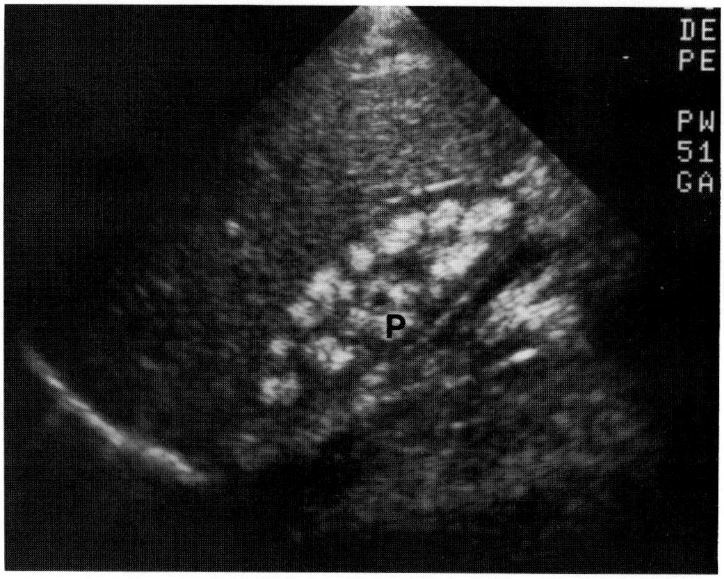

Figure 6.10. Longitudinal sonogram of right kidney. Highly echogenic pyramids (*P*) due to furosemide-induced calcinosis in a neonate.

cification. Sonographic features of acute cortical necrosis, nephrocalcinosis, and chronic nephritis are described elsewhere in this chapter.

Vascular Diseases

Compression or obstruction of both renal arteries in their extrarenal course may lead to chronic or acute renal failure (extrarenal renovascular disease). Obstruction or severe sclerosis of arteries or arterioles in the kidneys produces ischemia, hypertension, and acute or chronic renal failure (intrarenal renovascular disease).

HYPERTENSIVE NEPHROPATHY

Severe obliterative sclerosis of arteries and arterioles may accelerate renovascular hypertension (malignant hypertension) and produce chronic renal failure. In children, 75% of cases of hypertension are secondary to renal diseases (parenchymal or vascular) (18). The kidneys are small, shrunken, finely granular, and scarred. The cortex is atrophic and may show petechiae. On sonograms, the kidneys are small and highly echogenic and show brightly reflective sclerotic or calcified interlobar and arcuate arteries (19).

RADIATION NEPHRITIS

Mild radiation injury to the kidney manifests as proteinuria and hypertension. When severe, it may manifest in acute or chronic form (20). The renal changes are vascular sclerosis, interstitial fibrosis, and tubular necrosis and atrophy. Chronic renal failure occurs in 3 to 12 months after exposure to about 2000 rads over several weeks. In the acute stage, the kidneys are enlarged and edematous. In the chronic stage they are small, irregular, grayish, and fibrotic. On sonograms, the kidneys are small, irregular, and hyper- or hypoechoic.

BILATERAL RENAL ARTERY STENOSIS

Bilateral renal artery stenosis (RAS) can produce chronic renal failure. The most common causes of RAS are fibromuscular hyperplasia and intimal fibroplasia in the young and arteriosclerotic plaques in the older age group. In a trauma victim, renal artery thrombosis is often unilateral but, when bilateral, causes acute renal failure. Sonograms in RAS show a small echogenic kidney. Recently, Doppler sonography was found to be promising for the noninvasive diagnosis of RAS. However, false-positive studies due to turbulent flow in tortuous sclerotic vessels and false-negative studies due to multiple arteries and the inability to sample the entire artery may limit widespread application.

CHRONIC RENAL VEIN THROMBOSIS

Progressive invasion of renal veins by renal cell carcinoma may produce chronic renal failure. Sonograms show a hypo- or hyperechoic nonhomogeneous thrombus in the renal veins and the presence or lack of invasion of vena cava or right atrium (Fig. 6.11) (21, 22). Doppler sonography shows the absence of flow in the

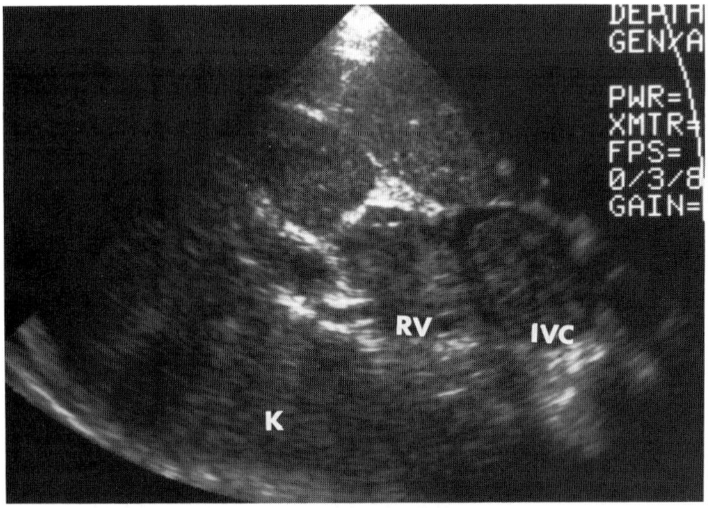

Figure 6.11. Transverse sonogram of right kidney. Enlarged, diffusely hypoechoic kidney (*K*) due to infiltrative renal cell carcinoma. The renal vein (*RV*) and inferior vena cava (*IVC*) are distended by a hypoechoic tumor thrombus.

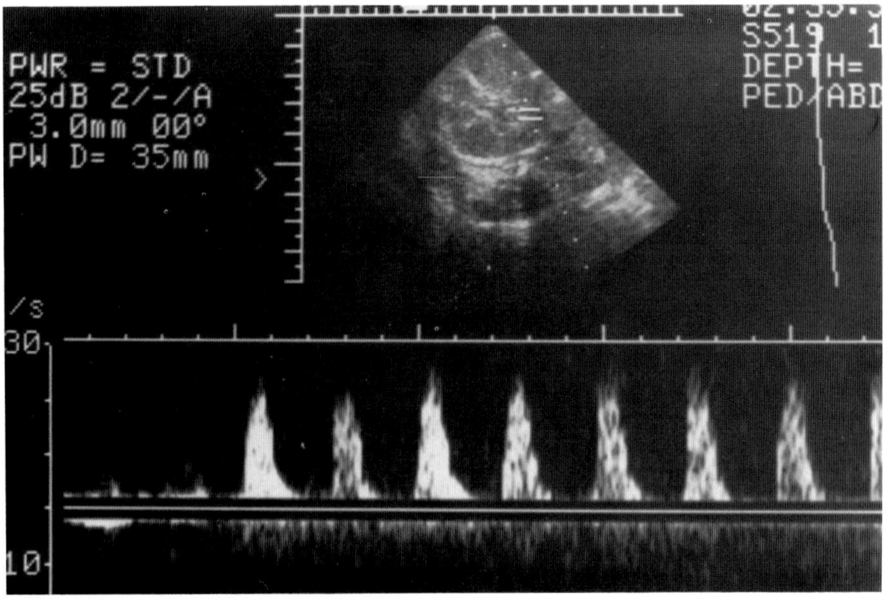

Figure 6.12. Doppler study of renal artery. Absence of diastolic flow with high-resistance systolic flow in a kidney with renal vein thrombosis.

renal vein and high-resistance systolic flow with or without reversed diastolic flow in arteries (Fig. 6.12).

Collagen Diseases

Progressive systemic sclerosis (PSS) (scleroderma), systemic lupus erythematosus (SLE), polyarteritis nodosa, Wegener's granulomatosis, and rheumatoid arthritis involve small arteries and produce chronic renal failure. The changes include arterial intimal thickening, necrotizing vasculitis, periarteritis, and glomerulonephritis. In PSS, the kidneys are usually normal in size and have a mottled reddish-yellow appearance with small hemorrhages or infarcts. In polyarteritis nodosa they are coarsely nodular and irregularly scarred and show thrombosed anuerysms at the corticomedullary junction. Sonographic findings are variable. On sonograms, the kidneys may be normal or small in size and show a thin cortex, loss of corticomedullary definition, and increased echogenicity.

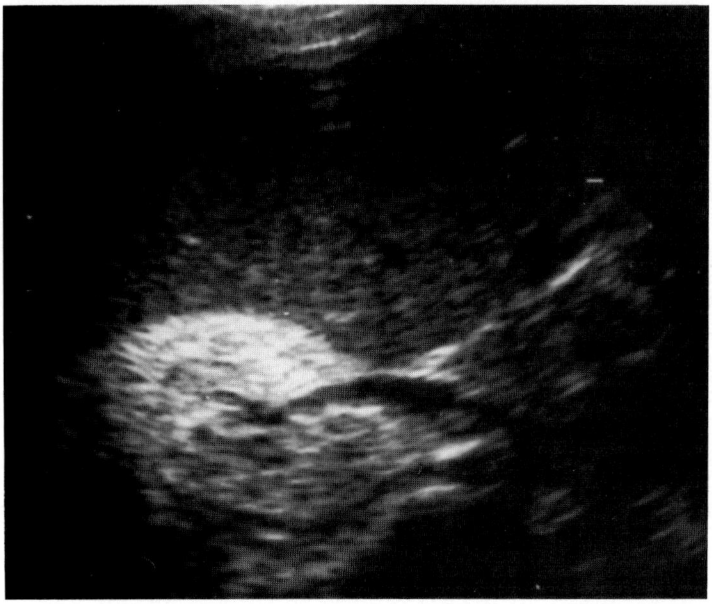

Figure 6.13. Transverse sonogram of right kidney. Intensely echogenic small kidney due to diffuse nephrocalcinosis in a hypercalcemic patient with renal sarcoidosis.

Metabolic Renal Diseases

Chronic hypercalcemic states (primary hyperparathyroidism, vitamin D intoxication, idiopathic hypercalcemia, sarcoidosis, metastatic bone disease, milk alkali syndrome), hyperurecemia, primary hyperoxaluria, and diabetes produce excessive excretion of physiologic substances such as calcium, uric acid, oxalic acid, etc. (Fig. 6.13). Their deposition in renal tubules and interstitium can lead to chronic renal failure. Sonographic findings of calcium nephropathy are described elsewhere.

In primary hyperoxaluria, excessive oxalic acid excretion in urine and calcium oxalate deposition in the tubules and tissues occurs. On sonograms, the renal cortex is intensely echogenic. When the medulla is involved, the kidneys are small and diffusely hyperechoic (Fig. 6.14) (11, 12). Primary uricemia produces uric acid crystalluria and calculi. The uric acid calculi are radiolucent on radiographs and tomograms. Sonography is highly sensitive for detection of radiolucent calculi and follow-up of their size during therapy (15, 23). Sonography is also useful to localize the site of obstruction and determine the renal cortical thickness.

DIABETIC NEPHROPATHY

The spectrum of renal changes in diabetes includes arterio- and arteriolosclerosis, glomerulosclerosis, presence of Armanni-Ebstein cells (glycogen-filled epithelial cells) in the proximal tubules, and interstitial nephritis due to infection. Sonography is usually normal in uncomplicated acute pyelonephritis but can be very useful in the diagnosis of emphysematous pyelonephritis, xanthogranulomatous pyelonephritis (XPN), acute bacterial nephronia, chronic pyelonephritis, renal or perirenal abscess, opportunistic infections, renal vein thrombosis, and chronic glomerulo-

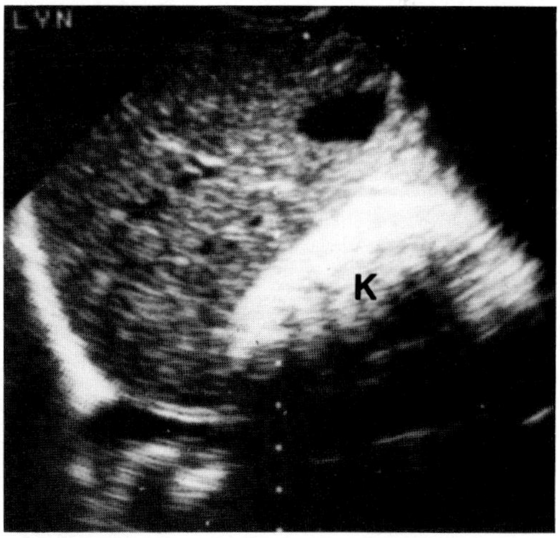

Figure 6.14. Longitudinal sonogram of right kidney. Intensely hyperechoic, small kidney (*K*) with corticomedullary calcinosis in a chronically uremic child with congenital hyperoxalosis.

nephritis. Chronic glomerulonephritis and vasculitis are the most common causes of chronic renal failure in a diabetic patient. The kidneys are small, irregular, and highly echogenic and show brightly reflective vascular calcifications (Fig. 6.3) (1, 2).

In acute pyelonephritis, sonograms may show an enlarged and hypoechoic kidney with enlarged pyramids and a mildly dilated pelvicaliceal system (Fig. 6.15) (24, 25). Brightly reflective clustered echoes due to air in the kidneys is pathognomonic of emphysematous pyelonephritis (Fig. 6.16) (26). Diffuse bilateral xanthogranulomatous pyelonephritis may produce chronic renal failure. On sonograms, the kidneys are enlarged and show multiple hypoechoic fluid-filled masses corresponding to debris-filled, dilated calices or areas of parenchymal destruction. The renal pelvis is not enlarged, due to extensive peripelvic fibrosis (27, 28). Acute nephronia is due to focal bacterial embolization involving a wedge-shaped renal segment and represents a preliquefaction stage of suppuration. On sonograms, it is seen as a hypoechoic focal mass with distal acoustic enhancement and poor corticomedullary definition (29, 30).

Infections

CHRONIC PYELONEPHRITIS

Chronic pyelonephritis represents an insidious infectious interstitial nephritis, which in late stages can produce chronic renal failure. Pathologically it is characterized by widespread interstitial inflammatory cellular infiltration, periglomerular fibrosis, tubular atrophy, tubular dilation with flattened epithelial cells, and arteriosclerosis. The kidneys are small, contracted, and coarsely granular. The capsule is thick and adherent to underlying parenchyma. The corticomedullary distinction is blurred and the pelvicaliceal system is dilated. On sonograms, the kidneys are very small and echogenic with loss of corticomedullary differentiation. The cortex is thin and shows hyper- or hypoechoic subcapsular scars (Fig. 6.17) (31). Often, echogenic foci of calcification are seen in the parenchyma. The renal pelvis and calices are dilated and may contain floating or layering pus debris.

TUBERCULOSIS OF KIDNEY

Tuberculosis of the kidney is almost always secondary to pulmonary disease, and advanced

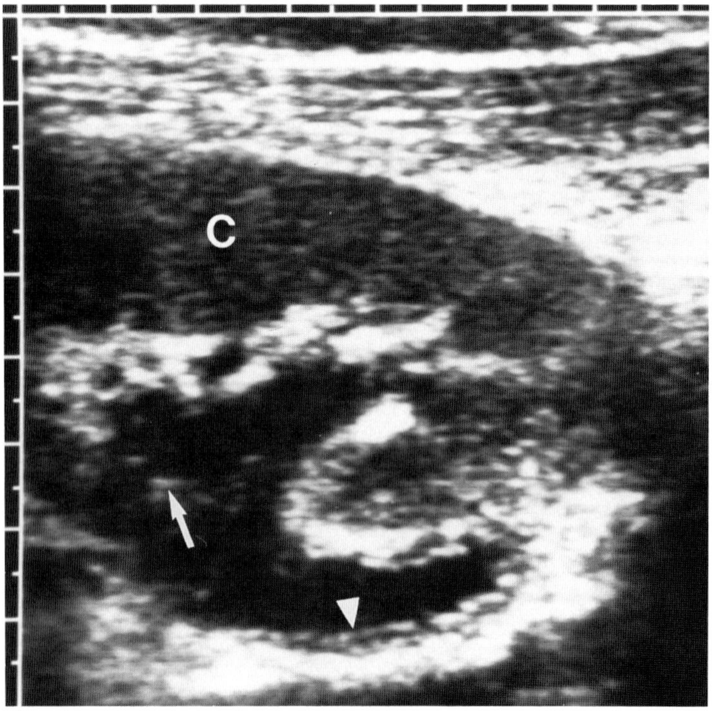

Figure 6.15. Longitudinal sonogram of right kidney. Slightly hypoechoic cortex (*C*), thickening of pelvicaliceal wall (*arrowhead*), and floating debris (*arrow*) in dilated calices in acute pyelonephritis.

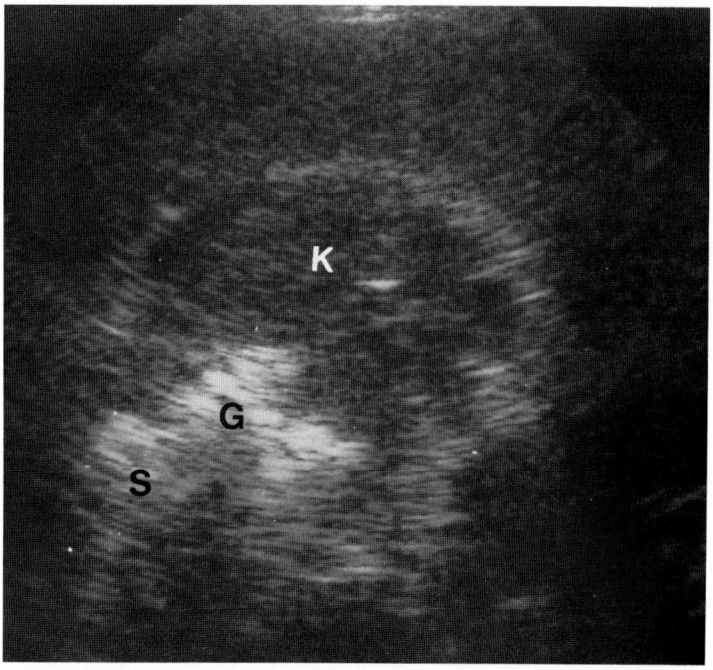

Figure 6.16. Transverse sonogram of right kidney. Irregular highly echogenic collections of gas (*G*) in the kidney (*K*) and perirenal space (*S*) in a diabetic with emphysematous pyelonephritis.

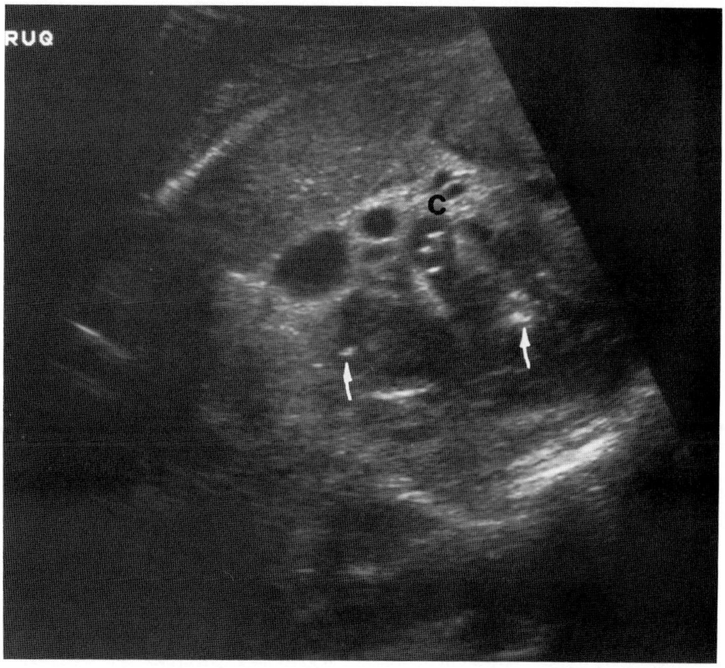

Figure 6.17. Transverse sonogram of right kidney. The cortex (*C*) is thin, irregular, and hyperechoic. Two peripheral cysts are seen. The dilated calices show echogenic pus debris and calculi (*arrows*).

bilateral miliary disease can produce chronic renal failure. Pathologically chronic granulomatous inflammation with caseation necrosis, cavitation, caliceal ulceration, fibrosis, and scarring occurs (32, 33). Early diagnosis of tuberculosis is made by culture of acid-fast bacilli from biological fluids. On sonograms, calcified granulomas, cavities, papillary necrosis, infundibular stenosis, and chronic pyelonephritis are late findings. Sonographic features are similar to those of chronic pyelonephritis. In addition, irregular caliceal dilation from infundibular stenosis, ureteral strictures, and a contracted bladder may be seen.

ACQUIRED IMMUNODEFICIENCY SYNDROME

Patients with acquired immunodeficiency syndrome (AIDS) may develop acute or chronic renal failure due to interstitial nephritis, acute tubular necrosis, focal nephrocalcinosis, opportunistic infections, and neoplasms such as Kaposi sarcoma and lymphoma (34). Pathologic findings in AIDS include focal segmental glomerulosclerosis, interstitial fibrosis, infiltrates, tubular atrophy, and hyaline tubular casts (35). AIDS patients are highly prone to infection by *Candida, Aspergillus,* and *Mycobacterium avium-intracellulare.* On sonograms, the kidneys are diffusely echogenic and show varying degrees of corticomedullary differentiation (36, 37). Corticomedullary calcinosis has been reported (38). Diffuse urothelial thickening, layering echogenic debris, and fungus balls in the calices, ureters, or bladder may be seen due to fungal infection (39). In the absence of sepsis, a focal hypoechoic renal mass in an AIDS patient should be considered a lymphoma or Kaposi sarcoma until proven otherwise (Fig. 6.18).

Infiltrative Processes

RENAL LYMPHOMA

Diffuse renal infiltration by lymphoma, leukemia, multiple myeloma, sarcoidosis, amyloidosis, and glycogen storage disease can lead to chronic renal failure. Sonography, like computed tomography, is more sensitive than urography for detection of early renal infiltrations (40). Sonography is useful for detection of focal lesions, their extrarenal extension, and their response to radiation or chemotherapy. Sonography is also useful for detecting vascular or ureteral compression by adjacent lymphadenopathy.

On sonograms, the kidneys show smooth or lobulated enlargement and a mildly nonhomogeneous hypoechoic texture (Figs. 6.19 and 6.20). The corticomedullary definition is preserved, but this is less obvious in the late stage. The central echo complex is distorted or lost. The pyramids are enlarged and hypoechoic (41, 42).

RENAL LEUKEMIA

On sonograms, kidneys diffusely infiltrated by leukemia show smooth enlargement with increased parenchymal echogenicity and poor corticomedullary definition (Fig. 6.21) (43). A few focal lesions may be scattered in a diffusely infiltrated parenchyma. Larger masses may infiltrate through the capsule into the peri- or pararenal space or adjacent muscles.

AMYLOIDOSIS OF THE KIDNEYS

Amyloidosis is characterized by deposition of a glycoprotein with distinct staining characteristics in multiple organs. It may be primary

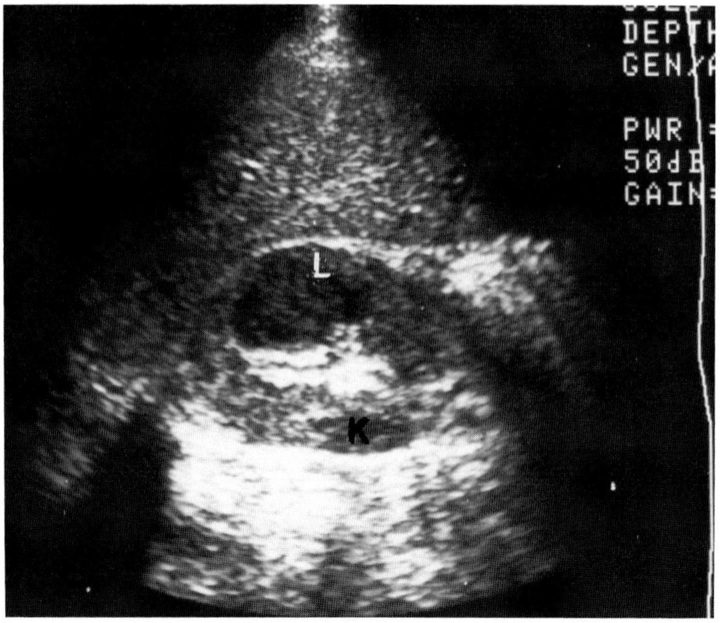

Figure 6.18. Transverse sonogram of right kidney. Increased echogenicity of kidney (*K*) with loss of corticomedullary distinction due to interstitial nephritis and a focal hypoechoic lymphoma (*L*) in the cortex in a patient with AIDS.

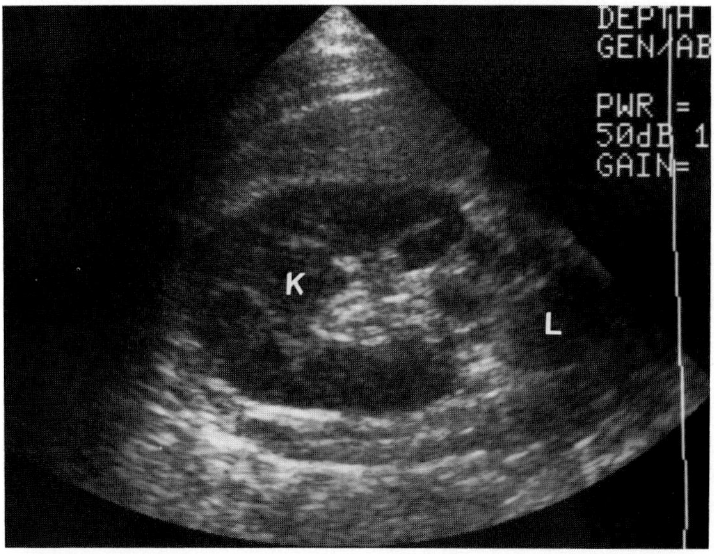

Figure 6.19. Transverse sonogram of right kidney. Diffusely hypoechoic, large kidney (*K*) with loss of corticomedullary distinction and perihilar lymphadenopathy (*L*) in a biopsy-proven lymphoma.

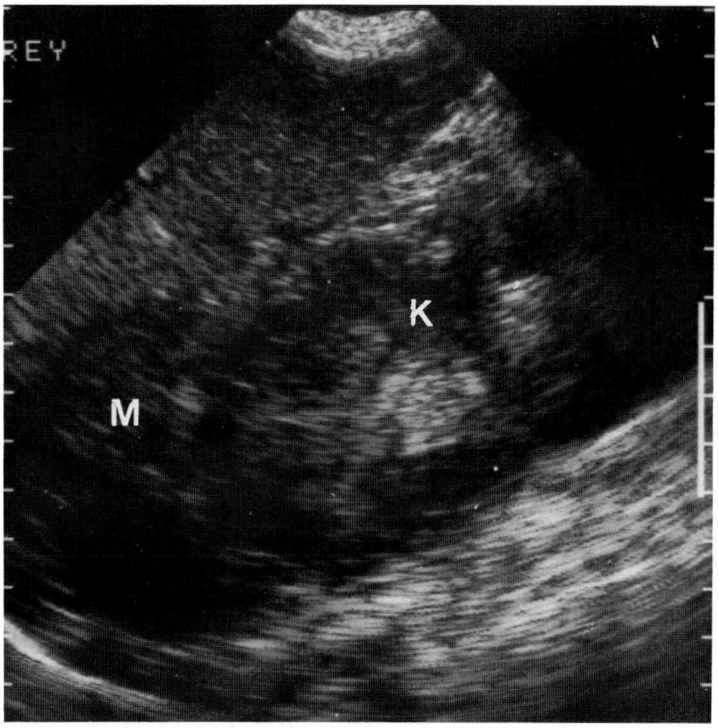

Figure 6.20. Longitudinal sonogram of right kidney. Large hypoechoic kidney (*K*) with loss of corticomedullary distinction and hypoechoic extrarenal mass (*M*) due to perirenal lymphomatous infiltration.

and heredofamilial or secondary to metabolic disease, neoplasm, chronic infection, or inflammation. Secondary amyloidosis is seen in diabetes, tuberculosis, bronchiectasis, osteomyelitis, rheumatoid arthritis and its variants, lymphoma, myeloma, renal cell carcinoma, medullary carcinoma of the thyroid, and several other diseases. Renal amyloidosis clinically manifests itself as nephrotic syndrome. On sonograms, the kidneys show smooth enlargement and diffusely increased echogenicity. The central sinus echoes and arcuate vessels are less distinct (Fig. 6.22). Sonography is useful for detection of bilateral renal vein thrombosis, which is known to occur commonly in nephrotic syndrome (44).

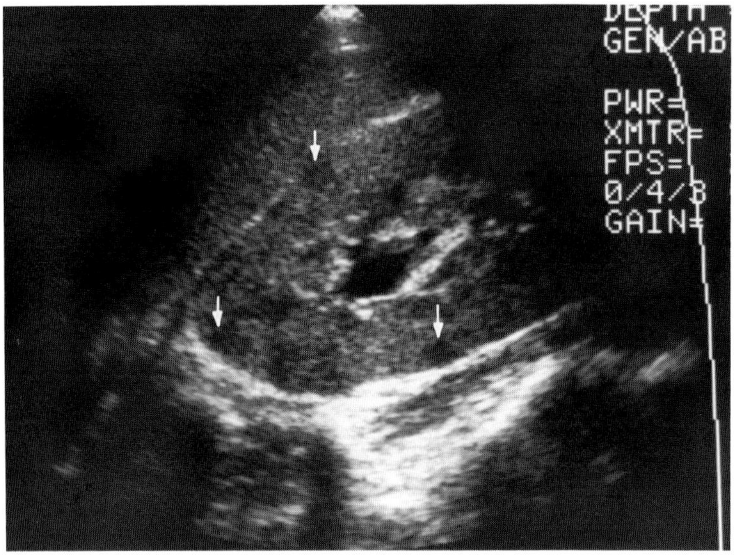

Figure 6.21. Longitudinal sonogram of right kidney. Enlarged kidney with hyperechoic cortex and poor corticomedullary distinction due to diffuse leukemic infiltration. Small hypoechoic foci (*arrows*) in peripheral cortex also represent leukemic deposits.

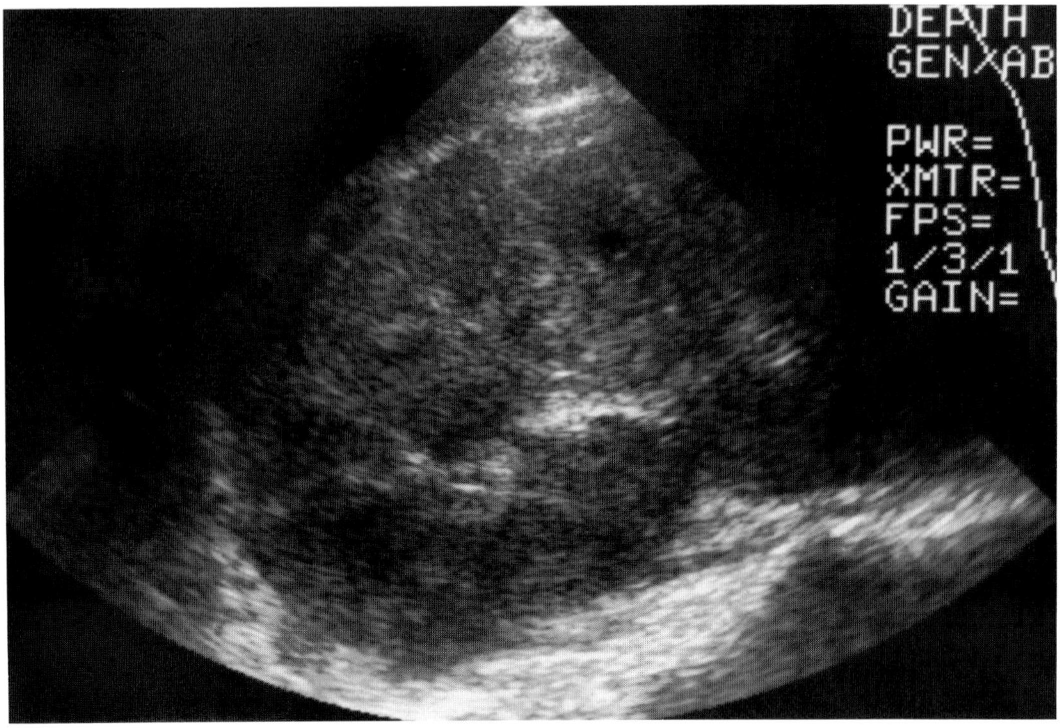

Figure 6.22. Longitudinal sonogram of right kidney. Hyperechoic kidney with loss of central sinus echoes and poor corticomedullary distinction in secondary amyloidosis in a patient with cystic bronchiectasis.

RENAL SARCOIDOSIS

Renal sarcoidosis manifests as hypercalcemia with nephrocalcinosis, lithiasis, or chronic pyelonephritis, and rarely as masses (45). On sonograms, the kidneys may be enlarged and show decreased echogenicity. In the late stage, they are small and shrunken and show increased echogenicity (Fig. 6.13). Rarely, focal hypoechoic masses may be present.

GLYCOGEN STORAGE DISEASES

Diffuse renal involvement is common in glycogen storage diseases. On sonograms, the kidneys show smooth enlargement and diffusely increased echogenicity, particularly around the calices and pyramids.

Congenital Renal Anomalies

HYPOPLASIA

Bilateral renal hypoplasia is a rare condition caused by the failure of normal development of metanephric blastema because of intrauterine ischemia. The kidneys are small and contain well-formed nephrons. Bilateral renal hypoplasia or unilateral hypoplasia with disease in the opposite kidney leads to renal failure. On sonograms the kidneys are very small and smooth and show normal echogenicity. Renal vessels are uniformly attenuated, and pyramids are few in number. The contralateral kidney shows compensatory hypertrophy.

MULTICYSTIC DYSPLASTIC KIDNEYS

Bilateral multicystic dysplasia of kidneys (MCDK) is incompatible with life. However, unilateral MCDK with disease (often cystic dysplasia or obstruction) in the other kidney leads to renal failure. Based on the site of obstruction, MCDK occurs in infundibulopelvic atretic or hydronephrotic forms (46).

In general, cystic dysplasia is severe if obstruction occurs early in fetal life. Multicystic dysplastic kidney is presumably due to intrauterine ischemia during nephrogenesis before 8 to 10 weeks. Ischemia leads to atresia of the infundibulopelvic region and proximal ureter, and the resulting lack of fusion between the ureteric bud and metanephric blastema produces renal cystic dysplasia. Large cysts, separated by septa containing fibrous and dysplastic tissue, replace renal parenchyma. A hydronephrotic form of MCDK occurs due to obstruction at the ureteropelvic junction in intrauterine life.

On sonograms, the kidneys show asymmetric enlargement with an irregular contour due to multiple cysts, which vary in size and shape. The cysts do not communicate with each other or with calices, and a dilated renal pelvis is not identifiable at the hilum (Fig. 6.23). A thin rim of parenchyma, renal vessels, renal pelvis, and proximal ureter are not identifiable. In the hydronephrotic form of MCDK, a large central cyst representing distended renal pelvis is seen at the hilum (Fig. 6.24) (47, 48). Other sonographic features are similar to those seen in the infundibulopelvic form. Occasionally, hyperechoic parenchyma with small peripheral cysts and a distended central pelvis may be seen (Fig. 6.25). A thin cortical rim with relatively uniformly dilated calices communicating with a central distended pelvis differentiate congenital ureteropelvic obstruction from the hydronephrotic form of MCDK, although the two entities may be occasionally indistinguishable (Fig. 6.26) (48).

POLYCYSTIC KIDNEYS

Polycystic disease (PCD) is classified into infantile, juvenile, and adult types on the basis of differences in hereditary, morphologic, and clinical features. Rarely, infantile PCD in an adult and adult PCD in a neonate may be seen (49).

Autosomal Dominant Polycystic Disease

Adult PCD is an autosomal dominant disease with high penetrance, and a family history of PCD is often present. Polycystic kidneys are often an incidental finding during the workup of renal failure, hypertension, or urinary tract infection in the 30- to 50-year age group. Rarely, pain due to rupture, infection, or bleeding in or around the kidney is the presenting symptom. On sonograms, the kidneys are asymmetrically enlarged and their parenchyma is replaced by numerous cysts of varying sizes and shapes (Fig. 6.27). The cysts may show low- or medium-level echoes, fluid debris level, or echogenic calcification in the wall or septa (50–52). Echogenic material in a cyst may be due to pus, blood, organized clot, or a tumor (Fig. 6.28). Cysts may be found in the liver, pancreas, and spleen. Sonography is useful to detect a hematoma around the kidney. In general, sonographic detection of a new bleed, infection, or carcinoma in a cyst in PCD is difficult due to the extensive search involving numerous cysts.

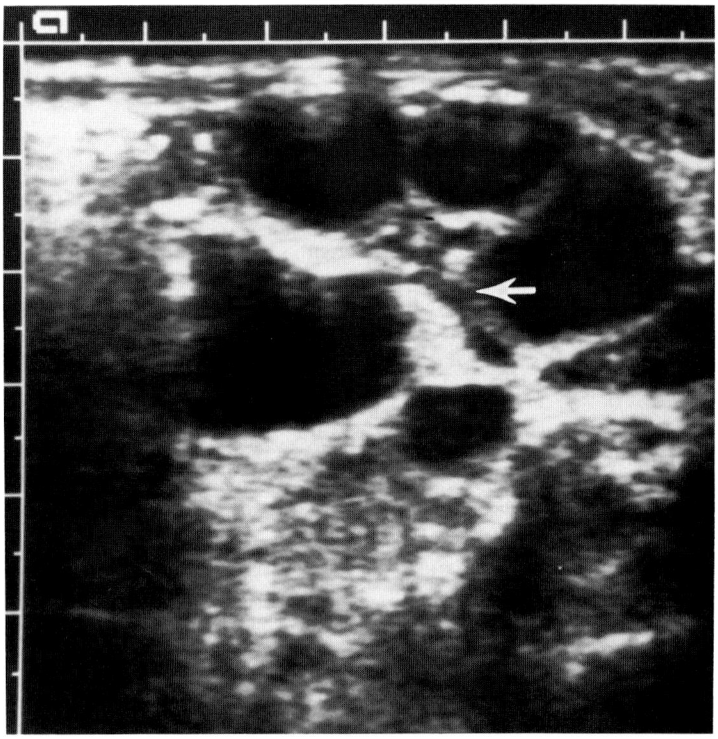

Figure 6.23. Transverse sonogram of right kidney. Multiple noncommunicating cysts replace parenchyma, and renal pelvis is not dilated (*arrow*) in infundibulopelvic atretic form of multicystic dysplastic kidney.

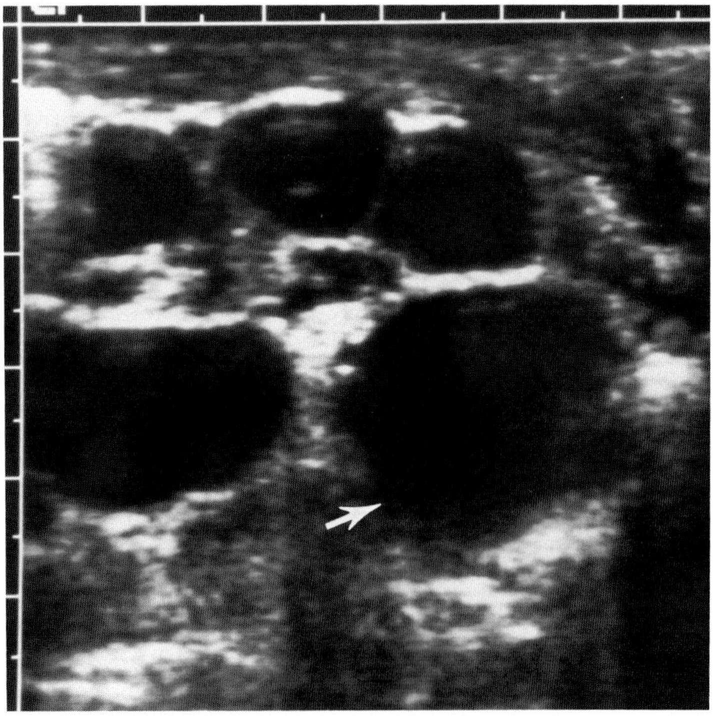

Figure 6.24. Transverse sonogram of right kidney. Multiple noncommunicating cysts replace parenchyma and renal pelvis is distended (*arrow*) in hydronephrotic form of multicystic dysplastic kidney.

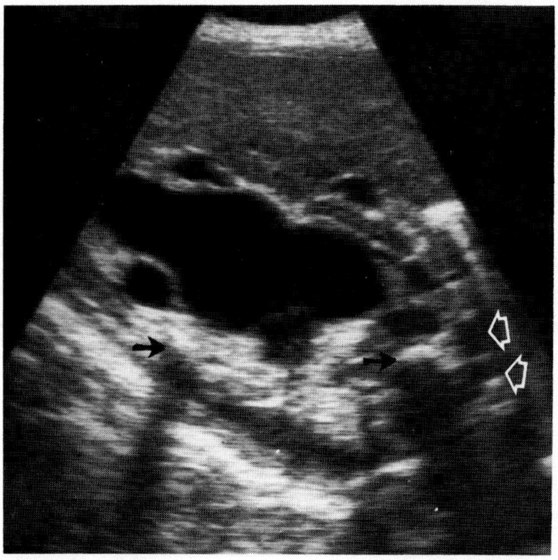

Figure 6.25. Longitudinal sonogram of right kidney. Markedly distended pelvis communicating with dilated calices, and a few peripheral cysts (*arrowheads*) and calcifications (*arrows*) in a slightly hyperechoic parenchyma are seen in dysplastic kidneys due to lower urinary tract obstruction.

Autosomal Recessive Polycystic Disease

Autosomal recessive PCD (infantile) is seen in the newborn as smooth enlargement of kidneys in which the renal tubules and collecting ducts are diffusely dilated. On sonograms, the kidneys are markedly enlarged and highly echogenic and show smooth contour (53).

An anechoic subcapsular rim due to cystic dilation of tubules, a central anechoic renal pelvis, and poor corticomedullary definition are seen (Fig. 6.29). A few small macroscopic cysts and occasional parenchymal calcification may be present.

Juvenile Polycystic Disease

Juvenile PCD is seen in children in the 2- to 6-year age group with renal tubular ectasia, hepatic fibrosis, and bile ductal dilation. The renal tubules and collecting ducts are diffusely dilated. Due to hepatic fibrosis, portal hypertension, hepatosplenomegaly, and gastrointestinal bleeding are more prominent features, and renal disease is less severe. Sonographic features are similar to those seen in autosomal recessive PCD. An enlarged liver with coarse echo texture, distended portal veins, portal-systemic collaterals, and splenomegaly may be seen (54, 55).

MEDULLARY CYSTIC DISEASE

Medullary cystic disease is a rare cause of renal failure in young adults and adolescents. On sonograms, the kidneys are small or normal in size and contain cysts in the medulla, which vary in size from 1 mm to several centimeters (56). Most cysts are scattered near the base of renal pyramids. The kidneys are more echogenic, and corticomedullary definition is poor (Fig. 6.30) (57).

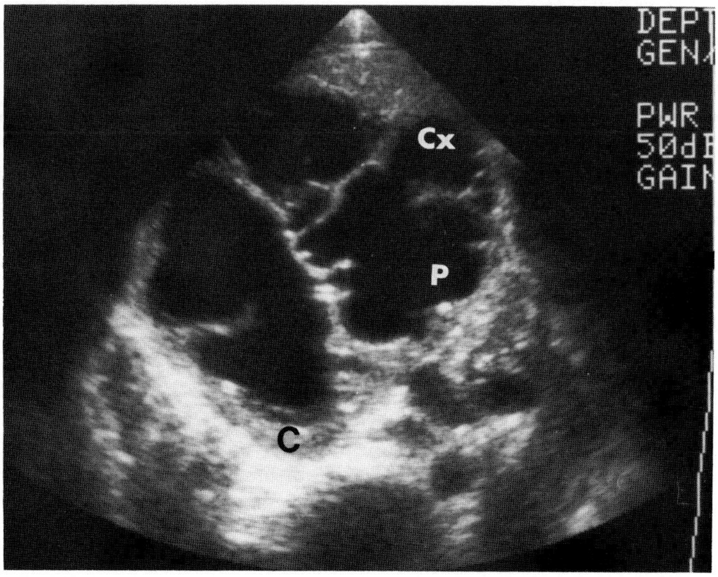

Figure 6.26. Transverse sonogram of right kidney. Thin peripheral rim of cortex (*C*), preserved reniform shape with smooth outline, and communication between dilated calices (*Cx*) and pelvis (*P*) are seen in congenital ureteropelvic junction obstruction.

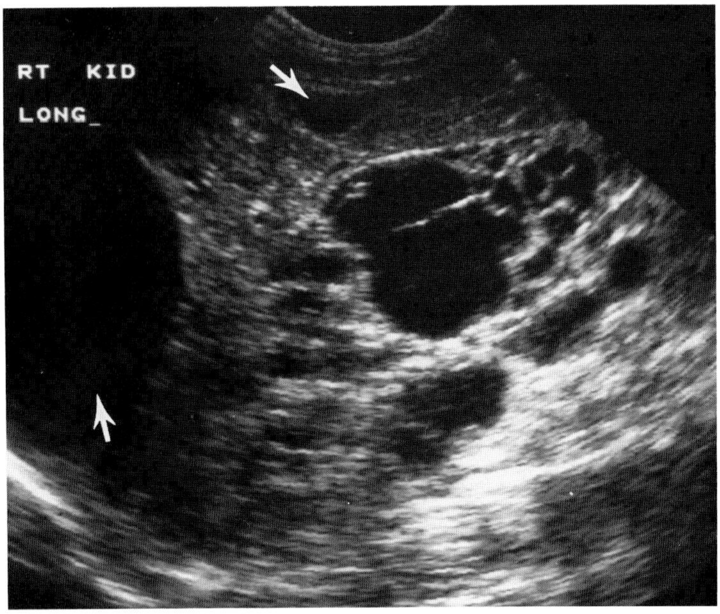

Figure 6.27. Longitudinal sonogram of right kidney. Two hepatic cysts (*arrows*) and several renal cysts of varying sizes and shapes separated by septa and islands of parenchyma are seen in autosomal dominant polycystic disease.

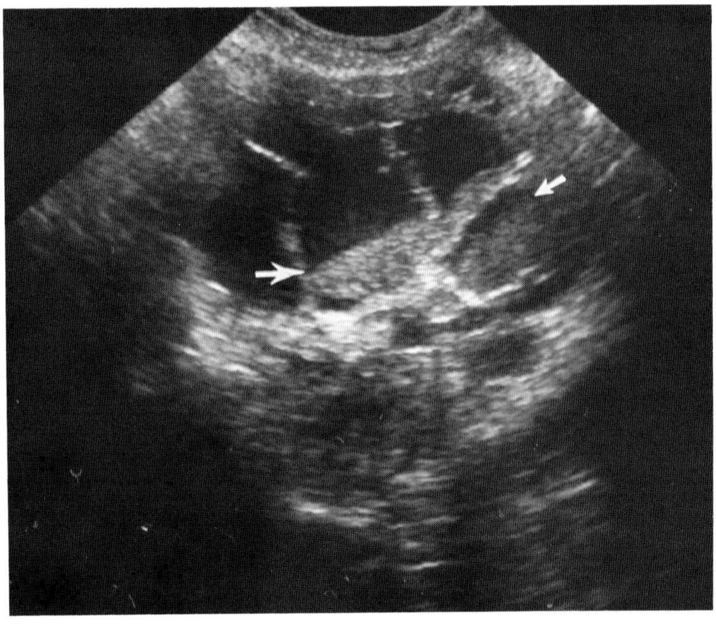

Figure 6.28. Transverse sonogram of left kidney. Dependent layering of echogenic pus debris (*arrows*) in infected cysts in autosomal dominant polycystic kidneys.

MEDULLARY SPONGE KIDNEY

Medullary sponge kidney is seen in young adults who present with recurrent infections or hematuria and rarely with chronic renal failure. The collecting ducts and tubules in renal pyramids are ectatic and may show radiopaque linear calcifications (58). On sonograms, a diffuse or focal increase in echogenicity is seen at sites of calcification in pyramids (59).

ACQUIRED RENAL CYSTIC DISEASE

Sonography is useful to detect changes in patients with chronic renal failure on long-term dialysis. The native kidneys show cysts and, in 5 to 6% of cases, renal cell carcinoma (60). On sonograms, features of "end-stage" parenchymal disease described earlier and several cysts, mostly scattered in the cortex, are seen. The cysts are often uniformly small, in

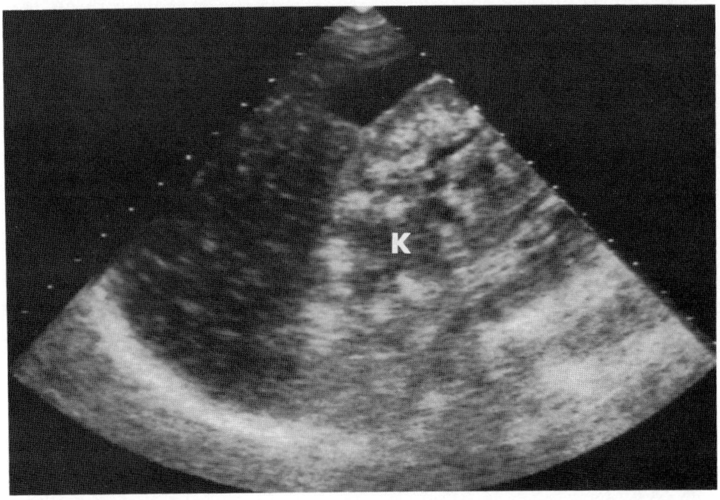

Figure 6.29. Longitudinal sonogram of right kidney. Smooth enlargement of kidney (*K*) with diffuse hyperechogenicity and subcortical hypoechoic rim (dilated tubules and collecting ducts) in a neonate with autosomal recessive polycystic disease.

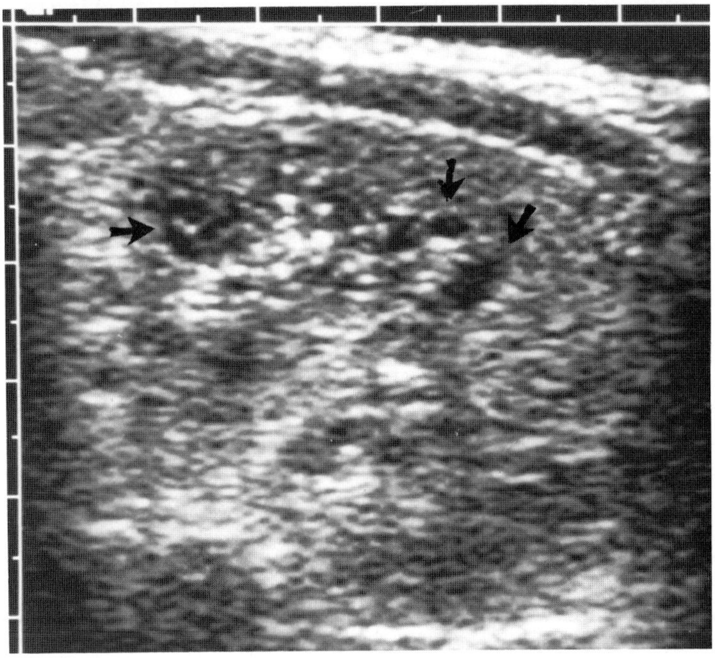

Figure 6.30. Longitudinal sonogram of right kidney. Echogenic kidney with multiple cysts in renal pyramids (*arrows*) in an adolescent with chronic azotemia and salt loss due to medullary cystic disease.

the 2- to 4-mm range, but may be up to 2 cm or more in diameter (Figs. 6.2 and 6.3) (61).

Obstructive Uropathy

Urinary tract obstruction can produce acute or chronic renal failure depending on the duration, completeness, site, and cause of obstruction. A variety of diseases can cause obstruction to urine flow from the level of renal tubules to the external urethral meatus and produce renal failure. Chronic renal failure can result from incomplete obstruction to the lower urinary tract or the solitary functioning kidney (when the other kidney is absent, hypoplastic, functioning poorly, or nonfunctioning). Rarely, "horseshoe" kidneys may be obstructed by calculi or vessels and produce chronic or acute renal failure (Fig. 6.31). Hydronephrosis denotes an enlarged pelvicalyceal system due to obstructive or nonobstructive causes. Chronic obstruction produces cortical atrophy, while acute obstruction produces marked pelvicalyceal dilation without atrophy. The extent of pelvicaliceal dilation depends on the following

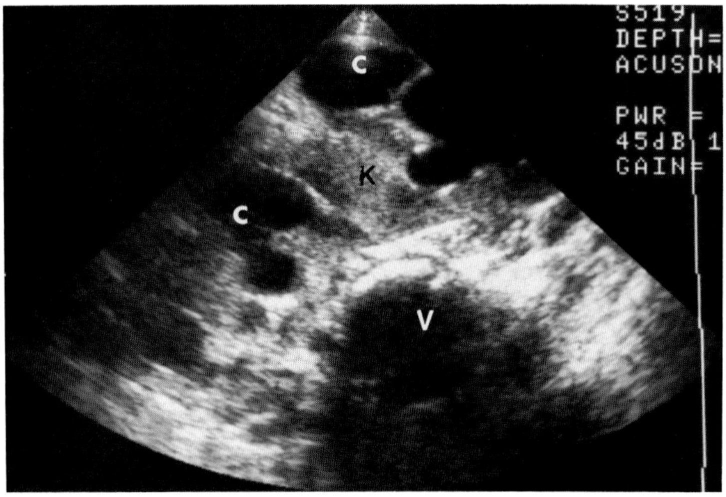

Figure 6.31. Transverse sonogram of mid-abdomen. Dilated calices (*C*) and renal parenchyma anterior to the lumbar vertebra (*V*) in a "horseshoe" kidney (*K*) with obstruction.

factors: (*a*) duration of obstruction, (*b*) completeness of obstruction, (*c*) intra- or extrarenal pelvis, (*d*) compliance of renal parenchyma, (*e*) spontaneous decompression by caliceal rupture, (*f*) state of hydration, and (*g*) renal function. Therefore, several false-positive and false-negative causes for obstruction can lead to inaccurate sonographic diagnosis (Tables 6.7 and 6.8) (62).

The causes of obstructive hydronephrosis leading to renal failure are numerous and can be divided into congenital or acquired, and intrinsic or extrinsic. The congenital causes include meatal stenosis, urethral stricture, webs, posterior urethral valves, bladder neck obstruction, and bilateral ureterovesical and ureteropelvic junction obstruction. The acquired conditions include urethral stricture, prostatomegaly of various causes, calculus, clot, cancer, and obstruction of the urethra, bladder neck, or ureters. The intrinsic causes include calculus, clot, foreign body, benign or malignant tumor, ureterocele, caustic chemicals, and sloughed papilla. The extrinsic causes include space-occupying lesions in the pelvis, prostatomegaly, bladder compression, gynecologic masses compressing or invading the lower urinary tract, pelvic masses (including the gravid uterus), and retroperitoneal processes such as fibrosis, hematoma, or tumor. Nonobstructive dilation of the pelvicaliceal system can be seen in patients with myelodysplasia, ureterovesical reflux nephropathy, congenital megacalices, primary megaureters, infection, residual dilation from previous obstruction, retroperitoneal fibrosis, and prune belly syndrome.

In mild hydronephrosis, the central echo complex is separated by a large anechoic pelvis that communicates with dilated calices, and the cortex remains intact (Fig. 6.32). In moderate and severe hydronephrosis, variable degrees of cortical atrophy are seen (Figs. 6.33 and 6.34). When dilated ureters are seen posterior to the bladder, obstruction at or below the vesicoureteral junction must be considered (Figs. 6.35 and 6.36). A patulous ureterovesical opening is due to reflux, infection, or severe

Table 6.7.
Causes of False-Positive Sonograms for Obstruction

Large extrarenal pelvis
High-urine-output states
Nonobstructive dilation
Congenital megacalices
Reflux nephropathy
Severe papillary necrosis
Parapelvic cyst

Table 6.8.
Causes of False-Negative Sonograms for Obstruction

Early stage of obstruction
Partial or intermittent obstruction
Decompressed pelvicaliceal system
Retroperitoneal fibrosis
Hypovolemia or dehydration
Severe parenchymal disease
Scarred kidney

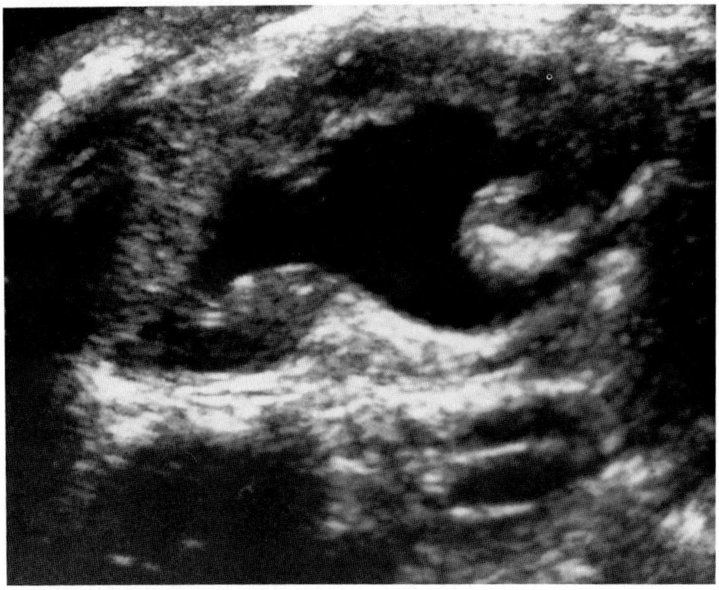

Figure 6.32. Longitudinal sonogram of left kidney. Mild pelvicaliceal dilation without cortical atrophy due to ureterovesical junction calculus.

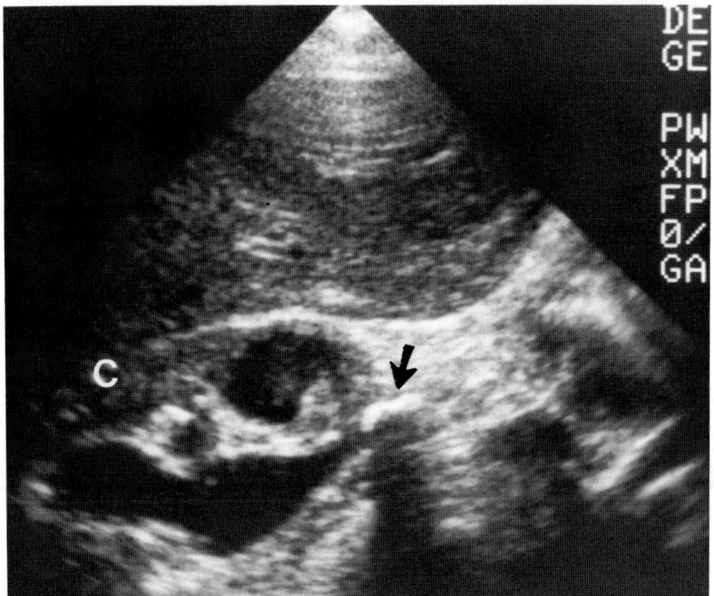

Figure 6.33. Transverse sonogram of right kidney. Cortical atrophy (*C*) and pelvicaliceal dilation due to impacted stone (*arrow*) at ureteropelvic junction.

distal obstruction (Fig. 6.37). In chronic obstruction below the level of the bladder neck, trabeculation of the bladder wall is seen.

Transrectal sonography is useful for the diagnosis of obstructive diseases of the bladder, proximal urethra, and prostate. Duplex Doppler sonography appears to be promising for differentiating early obstructive and nonobstructive dilation of the pelvicaliceal systems (63). Duplex Doppler sonography and Lasix-stimulated isotope renography are complementary in the early diagnosis of minimal ureteropelvic junction obstruction. Sonography is slightly more sensitive and specific in obstruction in the presence of chronic renal failure than radioisotope studies (64).

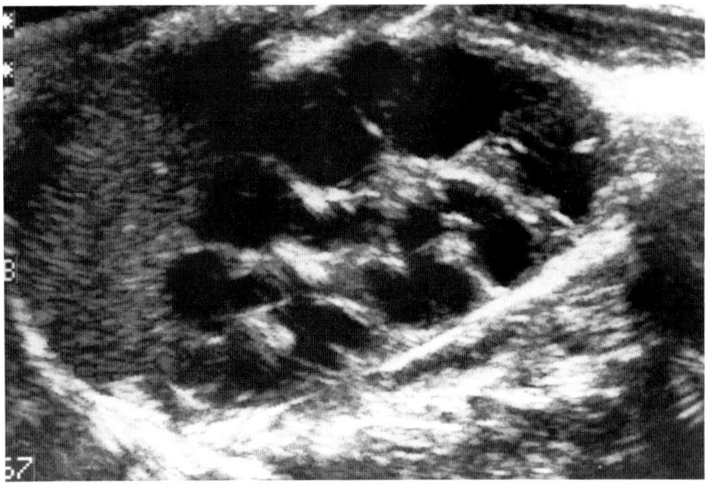

Figure 6.34. Longitudinal sonogram of left kidney. Severe caliceal dilation and cortical atrophy due to chronic obstruction.

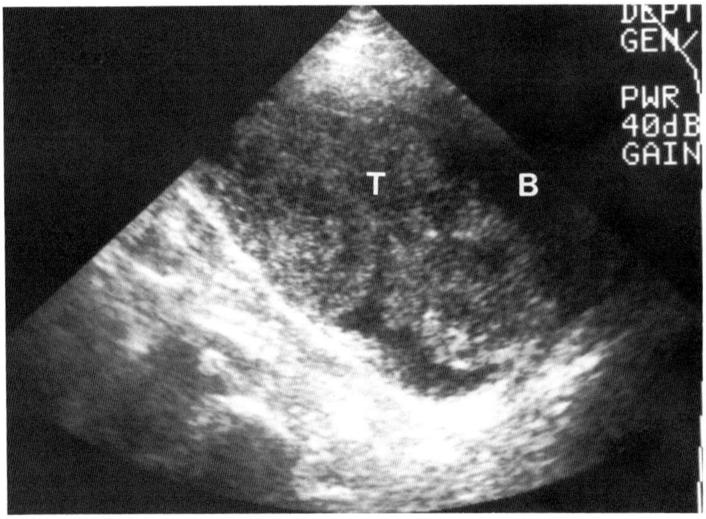

Figure 6.35. Longitudinal sonogram of urinary bladder. Large, irregular, and nonhomogeneously echogenic tumor (*T*) in the bladder (*B*) is the cause of bilateral ureteric obstruction in a patient with chronic renal failure.

ACUTE RENAL FAILURE

Acute renal failure is an abrupt reduction in renal function that is incompatible with life if continued. Acute ischemia, tubular necrosis, and tubular obstruction are the primary mechanisms in the pathogenesis of acute renal failure (65). The causes of acute renal failure are classified into prerenal, renal, and postrenal groups (Table 6.2).

Prerenal Diseases

Acute hypovolemia, hypotension, salt depletion, and arterial occlusion of any cause can produce acute cortical ischemia and renal failure. Although the primary diagnosis is established by clinical and biochemical profiles, sonography is useful to exclude obstruction and direct attention to specific groups of causes such as renal arterial or venous obstruction, cortical or tubular necrosis, and nephrotoxicity. If dehydration is severe in patients with acute renal failure, sonography may be suboptimal for echo texture analysis due to poor ultrasonic beam transmission.

ACUTE RENAL ARTERIAL OCCLUSION

Bilateral renal arterial occlusion is a rare cause of acute renal failure. Acute arterial occlusion produces renal cortical ischemia, tubular necrosis, and infarction. The most common

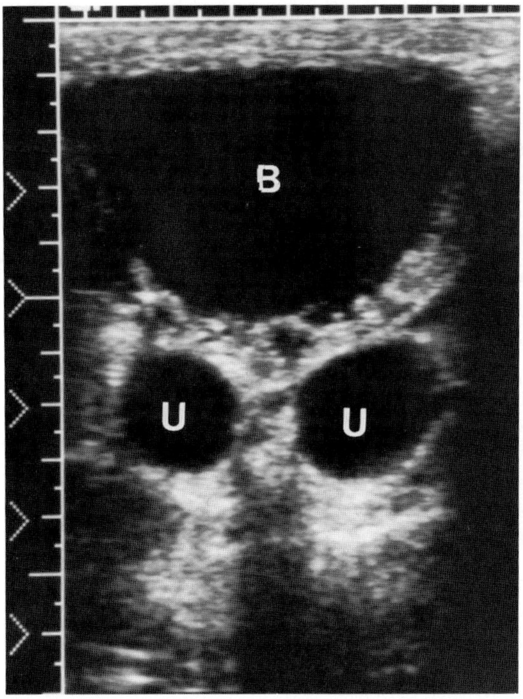

Figure 6.36. Transverse sonogram of pelvis. Heavily trabeculated bladder (*B*), mucosa, and dilated ureters (*U*) in a child with chronic obstruction due to posterior urethral valves.

cause of renal infarction is embolism from cardiac disease (66). Other causes include posttraumatic avulsion, thrombosis, and aortic dissection. Global renal infarction occurs if the main renal artery is occluded for longer than 1.5 hr (67). The subcortical layers become ischemic but not necrotic, presumably due to collateral flow through capsular vessels, while central corticomedullary layers become necrotic. The subcapsular zone shows reactive hyperemia around focal infarcts. The infarcted areas shrink after a week, and cortical depressions form in about 4 weeks (Fig. 6.38). Calcification occurs in necrotic tubules after 72 hr.

Diagnosis of renal infarction is made when nephrotomograms or dynamic computed tomograms after a bolus contrast injection show a 2- to 3-mm subcapsular rim of contrast enhancement around nonopacified parenchyma (66). The retrograde urogram is normal, and an angiogram confirms the diagnosis. Doppler evaluation of renal arteries is useful for noninvasive diagnosis of infarction. On color Doppler study, nonvisualization of flow in the renal artery and its branches is diagnostic.

In animal models the cortical rim sign was not seen on sonograms. Spies et al. found no obvious changes in cortical echogenicity after renal artery ligation in a dog model (68). This could be due to differences in cortical perfusion

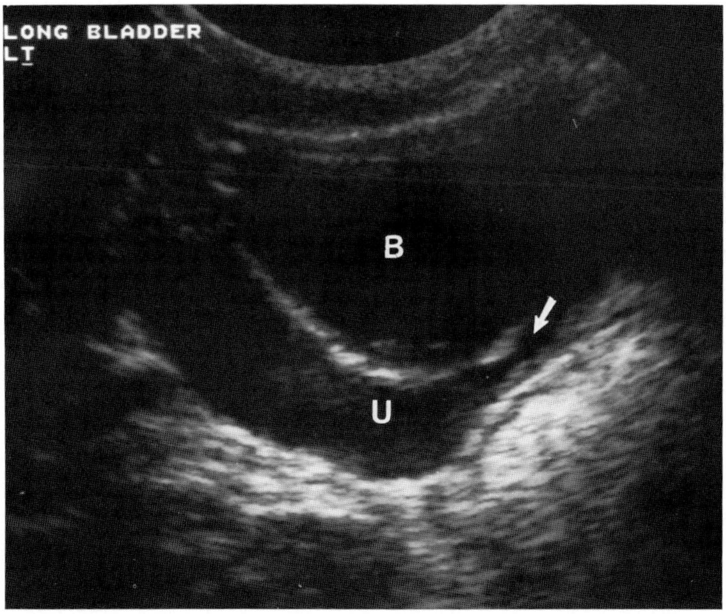

Figure 6.37. Longitudinal sonogram of left ureter and bladder. Patulous ureterovesical junction (*arrow*) with dilated ureter (*U*) in a child with reflux nephropathy. *B,* bladder.

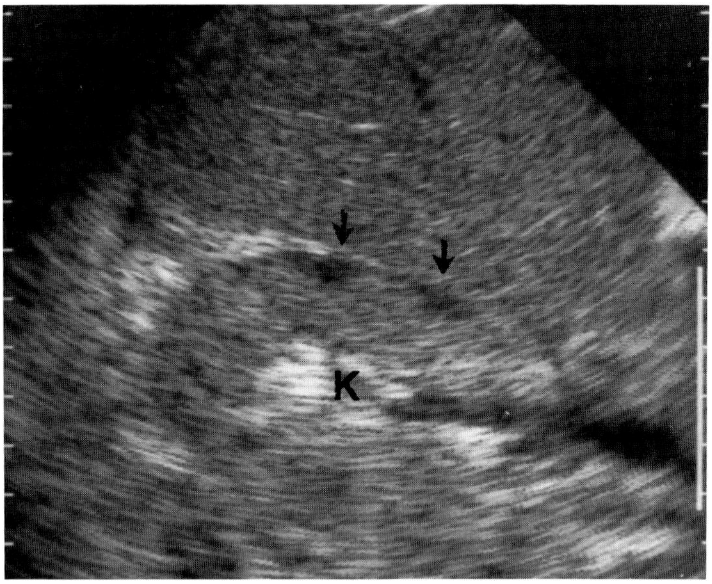

Figure 6.38. Transverse sonogram of right kidney. Diffusely hyperechoic kidney (*K*) with loss of corticomedullary distinction in a patient with sickle cell crisis. Peripheral subcortical infarcts are seen as wedge-shaped hypoechoic areas (*arrows*).

by collateral flow. Other sonographic findings due to acute renal cortical necrosis are described below.

Parenchymal Causes

Acute disease of either glomeruli, tubules, vessels, or a combination can result in acute renal failure. The most common processes include (*a*) acute cortical necrosis, (*b*) acute tubular necrosis, (*c*) acute tubular obstruction, and (*d*) acute inflammation.

ACUTE RENAL CORTICAL NECROSIS

Renal cortical necrosis is an important cause of acute renal failure, particularly in newborns and infants. It occurs under conditions of severe stress such as asphyxia neonatorum, septicemia, hemorrhage, gastroenteritis, hemolytic-uremic syndrome, feto-maternal transfusion, and renal vein thrombosis. In adults, acute cortical necrosis is associated with hemorrhagic shock, placental abruption, trauma, sepsis, dehydration, transfusion reaction, and toxemias (e.g., snake venom) (69). Sonograms in the early stage show only mild nephromegaly. Later on, the renal cortex shows increased echogenicity, probably due to collagen deposition and linear or punctate calcification. In the late stage, the kidneys are small and hyperechoic and show calcification (70).

ACUTE TUBULAR NECROSIS

Several causes produce acute tubular necrosis (ATN) and acute renal failure. Acute ischemia, nephrotoxic insult (e.g., ethylene glycol poisoning), and acute tubular obstruction by precipitation of proteins, calcium, or myoglobin result in ATN. Ischemic ATN is commonly seen in transplanted kidneys and in native kidneys after renal arterial occlusion. In ischemic ATN, the renal size is increased slightly without change in cortical or pyramidal echo texture. In nephrotoxic ATN, the cortical echogenicity is increased and corticomedullary distinction is more prominent (71, 72).

ACUTE TUBULAR OBSTRUCTION

In rhabdomyolysis, irrespective of the cause, myoglobinuria produces acute tubular obstruction and acute renal failure. In trauma victims with myoglobinuria, the renal cortex is hyperechoic and the corticomedullary distinction is preserved (73). In multiple myeloma the kidneys are enlarged and show a diffuse increase in cortical echogenicity with poor corticomedullary distinction (Fig. 6.39). In acute renal failure due to precipitation of Tamm-Horsfall proteins in tubules, the renal pyramids are hyperechoic (71).

HEMOLYTIC-UREMIC SYNDROME

Hemolytic-uremic syndrome consists of hemolytic anemia, thrombocytopenia, hypertension, and nephropathy due to fibrinous deposition in glomeruli and thrombotic microangiopathy (arteriolar thrombosis and capillary wall thickening) (74). Between 70 and 80% of cases occur in children below 5 years of age (75).

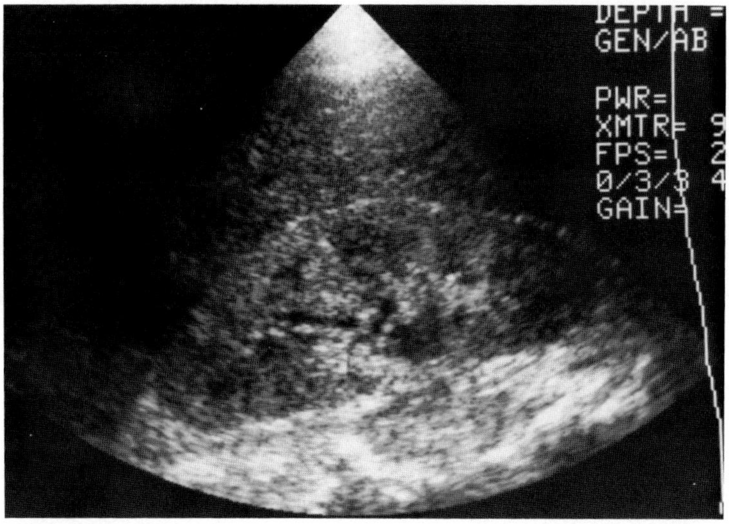

Figure 6.39. Transverse sonogram of right kidney. Enlarged and diffusely hyperechoic kidney with poor corticomedullary distinction in a patient with acute renal failure due to multiple myeloma.

Hemolytic-uremic syndrome may be idiopathic or secondary to complications of pregnancy or delivery (abruption, amniotic fluid embolism, fetal demise, eclampsia, etc.), malignant hypertension, disseminated carcinomatosis, and severe inflammation. In the acute stage, the kidneys are enlarged and edematous. In severe cases, grayish-yellow necrotic areas surrounded by hyperemia are seen diffusely or in patches. On sonograms, the cortex is hyperechoic, while pyramids remain hypoechoic and the corticomedullary differentiation is markedly accentuated (76, 77).

ACUTE PYELONEPHRITIS

Bilateral acute pyelonephritis is a rare cause of acute renal failure. Acute pyelonephritis due to *Escherichia coli* is most common in young women and occurs in association with diabetes, calculi, reflux, obstruction, trauma, intravenous drug abuse, and bacterial endocarditis. Acute pyelonephritis may occur in the diffuse or focal form. On sonograms, the kidneys show asymmetric enlargement and diffusely reduced echogenicity. The pelvicaliceal system is dilated and may show a thickened wall (suburothelial edema) and floating or layering echogenic debris (Fig. 6.15) (24, 25). The ureters and bladder may show the same findings. After recurrent episodes of acute pyelonephritis, the kidneys show focal scarring and caliceal clubbing as seen in chronic pyelonephritis (31, 78).

Sonographic features of acute toxic nephropathy and acute glomerulonephritis are discussed elsewhere in the chapter.

Postrenal Diseases

Acute venous, ureteral, or urethral obstruction of a solitary functioning kidney or both kidneys can produce backpressure effects that reduce glomerular filtration and effective renal plasma flow and lead to acute renal failure. Acute bilateral renal vein thrombosis and acute bilateral renal obstruction, irrespective of the cause, can produce acute renal failure.

ACUTE RENAL VEIN THROMBOSIS

Bilateral acute renal vein thrombosis (RVT) is a rare cause of acute renal failure. RVT occurs because of hypercoagulability, hyperviscosity, hemostasis, and venous intimal injury. In the neonate, birth trauma, dehydration, hypotension, anemia, intravascular catheters, cyanotic heart disease, maternal diabetes, and maternal diazide ingestion predispose to RVT (79). In adults, diabetes, sickle cell disease, membranous glomerulonephritis, nephrotic syndrome, amyloidosis, polyarteritis nodosa, systemic lupus erythematosus, burns, pregnancy, trauma, and extrinsic compression by tumor, hematoma, aneurysm, etc. are associated with RVT (80).

Several experimental studies reported the sonographic findings in acute renal vein thrombosis (81–83). In the acute stage (1 to 7 days), when congestion and edema predominate, sonograms show mild to moderate renomegaly, a subtle increase in cortical echogenicity, prominence of corticomedullary differentiation, and anechoic areas from infarction and hemorrhage (Fig. 6.40). In the subacute stage (1 to 3 weeks), the cortical echogenicity is decreased and cor-

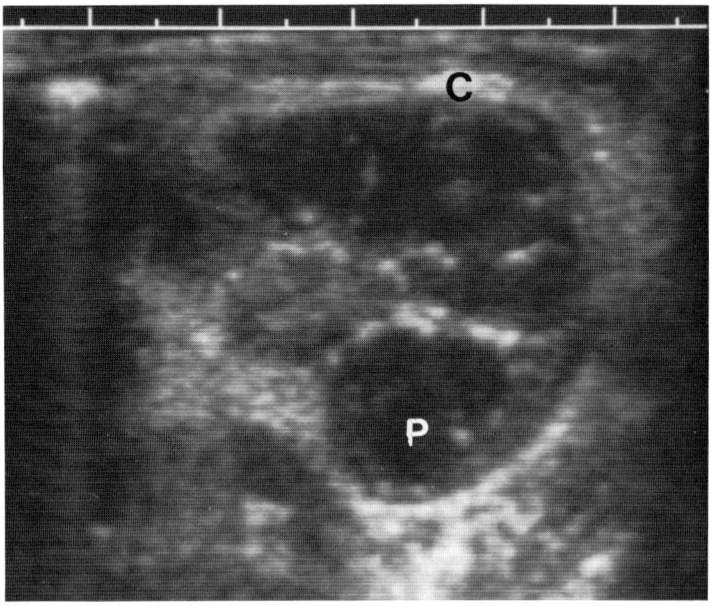

Figure 6.40. Transverse sonogram of left kidney. Enlarged kidney with large hypoechoic pyramids (*P*) and mildly hyperechoic cortex (*C*) in a neonate with acute renal vein thrombosis.

ticomedullary boundaries are less sharp. Calcifications may be seen at the corticomedullary junction sites (Fig. 6.41). Focal hemorrhages are seen as hyperechoic areas (Fig. 6.42) (83, 84). In the chronic stage (3 to 6 weeks), when interstitial fibrosis is prominent, the kidneys are small and show increased echogenicity with blurred corticomedullary borders (Fig. 6.43). The renal veins are distended and lack normal respiratory variation in size. An acute thrombus is hypoechoic, and a chronic thrombus is echogenic, with or without calcification.

On Doppler sonography, renal venous flow is absent and renal arterial signals show high-resistance nonpropulsive flow consisting of sharp systolic spikes that descend to the baseline without the normal sigmoid shape. Retrograde flow may be seen as an inverted peak or plateau during diastole (85, 86).

DOPPLER VASCULAR STUDIES IN ACUTE RENAL FAILURE

Doppler studies of renal blood flow in patients with acute renal failure from parenchymal disease show absence of flow in late diastole or throughout diastole (Fig. 6.44) (87). Doppler evaluation in renal artery stenosis shows increased turbulence at the site of stenosis, increase in peak systolic and diastolic velocities, and abnormal waveform with spectral broadening (88). In renal artery occlusion, loss of flow in the main artery and its small branches and loss of venous return are seen (89). In renal vein thrombosis, loss of venous flow, high-resistance arterial spikes in systole, and reversed flow during diastole in the renal arteries are highly suggestive (83–85). When the kidney is edematous, as in acute pyelonephritis, glomerulonephritis, and acute tubular necrosis, high-resistance arterial flow is also seen. High arterial resistive indices are nonspecific and are seen in acute renal edema (irre-

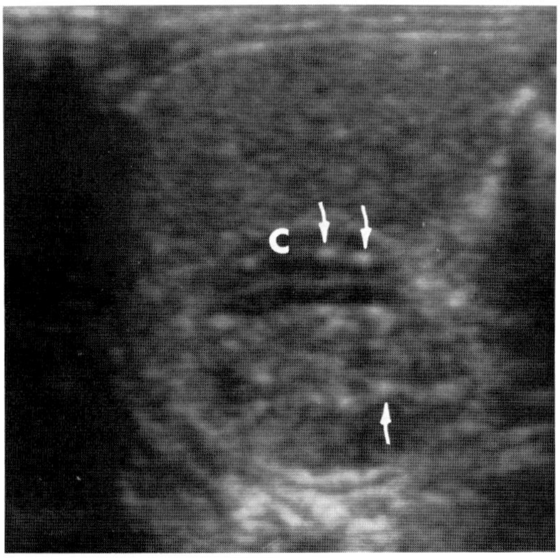

Figure 6.41. Transverse sonogram of right kidney. Enlarged kidney with slightly hypoechoic cortex (*C*), large pyramids, and calcification at corticomedullary junction (*arrows*) in subacute phase of renal vein thrombosis.

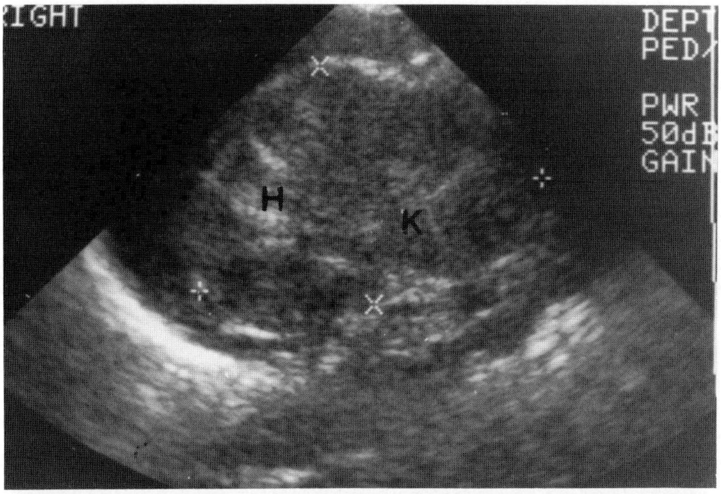

Figure 6.42. Oblique sonogram of kidney. Nonhomogeneous echo texture of kidney (*K*) with hyperechoic patches representing hemorrhagic areas (*H*) in renal vein thrombosis with parenchymal hemorrhages.

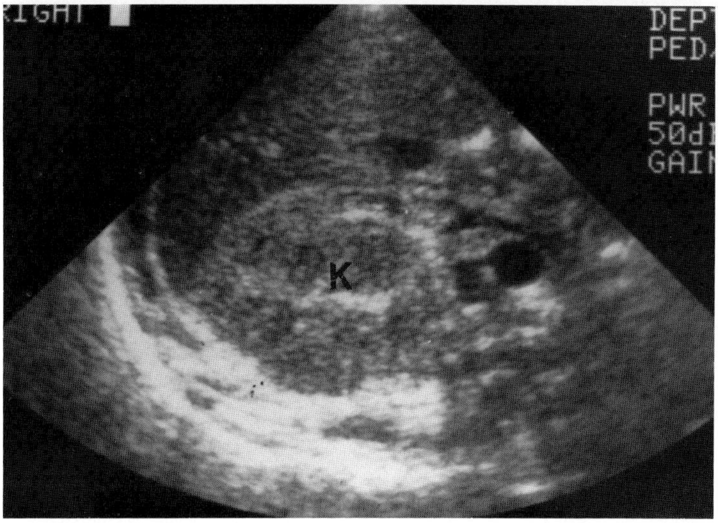

Figure 6.43. Transverse sonogram of right kidney. Diffusely hyperechoic kidney (*K*) with loss of corticomedullary differentiation due to fibrosis in the chronic stage of renal vein thrombosis.

spective of the cause), acute tubular necrosis, venous compression or obstruction, and ureteral obstruction.

ACUTE OBSTRUCTIVE UROPATHY

Abrupt and complete obstruction to a solitary functioning kidney or lower urinary tract obstruction leads to acute renal failure. Often, acute failure is superimposed over chronic renal insufficiency, when partial or intermittent obstruction becomes complete. Following complete obstruction, the renal blood flow and glomerular filtration rate are markedly reduced and intraluminal pressure in tubules and the pelvicaliceal system is increased. Glomerular and tubular function is reduced or lost due to ischemia and pressure atrophy. Acute obstruction can be due to calculus, trauma, or inflammation or clot in the urethra, bladder, or both ureters. Nonobstructive dilation of the pelvicaliceal system can occur in patients with myelodysplasia, reflux nephropathy, congenital megacalices, megaureters, infection, retroperitoneal fibrosis, and prune belly syndrome (90). On sonograms, the kidney is mildly enlarged and is normal, hyper-, or hypoechoic, depending on preexisting disease. The pelvicaliceal system is markedly dilated without cortical atrophy.

SONOGRAPHICALLY GUIDED INVASIVE PROCEDURES

Renal Biopsy

When obstruction is excluded as a cause of acute or chronic renal failure, percutaneous bi-

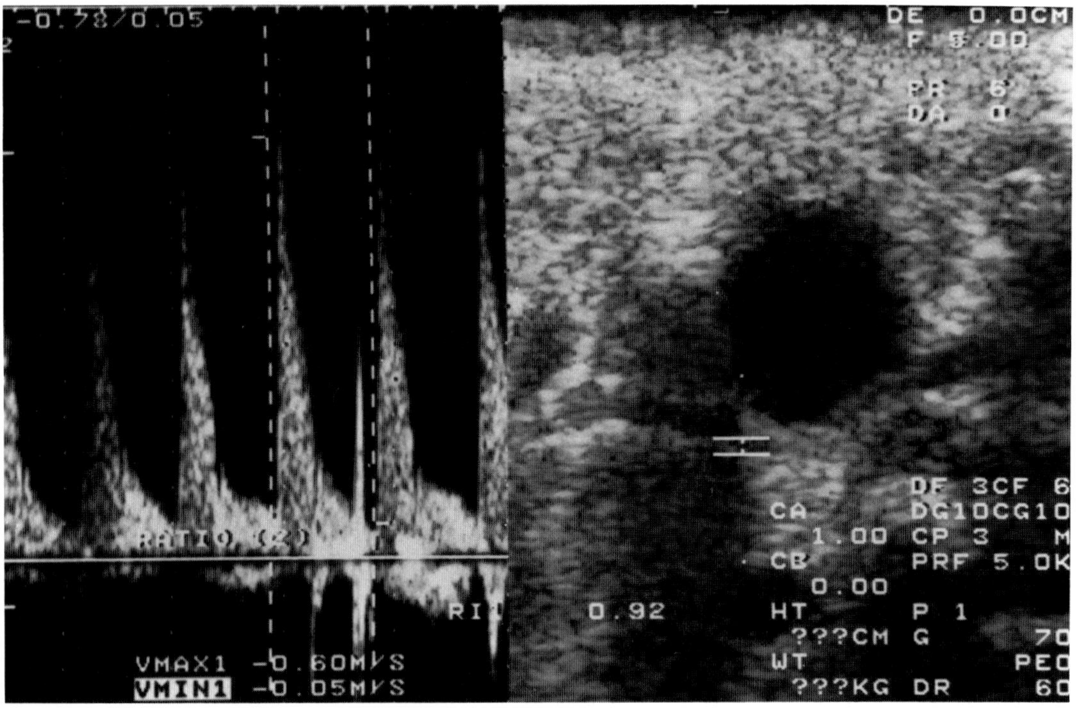

Figure 6.44. Doppler study of renal artery. Reduction in flow during diastole and high-resistance flow pattern during systole in a dysplastic kidney.

opsy is performed to establish a histologic diagnosis. During the biopsy sonography is used to (*a*) mark the optimal site of entry over the skin, (*b*) obtain the approximate depth from skin to renal capsule, (*c*) guide the needle to the desired site of the renal cortex, and (*d*) establish the presence or lack of a hematoma at biopsy site.

Biopsy may be performed with or without a guide attached to the sonographic probe. The complications include hematuria, subcapsular or perirenal hematoma, abscess, and arteriovenous fistula formation at the biopsy site. The rate of complications is between 1 and 8%, and adequate samples are obtained in about 95% of cases under sonographic guidance (91, 92).

Percutaneous Nephrostomy

When renal obstruction is confirmed, nephrostomy may be performed for permanent or temporary urinary diversion. Sonography is useful to (*a*) locate the optimal site for skin puncture, (*b*) estimate the depth from skin to renal surface, (*c*) guide the needle and trocar to the desired site of entry in the kidney, (*d*) confirm the placement of the catheter in the correct position, and (*e*) detect local complications. The rate of complications is around 4% and the success rate is over 95% (93).

SUMMARY

Sonography plays an important role in the diagnosis and therapy of acute or chronic renal failure. Sonography is useful to (*a*) differentiate between obstructive and nonobstructive causes, (*b*) determine the site and cause of obstruction, (*c*) guide invasive procedures (e.g., biopsy, nephrostomy), (*d*) identify patterns of parenchymal disease to limit the differential diagnosis, (*e*) detect vascular causes by Doppler study, and (*f*) provide frequent noninvasive follow-up information during and after therapy. Spectral and color flow Doppler studies and imaging across the rectum, vagina, urethra, and urinary bladder will further expand the sonographic applications in the investigation of renal failure.

References

1. Rosenfield AT, Siegel NJ. Renal parenchymal disease: histopathologic-sonographic correlation. AJR 1981;137:793.
2. Hricak H, Cruz C, Romanski R, et al. Renal pa-

renchymal disease: sonographic-histologic correlation. Radiology 1982;144:141.
3. Platt JF, Rubin JM, Bowerman RA, Marn CS. The inability to detect kidney disease on the basis of echogenicity. AJR 1988;151:317.
4. Haller JO, Berdon WE, Friedman AP. Increased renal cortical echogenicity: a normal finding in neonates and infants. Radiology 1982;142:173.
5. Sanders RC, Conrad MR. The ultrasonic characteristics of the renal pelvocalyceal echo complex. J Clin Ultrasound 1977;5:371.
6. Winkler P, Altrogge H. Sonographic signs of nephritis in children. A comparison of renal echogenicity with clinical evaluation, laboratory data and biopsy. Pediatr Radiol 1985;15:231.
7. Rochester D, Aronson AJ, Bowie JD, et al. Ultrasonic appearance of acute poststreptococcal glomerulonephritis. J Clin Ultrasound 1978;6:49.
8. Evans JB, Shapeero LG, Roscelli JD. Infantile glomerulonephritis mimicking polycystic kidney disease. J Ultrasound Med 1988;7:29.
9. Shuman WP, Mack LA, Rogers JV. Diffuse nephrocalcinosis: hyperechoic sonographic appearance. AJR 1981;136:830.
10. Alon U, Brewer WH, Chan JCM. Nephrocalcinosis: detection by ultrasonography. Pediatrics 1983;71:970.
11. Brennan JN, Diwan RV, Makker SP, et al. Ultrasonic diagnosis of primary hyperoxaluria in infancy. Radiology 1982;145:147.
12. Wilson DA, Wenzl JE, Altshuler GP. Ultrasound demonstration of diffuse cortical nephrocalcinosis in a case of primary hyperoxaluria. AJR 1979;132:659.
13. Glazer GM, Callen PW, Filly RA. Medullary nephrocalcinosis: sonographic evaluation. AJR 1982;138:55.
14. Manz F, Jaschke W, Van Kaick G, et al. Nephrocalcinosis in radiography, computed tomography, sonography and histology. Pediatr Radiol 1980;9:19.
15. Pollack HM, Arger PH, Goldberg BB, Mulholland SG. Ultrasonic detection of non-opaque renal calculi. Radiology 1978;127:233.
16. Glasier CM, Stoddard RA, Ackerman NB, McCurdy FA, Null DM Jr, deLemos RA. Nephrolithiasis in infants: association with chronic furosemide therapy. AJR 1983;140:107.
17. Hoffman JC, Schnur MJ, Koenigsberg M. Demonstration of renal papillary necrosis on sonography. Radiology 1982;145:785.
18. Stanley P, Gyepes MT, Olson DL, Gates GF. Renovascular hypertension in children and adolescents. Radiology 1978;129:123.
19. Garel LA, Pariente DM, Gubler MC, Broyer MC, Sauvegrain JH. The dotted corticomedullary junction: a sonographic indicator of small-vessel disease in hypertensive children. Radiology 1984;152:419.
20. Willett CG, Tepper JE, Orlow EL, et al. Renal complications secondary to radiation treatment of upper abdominal malignancies. Int J Radiat Oncol Biol Phys 1986;12:1601.
21. Thomas JL, Bernardino ME. Neoplastic-induced renal vein enlargement: sonographic detection. AJR 1981;136:75.
22. Schwerk WB, Schwerk WN, Rodeck G. Venous renal tumor extension: a prospective US evaluation. Radiology 1985;156:491.
23. Edell S, Zegel H. Ultrasonic evaluation of renal calculi. AJR 1978;130:261.
24. Edell SL, Bonavita JA. The sonographic appearance of acute pyelonephritis. Radiology 1979; 132:683.
25. Morehouse HT, Weiner SN, Hoffman JC. Imaging the inflammatory disease of the kidney. AJR 1984;143:135.
26. Allen HA, Walsh JW, Brewer WH, Vick CW, Haynes JW. Sonography of emphysematous pyelonephritis. J Ultrasound Med 1984;3:533.
27. Hartman DS, Davis CJ, Goldman SM, Isbister SS, Sanders R. Xanthogranulomatous pyelonephritis: sonographic-pathologic correlation of 16 cases. J Ultrasound Med 1984;3:481.
28. Van Kirk OC, Go RT, Wedel VJ. Sonographic features of Xanthogranulomatous pyelonephritis. AJR 1980;134:1035.
29. Rosenfield AT, Glickman MG, Taylor KJW, Crade M, Hodson J. Acute focal bacterial nephritis (acute lobar nephronia). Radiology 1979; 132:553.
30. Lee JKT, McClennan BL, Melson GL, Stanley RJ. Acute focal bacterial nephritis: emphasis on gray scale sonography and computed tomography. AJR 1980;135:87.
31. Kay CJ, Rosenfield AT, Taylor KJW, Rosenberg MA. Ultrasonic characteristics of chronic atrophic pyelonephritis. AJR 1979;132:47.
32. Narayana AS. Overview of renal tuberculosis. Urology 1982;19:236.
33. Gow JG. Genitourinary tuberculosis: A 7-year review. Br J Urol 1979;51:239.
34. Vaziri ND, Barbari A, Licorish K, Cesario T, Gupta S. Spectrum of renal abnormalities in acquired immune-deficiency syndrome. J Natl Med Assoc 1985;77:369.
35. Gardenswartz MH, Lerner CW, Seligson GR, et al. Renal disease in patients with AIDS: a clinicopathologic study. Clin Nephrol 1984;21:197.
36. Schaffer RM, Schwartz GE, Becker JA, Rao TKS, Shih YH. Renal ultrasound in acquired immune deficiency syndrome. Radiology 1984;153:511.
37. Hamper UM, Goldblum LE, Hutchins GM, et al. Renal involvement in AIDS: sonographic-pathologic correlation. AJR 1988;150:1321.
38. Falkoff GE, Rigsby CM, Rosenfield AT. Partial, combined cortical and medullary nephrocalcinosis: US and CT patterns in AIDS-associated MAI infection. Radiology 1987;162:343.
39. Stuck KJ, Silver TM, Jaffe MH, Bowerman RA. Sonographic demonstration of renal fungus balls. Radiology 1981;142:473.
40. Hartman DS, Davidson AJ, Davis CJ JR, Goldman SM. Infiltrative renal lesions: CT-sonographic-pathologic correlation AJR 1988;150: 1061.
41. Hartman DS, Davis CJ, Goldman SM, Friedman AC, Fritzsche P. Renal lymphoma: radiologic-pathologic correlation of 21 cases. Radiology 1981;144:759.
42. Gregory A, Behan M. Lymphoma of the kidneys: unusual ultrasound appearance due to infiltration of the renal sinus. J Clin Ultrasound 1981; 9:343.

43. Kumari SS, Lee WJ, Festa R, et al. Sonographic findings in leukemic renal disease. J Clin Ultrasound 1984;12:465.
44. Subramanyam BR. Renal amyloidosis in juvenile rheumatoid arthritis: sonographic features. AJR 1981;136:411.
45. Hughes JJ, Wilder WM. Computed tomography of renal sarcoidosis. J Comput Assist Tomogr 1988;12:1057.
46. Walker D, Fennell R, Garin E, Richard G. Spectrum of multicystic renal dysplasia: diagnosis and management. Urology 1978;11:433.
47. Stuck KJ, Koff SA, Silver TM. Ultrasonic features of multicystic dysplastic kidney: expanded diagnostic criteria. Radiology 1982;143:217.
48. Sanders RC, Hartman DS. The sonographic distinction between neonatal multicystic kidney and hydronephrosis. Radiology 1984;151:621.
49. Walker FC Jr, Loney LC, Root ER, et al. Diagnostic evaluation of adult polycystic kidney disease in childhood. AJR 1984;142:1273.
50. Lawson TL, McClennan BL, Shirkhoda A. Adult type of polycystic disease: ultrasonographic and computed tomographic appearance. J Clin Ultrasound 1978;6:297.
51. Kelsey JA, Bowie JD. Gray-scale ultrasonography in the diagnosis of polycystic kidney disease. Radiology 1977;122:791.
52. Rosenfield AT, Lipson MH, Wolf B, et al. Ultrasonography and nephrotomography in the presymptomatic diagnosis of dominantly inherited (adult onset) polycystic kidney disease. Radiology 1980;135:423.
53. Boal DK, Teele RL. Sonography of infantile polycystic kidney disease. AJR 1980;135:575.
54. Thaler MM, Ogta ES, Goodman JR, Piel CF, Korobkin MT. Congenital fibrosis and polycystic disease of liver and kidneys. Am J Dis Child 1973;126:374.
55. Rosenfield AT, Siegel NJ, Kappelman NB, Taylor KJW. Gray scale ultrasonography in medullary cystic disease of the kidney and congenital hepatic fibrosis with tubular ectasia: new observations. AJR 1977;129:297.
56. Rego JD Jr, Laing FC, Jeffrey RB. Ultrasonographic diagnosis of medullary cystic disease. J Ultrasound Med 1983;2:433.
57. Garel LA, Habib R, Pariente D, et al. Juvenile nephronophthisis: sonographic appearance in children with severe uremia. Radiology 1984; 151:93.
58. Lalli AF. Medullary sponge kidney disease. Radiology 1969;92:92.
59. Patriquin HB, O'Regan S. Medullary sponge kidney in childhood. AJR 1985;145:315.
60. Hughson MD, Buchwald D, Fox M. Renal neoplasia and acquired cystic kidney disease in patients receiving long-term dialysis. Arch Pathol Lab Med 1986;110:592.
61. Kutcher R, Amodia JB, Rosenblatt R. Uremic renal cystic disease: value of diagnostic screening. Radiology 1983;147:833.
62. Amis ES Jr, Cronan JJ, Pfister RC, Yoder IC. Ultrasonic inaccuracies in diagnosing renal obstruction. Urology 1982;19:101.
63. Platt JF, Rubin JM, Ellis JH, DiPetro MA. Duplex Doppler ultrasound of the kidney: differentiation of obstructive from nonobstructive dilation. Radiology 1989;171:515.
64. Malave SP, Neiman HL, Spies SM, et al. Diagnosis of hydronephrosis: comparison of radionuclide scanning and sonography. AJR 1980; 135:1179.
65. Levinsky NG. Pathophysiology of acute renal failure. N Engl J Med 1977;296:1453.
66. Glazer GM, Francis IR, Brady TM, Teng SS. Computed tomography of renal infarction: clinical and experimental observations. AJR 1983; 140:721.
67. Regan FC, Crabtree EG. Renal infarction: a clinical and possible surgical entity. J Urol 1948; 59:981.
68. Spies JB, Hricak H, Slemmer TM. Sonographic evaluation of experimental acute renal arterial occlusion in dogs. AJR 1984;142:341.
69. Sty JR, Starshak RJ, Hubbard AM. Acute renal cortical necrosis in hemolytic uremic syndrome. J Clin Ultrasound 1983;11:175.
70. Sefczek RJ, Beckman I, Lupetin AR, Dash N. Sonography of acute renal cortical necrosis. AJR 1984;142:553.
71. Rosenfield AT, Zeman RK, Ciccnetti DV, Siegel NJ. Experimental acute tubular necrosis: US appearance. Radiology 1985;157:771.
72. Nomura G, Kinoshita E, Yamagata Y, Koga N. Usefulness of renal ultrasonography for assessment of severity and cause of acute tubular necrosis. J Clin Ultrasound 1984;12:135.
73. Pardes JG, Yong HA, Kazam E. Sonographic findings in myoglobinuric renal failure and their clinical implications. J Ultrasound Med 1983; 2:391.
74. Fong JSC, deChadarevian JP, Kaplan BS. Hemolytic uremic syndrome: current concepts and management. Pediatr Clin North Am 1982; 29:835.
75. Loirat C, Sonsino E, Varga Mareno A, et al. Hemolytic uremic syndrome: an analysis of the natural history and prognostic features. Acta Paediatr Scand 1984;73:505.
76. Kenny PJ, Brinsko RE, Patel DV, et al. Sonography of the kidneys in hemolytic uremic syndrome. Invest Radiol 1986;21:547.
77. Choyke PL, Grant EG, Hoffer FA, Tina L, Korec S. Cortical echogenicity in the hemolytic uremic syndrome: clinical correlation. J Ultrasound Med 1988;7:439.
78. Filly R, Friedland GW, Govan DE. Development and progression of clubbing and scarring in children with recurrent urinary tract infections. Radiology 1974;113:145.
79. Gonzales R, Schwartz S, Sheldon CA, Fraley EF. Bilateral renal vein thrombosis in infancy and childhood. Urol Clin North Am 1982;9:279.
80. Clark RA, Colley DP. Radiological evaluation of renal vein thrombosis. CRC Crit Rev Diagn Imaging 1980;13:337.
81. Rosenfield AT, Zeman RK, Cronan JJ, Taylor KJW. Ultrasound in experimental and clinical renal vein thrombosis. Radiology 1980;137:735.
82. Hricak H, Sandler MA, Madrazo BL, et al. Sonographic manifestations of acute renal vein thrombosis: an experimental study. Invest Radiol 1981;16:30.

83. Paling MR, Wakefield JA, Watson LR. Sonography of experimental acute renal vein occlusion. J Clin Ultrasound 1985;13:647.
84. Rosenberg ER, Trought WS, Kirks DR, Sumner DE, Grossman H. Ultrasonographic diagnosis of renal vein thrombosis in neonates. AJR 1980; 134:35.
85. Avasthi PS, Greene ER, Scholler C, Fowler CR. Noninvasive diagnosis of renal vein thrombosis by ultrasonic echo-Doppler flowmetry. Kidney Int 1983;23:882.
86. Rifkin MD, Pasto ME, Goldberg BB. Duplex Doppler examination in renal disease: evaluation of vascular involvement. Ultrasound Med Biol 1985;11:341.
87. Wong SN, Lo RNS, Yu ECL. Renal blood flow pattern by noninvasive Doppler ultrasound in normal children and acute renal failure patients. J Ultrasound Med 1989;8:135.
88. Greene ER, Avasthi PS, Hodges JW. Noninvasive Doppler assessment of renal artery stenosis and hemodynamics. J Clin Ultrasound 1987; 15:653.
89. Martin KW, McAlister WH, Shakelford GD. Acute renal infarction: diagnosis by Doppler ultrasound. Pediatr Radiol 1988;18:373.
90. Maillet PJ, Pelle Francoz D, Laville M, Gay F, Pinet A. Nondilated obstructive acute renal failure: diagnostic procedures and therapeutic management. Radiology 1986;160:659.
91. Goldberg BB, Pollack HM, Kellerman E. Ultrasonic localization for renal biopsy. Radiology 1975;115:167.
92. Saitoh M. Selective renal biopsy under ultrasonic realtime guidance. Urol Radiol 1984;6:30.
93. Stables DP, Johnson ML. Percutaneous nephrostomy: the role of ultrasound. In: Rosenfield AT, ed. Clinics in diagnostic ultrasound—genitourinary ultrasound. New York: Churchill Livingston, 1979:73.

CHAPTER 7

Ultrasonography of Renal Trauma

R. BROOKE JEFFREY, JR., M.D.

BLUNT RENAL TRAUMA

Clinically significant renal trauma occurs in approximately 15 to 40% of all patients sustaining blunt abdominal injuries (1, 2). The incidence of renal trauma appears to be increasing with the greater frequency of motor vehicle accidents. The majority of patients with isolated blunt renal injuries can be successfully managed conservatively. However, it is essential to identify patients with major renal injuries early in their clinical course to determine if immediate surgical intervention is required to avoid complications such as ongoing hemorrhage, urinary extravasation, and posttraumatic renal infarction. Accurate radiologic assessment is crucial to stage renal trauma and to select patients for either nonoperative or operative management.

Indications for Uroradiologic Imaging

Following prompt clinical assessment, patients with blunt abdominal trauma can be classified into various risk categories for renal injuries. Clinical parameters generally determine the urgency and completeness of radiologic investigation. In patients with shock and obvious multiorgan trauma, a limited excretory urogram is performed prior to urgent laparotomy. The purpose of this limited study is to provide documentation of bilateral renal function and to determine if an underlying major renal injury is present. Because of time constraints, the radiologic investigation is often limited to several radiographic exposures 5 to 10 minutes after a bolus of intravenous contrast material.

In patients with relatively minor blunt trauma to the flank with microhematuria, the value of radiologic investigation is open to question. Reports by Nicolasien et al. (3) and Monstrey et al. (4) noted that patients with microhematuria and no evidence of shock may be safely observed without undergoing emergency radiologic investigation with urography. Of 287 hemodynamically stable patients with microhematuria, Monstrey et al. reported that all patients recovered without early complications or late sequelae (4). Thus, there is significant evidence that patients with only minimal clinical evidence of renal trauma are best observed nonoperatively. These patients need not undergo the expense and small but definite morbidity of excretory urography, since there is very little clinical likelihood that surgical intervention will be necessary.

The radiologic investigation of stable patients with more significant renal trauma, however, remains controversial. The diagnostic roles of ultrasound, computed tomography (CT), excretory urography, and angiography vary from institution to institution depending on availability, expertise, and clinical philosophy. In stable patients with isolated flank trauma and gross hematuria, excretory urography with nephrotomography remains an excellent diagnostic screening modality. Urography provides both anatomic and functional assessment of renal injuries and can accurately stage the extent of blunt renal trauma in approximately 75% of all patients (5). However, Cass and Viera have emphasized that in patients with more severe renal trauma the accuracy of excretory urography is substantially lower (5). In their series of 22 patients with clinically severe renal injuries 82% had indeterminate excretory urograms. There are several important limitations to excretory urography in patients with major renal trauma. These include (*a*) lack of multiorgan imaging, (*b*) limited diagnostic value due to poor patient preparation and overhydration, and (*c*) poor definition of perirenal hemorrhage.

Indications for CT and Ultrasound in Patients with Blunt Renal Trauma

CT is particularly valuable in hemodynamically stable patients with clinically significant multiorgan trauma. When technically adequate, CT can accurately diagnose and stage renal injuries. In addition, CT provides precise anatomic detail regarding other intra- and extraperitoneal traumatic lesions (6–9). Finally, CT can quantify the extent of associated visceral hemorrhage, which may be of significant prognostic value. Contrast enhancement with CT provides exquisite functional information about renal perfusion and excretion. In addition, contrast enhancement affords accurate diagnosis of caliceal extravasation.

At San Francisco General Hospital, CT rather than ultrasound or angiography is the primary diagnostic method for imaging stable patients with either suspected major renal or multiorgan trauma in whom further diagnostic information is required to assess the need for laparotomy. Contrast enhancement is essential for optimal CT diagnosis. Technical factors are also important, as significant patient motion or artifacts may degrade the diagnostic quality of the study. It should be emphasized that small arterial injuries such as intimal dissections, pseudoaneurysms, etc., cannot be reliably diagnosed by CT. Selective angiography remains the primary diagnostic technique in this regard. CT is generally performed when the findings on excretory urography are either nondiagnostic, incomplete, or inconclusive.

The role of ultrasound in the diagnosis of blunt renal trauma is not well defined at this time. To date, ultrasound has been used in combination with excretory urography primarily in pediatric patients (10, 11). There are a number of advantages of ultrasound in the assessment of renal trauma. It is readily available at most institutions, and the equipment is easily transportable. Ultrasound can be performed at the patient's bedside and can be repeated with little cost or discomfort. The study can generally be performed rapidly within minutes and provides additional diagnostic information regarding injuries to other parenchymal organs. Sonography does not require the use of intravenous injection of iodinated contrast material and thus can be performed in patients with an allergic history or in patients with severely impaired renal function. Because there is no ionizing radiation, it can be readily used in pregnant or pediatric patients.

It should be emphasized, however, that there are significant limitations to the use of ultrasound in blunt renal trauma that hamper its overall clinical usefulness. Currently, there is no clinically available contrast agent for renal sonography, and therefore it is impossible to obtain functional information regarding renal vascular perfusion, contrast material excretion, or extravasation. This information is of critical importance in patients with traumatic renal artery thrombosis, in whom sonography may be normal (9). Contrast material extravasation from the renal collecting system cannot be definitively diagnosed with sonography, because surrounding hemorrhage may have a similar sonographic appearance. Because of these significant limitations, it is recommended that ultrasonography should always be performed in conjunction with excretory urography in order not to misdiagnose traumatic renal artery occlusion or contrast material extravasation from deep cortical lacerations. Ultrasound may provide diagnostic images of injuries to the liver and spleen. However, when compared to CT, it does not always provide equivalent diagnostic information. This is particularly true for bowel and pancreatic injuries that may accompany renal trauma.

Classification of Blunt Renal Injuries

Accurate classification and staging of the extent of blunt renal injuries is essential for optimal patient management. Radiologic investigation is critical, as the clinical assessment alone is quite limited in determining the true extent of renal parenchymal injuries. The classification schemes of renal trauma are based on the status of the renal pedicle, the depth and extent of parenchymal cortical lacerations, and whether or not there is extravasation of contrast material from the renal collecting system. Approximately 90% of all blunt renal injuries may be classified as minor (1) (Fig. 7.1**A** and **B**). These include renal parenchymal contusions, superficial cortical lacerations, and small subcapsular and perirenal hematomas. Major renal injuries occur in only 10% of patients with blunt trauma and include deep cortical lacerations (with or without disruption of the collecting system), renal fractures, and renal vascular pedicle injuries (including avulsion, intimal dissection, or traumatic occlusion) (1) (Fig. 7.1**C** and **D**).

Ultrasound Diagnosis of Minor Renal Injuries

Sonographically, blunt renal injuries resulting in renal or perirenal hemorrhage demonstrate focal echogenic areas either within or adjacent to the normally hypoechoic renal pa-

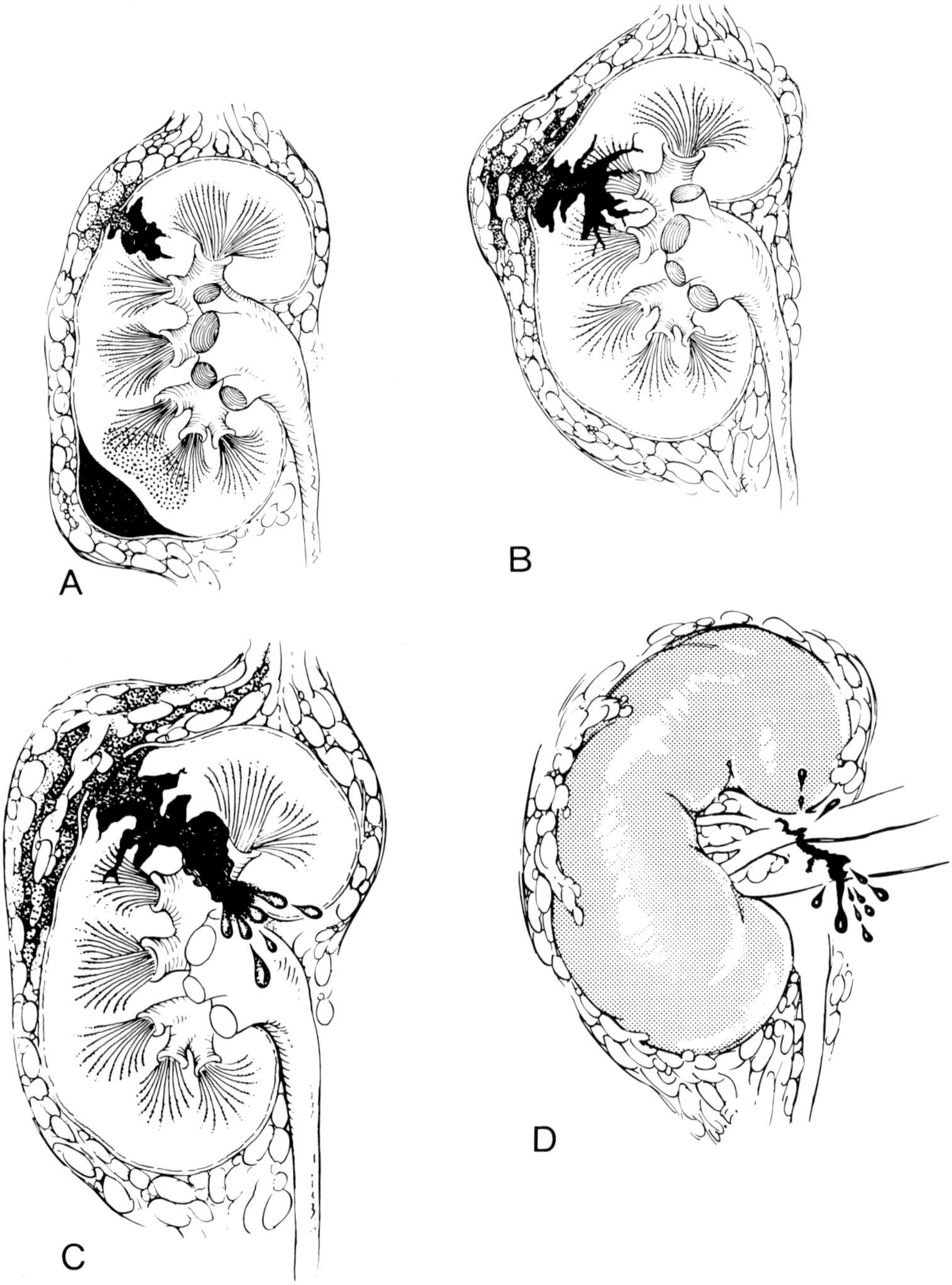

Figure 7.1. Schematic classification of the types of renal parenchymal and vascular injuries following blunt trauma. **A,** Minor parenchymal injuries such as small cortical laceration and subcapsular hematomas. **B,** Cortical laceration with adjacent perirenal hemorrhage. Major renal injuries include fractures (**C**) and renal pedicle injuries (**D**).

renchyma (Fig. 7.2). Clotted blood in particular may be relatively echogenic. The sonographic appearance often evolves with time, and areas of hemorrhage or hematoma formation become less echogenic and may be nearly isoechoic when compared to normal renal parenchyma (Figs. 7.3 and 7.4). The echogenicity of renal parenchymal lacerations in some patients may approximate the echogenic fat within the renal sinus. Thus, caution should be exercised to avoid misinterpreting areas of parenchymal hemorrhage for normal hyperechoic sinus fat. Unclotted blood, particularly in patients with subacute hemorrhage, may be relatively hypoechoic or even anechoic. This may be indistinguishable in appearance from extravasated urine. Renal subcapsular hematomas characteristically flatten the lateral contour of the kidney.

Follow-up sonograms in patients with renal parenchymal or perinephric hematomas successfully treated with conservative therapy generally reveal gradual diminution in size and echogenicity of the areas of hemorrhage (Fig. 7.4). It is not uncommon, however, for minor sonographic abnormalities to be present for 6 to 8 weeks in patients with extensive parenchymal injuries. Large areas of parenchymal laceration or infarction may heal with cortical scarring. Because of the ease of per-

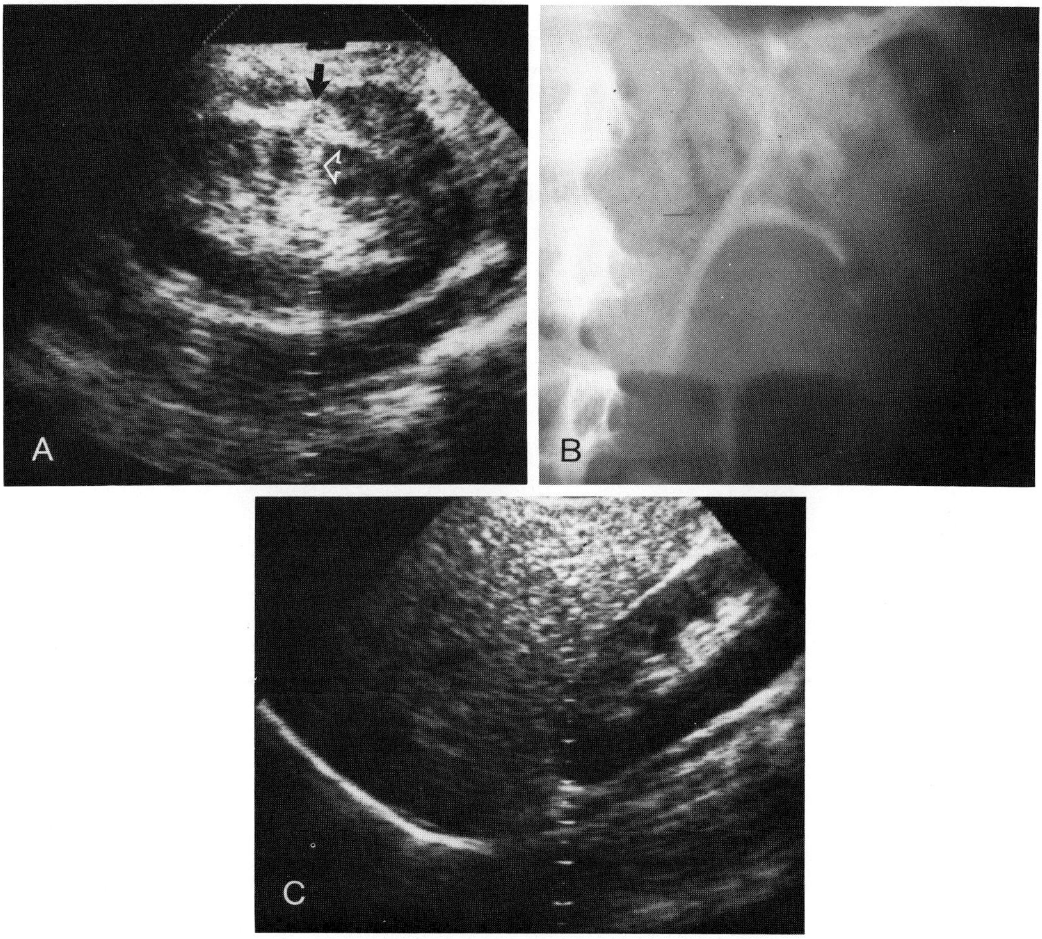

Figure 7.2. Echogenic renal and perirenal hemorrhage. **A,** Sagittal scan of the left kidney demonstrating echogenic hematoma within the renal parenchyma (*open white arrow*) and adjacent echogenic perirenal hemorrhage (*black arrow*). **B,** Excretory urogram (performed prior to the sonogram) that reveals little evidence of the extent of injury. **C,** Sagittal sonogram of contralateral normal right kidney for comparison. (From Jakse G, Furtschegger A, Egender G. Ultrasound in patients with blunt renal trauma managed by surgery. J Urol 1987;138:21–23.)

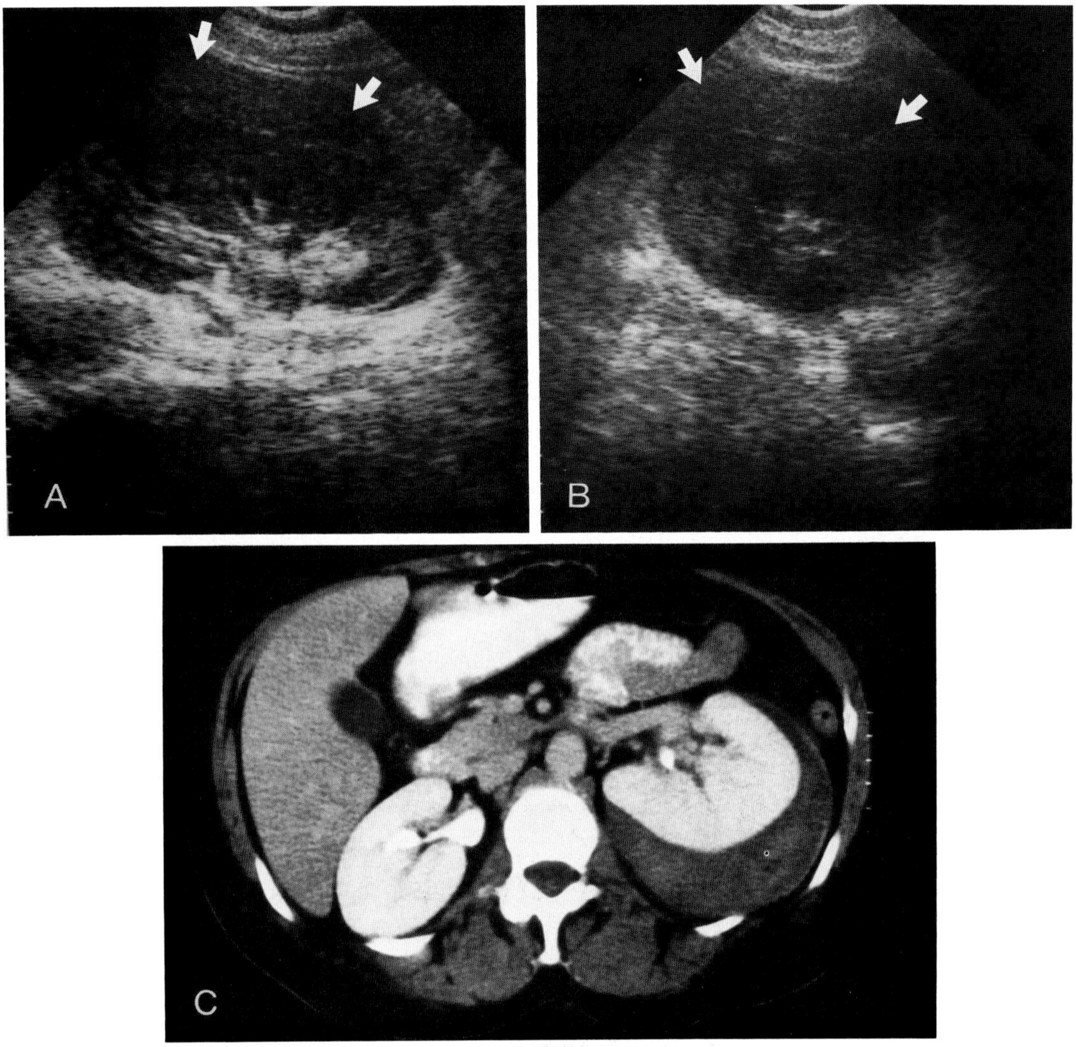

Figure 7.3. Isoechoic posttraumatic perirenal hematoma. Patient was traumatized 4 days previously. **A,** Sagittal scan of the left kidney demonstrating a nearly isoechoic perirenal hematoma (*arrows*). **B,** Transverse view of the kidney, again demonstrating the surrounding perirenal hematoma (*arrows*). **C,** Contrast-enhanced CT scan confirming the extensive perirenal hematoma.

forming follow-up examinations, sonography is a useful method to further evaluate minor parenchymal injuries treated nonoperatively to exclude increasing urine extravasation or an enlarging hematoma.

The majority of patients with minor renal parenchymal injuries following blunt trauma do not undergo surgical intervention. Thus, there is little direct pathologic correlation with sonography to judge its overall accuracy in staging of minor renal injuries. The report by Filiatrault et al. investigating blunt abdominal trauma in pediatric patients is an example of the lack of direct surgical correlation in this area (11). One hundred eighty-one pediatric patients with blunt renal trauma were evaluated with both ultrasound and excretory urography. Of the 122 renal injuries in this group of patients, the majority were minor parenchymal or perinephric hematomas. The surgical findings at exploration and the clinical outcome were used as the "gold standard" to

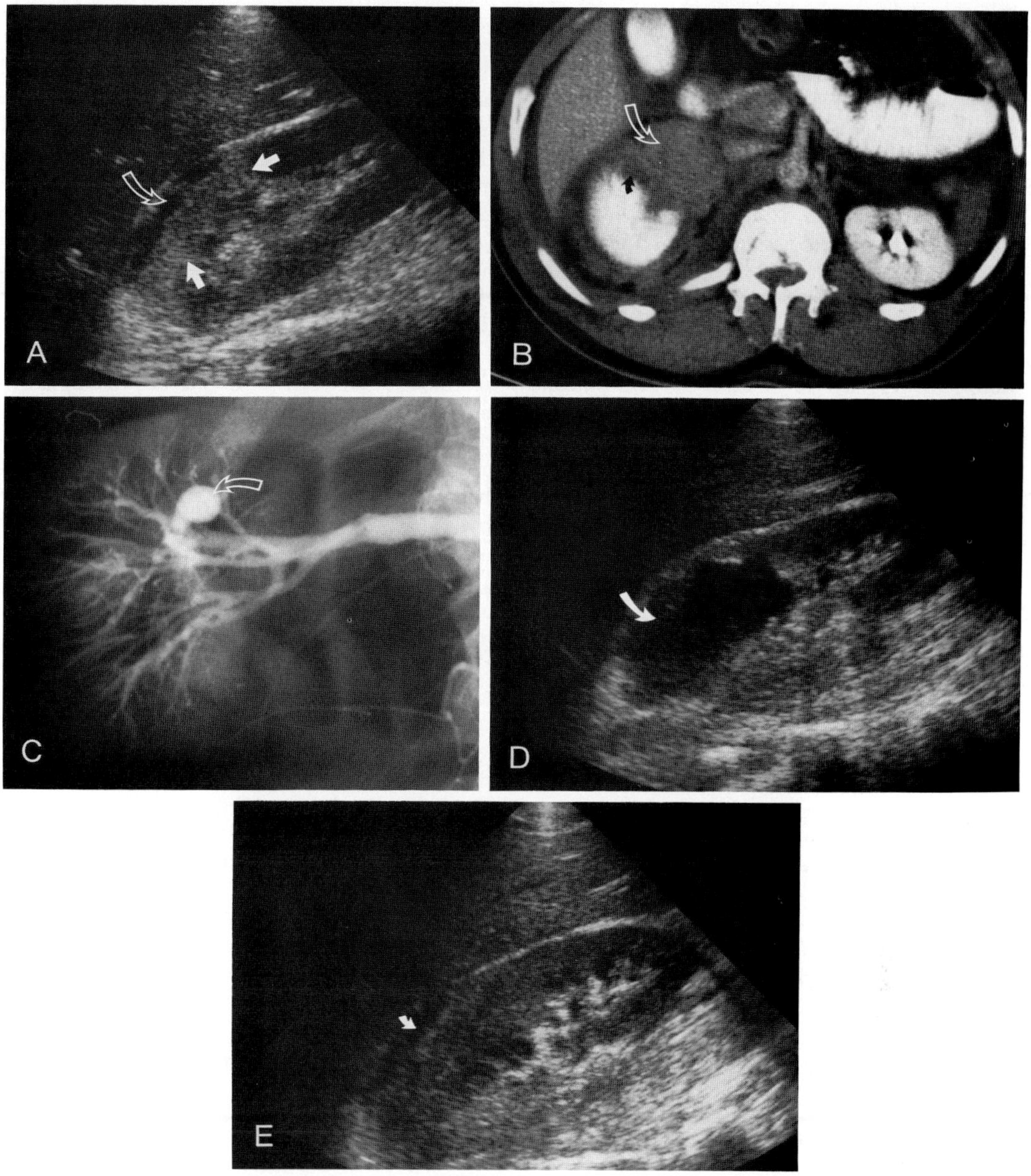

Figure 7.4. Deep cortical laceration with traumatic pseudoaneurysm formation. **A,** Sagittal scan of the right kidney demonstrating echogenic intraparenchymal renal hematoma involving the anterior cortex of the upper pole (*arrows*). Note the adjacent hypoechoic perirenal hemorrhage representing unclotted blood (*curved arrow*). **B,** Contrast-enhanced CT scan showing a large perirenal hematoma centered near the renal hilus (*white arrow*). There is a relatively small intraparenchymal area of nonenhancement indicating a laceration of the upper pole (*black arrow*). Because of the large hematoma near the renal hilum, an arteriogram was performed (**C**), which demonstrates a pseudoaneurysm of a segmental branch of the upper pole (*arrow*). Because no active extravasation was seen from the pseudoaneurysm, it was elected to treat this expectantly. A follow-up sonogram 10 days later (**D**) reveals a large hypoechoic renal and perirenal hematoma (*arrow*). The patient remained hemodynamically stable. A subsequent arteriogram (not shown) 6 weeks after injury demonstrated that the pseudoaneurysm occluded spontaneously. A follow-up sonogram at this time (**E**) demonstrates only minimal perirenal hematoma (*arrow*).

assess the accuracy of any individual imaging techniques. However, 95% of the patients were successfully treated nonoperatively and hence there was little surgical correlation. The clinical outcome suggested no false-negative examination by sonography. It is important to point out, however, that CT was used in only 8% of these patients. Thus, it is possible that some small contusions and parenchymal and perirenal hematomas that could have been detected by CT may have been missed by sonography. The authors emphasized that sonography should not be used alone in renal trauma and should always be performed in combination with excretory urography, as traumatic renal artery occlusions cannot be diagnosed by sonography alone.

Major Renal Injuries

To date, the experience with renal sonography in the assessment of major renal injuries is quite limited. Far more experience exists with computed tomography and angiography. The sonographic appearance of a renal fracture has been described as a "disorganized" kidney with extensive surrounding perirenal hemorrhage (10). The normal renal architecture of renal sinus echoes, hypoechoic renal pyramids, and renal cortex is replaced by heterogeneous echogenicity representing a combination of blood and extravasated urine. Traumatic renal artery occlusion, however, may have deceptively normal sonographic appearance with no surrounding perirenal hemorrhage and no alteration in renal echogenicity (10).

In attempting to assess the accuracy of ultrasound in patients with major blunt renal trauma, Jakse et al. compared both excretory urography and ultrasound to the surgical findings at exploration (10). Ultrasound correctly identified 16 of 18 patients with major parenchymal injuries (10). However, neither disruption of the pelvis or ureter nor injury to the renal pedicle was prospectively diagnosed by ultrasound alone. The diagnosis was established only in conjunction with excretory urography. There were no false-positive sonograms in this series. Of note is the fact that eight patients with renal fracture, four with polar avulsion, and two with fragmentation of the kidney were accurately diagnosed preoperatively by sonography alone (10).

Although there is little clinical information at present, the use of color flow Doppler may prove to be of clinical benefit in diagnosing renal pedicle injuries, particularly if the patency of the renal artery and vein can be determined with a high degree of accuracy. Renal parenchymal hemorrhage may cause avascular areas that potentially might be visualized with this technique. However, there is insufficient experience to date with color flow Doppler in renal trauma to judge its overall usefulness.

At many trauma centers, CT is the imaging method of choice for the radiologic investigation of suspected major renal injuries based on either clinical criteria or an abnormal excretory urogram (6–9). Traumatic renal artery occlusion can be confidently diagnosed by CT in patients demonstrating a lack of both renal enhancement and excretion (7) (Fig. 7.5). Traumatic renal artery occlusion is relatively rare and accounts for only 5% of patients with blunt trauma (12). However, renal salvage requires urgent revascularization of the kidney within 12 hr (12). Because the CT appearance of traumatic renal artery occlusion is so specific, the delay in performing angiography adds little to the diagnosis and, in our opinion, is unnecessary. Nevertheless, the role of angiography remains a controversial issue among trauma surgeons (7). In patients with partial intimal dissection of the main renal artery and partial obstruction to arterial flow, a diminished nephrogram of the affected kidney is noted with CT. There is also a delay in the excretion of contrast material. Emergency selective angiography is essential in these patients to define the site and extent of arterial injury and to plan the operative repair. Because there is still some arterial perfusion to the kidney, the time lapse required to perform arteriography in these patients is not as critical as with complete arterial occlusion.

Renal fractures can be confidently diagnosed by CT when a laceration is noted to extend completely through the renal cortex and hilum. The extent of corresponding perirenal hemorrhage is clearly depicted by CT. In numerous clinical series CT has proven to be quite accurate for diagnosing renal fractures and deep lacerations (6–9). It appears to be significantly more sensitive than excretory urography in identifying areas of contrast material extravasation, due to the exquisite density resolution of this technique (13).

Summary

At present sonography plays a rather limited role in the evaluation of most of patients with

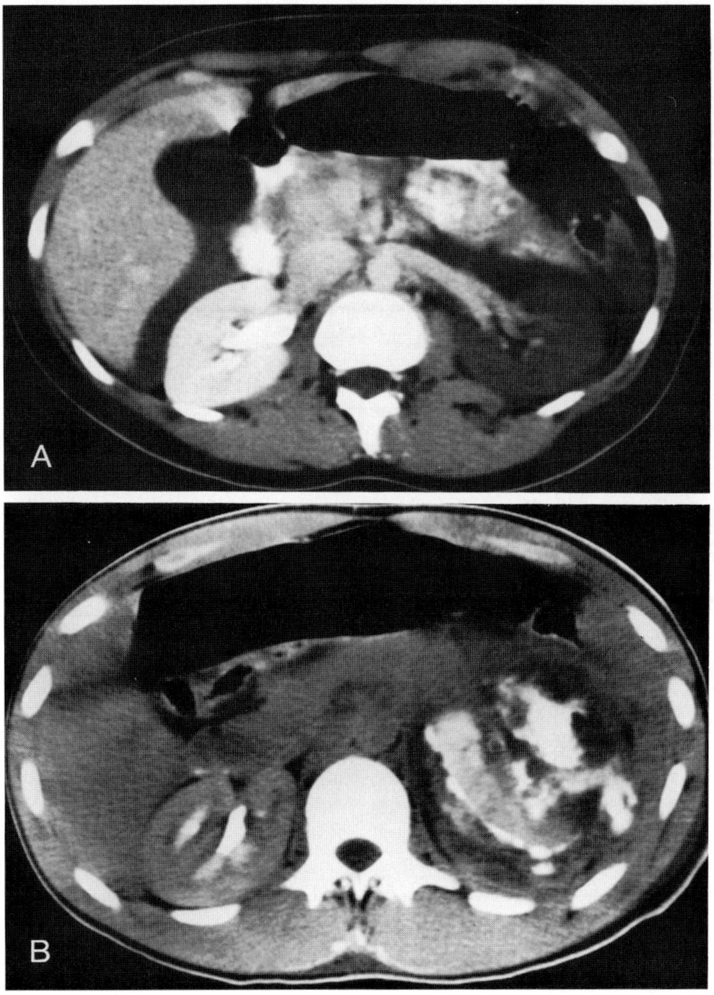

Figure 7.5. Examples of the superiority of CT in defining vascular perfusion and contrast material extravasation. **A,** An example of a surgically confirmed traumatic renal artery occlusion of the left kidney. There was no contrast enhancement or excretion from the kidney. Incidentally noted is contrast material refluxing into the renal vein via gonadal vein contributaries. Ultrasound alone in the absence of color flow Doppler or duplex sonography would undoubtedly have shown a normal kidney in the setting, since there was no intraparenchymal or perirenal hemorrhage. **B,** An example of extravasation of contrast material from a deep cortical laceration. Note the high-density contrast material extravasating into the perirenal space. Sonography in this setting cannot distinguish anechoic hemorrhage from extravasated urine. (Used by permission from Jeffrey RB Jr. CT and sonography of the acute abdomen. New York: Raven Press, in press.)

blunt renal trauma. Excretory urography, CT, and angiography are the mainstays of diagnosis. In combination with excretory urography, however, renal sonography may become a more important technique as experience with color flow Doppler increases. Sonography appears to be particularly useful in patients with relatively minor injuries, in pediatric patients, and in patients in whom noninvasive follow-up is considered helpful. The major limitation of sonography at this time is the lack of functional assessment of vascular perfusion and excretion. CT is preferred in most patients with major renal injuries at this time because of its superior multiorgan imaging and its ability to assess functional abnormalities of the kidney. Angiography is currently used less as an initial diagnostic technique and is being reserved primarily for suspected intimal tears of the renal artery and in patients in whom therapeutic embolization is considered.

PENETRATING RENAL TRAUMA

Penetrating renal trauma occurs in approximately 8% of all abdominal wounds and accounts for 20 to 30% of all renal injuries (14, 15). There is a high percentage of associated visceral injuries in patients with penetrating renal trauma. In some series this approximates 80% (15). In patients with anterior abdominal stab wounds, generally no radiologic assessment is required, since urgent laparotomy is performed due to the high probability of associated visceral injuries. In patients with isolated penetrating trauma to the flank, however, a mandatory policy of exploration of all stab wounds results in a high percentage of unneces-

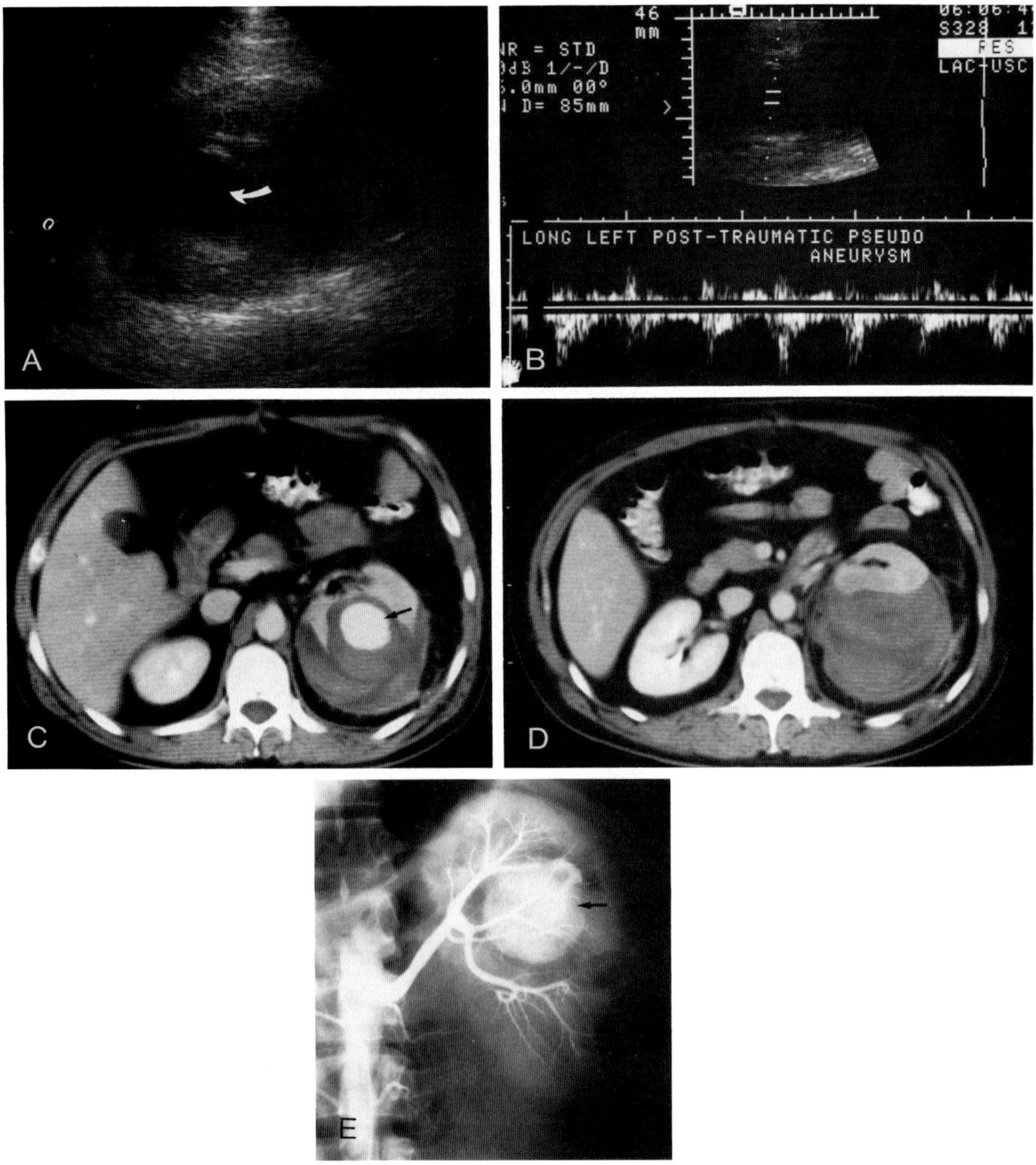

Figure 7.6. Examples of the value of duplex sonography in the diagnosis of posttraumatic pseudoaneurysm from penetrating trauma. **A,** A sagittal sonogram of the left kidney demonstrating no evidence of intraparenchymal hematoma or perirenal hematoma. A "cystic" anechoic area is seen centrally within the left kidney (*arrow*). **B,** A duplex sonogram demonstrating arterial flow within the cystic mass diagnostic of a pseudoaneurysm. **C,** Contrast-enhanced CT identifies a rounded area of intense arterial enhancement (*arrow*) corresponding to a pseudoaneurysm. **D,** CT scan at a more caudal level showing the extensive subcapsular hematoma that flattens the posterior contour of the kidney. **E,** A selective left renal arteriogram demonstrating the large pseudoaneurysm (*arrow*). This was satisfactorily treated by transcatheter embolization. (Case courtesy of Philip W. Ralls, M.D., Glendale, CA. Used by permission from Jeffrey RB Jr. CT and sonography of the acute abdomen. New York: Raven Press, in press.)

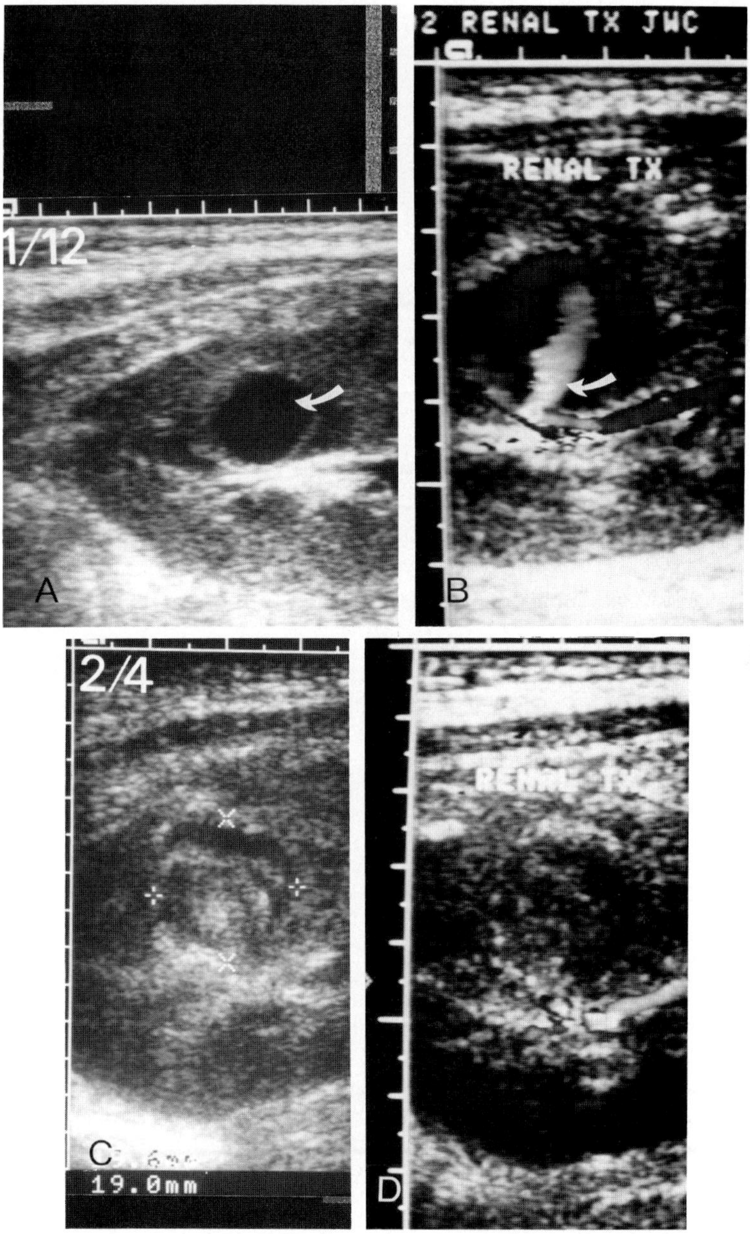

Figure 7.7. Color flow Doppler of pseudoaneurysm in transplanted kidney after renal biopsy (see color plate 1). **A,** Sonogram of a renal transplant kidney demonstrating a cystic mass near the upper pole (*arrow*). **B,** Color flow Doppler showing arterial flow and jet effect (*arrow*) into a pseudoaneurysm. A follow-up scan 3 weeks later (**C**) demonstrates an echogenic clot within the pseudoaneurysm. A color flow Doppler study done at this time (**D**) shows no evidence of arterial flow within the pseudoaneurysm diagnostic of spontaneous occlusion. (Case courtesy of E. Meredith James, M.D., Rochester, MN. Used by permission from Jeffrey RB Jr. CT and sonography of the acute abdomen. New York: Raven Press, in press.)

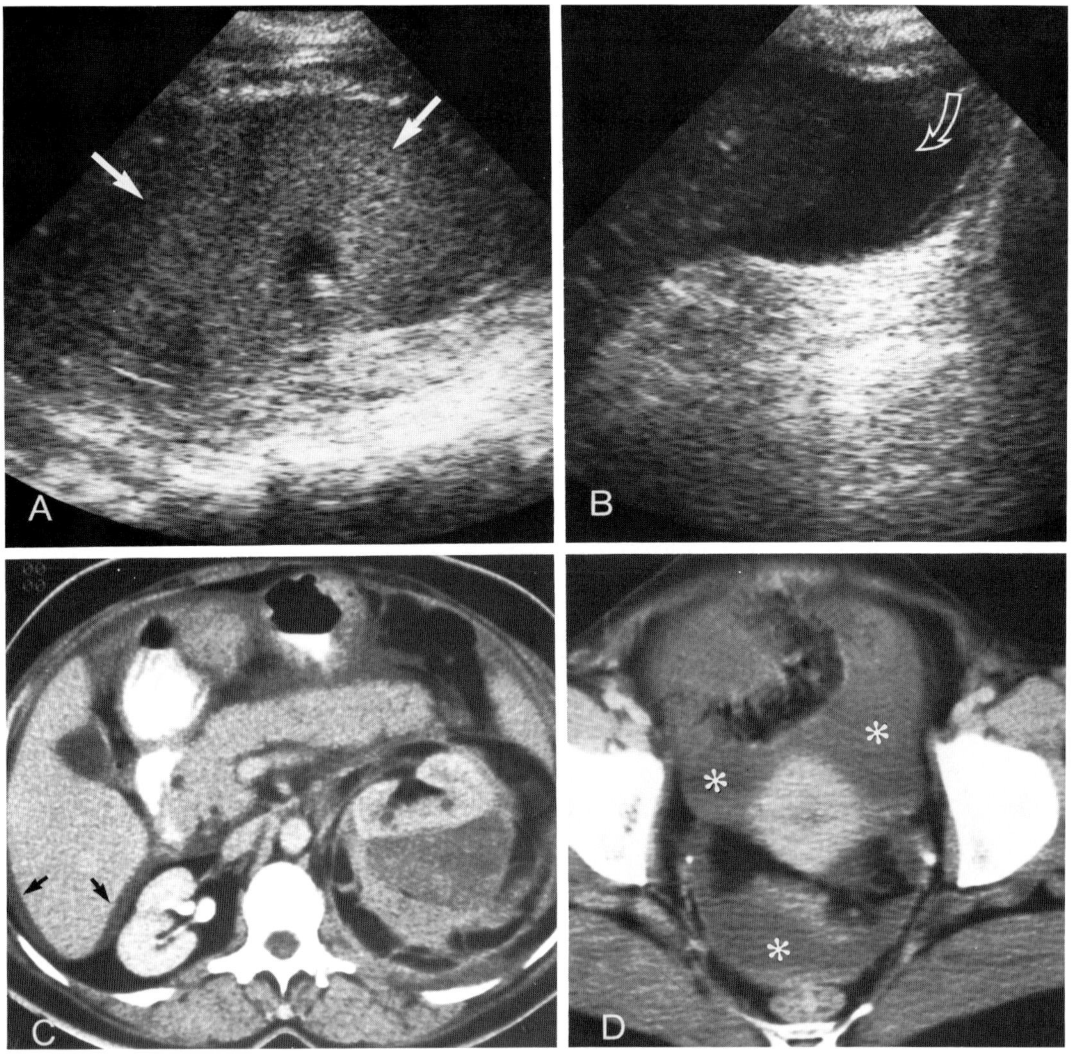

Figure 7.8. Massive retroperitoneal and intraperitoneal hemorrhage following renal biopsy in two different patients. **A,** Sagittal sonogram of the left flank demonstrating a large retroperitoneal hematoma (*arrows*) 6 days after attempted percutaneous renal biopsy. **B,** Sonogram showing associated hemoperitoneum (*arrow*) adjacent to the liver. Patient required urgent angiographic embolization for control of the lower-pole left renal artery extravasation. In another patient, a large left subcapsular hematoma is identified (**C**). Notice hemoperitoneum adjacent to the liver (*arrows*). **D,** CT scan demonstrating a large amount of hemoperitoneum in the pelvis. Patient required angiographic embolization of the lower-pole arteriovenous fistula. (**C** and **D** used by permission from Low RN, Jeffrey RB Jr. Intraperitoneal hemorrhage after renal biopsy: a grave prognostic sign. AJR 1988;151:113–114.)

sary or nontherapeutic laparotomies. Radiologic investigation can be of considerable clinical value in this subgroup of patients. It should be noted that the degree of hematuria in penetrating renal trauma is a poor predictor of the extent of parenchymal injury. Microhematuria may, in fact, be present in a relatively small percentage of patients with major renal penetrating injuries to the kidney (14–16).

Radiologic Investigation of Penetrating Trauma

As with blunt abdominal trauma, there is no universal consensus regarding the diagnostic evaluation of isolated stab wounds to the flank. Unless the stab wound has penetrated the renal collecting system or has produced a major renal hematoma, excretory urography is often of limited value. Another inherent limitation of excretory urography is that the integrity of the retroperitoneal colon cannot be assessed. CT performed with a combination of intravenous and rectal contrast may be of particular value in patients with isolated stab wounds to the flank (17). CT can accurately determine the depth of renal laceration and determine the extent of perirenal hemorrhage. In addition, when dilute contrast material is instilled into the rectum as an enema, colonic lacerations can be confidently diagnosed by CT (17). Laceration of the main renal artery and vein by penetrating trauma can be suggested by CT on the basis of several characteristic findings. These include the presence of a perihilar parenchymal injury, an extensive perirenal hemorrhage out of proportion to the size of the parenchymal injury, and a high-density hematoma located near the renal hilum. At some institutions, however, routine angiography is performed in all patients with suspected renal vascular injuries and cross-sectional imaging is never used.

Federle et al. reviewed the CT and surgical findings in 27 patients with isolated stab wounds to the flank (14). Only seven patients had deep cortical lacerations or renal pedicle injuries that required surgical intervention for control of hemorrhage. All seven of these patients had major renal hematomas identified by CT or had findings highly suggestive of renal pedicle injuries. The remaining 20 patients had small cortical lacerations diagnosed by CT and were successfully managed nonoperatively. Arteriography was rarely performed to further evaluate the CT findings.

To date, there have been a few reports of the use of ultrasound in the assessment of penetrating trauma. Duplex sonography may be of value in patients with suspected perirenal hemorrhage or pseudoaneurysms after renal biopsy (Figs. 7.6 to 7.9). In patients with massive hematuria or obvious major blood loss from renal biopsy, emergency angiography with embolization is clearly the method for both diagnosis and therapy. In patients with subacute hemorrhage—obvious clinical cases—either sonography or CT may be helpful in identifying major subcapsular or perirenal hematomas (18). Duplex sonography, particularly with color flow, may be helpful in identifying larger pseudoaneurysms; however, the overall sensitivity for this technique is not known at this time (Fig. 7.6).

Renal Trauma Following Extracorporeal Shock-Wave Lithotripsy

Renal extracorporeal lithotripsy has become the therapeutic method of choice in the fragmentation or pulverization of renal calculi. In patients with only single stones, 75% may be stone free within weeks to months after the shock-wave therapy (19). Although major complications are relatively few, renal and perirenal hemorrhage have been reported. Papanicolaou et al. reported identifying significant renal hemorrhage in five of 2149 patients undergoing shock-wave lithotripsy (19). The diagnosis of perirenal or renal hemorrhage may be readily established by sonography, CT, or MRI scanning (Fig. 7.9). In general, underlying tissue damage and secondary hemorrhage occur more often when the stone is intrarenal rather

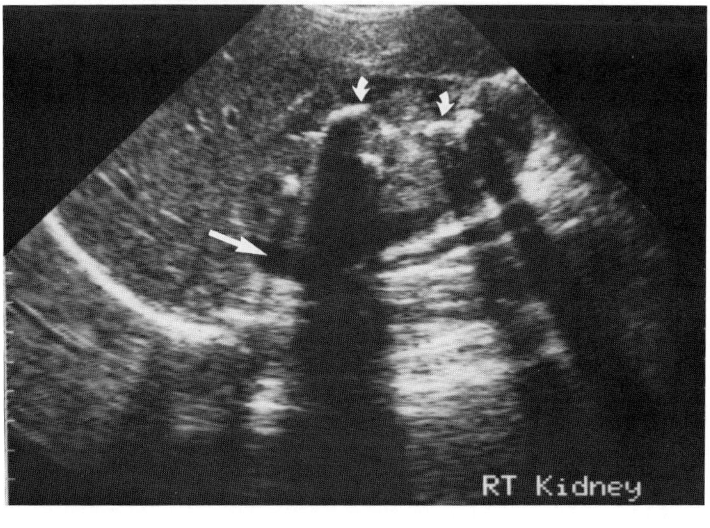

Figure 7.9. Perirenal hemorrhage following extracorporeal lithotripsy for renal calculi. A small perirenal hematoma (*arrow*) can be seen on the posterior aspect of the kidney. Note residual intravenous calculi (*curved arrows*).

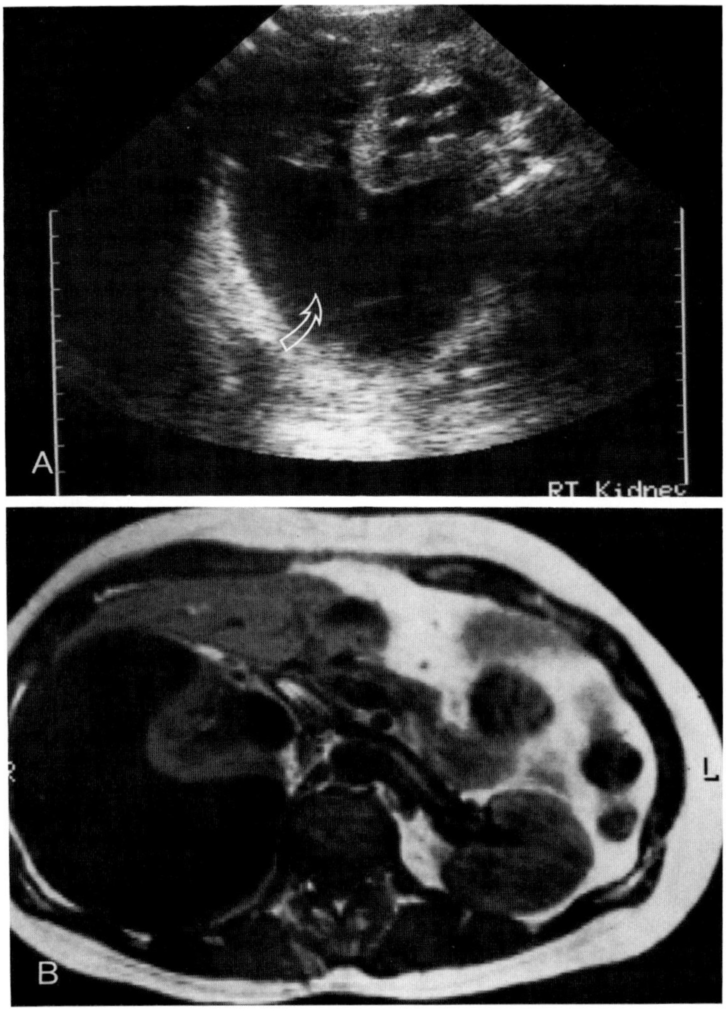

Figure 7.10. Large perinephric urinoma following percutaneous removal of renal calculi. **A,** Transverse sonogram of right kidney demonstrating large hypoechoic urinoma (*arrow*). **B,** A T1-weighted axial magnetic resonance image of the right kidney confirming urinoma isointense with urine in the renal pelvis.

than in the ureter or extrarenal pelvis. The composition of the stone may necessitate increasing the number of shock waves, thus predisposing to a greater possibility of hemorrhage. In a majority of instances, patients with perirenal hematomas can be treated expectantly with transfusion (19). In addition, perinephric urinomas from disruption of the collecting system can also be diagnosed with these same modalities (Fig. 7.10).

References

1. McAninch JW. Injuries to the urinary system. In: Blaisdell FW, Trunkey DD, eds. Trauma management. New York: Thieme-Stratton, 1982;1: 199–228.
2. Jend HH, Reiser M. Retroperitoneal injuries. In: Heller M, Jend HH, Genant HK, eds. Computed tomography of trauma. Stuttgart, Germany: Georg Thieme Verlag, 1986:82.
3. Nicolaisen GS, McAninch JW, Marshall GA, Bluth RF, Carrol PR. Renal trauma: re-evaluation of the indications for radiographic assessment. J Urol 1985;133:183–187.
4. Monstrey SJM, Vander Werken CHR, Debruyne FMJ, et al. Rational guidelines in renal trauma assessment. Urology 1988;31:469–473.
5. Cass AS, Luxenberg M, Gleich P, Smith CS. Clinical indications for radiographic evaluation of blunt renal trauma. J Urol 1986;136:370–373.
6. Bretan PN, McAninch JW, Federle MP, Jeffrey RB Jr. Computerized tomographic staging of renal trauma: 85 consecutive cases. J Urol 1986;136:561–565.
7. Steinberg DL, Jeffrey RB, Federle MP, McAninch JW. The computed tomographic appearance of renal pedicle injury. J Urol 1984;132: 1163–1166.
8. Ishikawa I, Matsura H, Onouchi Z, Suzuki M. CT appearance of the kidney in traumatic renal artery occlusion. J Comput Assist Tomogr 1982;6:1021–1024.
9. Jeffrey RB Jr. CT and sonography of the acute abdomen. New York: Raven Press, in press.

10. Jakse G, Furtschegger A, Egender G. Ultrasound in patients with blunt renal trauma managed by surgery. J Urol 1987;138:21–23.
11. Filiatrault D, Longpre D, Patriquin H, et al. Investigation of childhood abdominal trauma: a practical approach using ultrasound as the initial diagnostic modality. Pediatr Radiol 1987; 17:373–379.
12. Spirnak JP, Resnick MI. Revascularization of traumatic thrombosis of the renal artery. Surg Gynecol Obstet 1987;164:22–25.
13. Cass AS, Luxenberg M, Gleich P, Smith C. Type of blunt renal injury rather than associated extravasation should determine treatment. Urology 1985;26:249–251.
14. Federle MP, Brown TR, McAninch JW. Penetrating renal trauma: CT evaluation. J Comput Assist Tomogr 1987;11:1026–1030.
15. Carrol PR, McAninch JW. Operative indications in penetrating renal trauma. J Renal Trauma 1986;26:1–8.
16. Whitney RF, Peterson NE. Penetrating renal injuries. Urology 1976;7:7–11.
17. Sclafani SJA, Phillips TF, Scale T, Fleitcher J, Duncan AO, Atiweh N. Imaging penetrating trauma of the back and flank: the CT enema. Presented at 89th American Roentgen Ray Society Meeting, San Francisco, May 1988.
18. Low RN, Jeffrey RB Jr. Intraperitoneal hemorrhage after renal biopsy: a g rave prognostic sign. AJR 1988;151:113–114.
19. Papanicolaou N, Stafford SA, Pfister RC, Althausen AF, Pretter SP. Significant renal hemorrhage following extracorporeal shock wave lithotripsy: imaging and clinical features. Radiology 1987;163:661–664.

CHAPTER 8

Ultrasonography of the Urinary Bladder

DONALD R. BODNER, M.D.
MARTIN I. RESNICK, M.D.

With improvements in ultrasound technology, the bladder can now be examined in accurate detail using this imaging modality. Disorders of the bladder are not uncommon, and, due to its position deep within the pelvis, the bladder is often difficult to evaluate by other diagnostic techniques. Ultrasonography of the pelvis is of value in assessing diseases of the bladder. In addition, distortion or invasion of the bladder from tumors arising in contiguous organs can often be detected. Ultrasonography of the bladder has also proved to be of value in staging the depth of penetration of bladder neoplasms. Soft-tissue masses in the pelvis such as gynecologic neoplasms and enlarged lymph nodes can also be evaluated by this imaging modality. Finally, ultrasonography of the bladder provides an accurate, convenient, and comfortable means of determining post-void residuals that can be performed quickly in the office setting without the need for catheter insertion.

TECHNIQUES OF EXAMINATION

The bladder can be imaged with ultrasound using three different approaches: transabdominal, transrectal, and transurethral. It should be emphasized that ultrasonic examinations of the pelvis should be considered as one diagnostic procedure among many, and the data obtained should be correlated with physical examination, cystoscopy, urine cytology, and other imaging studies performed. The examiner should be aware of the clinical history and what pathology is suspected so that he or she can direct his or her attention to specific structures. When the bladder is imaged, it is advisable to study all of the pelvic structures. The prostate, seminal vesicles, rectum, and uterus should be imaged routinely. It should be remembered that disease processes involving one structure can involve other closely related organs.

Transabdominal Scanning

Bladder distention is the only preparation that is required for performing transabdominal ultrasonography of the pelvis. If the bladder is not distended, it can be catheterized and then filled with saline. No special diet or mechanical bowel preparation is required. Since barium can interfere with ultrasound scanning, it is advisable that pelvic ultrasonography be performed before imaging of the upper or lower intestinal tract. The patient is placed supine on the examining table. Mineral oil or another suitable coupling agent is placed on the skin surface. The bladder should be imaged in both the transverse and longitudinal directions (Fig. 8.1). A 3.5-, 4-, or 5-MHz transducer will generally provide good visualization of the bladder and other pelvic structures. Transverse scans are performed from the symphysis to the umbilicus in 1- to 2-cm intervals. Longitudinal scans are routinely performed from the umbilicus to the pubis at 1- to 2-cm intervals from the midline. The technique of transabdominal bladder ultrasonography is easily learned, and with the use of real-time ultrasonography a complete examination of the bladder can be performed in several minutes.

Transrectal Scanning

The basic technique for transrectal ultrasonography was developed by Watanabe and associates and consists of a transrectal transducer, radial scanner, and imaging screen (1, 2). While initially performed in the sitting position on a special chair that allows for the probe insertion, the technique can also be performed in the lithotomy position (3, 4). A major ad-

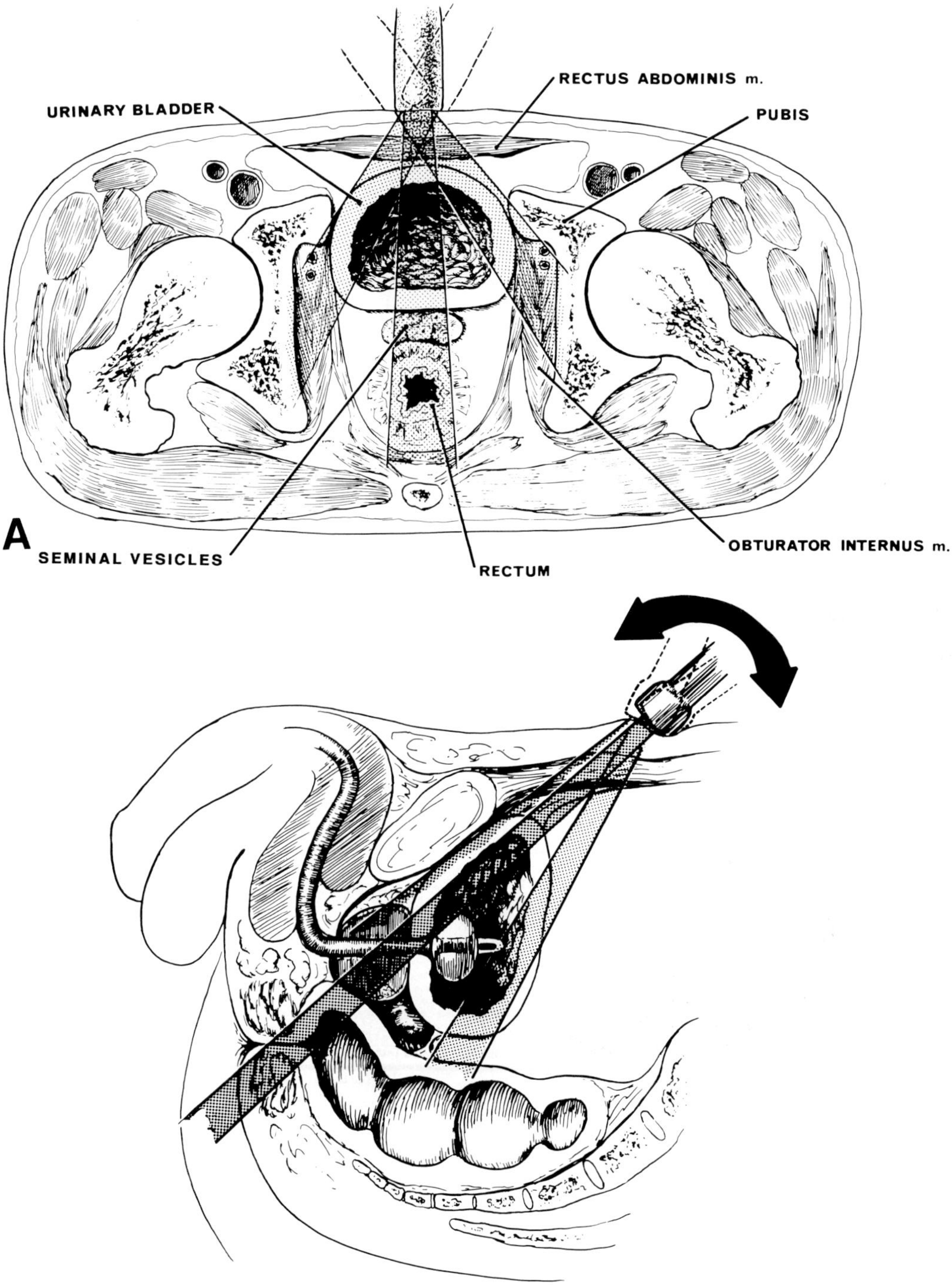

B

Figure 8.1. Transabdominal pelvic ultrasonography. **A,** Transverse scan. **B,** Longitudinal scan.

vance in transrectal scanning was the development of gray-scale and subsequent real-time imaging.

Present instrumentation consists of a two-part probe. The outer part is stationary, while the inner assembly is freely movable. The outer stationary unit provides inflow and outflow parts for the fluid interface and a polyethylene cover to protect the rectal mucosa. The inner assembly is free to move in longitudinal and rotational directions. Longitudinal movement provides an infinite number of serial sections of the bladder, and the rotational movement provides sonotomograms of it (Fig. 8.2). An

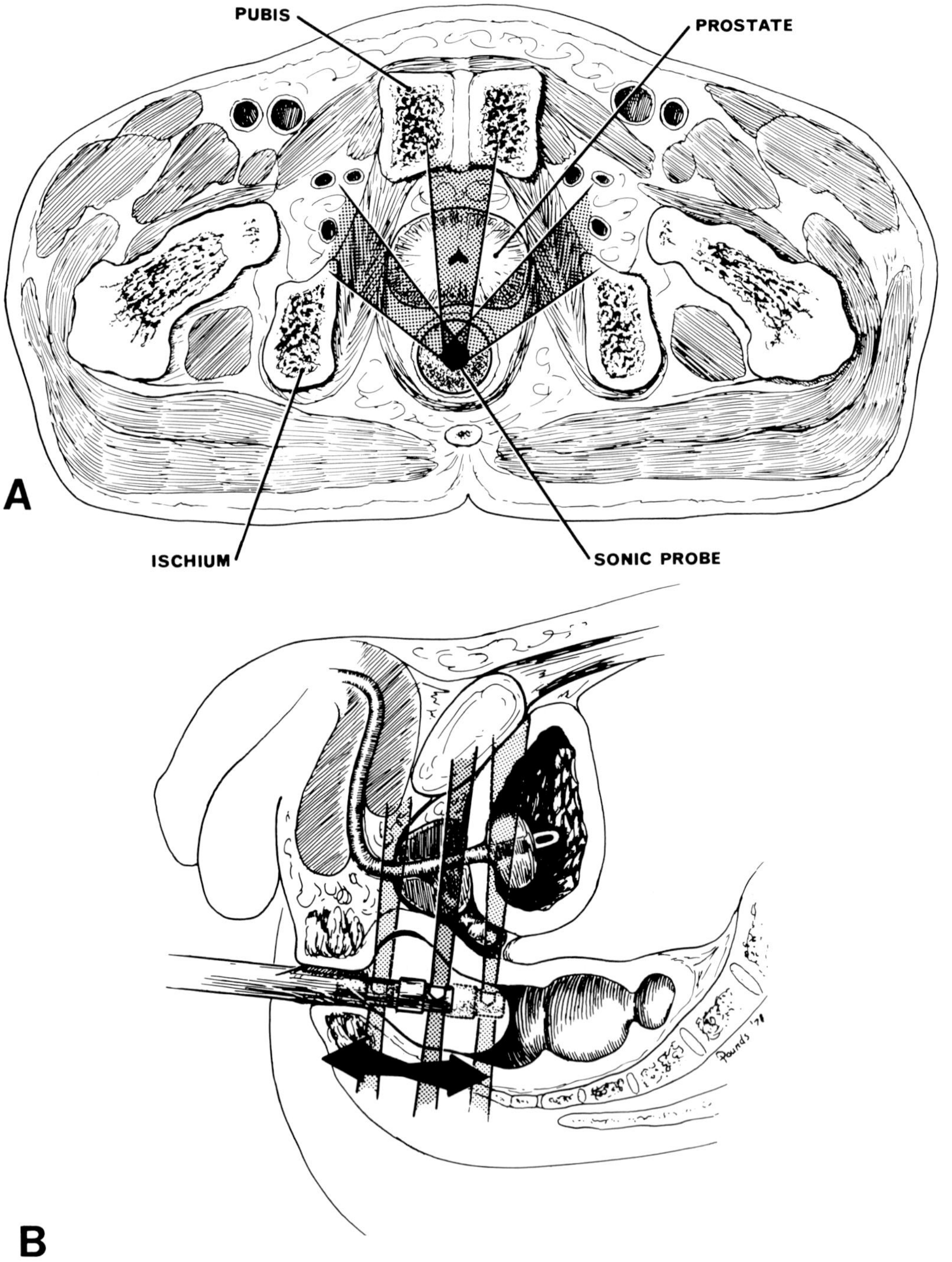

Figure 8.2. Transrectal pelvic ultrasonography. **A,** Transverse scan. **B,** Longitudinal scan.

ultrasonic beam is emitted at right angles to the probe, and the transducer receives the echoes and transmits them to the gray-scale unit.

In preparation for transrectal scanning, the patient is given an enema just prior to the study. If the patient has recently voided, a catheter can be inserted into the bladder and 200 ml of sterile saline infused. The catheter can be left indwelling during the study, as the catheter balloon is a useful landmark of the bladder neck. Prior to rectal insertion, the transducer is covered with a rubber condom. The probe is lubricated with a suitable coupling agent such as a water-soluble jelly and inserted 8 to 9 cm above the anal verge with the patient in the lithotomy or lateral decubutus position. After insertion, the condom is filled with approximately 100 ml of sterile saline until it is airtight with the rectum, taking care to eliminate all air bubbles. This procedure interposes an aqueous interface between the sonic disk and the rectum to ensure uniformity of the conducting media in the area. Serial transverse tomograms are then obtained beginning at the level of the bladder and progressing distally at 0.5- to 1.0-cm increments. The entire examination can be performed in 15 to 20 min with minimal patient discomfort. The main usage of transrectal ultrasonography has been in imaging the prostate. The bladder can be imaged, but the newer probes are particularly useful in scanning the prostate.

Transurethral Scanning

Holm and Northeved described the first transurethral ultrasound scanner in 1974 and postulated that this scanning method may provide an improved means of staging carcinoma of the bladder (5). Nakamura and Niijima improved on this instrument (6, 7). With increasing experience by other investigators, it has been shown that transurethral ultrasonography can add valuable information to the staging and management of bladder cancer (8–10). CT scans of the abdomen, on the other hand, have been of limited usefulness in staging bladder cancers (11). Papillary tumors are recognizable by CT, but normal bladder musculature, hypertrophy, and tumor infiltration all appear similar; tumors of the dome are also difficult to image because of the limitation of the transverse plane used in CT scanning (11). Transurethral ultrasonography is very helpful for differentiating stage A from stage C disease but is less helpful in defining stage B disease.

The scanner for transurethral ultrasonography consists of a motor that rotates a long rod which is connected at the opposite end to an interchangeable transducer. The scanner fits within a standard 24 F resectoscope sheath (Fig. 8.3). The transurethral probe can be ster-

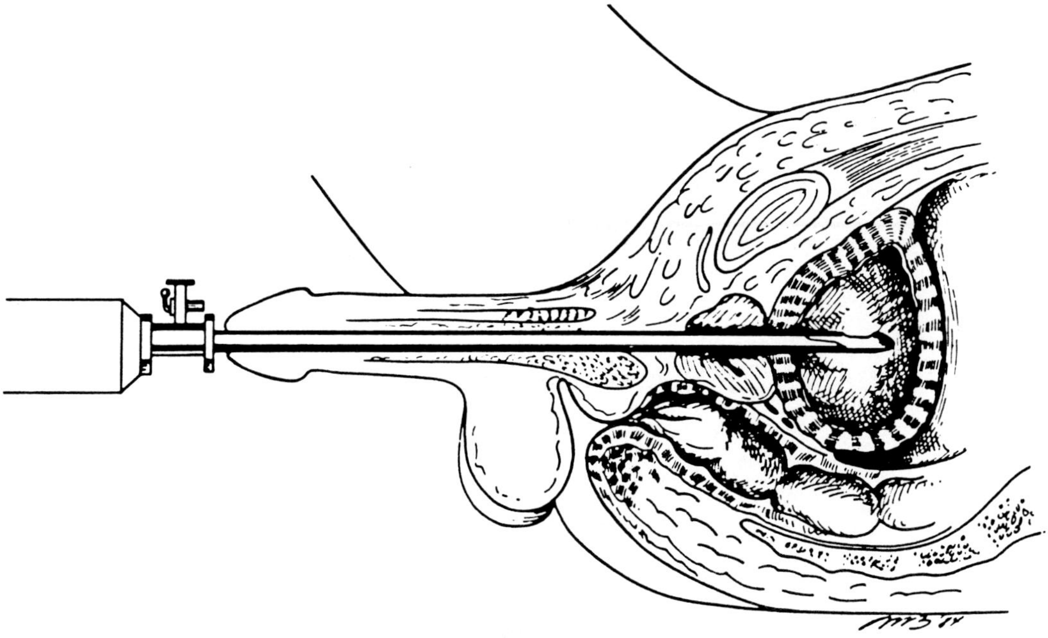

Figure 8.3. Transurethral ultrasonography. The transurethral transducer fits through a standard resectoscope sheath.

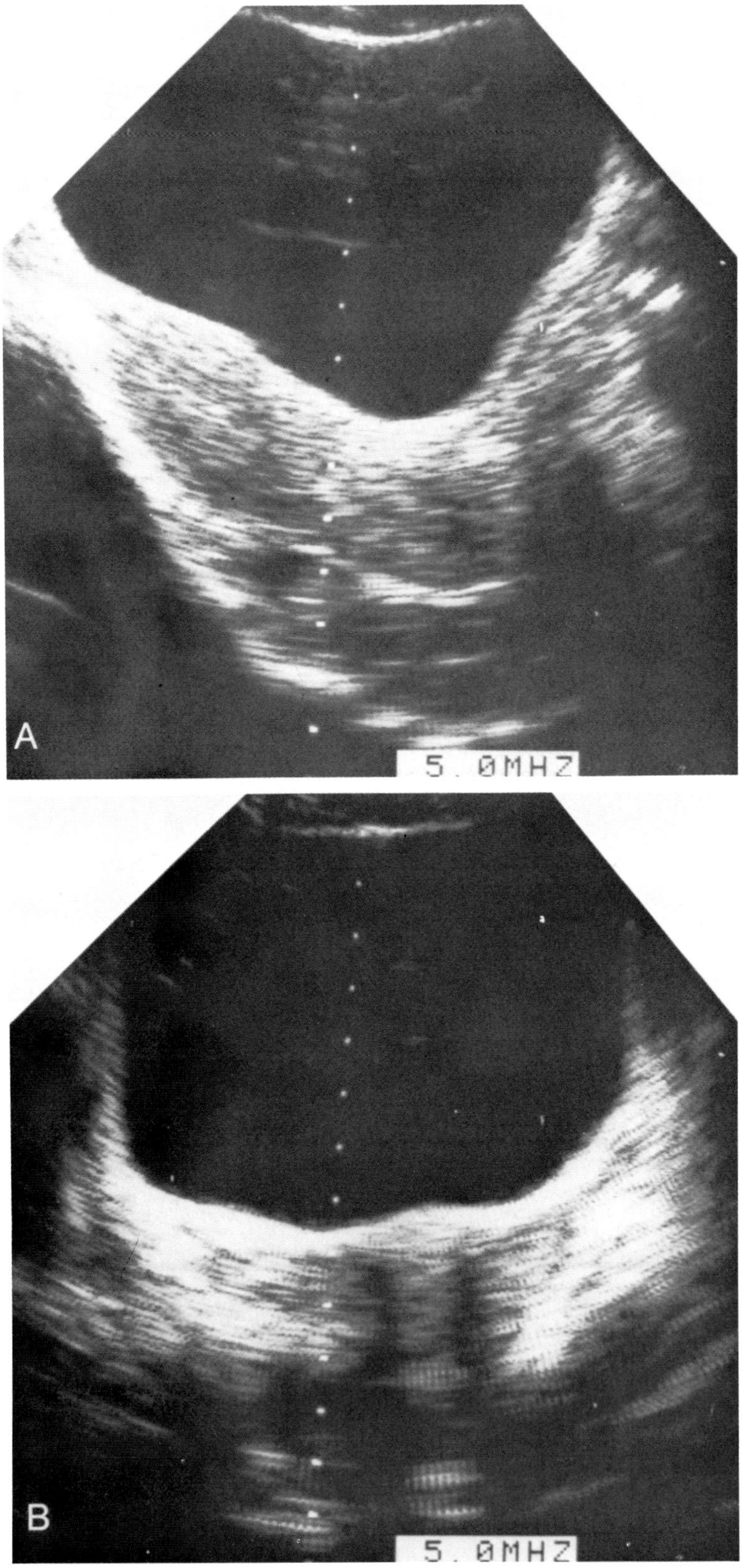

Figure 8.4. Transabdominal real-time sonogram of a normal female bladder. **A,** Longitudinal scan. **B,** Transverse scan.

ilized before use. When further information is desired during cystoscopy, the optics can be removed from the sheath and replaced with the transurethral scanner. The bladder is distended with sterile water infusion and the motor is activated. Dynamic scans of the bladder are obtained at different angles, positions, and degrees of inflation to view all surfaces of the bladder. The seminal vesicles in males, the bladder neck, and the ureteral orifices serve as landmarks in localizing abnormalities in the bladder. The procedure need not be performed under general anesthesia if the cystoscopy can be obtained under local anesthesia. The procedure is sterile and rapid and can greatly enhance the information gained at cystoscopy.

NORMAL BLADDER

The bladder should appear as a sonolucent structure with sharply demarcated walls. Typically, the bladder is seen as a global structure, and the interface between the fluid medium and bladder wall is distinct. The bladder wall normally appears as a symmetrical, smooth, gently curved surface. Scans obtained during different phases of filling clearly reveal the distensibility of the walls, and areas of fixation are readily identifiable.

When viewed abdominally the bladder shows some variability in shape depending on the amount of fluid present, changes in intrapelvic pressure, patient position, and the position of the probe (Fig. 8.4). The seminal vesicles and prostate can be imaged abdominally but not as precisely as with a transrectal probe (Fig. 8.5). Longitudinal scans reveal there to be a tapering of the bladder anteriorly with an orientation toward the umbilicus. Frequently, parallel reverberation echoes arise from the interface of the bladder wall and urine and are readily dis-

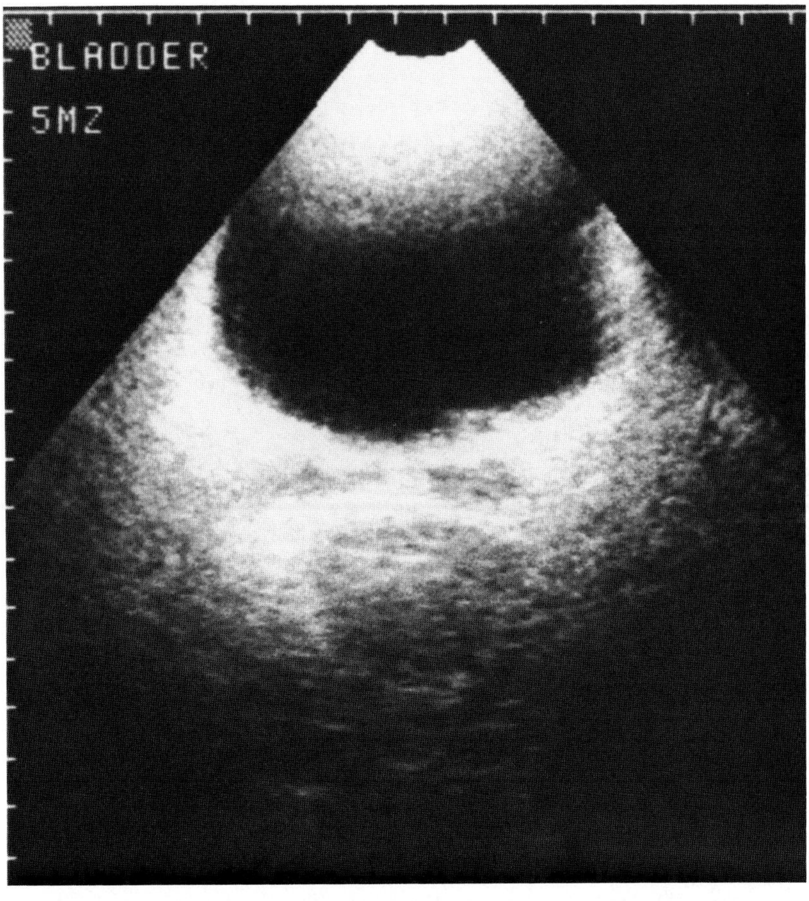

Figure 8.5. Transabdominal real-time sonogram of a normal male bladder. The seminal vesicles and prostate can be seen.

tinguishable from echo patterns arising from tumors. Transverse scans reveal variations in the shape of the bladder ranging from almost circular to nearly square; but, as with the longitudinal scans, they are also affected by the degree of filling and intrapelvic pressures. Real-time sonography has allowed visualization of urine as it enters the bladder from the ureters (Fig. 8.6). Urine normally squirts into the bladder intermittently, forming the "jet" effect (12, 13). If a Foley catheter is in place, it can easily be visualized transabdominally, and the balloon serves as a useful landmark to identify the bladder neck (Fig. 8.7).

Transrectal scans provide similar information about the bladder contour to the transabdominal study (Fig. 8.8). Reverberation echoes are also frequently seen but are located posteriorly. Experience reveals that the methods of scanning are comparable. Abdominal scanning does, however, offer the advantage of assessing pelvic lymph nodes, psoas muscle, and other intraabdominal and pelvic structures that are not accessible by the transrectal technique (14, 15).

Transurethral scans provide similar information to transabdominal and transrectal scans. A normal bladder imaged by transurethral ultrasound is shown in Figure 8.9. Recent experience suggests that the bladder is best imaged using a transurethral ultrasound transducer. Since the ultrasound probe is in the center of the bladder and images the bladder at right angles circumferentially, the best detail of the bladder wall can be obtained (9–11, 16).

BLADDER TUMORS

Successful management of patients with transitional cell carcinoma of the bladder depends on accurate staging of the tumor. Understaging of bladder cancer is a common problem. The methods currently available for staging bladder cancers include bimanual examination under anesthesia, excretory urography, cystoscopy and transurethral biopsy, pelvic computed tomography, and magnetic resonance imaging

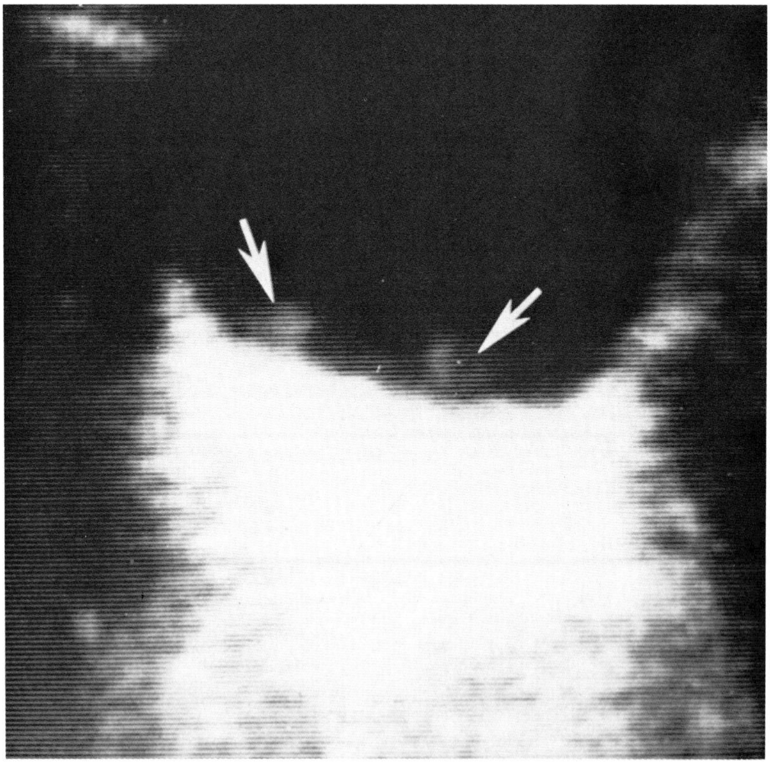

Figure 8.6. Urine jets (*arrows*) are seen emerging from the ureteral orifices on this real-time scan. Echoes from such urine jets are frequently seen on real-time studies. The echoes are thought to be due to an acoustic mismatch caused by propulsion of the urine emerging from the ureters compared to the urine already in the bladder in patients who have been given a water load.

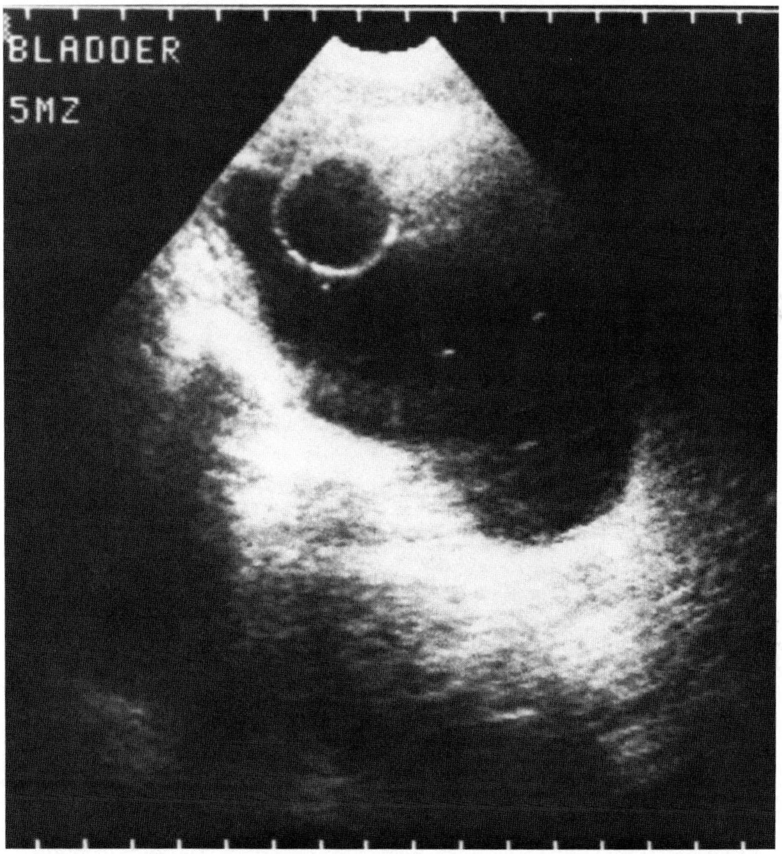

Figure 8.7. Transabdominal real-time sonogram of a bladder with an indwelling catheter present. The catheter balloon is easily identifiable.

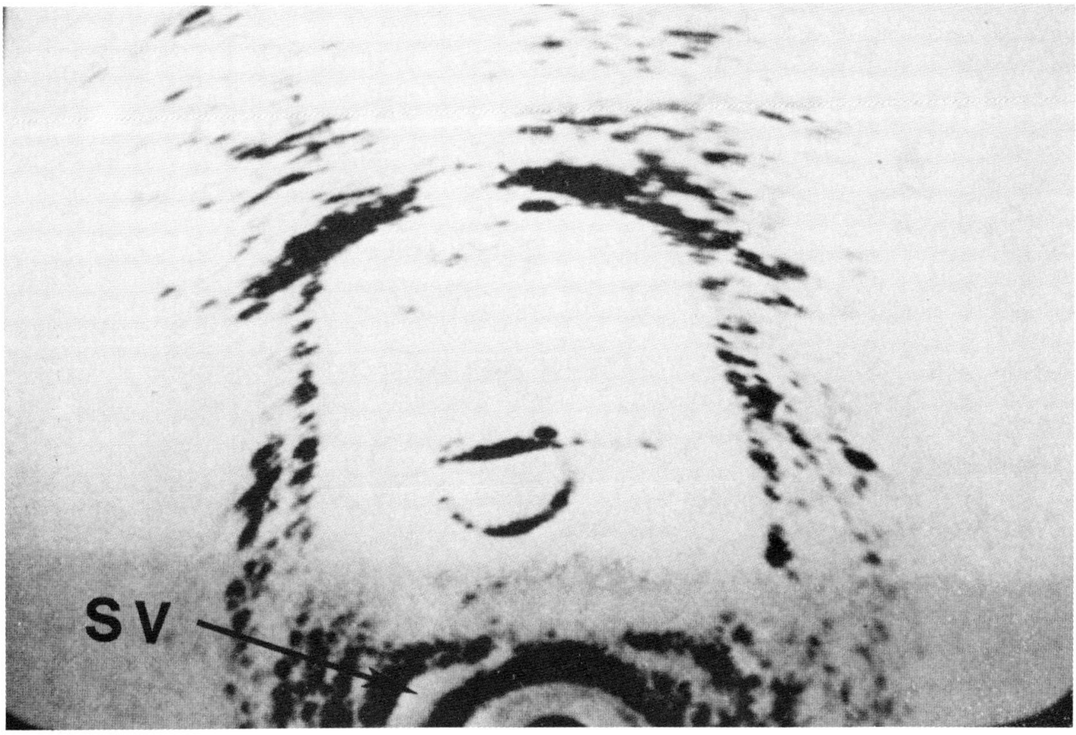

Figure 8.8. Transrectal gray-scale sonogram of a normal bladder. The seminal vesicles (*SV*) are visualized posteriorly.

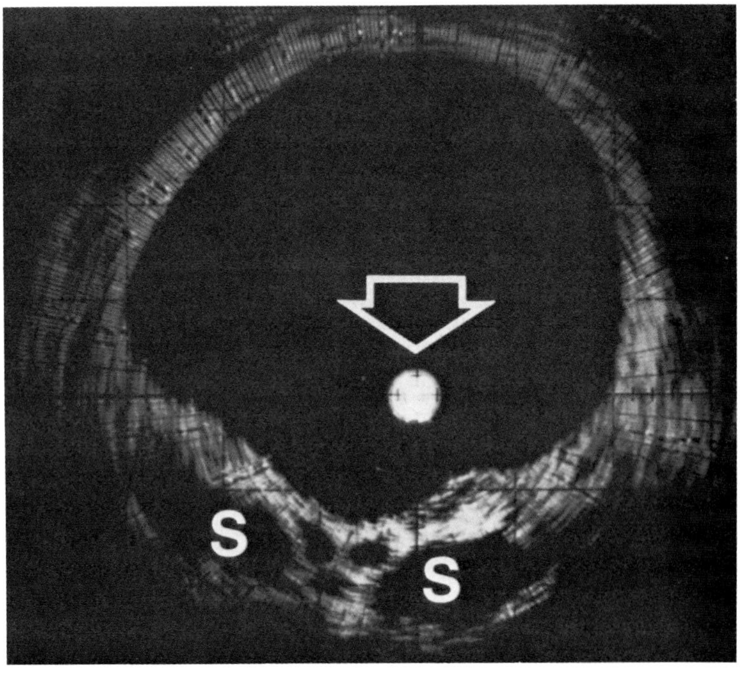

Figure 8.9. Transurethral sonogram of a normal bladder. The seminal vesicles (*S*) are visualized posteriorly. The transducer is present in the center of the bladder (*arrow*).

(9, 10, 17). Various investigators report an error in the staging of bladder tumors that approaches 50%, mainly due to understaging of superficial and deeply invasive bladder carcinomas (15, 17–19). Although not unassociated with false-negative studies, ultrasonography has been shown to improve the estimation of local tumor involvement (3, 18, 20–24). Small, superficial, noninfiltrating bladder tumors are difficult to visualize ultrasonically, and direct endoscopic visualization continues to be the most accurate diagnostic modality in the assessment of patients with this condition. Larger bladder tumors appear ultrasonically as echogenic masses projecting into the lumen of the echo-free urinary bladder. These areas are fixed to the wall and, unlike blood clots or stones, do not alter their location with changes in patient position (Fig. 8.10).

Transabdominal ultrasound has been used in bladder carcinoma detection and staging. Itzchuk and associates reported their experience in diagnosing and staging 71 known bladder tumors (23). Twenty-one of the tumors could not be confirmed with ultrasound because of the tumor size being less than 0.5 cm or the location being on the dome or bladder neck. Transabdominal ultrasound was accurate in differentiating stages B2, C, and D disease as a whole but was less specific in differentiating

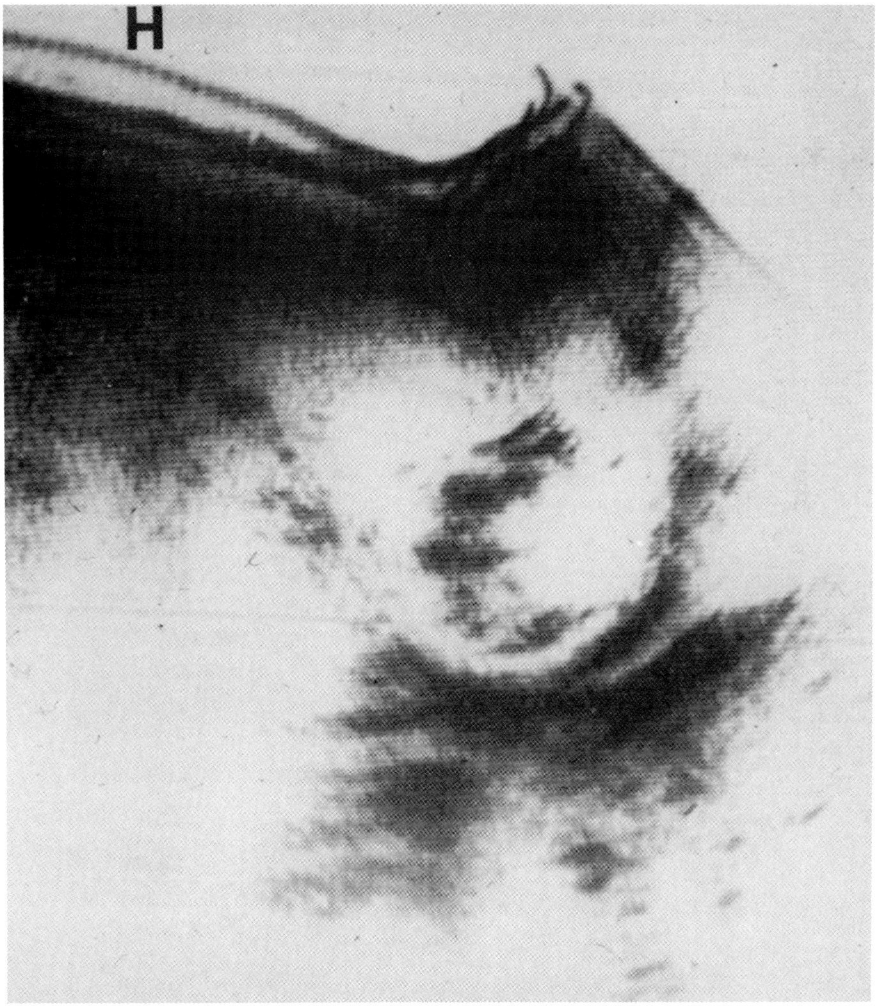

Figure 8.10. Transabdominal (longitudinal) gray-scale sonogram demonstrating blood clots in the bladder. The clots are not fixed to the bladder wall and change location with alteration in patient position. *H*, toward the head.

stage A and B tumors. Others have found similar findings but have also noted false-positive studies secondary to cystitis, bladder trabeculation, and prostatic median lobe hyperplasia and false negatives in very obese patients (26, 27).

Superficial and noninvasive bladder tumors have a well-defined base (Figs. 8.11 and 8.12). There is no distortion of the bladder wall. Although they are fixed to the bladder wall, ureteroceles can easily be differentiated from tumors by their lack of echogenicity and identification of their thin wall (Fig. 8.13). It is important to be able to distinguish bladder tumors from reverberation patterns, which can usually be eliminated by altering the angle of the transducer and which are usually parallel to the bladder wall (Fig. 8.14). If multiple scans are obtained during the filling phase, normal contour will be preserved and movement of the bladder wall with increasing intraluminal volume will be appreciated.

Infiltrative tumors tend to have a broader base that can be visualized ultrasonically (Figs. 8.14 to 8.18). Often the bladder wall will be fixed and the natural contour distorted when the bladder is full. Tumors that have completely extended through the bladder wall can be identified by the presence of an extravesical mass. With extensive extravesical invasion, the bladder wall becomes fixed and is often markedly distorted.

Transurethral ultrasonography has greatly improved the urologist's clinical ability to accurately stage bladder cancers. Salo and Alfthan reported that only one of 45 bladder tumors was missed by transurethral scanning in their series, and the technique was correct in 95% of the cases in differentiating superficial (Ta, T1) from intramural (T2, T3a) and extravesical (T3b, T4) tumors (28). Pavone and associates also noted that local staging was improved with transurethral ultrasonography (29). Devonel and associates reported an 80% correlation between transurethral ultrasonography staging and actual pathological stage (30). Braeckman

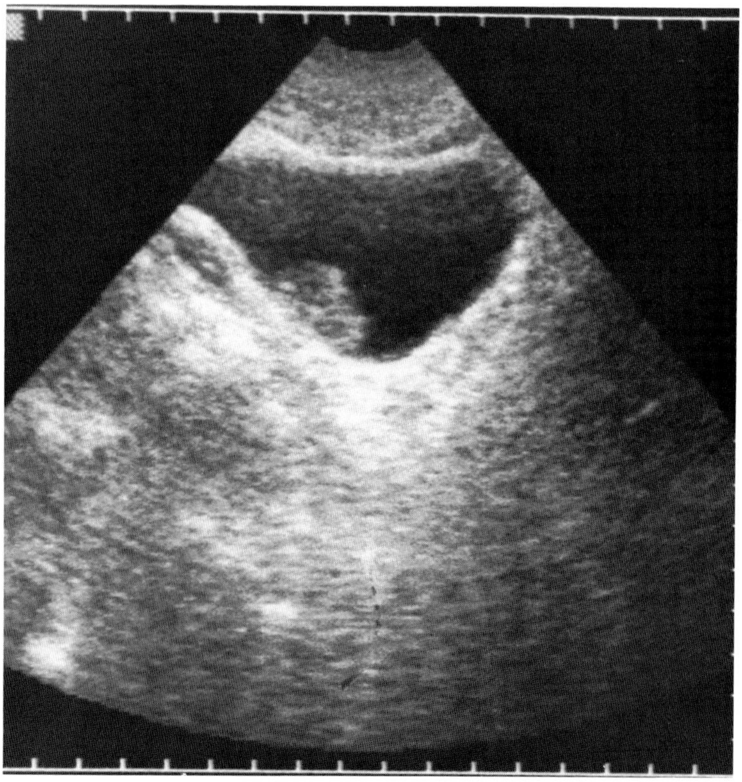

Figure 8.11. Transabdominal sonogram demonstrating a superficial tumor located on the lateral wall of the bladder. The bladder muscle is not involved.

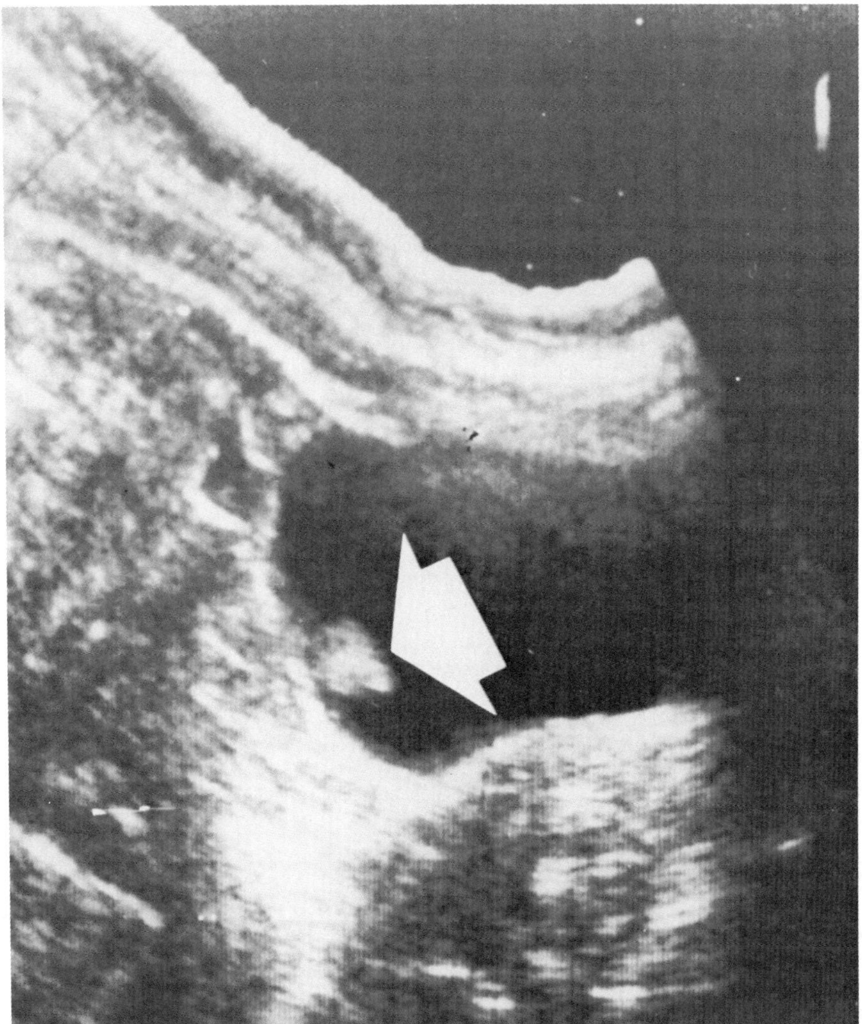

Figure 8.12. Transabdominal (longitudinal) gray-scale sonogram of the bladder demonstrating a superficial tumor located on the dome (*arrow*). The bladder wall is free of distortion and is not fixed.

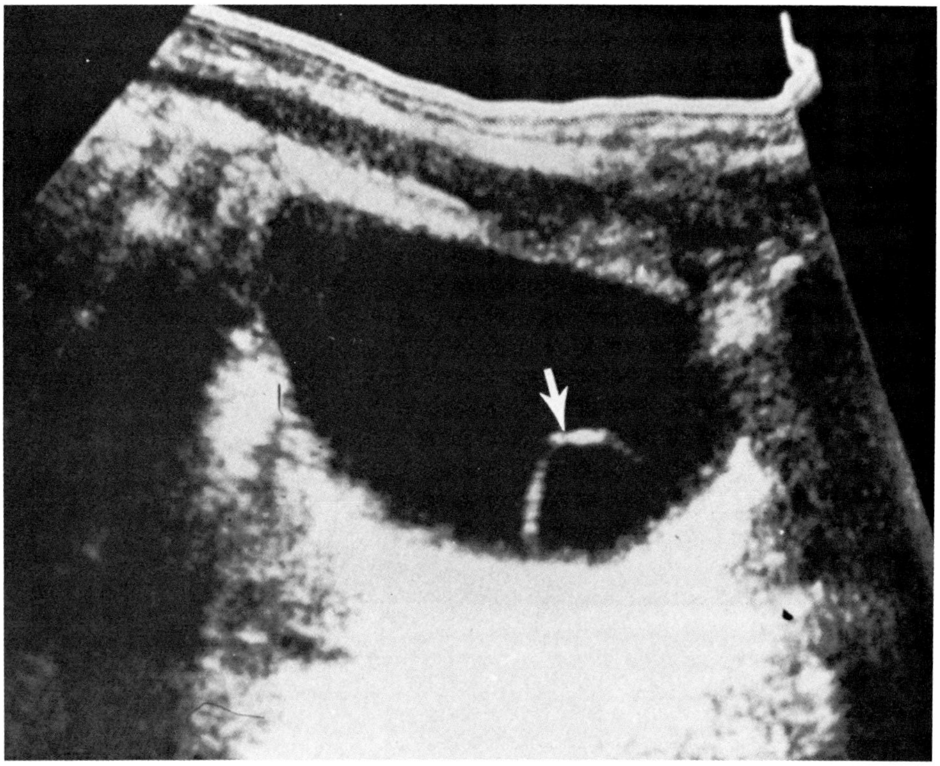

Figure 8.13. Transabdominal sonogram demonstrating a walled ureterocele (*arrow*) projecting into the bladder lumen.

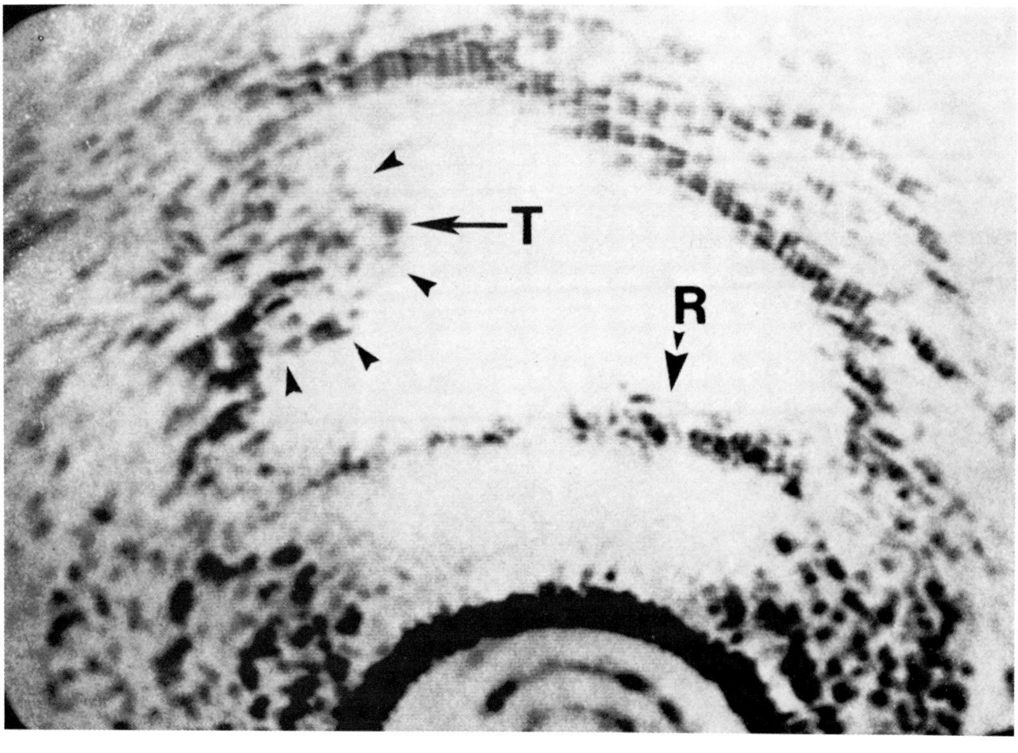

Figure 8.14. Transrectal gray-scale sonogram of the bladder demonstrating tumor involvement of the wall. The depth of invasion cannot be determined. *T,* tumor; *R,* reverberation echo.

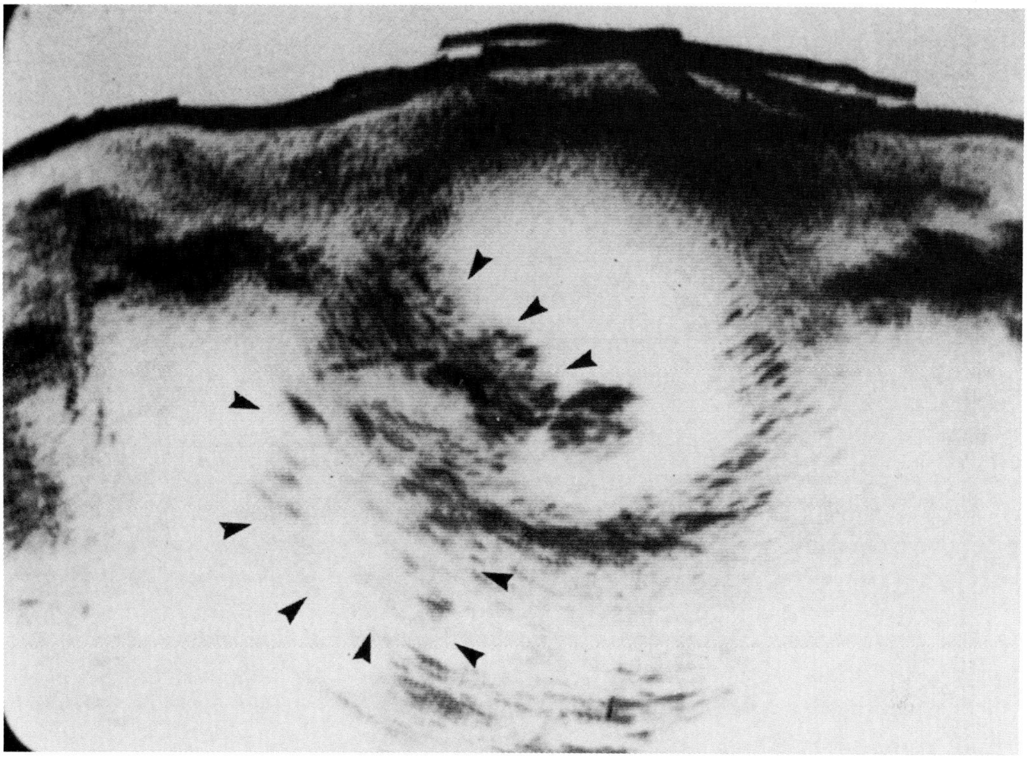

Figure 8.15. Transabdominal (transverse) gray-scale sonogram of the bladder demonstrating a tumor (*arrows*) distorting the bladder wall and invading the perivesical space.

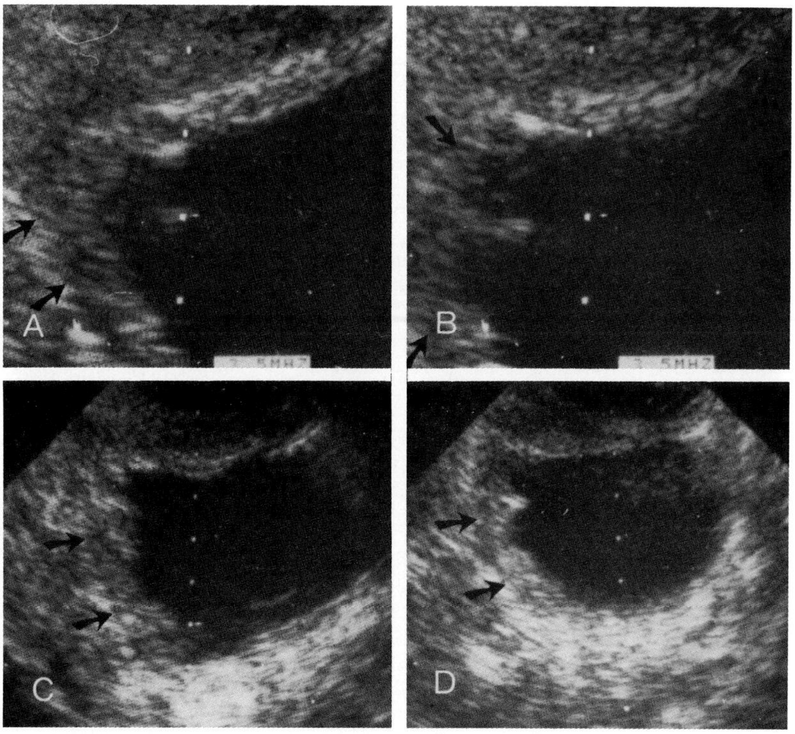

Figure 8.16. Irregular plaque-like bladder carcinoma. Four scans at different levels show irregular thickening of the right wall of the bladder (*arrows*). There is no evidence of extension of tumor beyond the bladder wall into perivesical fat.

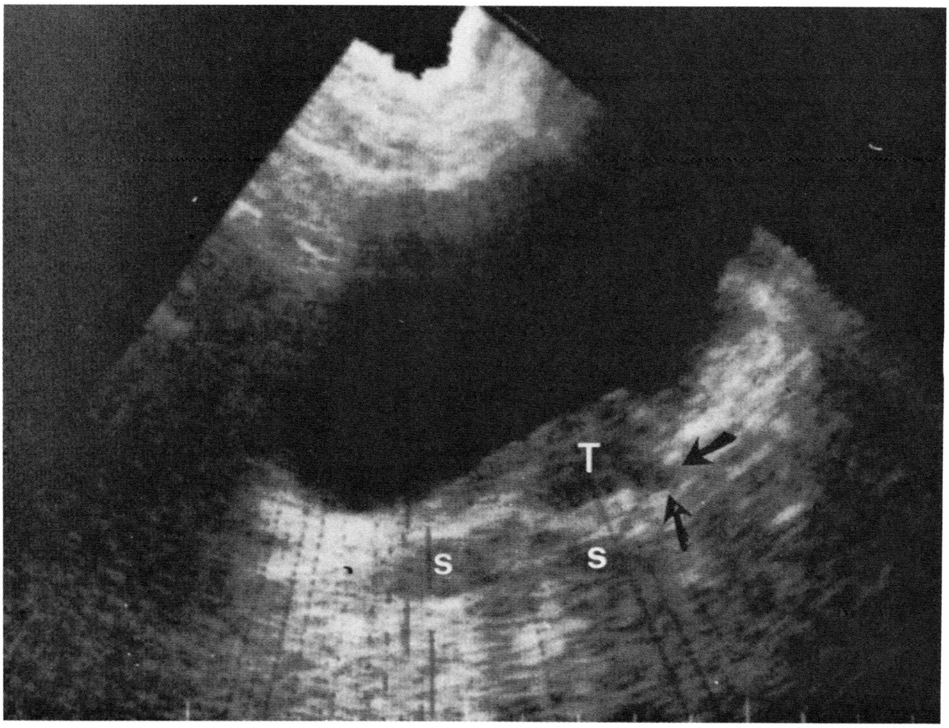

Figure 8.17. Bladder carcinoma (*T*) with extension of the tumor beyond the confines of the bladder wall into the perivesical fat (*arrows*). This indicates that the tumor is at least a stage C. *S*, seminal vesicles.

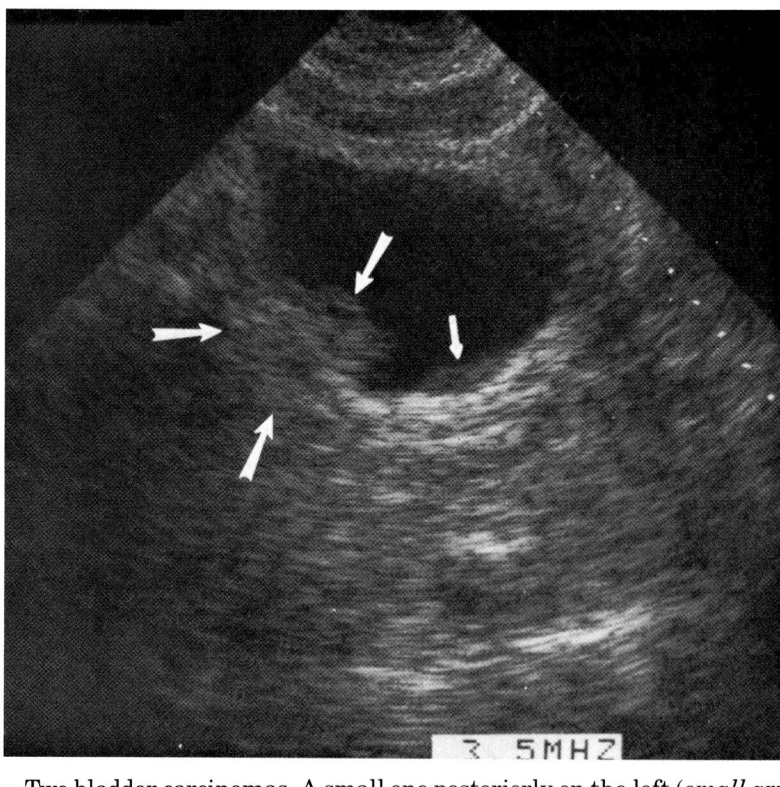

Figure 8.18. Two bladder carcinomas. A small one posteriorly on the left (*small arrow*) does not extend beyond the bladder wall, but the larger one on the right side does extend into the perivesical fat (*large arrows*), indicating that this is a stage C tumor.

reported a 97% accuracy in differentiating Ta-T1 disease from T2-T3, with only 5% of patients being understaged because of the pathologic finding of microscopic invasion that was not visualized by ultrasonography (31).

Transurethral scanning offers the potential to differentiate stage B1 and B2 tumors and tumors with only minimal extravesical involvement from those with muscle involvement, which is a great advantage (Figs. 8.19 to 8.22). Ultrasonography has been found to be of value in the assessment of bladder tumor patients following radiation therapy or chemotherapy. Ultrasound is a useful noninvasive method of assessing response to treatment and assessing tumor staging prior to surgery so that appropriate therapy may be instituted (Fig. 8.23). If extravesical tumor involvement persists following an appropriate course of preoperative radiotherapy or chemotherapy, extensive operative procedures could be avoided in patients who would not benefit from such treatment. Computed tomography gives similar information to that provided by ultrasonography. Extension of tumor into the perivesical fat is more obvious on computed tomography (CT), and CT is also superior to ultrasonography in demonstrating metastatic involvement of pelvic and abdominal lymph nodes.

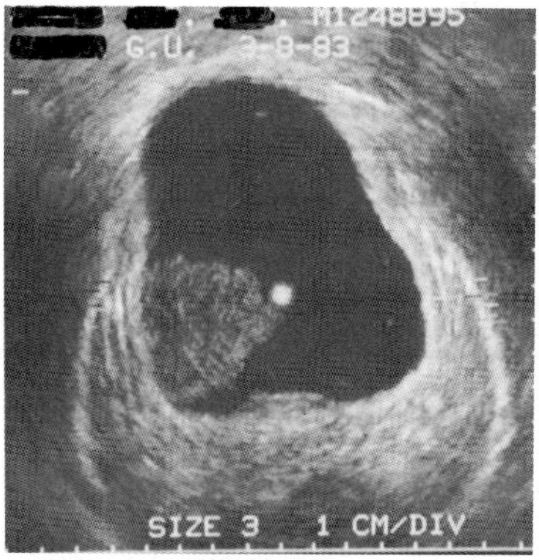

Figure 8.19. Transurethral scan demonstrating a superficial bladder tumor. The bladder wall is preserved. No invasion of the lamina propria was detected histologically following resection.

BLADDER DIVERTICULA

Bladder diverticula are usually associated with diseases resulting in bladder outlet obstruction (such as benign prostatic hyperplasia) or neurogenic conditions resulting in abnormalities in the bladder or sphincter function. Diverticula resulting from these processes do not possess muscular coatings and can often be differentiated from the thickened and irregular bladder wall. Diverticula greater than 2 cm in diameter can usually be seen ultrasonically, and with multiple scans often the narrow communication between a diverticulum and the bladder can be demonstrated (Fig. 8.24). Since tumors and stones can occur in diverticula, they should be sought by ultrasonography. Postvoiding scans are helpful, since often diverticula will not empty and occasionally they will actually increase in size. Diagnosis should be confirmed by cystography or cystoscopy, which are necessary procedures in the evaluation of patients with conditions that lead to diverticula formation. Pelvic ultrasonography is also of value in detecting the presence of urachal remnants (Fig. 8.25) and bladder duplication (32, 33).

BLADDER CALCULI

Bladder stones are usually seen in association with bladder outlet obstruction, chronic indwelling urinary catheters, and neurogenic diseases resulting in bladder dysfunction. Like stones in the kidney, bladder stones are strongly echogenic and are highly reflective of the ultrasonic beam. Due to their extreme density, echo shadows are often produced because of the inability of the sound waves to penetrate the stone (Fig. 8.26).

MEASUREMENT OF RESIDUAL URINE

The measurement of a postvoiding residual plays an important role in the management of many urologic patients. Postvoiding residuals are helpful in confirming the diagnosis of bladder outlet obstruction and establishing when surgical intervention may be appropriate. The effectiveness of bladder management in patients with neurogenic bladder is also established in part by measuring postvoid residuals. Traditionally, such measurements have been made by passing a catheter into the bladder after the patient has made an optimal effort to void. Indirect estimates of postvoid residuals can be obtained from an excretory urogram or

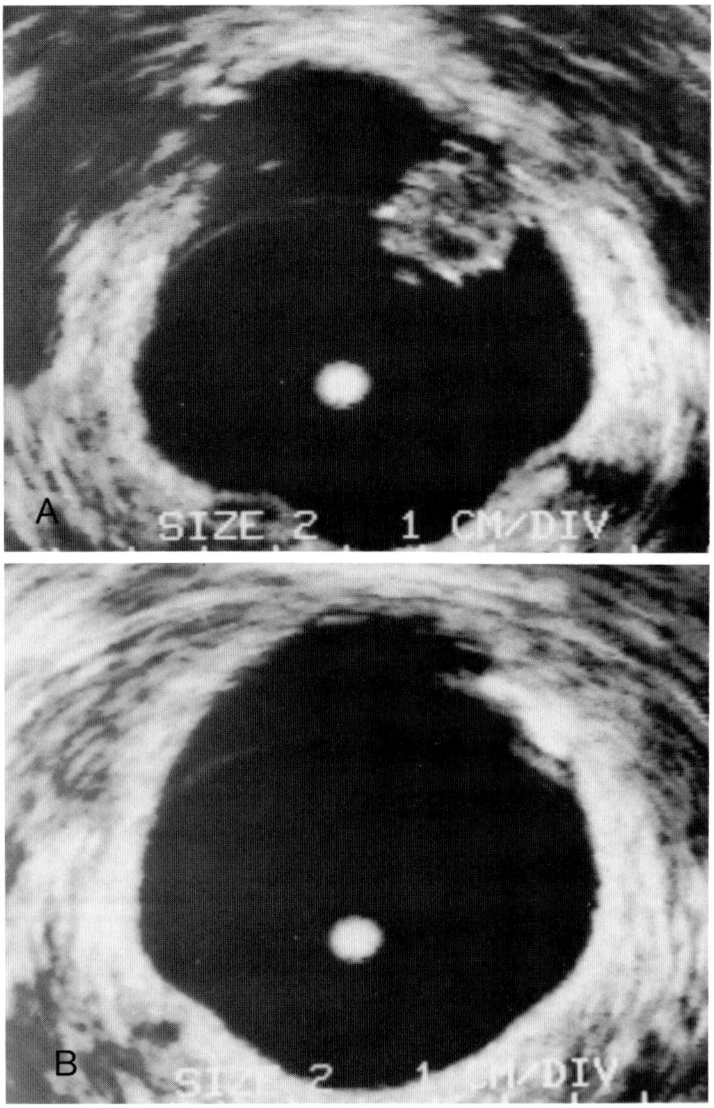

Figure 8.20. **A,** Transurethral scan demonstrating a superficial bladder tumor before transurethral resection. **B,** After resection, the tumor is no longer seen and the bladder wall remains intact.

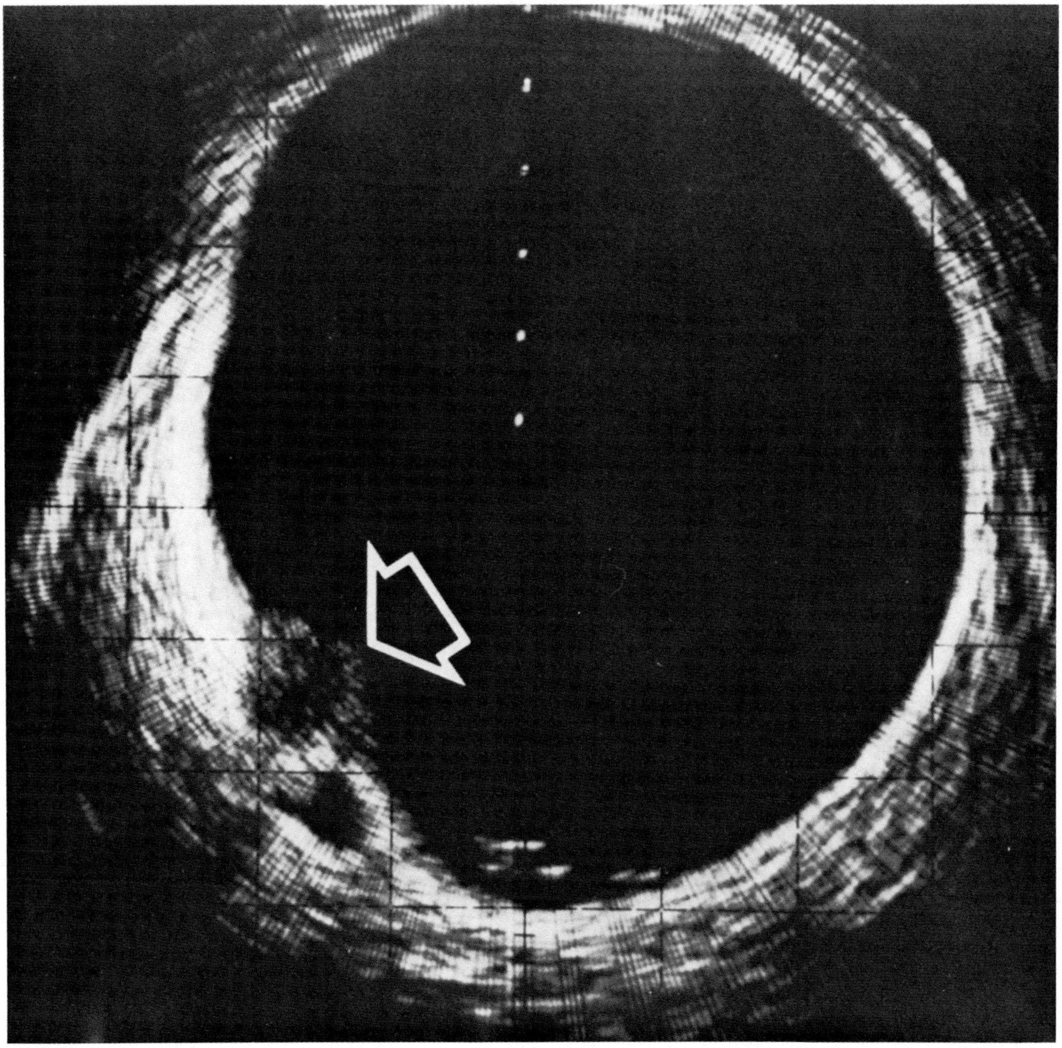

Figure 8.21. Transurethral scan demonstrating a bladder tumor invading into but not through muscle.

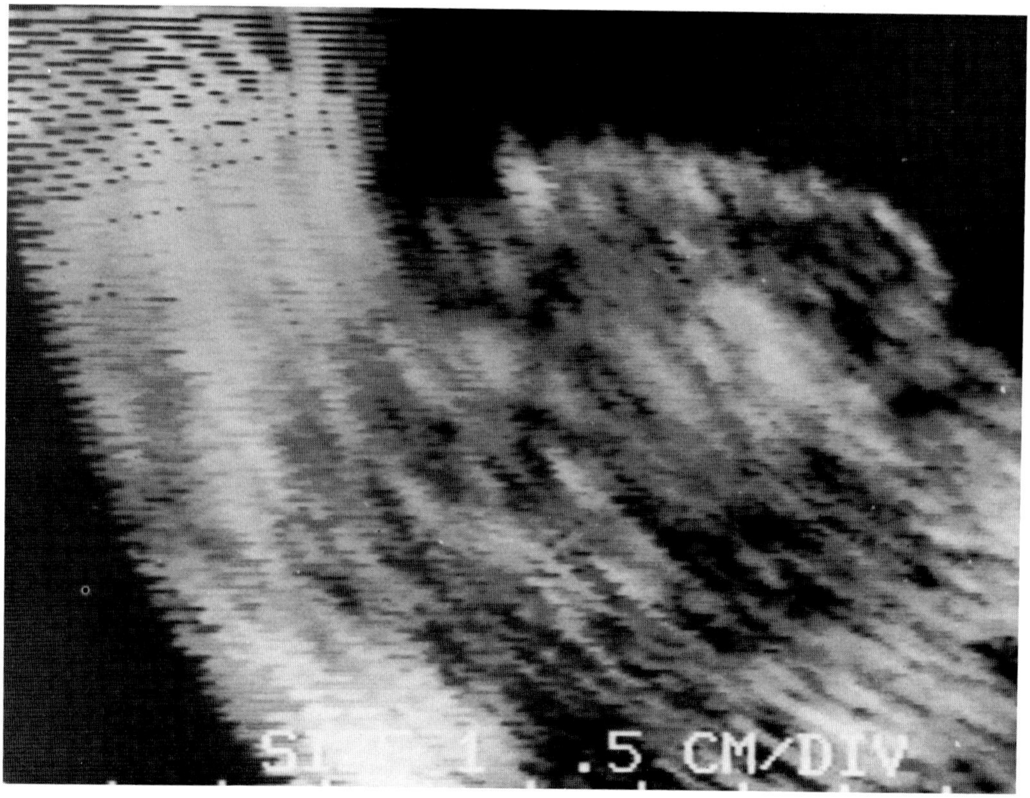

Figure 8.22. Transurethral scan under magnification demonstrates a bladder tumor with deep invasion into the bladder wall.

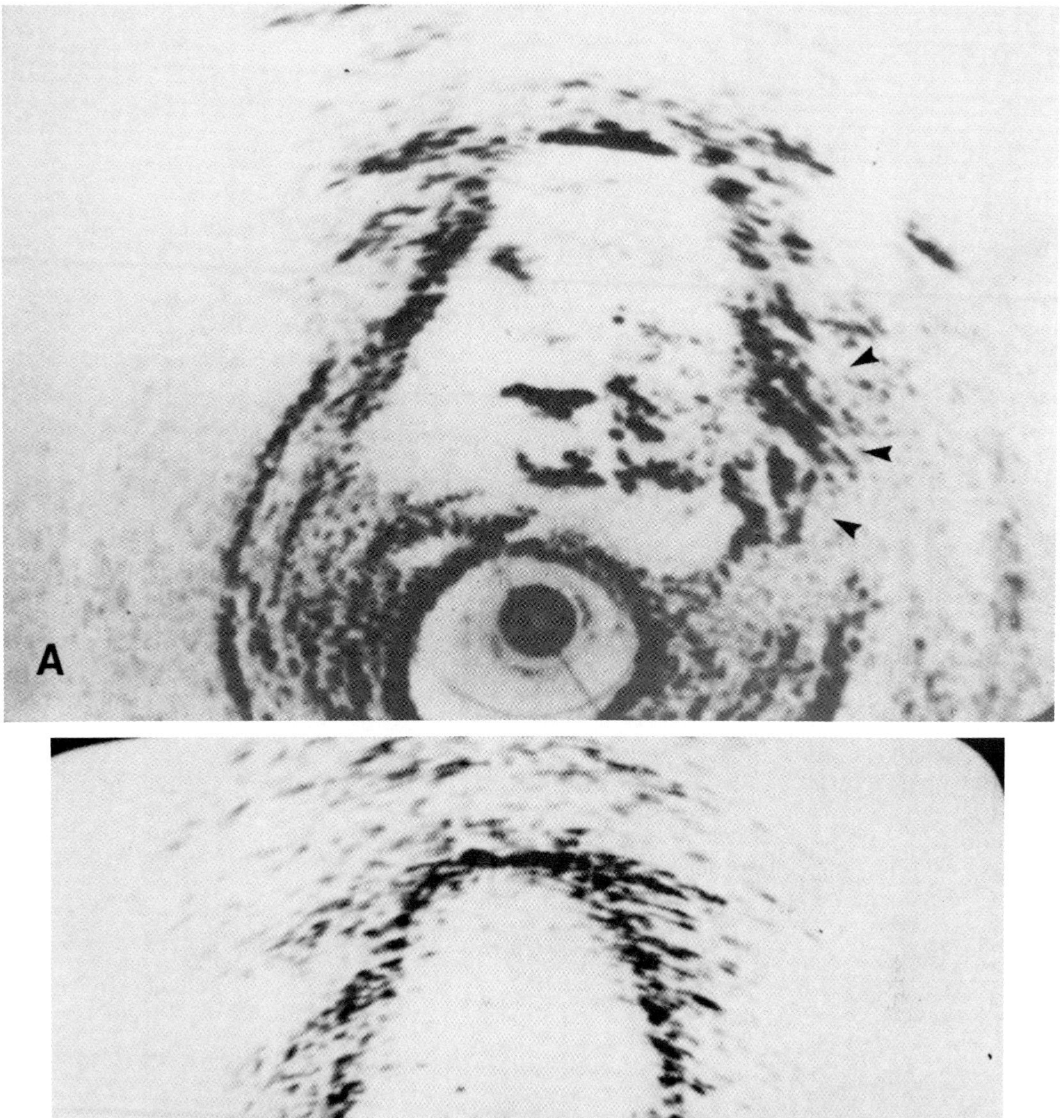

Figure 8.23. Transrectal gray-scale sonogram in a patient with an invasive bladder tumor treated with preoperative irradiation. **A,** Preradiation scan demonstrating a large tumor on the left lateral wall of the bladder invading the perivesical space (*arrows*). **B,** Postradiation scan showing no evidence of tumor. The cystectomy specimen was negative for tumor.

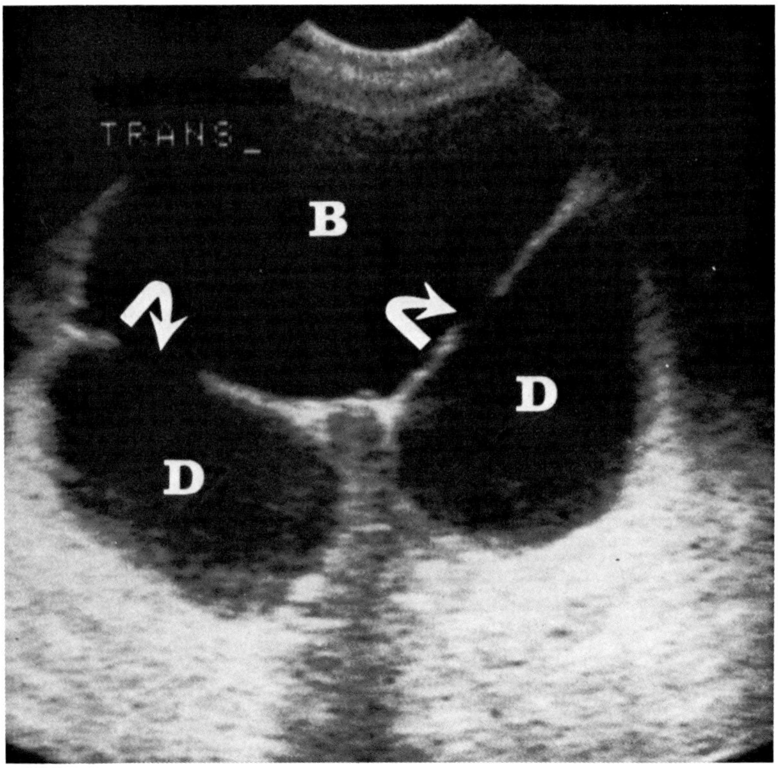

Figure 8.24. Transverse scan showing two large diverticula (*D*). Note the large diverticular orifices (*curved arrows*). *B,* bladder.

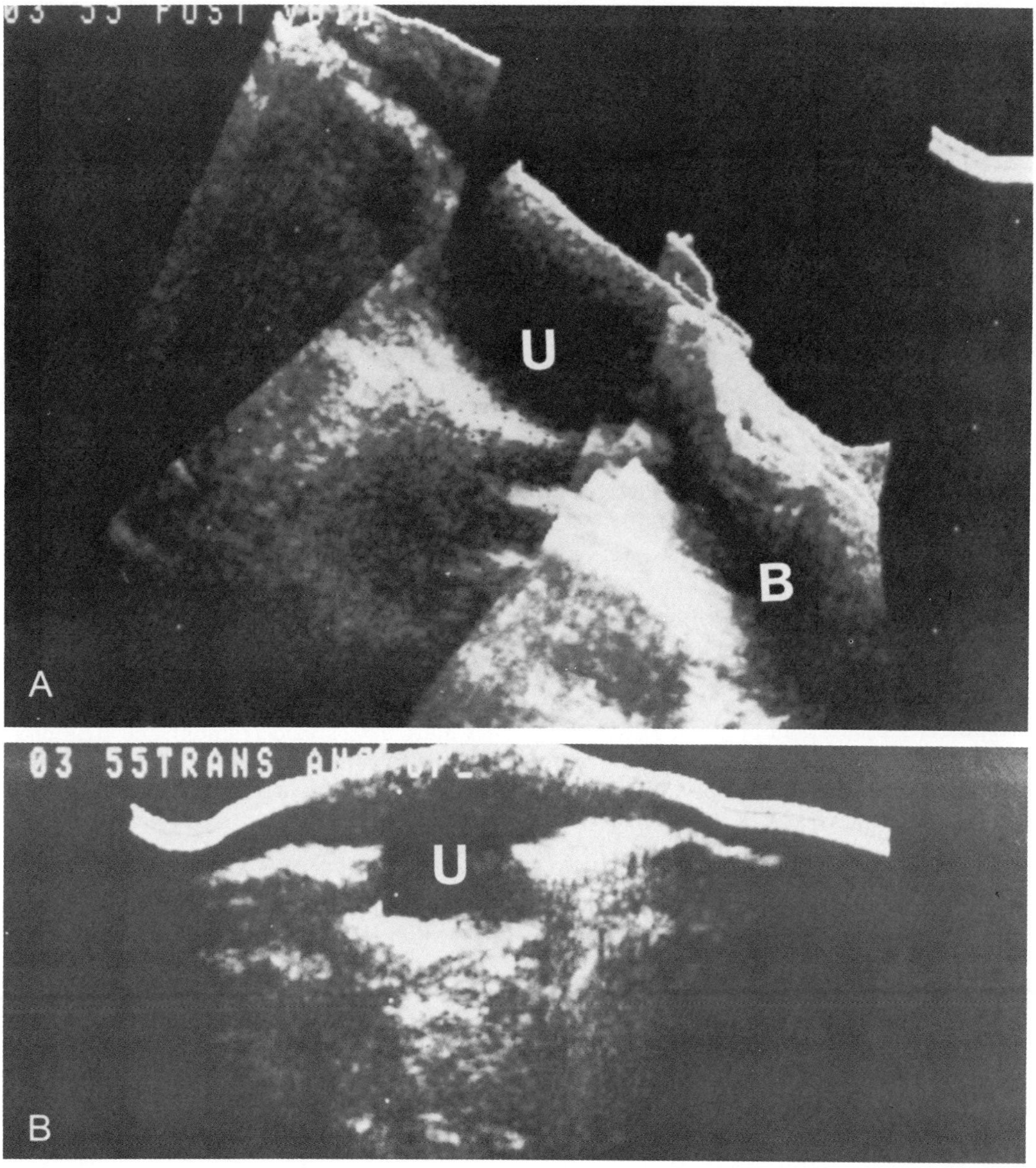

Figure 8.25. **A,** Transabdominal (longitudinal) sonogram demonstrating a normal bladder (*B*) and a urachal cyst (*U*) superior to the bladder. **B,** Transverse view shows that the urachal cyst invades the abdominal wall and intraperitoneal area.

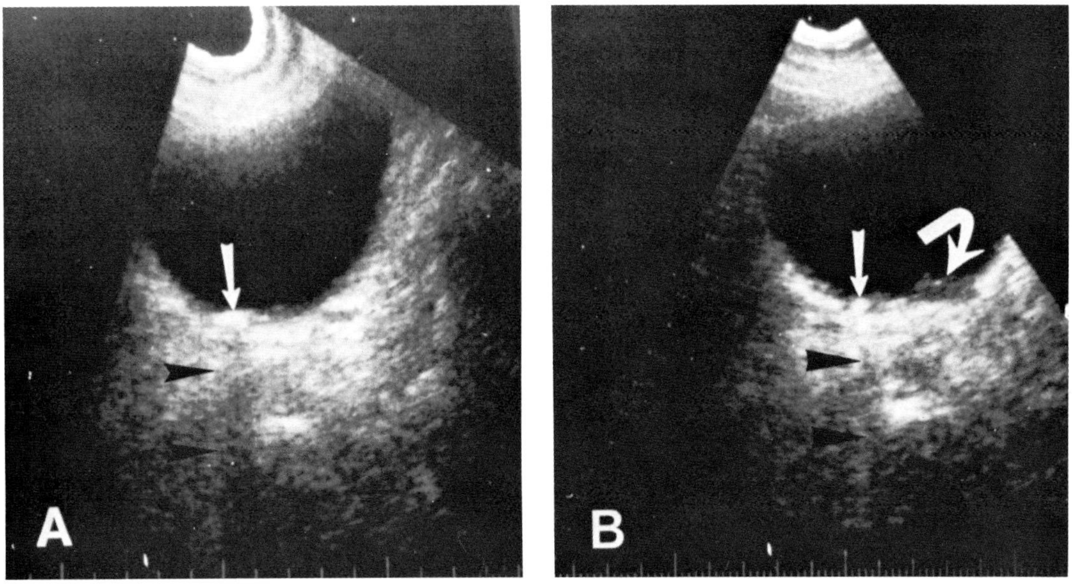

Figure 8.26. **A** and **B,** Two scans of the bladder showing calculi (*straight arrows*) with posterior acoustic shadowing (*arrowheads*). There is a coexisting small bladder carcinoma (*curved arrow*).

radionuclide study, but these methods are inaccurate (34).

Early studies with ultrasonography revealed that the technique offered a good qualitative estimate of bladder volume (35–37). With refinement of the technique, quantitative errors were reduced to 15 to 20% of the actual volume (38–41). Roehrborn and Peters recently reported that for calculation of bladder volume by ultrasound, the formula for an ellipsoid ($V = \frac{4}{3}\pi \times r1 \times r2 \times r3$) was the most accurate method to determine the actual volume measured by straight catheterization, with a correlation coefficient of 0.982 (42). They noticed the highest error in the low volume range (20 to 100 ml), but the absolute difference between actual and estimated postvoid residuals was always low (42). Ultrasound is therefore an inexpensive, accurate, quick, and well-tolerated method of determining postvoiding residuals (Figs. 8.27 and 8.28).

The application of ultrasound to determine bladder residuals in the spinal cord–injured population has also recently been reported (43, 44). Residual urine can be estimated by obtaining scans prior to and after voiding. The presence of residual urine can easily be seen and the volume accurately estimated. The presence of residual urine often indicates bladder dysfunction and decompensation, and its determination is an important part of the examination of patients with urinary tract disorders. Since ultrasound provides an accurate and inexpensive estimate of postvoid residual and it is better tolerated by the patient than catheterization, it will continue to be used more frequently for this purpose.

EXTRINSIC MASSES

Disorders of structures adjacent to the bladder will at times deform it and cause distortion and fixation of its walls. Cervical, colonic, and prostatic carcinomas are common malignancies that frequently will extend locally into the bladder musculature (Figs. 8.29 to 8.31). Although an intraluminal mass may not be present, often the involved wall will be fixed and associated with the mass produced by the primary tumor. As is seen with primary malignancies of the bladder, scans obtained following surgery or radiotherapy are useful in the assessment of tumor response and in the detection of tumor recurrence. It is often very helpful to know the extent of bladder involvement prior to initiating surgical exploration, radiation therapy, or (more recently) chemotherapy. Other perivesical benign processes or diseases that may distort the bladder include müllerian

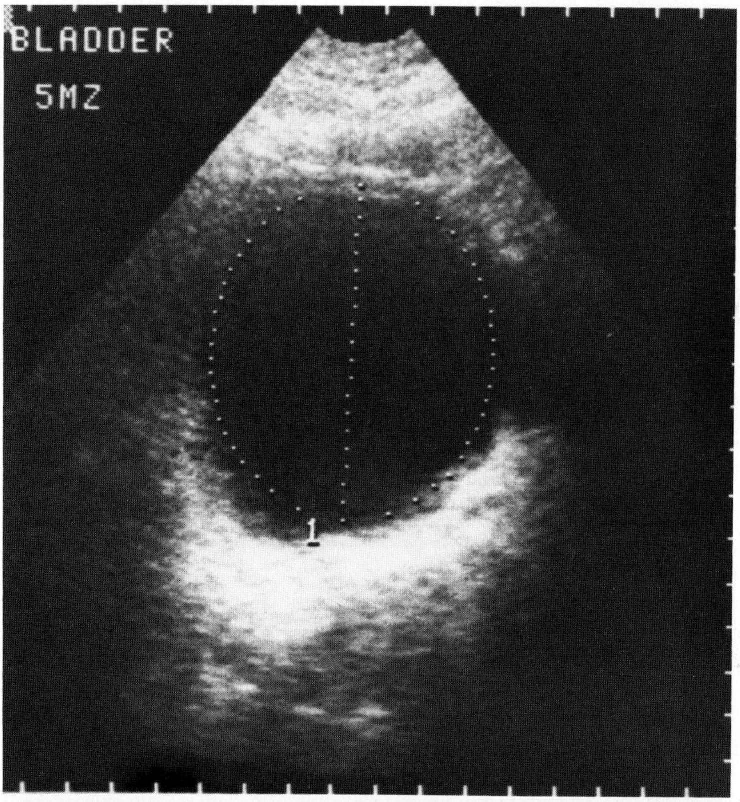

Figure 8.27. Transabdominal ultrasound used to estimate bladder volume. An ellipse can be used to estimate the bladder volume when the bladder is distended and most like an ellipse in shape.

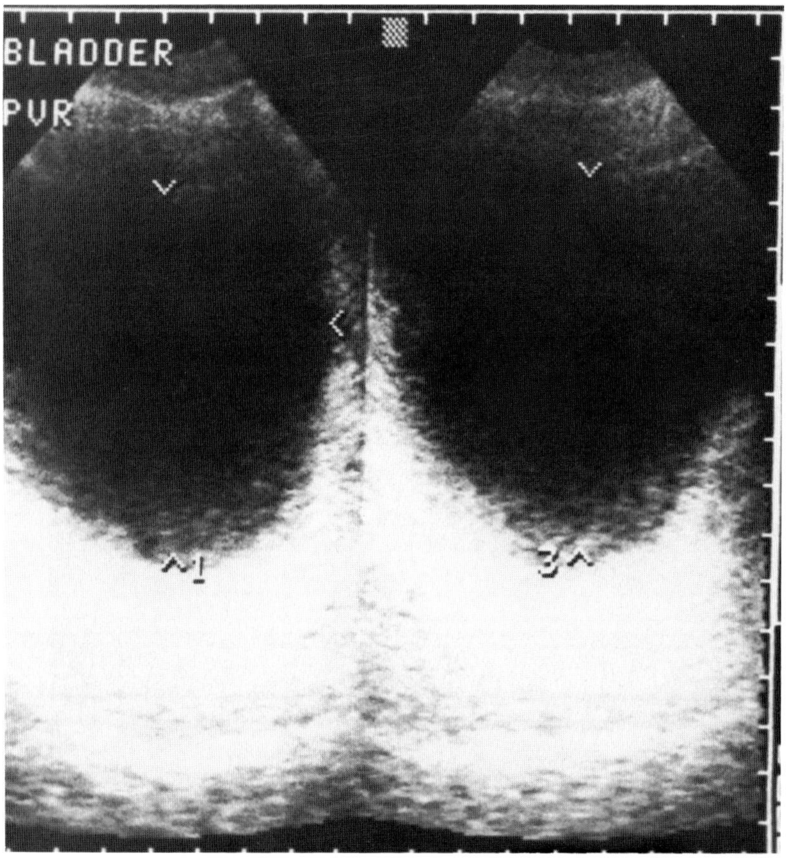

Figure 8.28. Bladder volume is most accurately determined by the formula for an ellipsoid ($V = \frac{4}{3} \pi \times r1 \times r2 \times r3$). The length, width, and height of the distended bladder can be obtained by obtaining a transverse and a longitudinal scan.

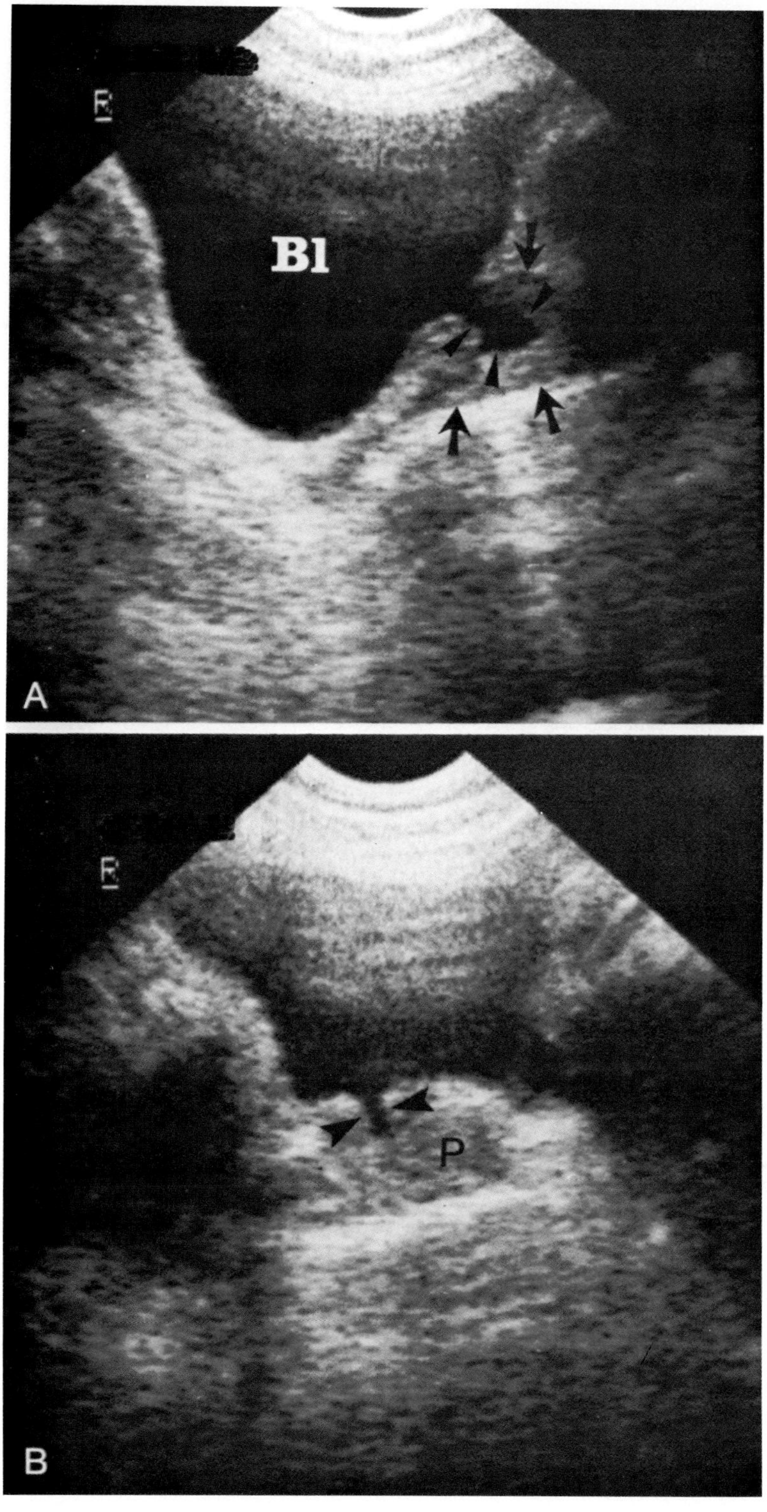

Figure 8.29. **A,** Midsagittal scan showing the prostate (*arrows*) at the base of the bladder. There is a fluid-filled defect in the prostate (*arrowheads*) following previous prostatectomy. **B,** Transverse scan, angled caudally, showing postprostatectomy defect at the urethral orifice (*arrowheads*). Note the numerous reverberation echoes anteriorly in the bladder. **C,** Scan in the same plane as **B** but slightly caudally, showing the dilated prostatic urethra (*arrowheads*). *Bl,* bladder; *P,* prostate.

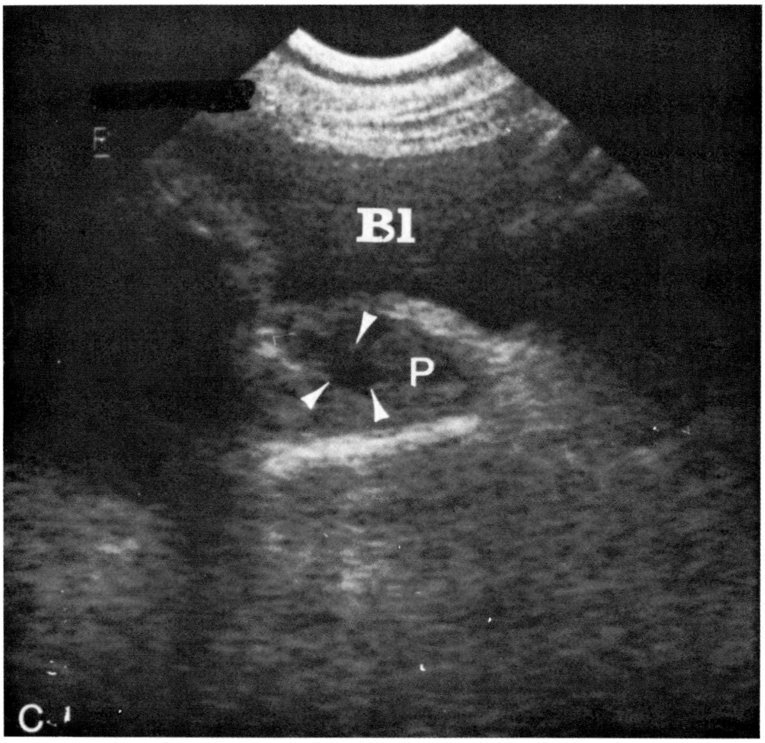

Figure 8.29. C.

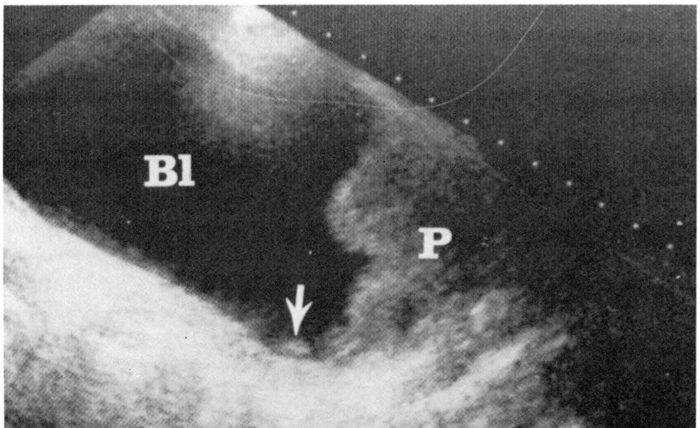

Figure 8.30. **A,** Sagittal scan showing a dilated bladder (*Bl*) with enlarged, irregular prostatic carcinoma (*P*). Note the metastatic lesion in the bladder wall (*arrow*). **B,** Transverse scan showing two small metastases on the bladder wall from the prostatic carcinoma (*arrows*). The ureters (*arrowheads*) are dilated due to obstruction by the bladder carcinoma. **C,** CT scan showing metastatic lesions in the bladder walls (*arrows*). The dilated ureters (*arrowheads*) are also seen on the CT scan.

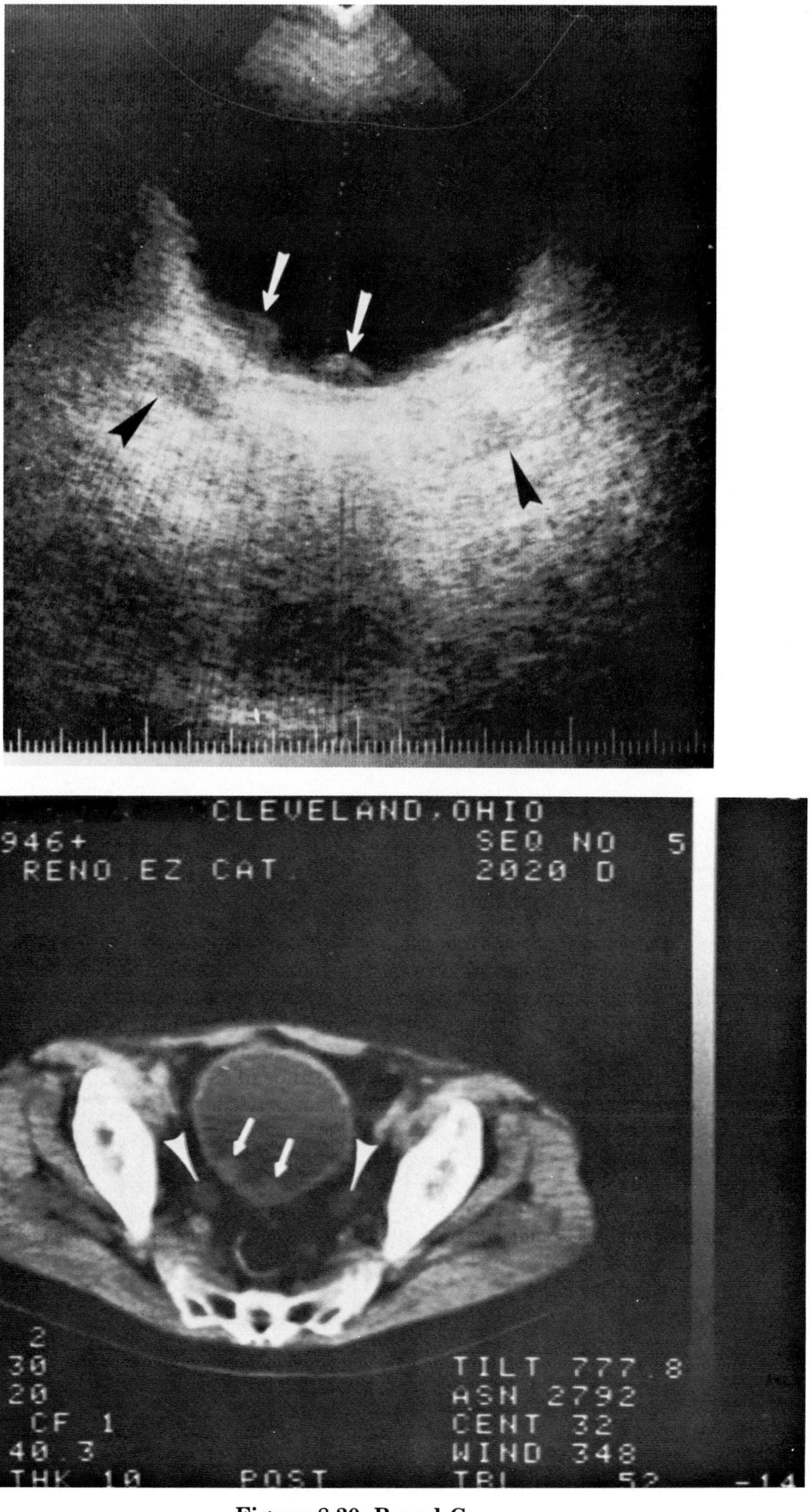

Figure 8.30. B and C.

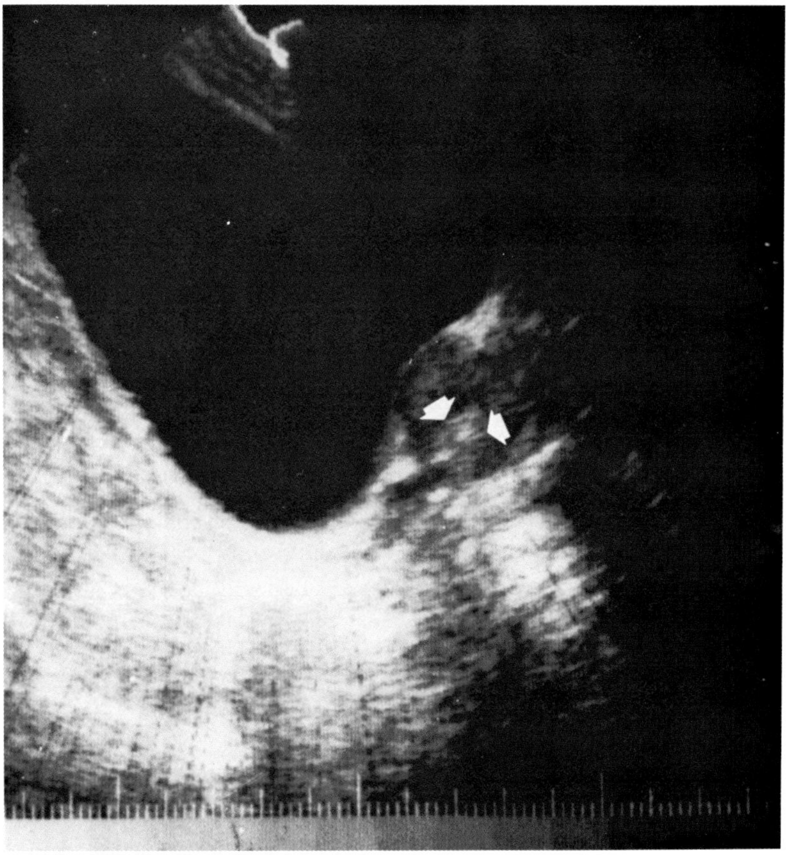

Figure 8.31. Carcinoma of the prostate. A somewhat irregular echogenic focus representing the carcinoma is seen within the prostate (*arrows*) on this sagittal transabdominal scan.

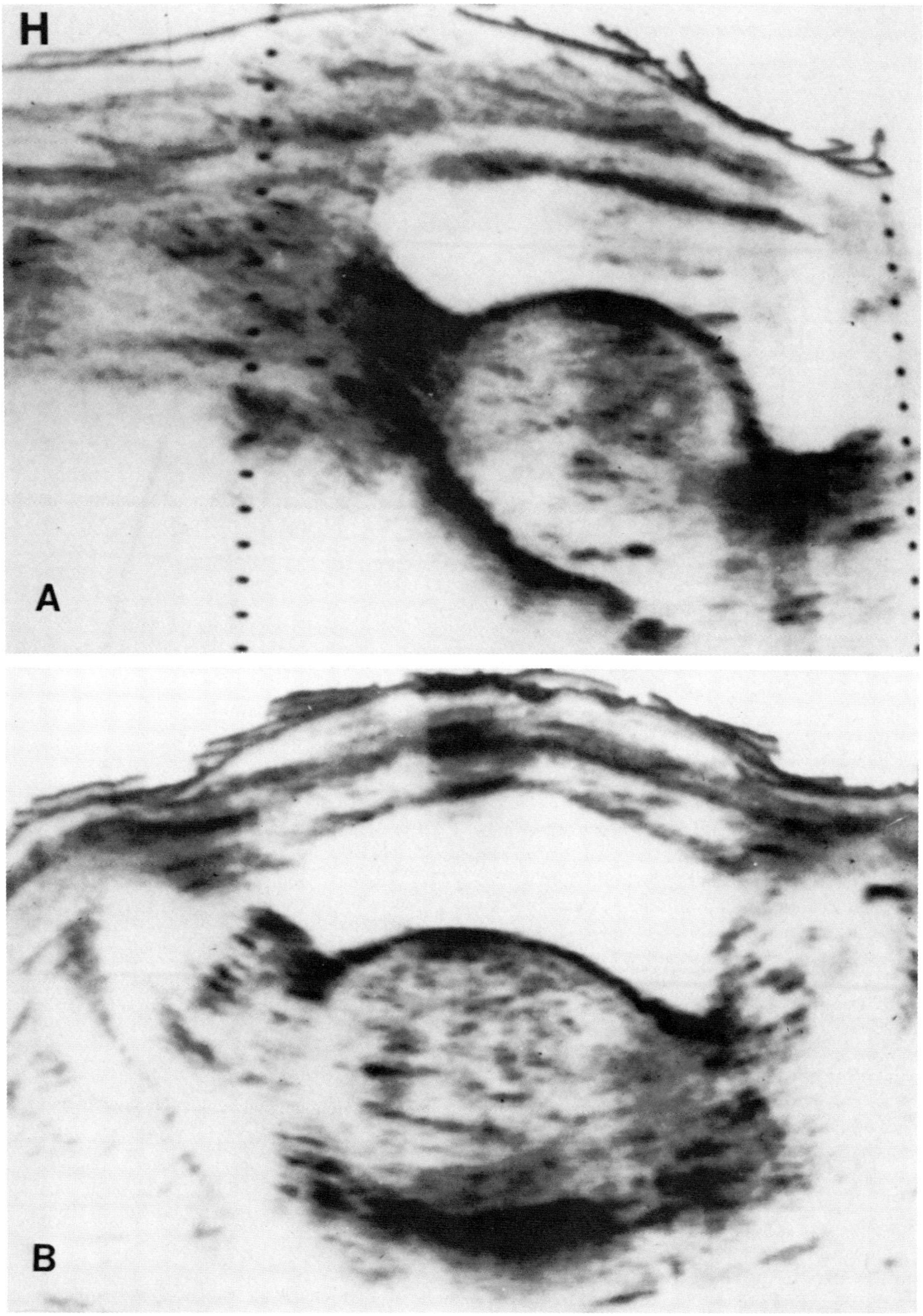

Figure 8.32. Transabdominal sonogram demonstrating a large uterine leiomyoma (fibroid) posterior to the bladder. **A,** Longitudinal scan. *H,* toward the head. **B,** Transverse scan.

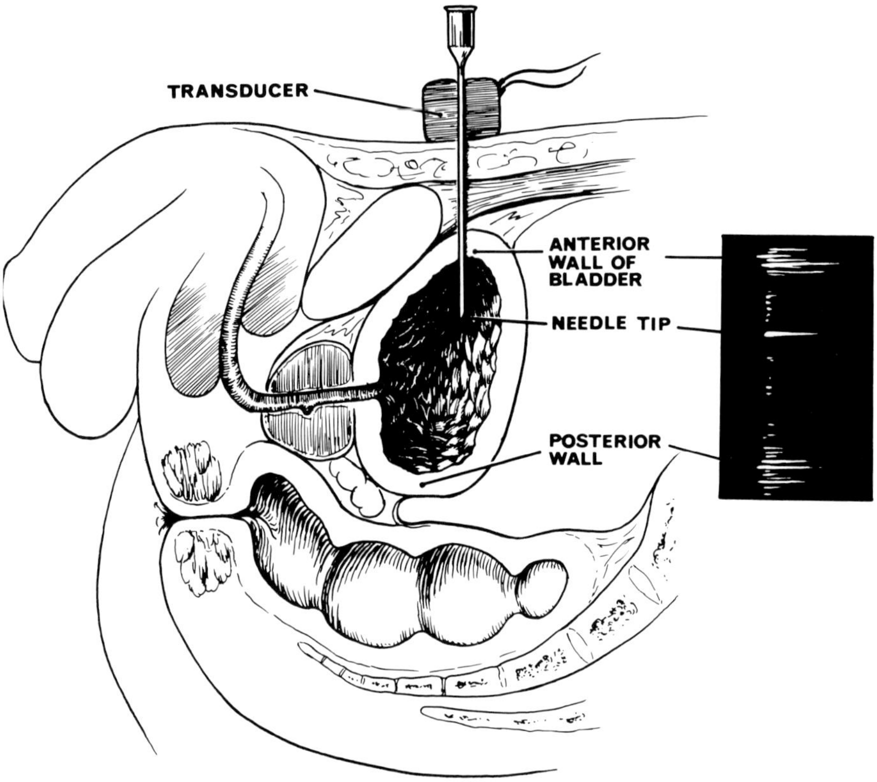

Figure 8.33. Anatomic drawing demonstrating the use of an aspiration transducer and A mode for percutaneous aspiration of the urinary bladder.

duct remnants, abscesses, urinary extravasation, uterine fibroids, and ovarian cysts (Fig. 8.32). Ultrasound can also be helpful in differentiating a distended bladder from another type of pelvic mass (45).

SUPRAPUBIC ASPIRATION

The techniques employed in percutaneous aspiration of the urinary bladder are similar to those used in renal cyst aspiration. The presence of urine in the bladder can be confirmed by ultrasonography, and a needle can be directed into the bladder with ultrasound guidance (Fig. 8.33). Ultrasound can also be helpful in the placement of a percutaneous cystostomy tube. The position of the distended bladder is determined and the punch tube is then placed directly into the bladder. This technique is helpful in children and obese patients, in whom the distended bladder may be more difficult to percuss.

References

1. Watanabe H, Kaiho H, Tanaka M, Terasawa Y. Diagnostic application of ultrasonography to the prostate. Invest Urol 1971;8:548.
2. Watanabe H, Igari D, Tanahasi Y, Harada K, Saitoh M. Development and application of new equipment for transrectal ultrasonography. J Clin Ultrasound 1974;2:91.
3. Resnick MI, Willard JW, Boyce WH. Recent progress in ultrasonography of the bladder and prostate. J Urol 1977;117:444.
4. Hallemans E, Declercq G, Denis L. Transrectal ultrasonotomography. Eur Urol 1977;3:37.
5. Holm HH, Northeved A. A transurethral ultrasonic scanner. J Urol 1974;111:238.
6. Nakamura S, Niijima T. Transurethral real-time scanner. J Urol 1981;125:781.
7. Nakamura S, Niijima T. Staging of bladder cancer by ultrasonography: a new technique by transurethral intravesical scanning. J Urol 1980;124:341.
8. Braeckman J, Denis L. The practice and pitfalls of ultrasonography in the lower urinary tract. Eur Urol 1983;9:143.
9. Resnick MI, Kursh ED. Transurethral ultrasonography in bladder cancer. J Urol 1986;135:253.

10. Resnick MI, Kursh ED. Transurethral ultrasonography of the urinary bladder. World J Urol 1988;6:22.
11. Hricak H. Urologic cancer, methods of early detection and future developments. Cancer 1987;6:677.
12. Kremer H, Dobrinski W, Mikyska M, Baumgartner M, Zollner N. Ultrasonic in vivo and in vitro studies on the nature of the ureteral jet phenomenon. Radiology 1982;142:175.
13. Dubbins PA, Kurtz AB, Darby J, Goldberg BB. Ureteric jet effect: the echographic appearance of urine entering the bladder. Radiology 1981; 140:513.
14. Wenzel WW, Carson PL, Johnson FB. Prostatic localization using ultrasound B-mode in scanning. In: White D. Ultrasound in medicine. New York: Plenum Press, 1975:149.
15. Schmidt JD, Weinstein SH. Pitfalls in clinical staging of bladder tumors. Urol Clin North Am 1976;3:107.
16. Gammelgaard J, Holm HH. Transurethral and transrectal ultrasonic scanning in Urology. J Urol 1980;124:863.
17. Choyre PL, Thickman D, Kressel MY, et al. Controversies in the radiologic diagnosis of pelvic malignancies. Radiol Clin North Am 1985;23: 530.
18. McLaughlin IS, Morley P, Deane RF, Barrett E, Graham AG, Kyle KF. Ultrasound in the staging of bladder tumors. Br J Urol 1975;47:51.
19. Wittenberger AR, Murphy GP. Correlation of B-scan ultrasonic laminography with bilateral selective hypogastric arteriography and lymphography in bladder tumors. Vasc Surg 1974;8:169.
20. Kyle KF, Deane RF, Morley P, Barrett E. Ultrasonography of the urinary tract. Br J Urol 1971; 43:709.
21. Bree RL, Silver TM. Sonography of bladder and perivesical abnormalities. AJR 1981;136:1101.
22. Cronan JJ, Simeone JF, Pfister RC, Newhouse JH, Ferrucci JT. Cystosonography in the detection of bladder tumors: a prospective and retrospective study. J Ultrasound Med 1982;1:237.
23. Itzchak Y, Singer D, Fischelovitch Y. Ultrasonographic assessment of bladder tumors. Part I. Tumor detection. J Urol 1981;126:31.
24. Singer D, Itzchak Y, Fischelovitch Y. Ultrasonographic assessment of bladder tumors. II. Clinical staging. J Urol 1981;126:34.
25. Deleted in proof.
26. Abu-Yousef MM, Narayana AS, Franken EA, et al. Urinary bladder tumors studied by cystosonography. Part I: Detection. Radiology 1984; 153:223.
27. Abu-Yousef MM, Narayana AS, Brown RC, et al. Urinary bladder tumors studied by cystosonography. Part II. Staging. Radiology 1984; 153:227.
28. Salo J, Alfthan O. Transurethral ultrasound versus CT scan. In: Smith PH, Pavone-Mancuso M, eds. Management of advanced cancer of prostate and bladder (Progress in Clinical and Biological Research series, vol 260). New York: Alan R. Liss, 1988:237.
29. Pavone C, DiTrapani D, Serruetta V, et al. Transurethral ultrasonography, CT scan, nuclear magnetic resonance (NMR) imaging and pathological control in staging and follow-up of invasive bladder carcinoma. In: Smith PH, Pavone-Mancuso M, eds. Management of advanced cancer of prostate and bladder (Progress in Clinical and Biological Research series, vol 260). New York: Alan R. Liss, 1988:251.
30. Devonel M, Chapelon JY, Codas M, et al. Evaluation of bladder cancer with a miniature high-frequency transurethral ultrasonography probe. Br J Urol 1987;59:550.
31. Braeckman J, Keuppens F, Denis L. Transurethral echography. In: Smith PH, Pavone-Mancuso M, eds. Management of advanced cancer of prostate and bladder (Progress in Clinical and Biological Research series, vol 260). New York: Alan R. Liss, 1988:231.
32. Sanders RC, Oh KS, Dorst JP. B-scan ultrasound: positive and negative contrast material evaluation of congenital urachal anomaly. AJR 1974;120:448.
33. Richman TS, Taylor KJW. Sonographic demonstration of bladder duplication. AJR 1982;139: 604.
34. Bear E. Visualization of amount of residual urine. JAMA 1936;107:1886.
35. Pedersen JF, Bartrum RJ, and Grytter C. Residual urine determination by ultrasonic scanning. AJR 1975;125:474.
36. Harrison NW, Parks C, Sherwood T. Ultrasound assessment of residual urine in children. Br J Urol 1975;47:805.
37. McLean GK, Edell SL. Determination of bladder volumes by gray scale ultrasonography. Radiology 1978;128:181.
38. Rageth JC, Langer K. Ultrasonic assessment of residual urine volume. Urol Res 1982;10:57.
39. Hackenberg OW, Ryall RL, Langlois SL, Marshall VR. The estimation of bladder volume by sonocystography. J Urol 1983;130:249.
40. Poston GJ, Joseph AEA, Riddle PR. The accuracy of ultrasound in the measurement of changes in bladder volume. Br J Urol 1983;55:361.
41. Griffiths CJ, Murray A, Ramsden PD. Accuracy and repeatability of bladder volume measurement using ultrasonic imaging. J Urol 1986; 136:808.
42. Roehrborn CG, Peters PC. Can transabdominal ultrasound estimation of postvoiding residual (PVR) replace catheterization? Urology 1988; 31(5):445.
43. Cardenas DD, Kelly E, Krieger JN, Chapman WH. Residual urine volumes in patients with spinal cord injury: measurement with a portable ultrasound instrument. Arch Phys Med Rehabil 1988;69(7):514.
44. Kjeldsen-Kragh J. Measurement of residual urine volume by means of ultrasonic scanning: a comparative study. Paraplegia 1988;26(3):192.
45. Lee TG, Reed TA. Ultrasonic diagnosis of the bladder as a symptomatic pelvic mass. J Urol 1977;144:283.

CHAPTER 9

Use of Ultrasound in Dynamic Evaluation of the Lower Urinary Tract

INDER PERKASH, M.D.
GERALD W. FRIEDLAND, M.D.

Abnormalities of function of the bladder and urethra are common in all age groups. In children, they are usually due to congenital anomalies, especially spinal dysraphism, of which there are about 4,000 cases per year in the United States (1). In young adults, especially young males, problems of function are commonly due to spinal cord injuries, most often the result of automobile or diving accidents (2). There are estimated to be 10,000 to 20,000 such surviving patients per year in the United States, which indicates that there may be between 500,000 and 1.5 million persons currently living with such lesions (2).

Abnormalities of function of the bladder and urethra become more common with slightly older patients, because millions of people suffer from diabetes mellitus or multiple sclerosis. Almost half of all patients with diabetes over the age of 50 years have a hypotonic or atonic bladder, which means they can void only when they are upright; as soon as they are in the hospital, reclining or supine, problems with voiding occur (3).

In addition, there is a growing population of people over the age of 80 years in the United States. Of these, about 50% are institutionalized before they die, primarily in nursing homes. Forty percent of this number are institutionalized because of incontinence (4).

This is no insignificant problem. The Surgeon General of the United States currently spends $8 billion per year on incontinence pads alone (5). This is more than is spent on kidney dialysis or coronary artery bypass procedures combined. As this figure reflects only one aspect of the costs involved, the true costs are clearly astronomical (4).

The majority of these cases of incontinence in older people are due to detrusor overactivity, involving voluntary detrusor contractions before the patient can reach the toilet (4). A significant number of these cases are due to detrusor hyperreflexia (6), due to an upper motor neuron lesion, caused typically by stroke, Alzheimer's disease, or Parkinsonism (4, 7).

There is a widespread misconception that problems of function of the bladder and urethra are relatively unimportant and uncommon, perhaps because these problems are not usually life threatening. The true situation, however, is that abnormalities of function of the bladder and urethra are among the most important, and certainly among the most costly, problems in medicine today.

Until recently, the standard investigation in such patients was a radiological study, often an intravenous urogram, a voiding cystourethrogram, or scintigraphy, with or without urodynamic studies. It was then found that transrectal sonography, using a linear array transducer, could produce exquisite images of the bladder and urethra (2, 3, 8–16). For this reason it has become the standard method of investigating such patients in our institution. Transrectal sonography has many advantages; it is cheap, simple to use, and involves no radiation either to the patient or to the observer. This means that the observer can watch a process for long periods of time and repeat examinations as necessary. This new technique has provided us with vast amounts of data not before available from any other source.

SONOGRAPHIC AND URODYNAMIC EQUIPMENT AND TECHNIQUES

It is best to use either a 3.5-MHz or a 5-MHz linear array transducer. Each transducer contains between 64 and 110 piezoelectric elements arranged in a straight line near the tip of a probe. The probe is surrounded by a water-filled bag, and then acoustic jelly, and is introduced intrarectally with the window facing anteriorly. This will yield sagittal pictures of the bladder and urethra, allowing the urethra to be visualized, in the male, as far distally as the bulbous urethra (Fig. 9.1).

When the patient is not paralyzed, he is placed on one side, usually the left side. If the patient is paralyzed, the lithotomy position works best. Patients with or without neurological problems can void with the transducer in the rectum, although those without neurological problems find it more difficult to do so.

Patients with lower motor neuron lesions and a wide bladder neck and urethra can initiate voiding with the Credé maneuver. If the patient has an upper motor neuron lesion, it is best to use suprapubic tapping (Fig. 9.2) (13); paraplegic patients can tap themselves, but quadriplegics will need help. This should be done 15 to 20 times, rapidly, with the ulnar side of the hand, in the immediately suprapubic region. With each tap, the periurethral striated sphincter contracts, but since this is striated muscle, it eventually tires and relaxes, allowing voiding to occur.

If simultaneous urodynamic studies are desired, a coaxial cable from the sonographic machine can be connected directly to the urodynamic studies equipment, which will enable the urodynamic studies and the ultrasound image to be displayed on a single monitor (Fig. 9.3). The combined study can then be videotaped, and hard copies can be obtained as necessary, either directly or from the videotape.

MAJOR FINDINGS

Transrectal sonography can, first, demonstrate problems at the bladder neck (10, 11). These may include posterior ledges, detrusor–bladder neck dyssynergia, isolated bladder neck obstruction in males, benign prostatic

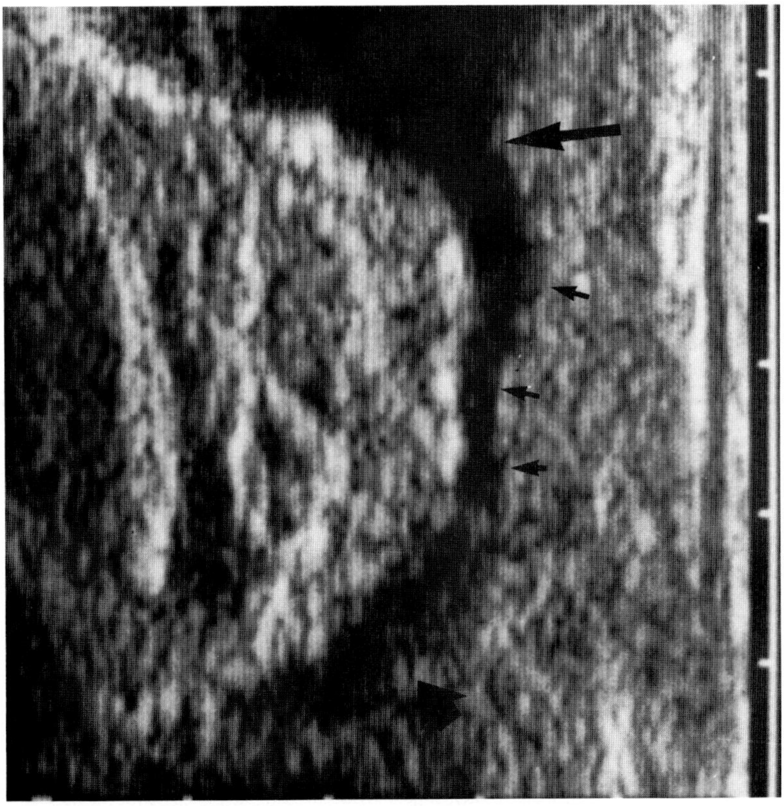

Figure 9.1. Normal sonographic voiding cystourethrogram in a male. The *long arrow* points to the bladder neck, the *short arrows* point to the verumontanum, and the *broad arrow* points to the bulbous urethra.

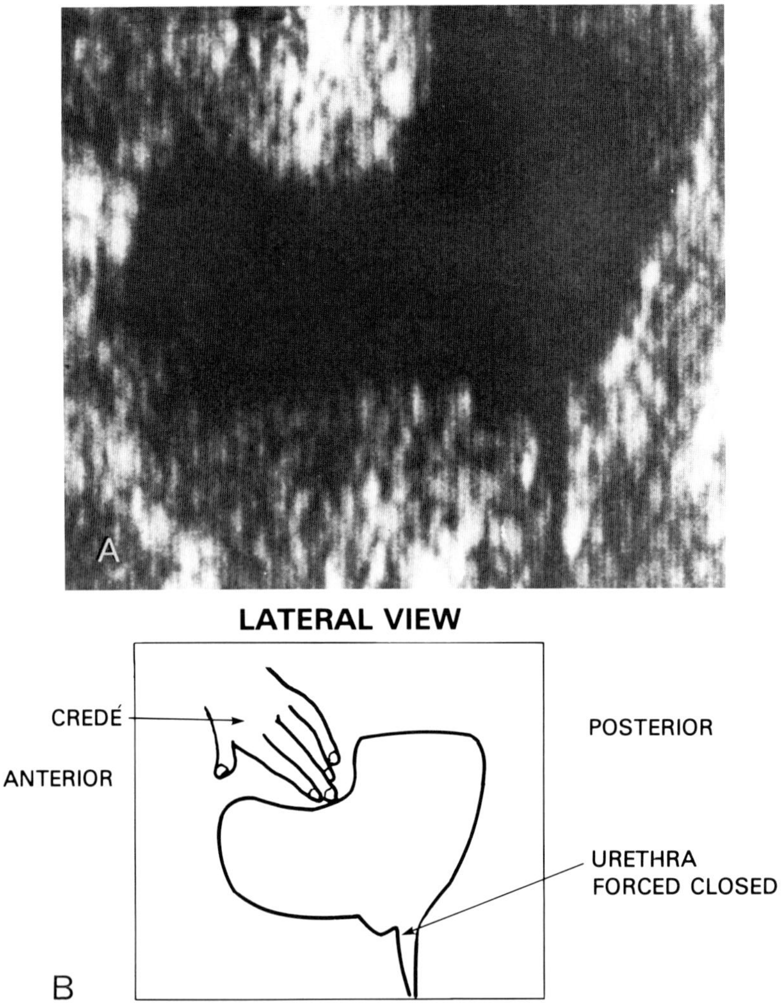

Figure 9.2. Patient with an upper motor neuron lesion. The Credé maneuver (**A** and **B**) closes the bladder neck. After suprapubic tapping (**C** and **D**) the urethra opens widely, and the bladder empties. (Reproduced with permission from Perkash I, Friedland GW. Using transrectal sonography to teach patients with spinal cord injury to retrain their bladders. Radiology 1984;152:228.

hyperplasia, and bladder neck strictures. It is particularly useful in the differential diagnosis of these entities.

Posterior Ledges at the Bladder Neck

A surprising number of spinal cord injury patients receiving long-term intermittent catheterization develop long ledges posteriorly at the bladder neck (Fig. 9.4) (10). These ledges are composed of muscle hypertrophy, muscle atrophy, and fibrosis and are the cause of two kinds of problems (10). First, the prostatic urethra angulates 45° anteriorly at its midpoint (17), so that as the slightly rigid catheter passes the angulation, it travels on the posterior side of the urethra (10). Thus, any abnormally long posterior ledge causes some degree of obstruction of the catheter. A small ledge, up to 5 mm in length, is normal; longer ledges begin to obstruct the passage of the catheter, and the longer the ledge, the more the degree of obstruction. Initially this may not be long enough to obstruct the flow of urine, but as the ledge becomes longer, there is an increased pressure gradient between the bladder and the bladder neck, and the ledge begins to obstruct the flow of urine as well (10). This occurs typ-

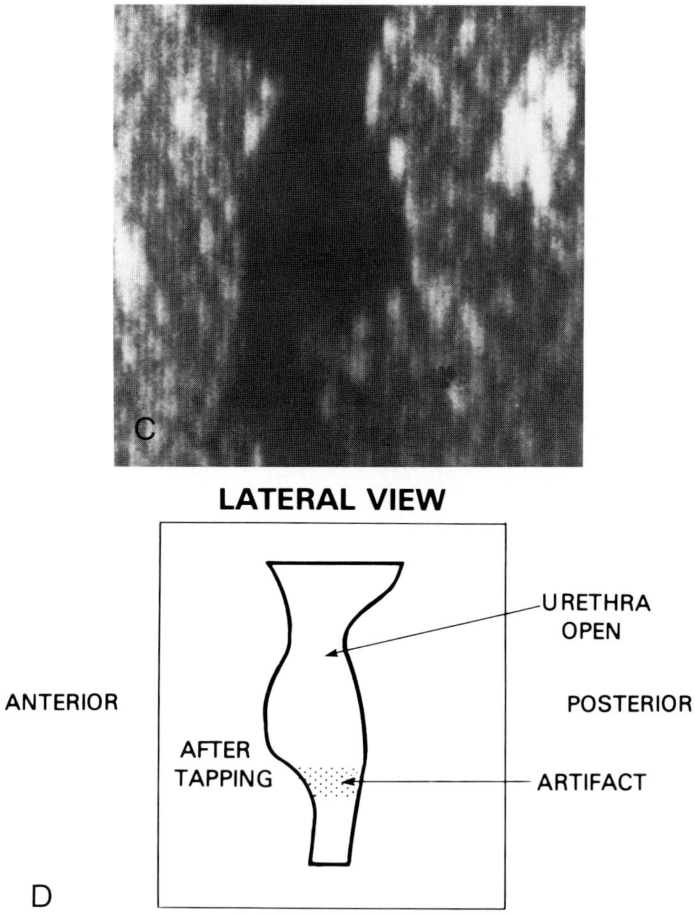

Figure 9.2. **C** and **D.**

ically when the pressure gradient between the bladder and the bladder neck begins to exceed 3 cm of water (10, 18).

Two factors have been shown to be statistically significant regarding the formation of these longer ledges (10): (*a*) How long the patient has been receiving intermittent catheterization (the longer the time, the more likely the longer ledge). This may occur because of chronic irritation. (*b*) The duration of detrusor-sphincter dyssynergia.

Detrusor–Bladder Neck Dyssynergia

The area of the bladder neck is heavily supplied with α-adrenergic receptors (1). When a patient has a lesion above T5, one result is detrusor-bladder neck dyssynergia, in which the bladder neck does not open when the detrusor contracts (1). As a result of stretching of the bladder neck against resistance, a large amount of norepinephrine is released (which raises the blood pressure because of peripheral vasoconstriction, causing a headache) and causes sweating and, through stimulation of the baroreceptors, bradycardia (1). In such patients there is a danger of cerebral hemorrhage.

But if an α-adrenergic blocker, such as phentolamine, is injected intravenously in doses of 5 to 10 mg, it will cause the bladder neck to open in such patients within 5 min (1). This opening of the bladder neck can be easily observed under sonographic control (Fig. 9.5) (2); in these circumstances, the complete opening of the bladder neck after the intravenous administration of 5 to 10 mg of phentolamine has been shown to be diagnostic of detrusor–bladder neck dyssynergia (2).

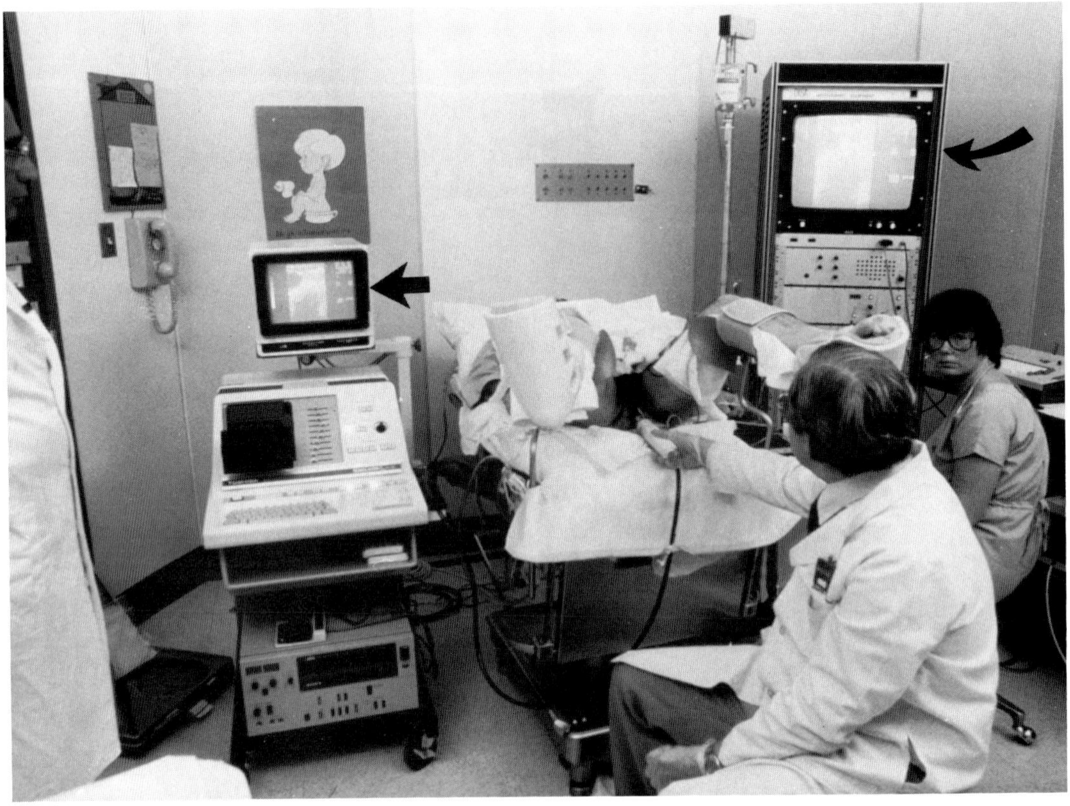

Figure 9.3. Simultaneous sonographic and urodynamic studies. A coaxial cable from the monitor of the sonographic machine (*arrow*) is connected directly to the urodynamics equipment, enabling the urodynamic studies and ultrasound image to be displayed on a single monitor (*curved arrow*).

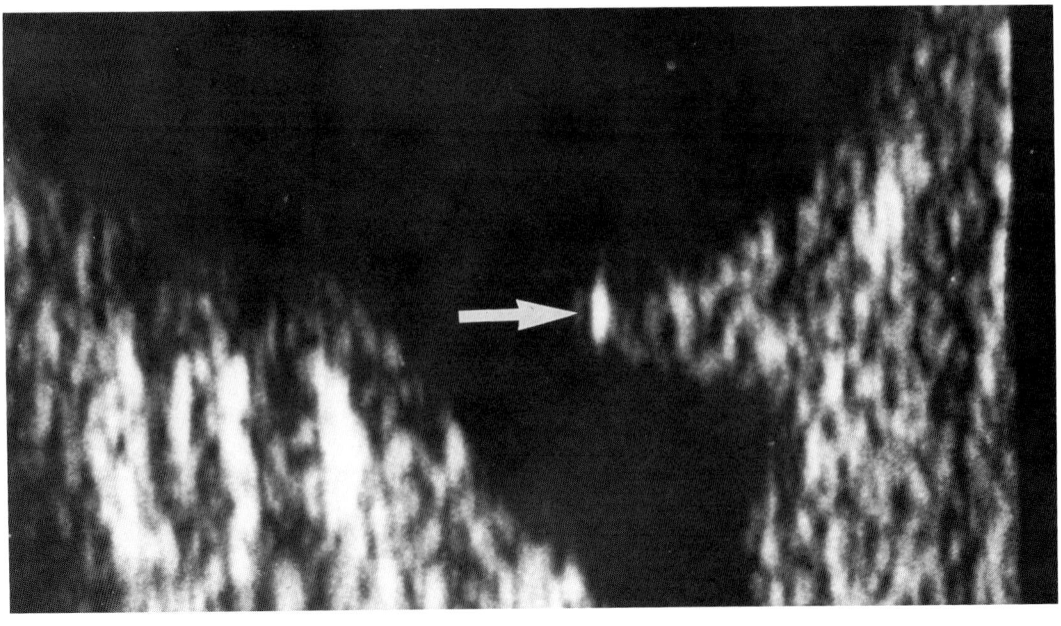

Figure 9.4. Long ledge at the bladder neck posteriorly (*arrow*).

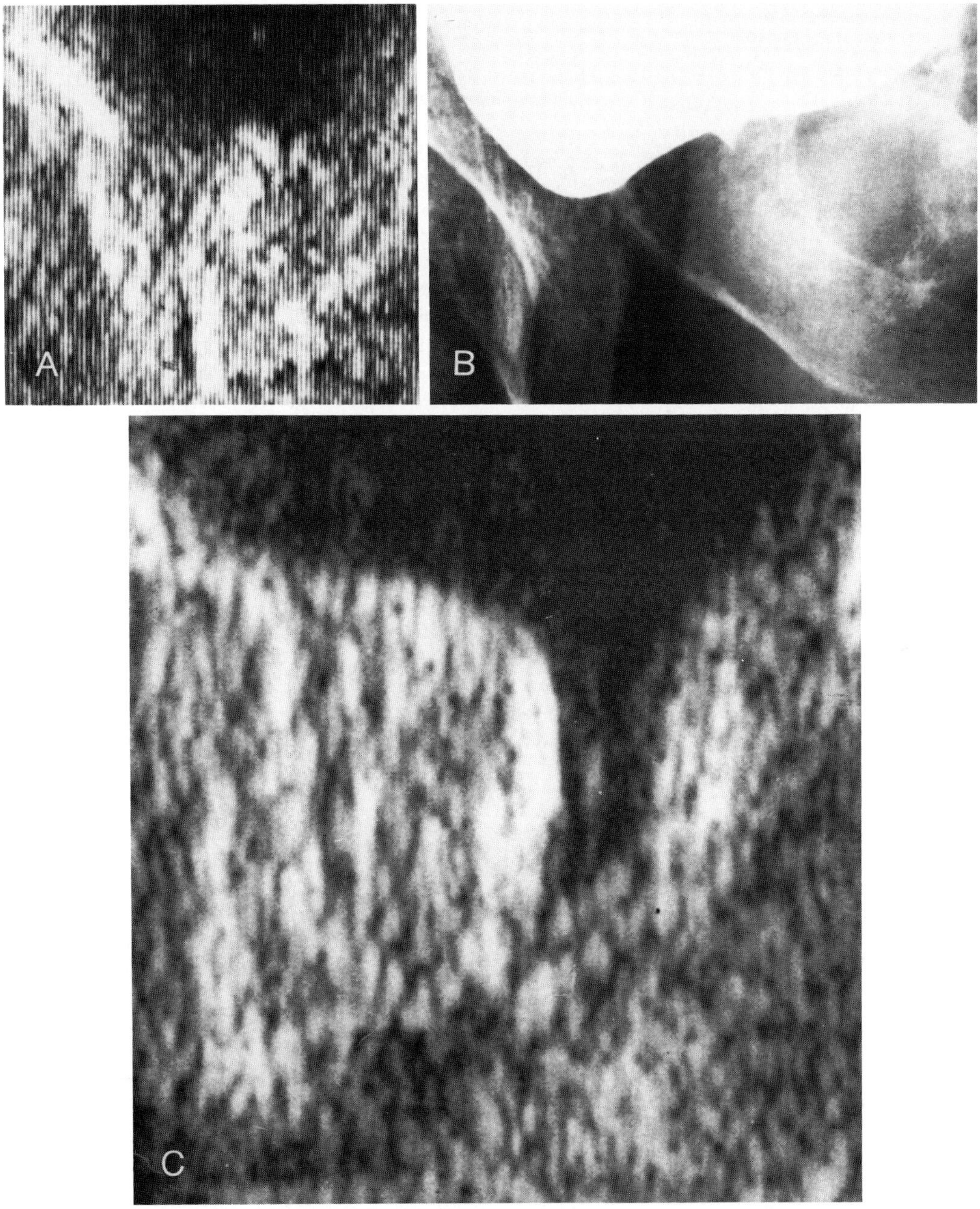

Figure 9.5. Detrusor–bladder neck dyssynergia. Sonographic (**A**) and radiological (**B**) cystograms prior to the administration of phentolamine. The patient is attempting to void, but the bladder neck remains closed. After the administration of 10 mg phentolamine intravenously (**C**), the bladder neck opens. (Reproduced with permission from Shapeero G, Friedland GW, Perkash I. Transrectal sonographic voiding cystourethrography. Studies in neuromuscular dysfunction. AJR 1983;141:83. Copyright by The American Roentgen Ray Society.)

Isolated Bladder Neck Obstruction in Males

We have seen two neurologically intact patients with longer ledges, one with a lifelong history (from birth) of difficulty with voiding (Fig. 9.6), the other with problems that developed more recently (10).

Other authors have seen an identical appearance on radiological voiding cystourethrograms and called the entity isolated bladder neck obstruction in men (19). They hypothesized that this is the disease previously known as Marion's disease or, despite the fact that there is no neurological lesion, isolated detrusor–bladder neck dyssynergia (19).

Previous authors have described three clinical grades, ranging from mild to severe (19). Mild forms have symptoms including frequency, hesitancy, and postvoid dribbling; moderate grades involve a decreased stream and sensations of fullness after voiding; severe grades involve episodes of acute urinary retention. In all patients, however, peak voiding flow rates are reduced; the worse the grade, the greater the reduction.

Manolin (20) has given the normal diameter at the bladder neck as 6 mm or more, the intermediate diameter as 4 to 6 mm, and a diameter of less than 4 mm as abnormal. A more physiological measurement is the pressure gradient between the bladder and the bladder neck; a normal resting gradient is up to 3 cm of water, while anything greater indicates obstruction (18).

The etiology is unknown; it has been suggested that it is due to α-adrenergic overactivity (19). It is claimed that voiding is much improved with the administration of α-adrenergic blockers, but thus far there are no published radiological or sonographic illustrations of this posterior ledge before and after the administration of α-adrenergic blockers. If α-adrenergic blockers help, such evidence ought to be forthcoming. In our two patients, there was no change in the appearance after intravenous administration of phentolamine.

Benign Prostatic Hyperplasia

Benign prostatic hyperplastic nodules may develop in the periurethral zone in the fourth decade. They are usually small nodules, which in the aggregate form a cylindrical mass surrounding the urethra from the bladder neck to the verumontanum, projecting into the bladder neck posteriorly (17).

This projection has been called, incorrectly,

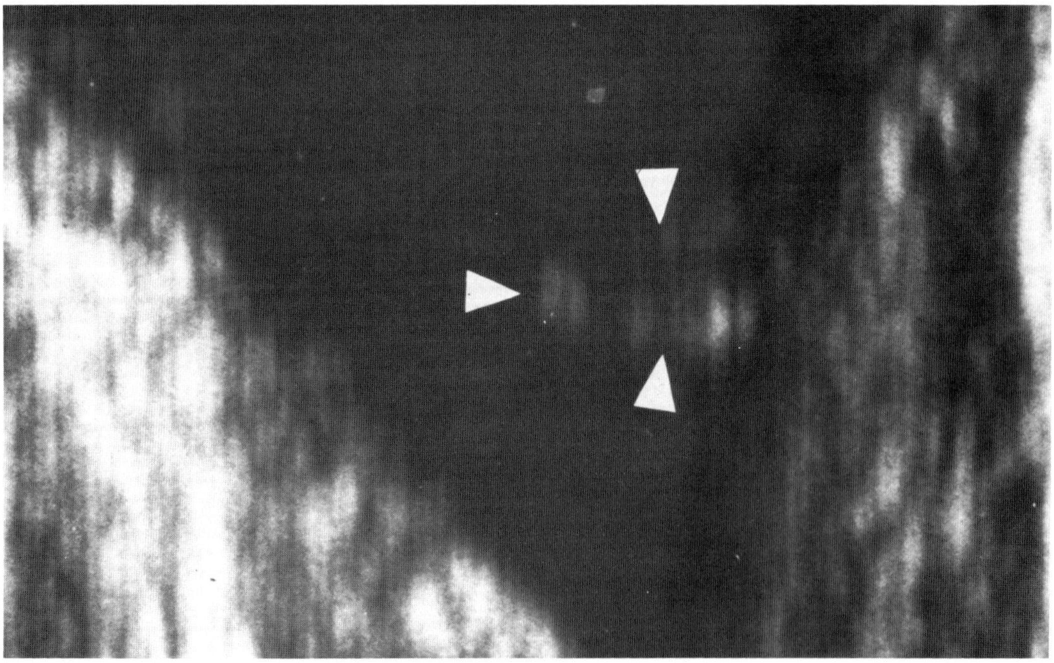

Figure 9.6. Isolated bladder neck obstruction in a neurologically intact male. There is a ledge protruding from the bladder neck posteriorly (*arrowheads*).

the median lobe of the prostate. This so-called median lobe is not an isolated mass; rather, it is the largest and most cephalad of a string of nodules extending proximally from the verumontanum (17).

In younger men, this string of nodules can reach an enormous size, usually with little or no enlargement in the transitional zone of the prostate (17).

On a sonographic voiding cystourethrogram, benign hyperplasia of the periurethral zone is seen as a rounded mass, not straight or ledge-like, projecting into the bladder neck posteriorly (2, 11). Unlike the posterior ledge, it bulges upwards into the bladder lumen itself (Fig. 9.7).

Stricture

Patients with long-term indwelling catheters may develop infection which, together with chronic irritation, can lead to submucosal fibrosis and stricture at the bladder neck. Unlike the posterior ledge, however, these strictures are circumferential. Unlike detrusor–bladder neck dyssynergia, they do not widen when phentolamine is administered intravenously (11).

THE POSTERIOR URETHRA

The proximal portion of the urethra up to the verumontanum is usually surrounded by smooth muscle; the distal half is surrounded by striated muscle. There is much variation between persons; some have striated muscle up to the bladder neck (1).

Detrusor-Sphincter Dyssynergia

A person with an upper motor neuron lesion between the pons and the conus usually develops detrusor-sphincter dyssynergia, in

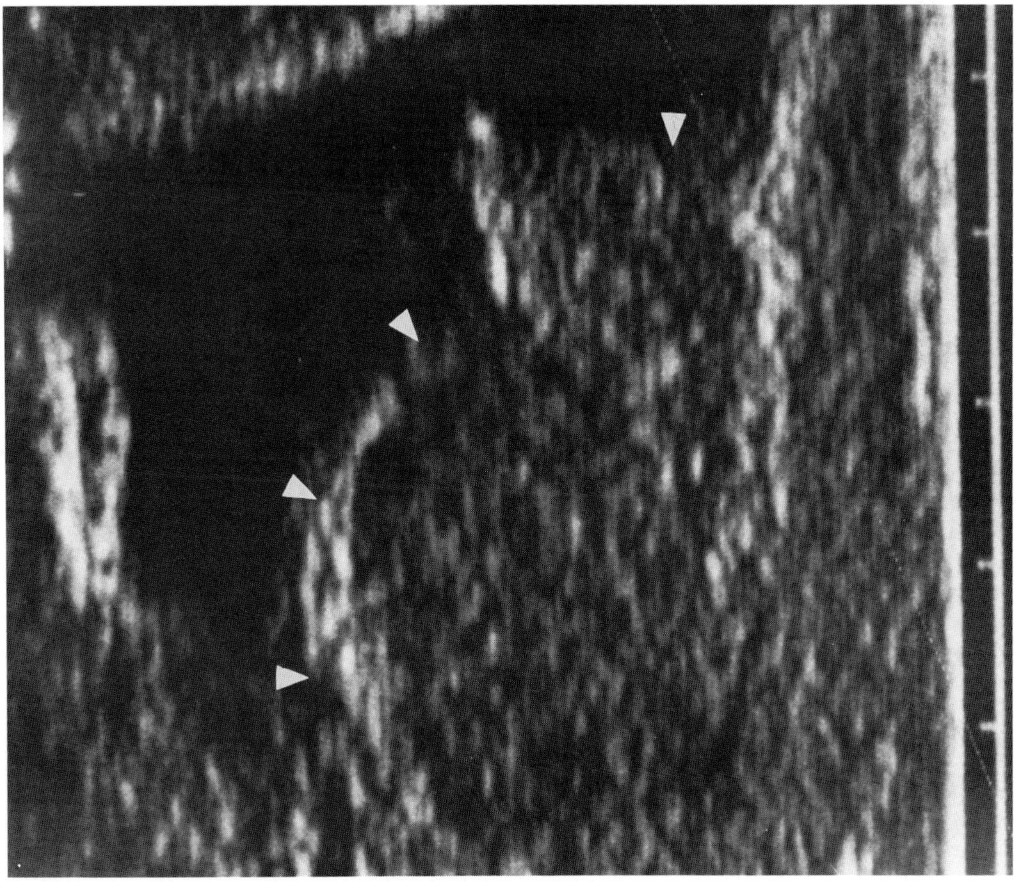

Figure 9.7. Benign hyperplasia of the periurethral zone of the prostate. A rounded mass (*arrowheads*) projects into the lumen of the bladder.

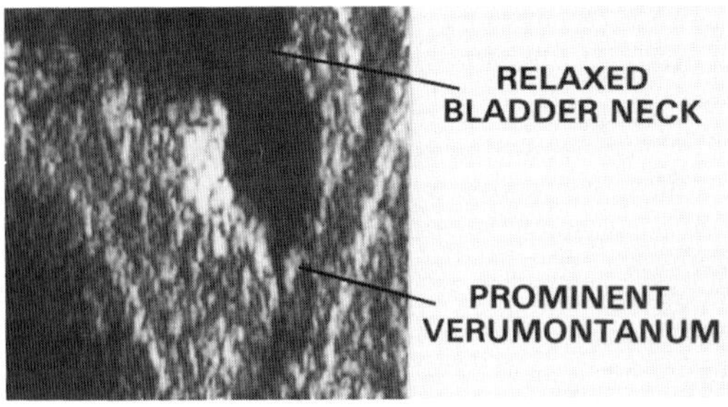

Figure 9.8. Detrusor-sphincter dyssynergia. The periurethral striated sphincter has failed to relax and the verumontanum is prominent. (Reproduced with permission from Shapeero G, Friedland GW, Perkash I. Transrectal sonographic voiding cystourethrography. Studies in neuromuscular dysfunction. AJR 1983; 141:83. Copyright by The American Roentgen Ray Society.)

which the periurethral striated sphincter does not relax when the detrusor contracts. This may have two results: the distal half of the prostatic urethra narrows, and the verumontanum is forced into the lumen and becomes prominent (1). Both features are well seen on a sonographic voiding cystourethrogram (Fig. 9.8).

DIFFERENTIAL DIAGNOSIS

Stricture

The main differential diagnosis is a stricture (Fig. 9.9) (1, 2). An electromyogram (EMG) will be necessary to differentiate the two: a patient with detrusor-sphincter dyssynergia but no stricture will have increased electrical activity in the periurethral striated sphincter when the bladder contracts as the patient attempts to void (Fig. 9.10). With stricture but no detrusor-sphincter dyssynergia, there will be no electrical activity in the periurethral striated sphincter when the patient attempts to void.

Functional Abnormalities of the Periurethral Striated Sphincter of Psychological Etiology

Detrusor-sphincter dyssynergia must also be differentiated from other entities of psychological etiology. Again, an EMG of the periurethral striated sphincter is helpful in the differential diagnosis (21). With detrusor-sphincter dyssynergia, electrical activity increases as the patient voids or attempts to void; at no time is it absent (Fig. 9.10) (1, 21). With the psychological entities, the electrical activity in the periurethral striated sphincter is momentarily absent (21); then, for psychological reasons, the patient contracts the periurethral striated sphincter, and electrical activity is present during the rest of the voiding process (21).

The *Hinman syndrome* (22) involves children with unstable bladders who learn to contract their periurethral striated sphincters when their bladders contract, even during voiding. As a result, they may develop bladder hypertrophy and trabeculation, vesicoureteral reflux, and even renal failure. The problem is cured with appropriate psychotherapy.

A similar phenomenon occurs in some women with unstable bladders, who may similarly contract their sphincters when voiding. This phenomenon has been called *the spastic external sphincter syndrome* (23).

Finally, the periurethral striated sphincter may be contracted during voiding for psychological reasons even with stable bladders (24). This can lead to acute retention and even renal failure, though these problems have been treated successfully with psychotherapy (25).

False Passages

The second major problem in the posterior urethra that is well demonstrated by transrectal sonography is false passages (12). Given that the posterior urethra angulates 45° anteriorly at its midpoint (Fig. 9.11) (17), and that there is also an angle where the bulbous and the posterior urethra unite, any catheter, no matter how flexible, will advance against the points of angulation and against the small ledge at the posterior bladder neck. As it does so, it may tear the mucosa and lift up a flap in the urethra; with each succeeding catheterization, this false passage may extend further (12).

When the patient voids, the flap is forced closed, and so may not cause difficulty with voiding, although it will with catheterization (12). It can easily be missed on a radiological voiding cystourethrogram, precisely because the flap is forced closed during voiding (Fig. 9.12**A**).

When the tip of the catheter is advanced under sonographic control, however, the examiner can see the catheter enter the false passage in real time (Fig. 9.12**B**) (12). Thus, transrectal sonography is the examination mode of choice for the detection of false passages (12).

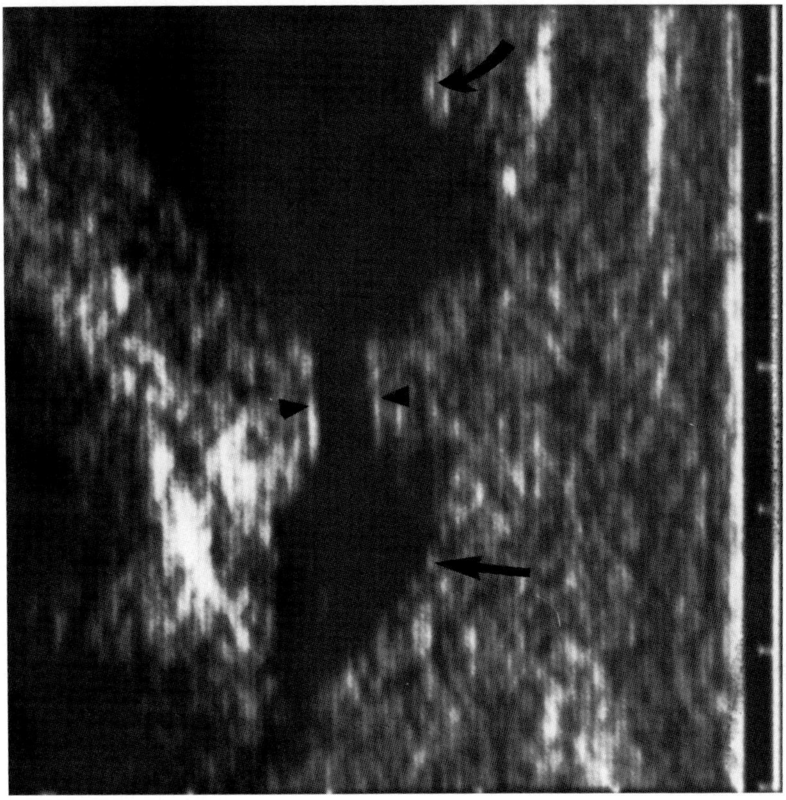

Figure 9.9. Stricture of the midprostatic urethra (*arrowheads*). The *curved arrow* points to the bladder neck; the *straight arrow* points to the distal prostatic urethra.

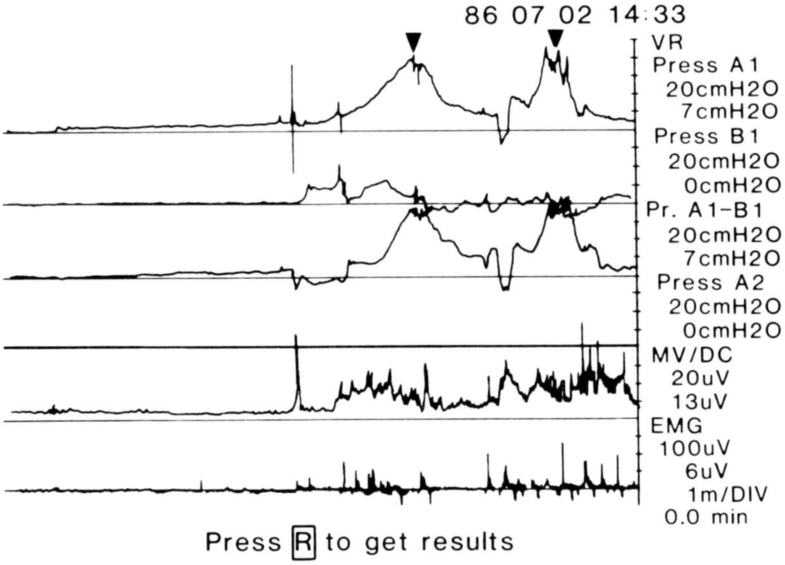

Figure 9.10. Urodynamic study in a patient with detrusor-sphincter dyssynergia. There are two detrusor contractions (*arrowheads*). With each contraction the electrical activity in the periurethral striated sphincter increases. (Reproduced with permission from Perkash I, Friedland GW. Principles of modern urodynamic studies. Invest Radiol 1987;22:279.)

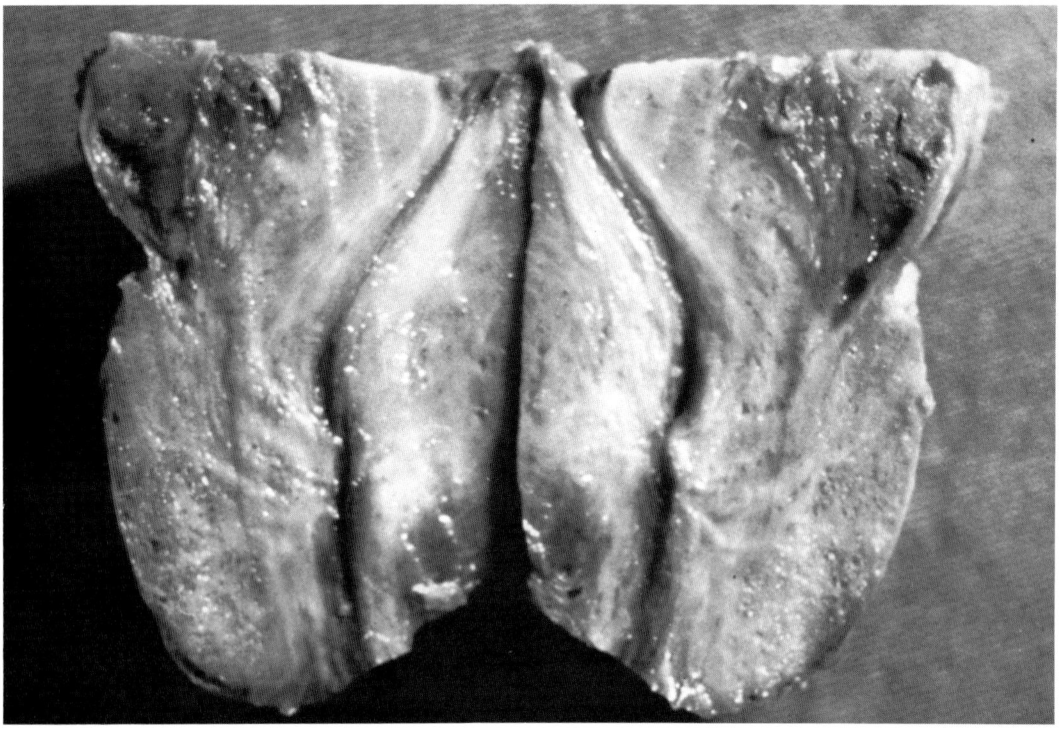

Figure 9.11. Specimen of prostate from a 22-year-old man, opened longitudinally. The prostatic urethra angulates 45° anteriorly at its midpoint. (Reproduced with permission from Perkash I, Friedland GW. Posterior ledge of the bladder neck: the crucial diagnostic role of ultrasonography. Urol Radiol 1986;8:175. Photo originally provided by John McNeal, M.D., Division of Urology, Stanford University.)

CATHETER-INDUCED PRECIPITOUS BLADDER CONTRACTIONS

In some spinal cord injury patients with an upper motor neuron lesion, a precipitous bladder contraction may occur if the tip of the catheter irritates the bladder wall (9). Should this occur with a small volume of urine in the bladder (125 ml or less has been arbitrarily chosen for the diagnosis), catheter-induced precipitous bladder contraction is the diagnosis (9). A similar phenomenon can occur without catheterization in patients with an upper motor neuron spinal cord lesion, either spontaneously or because of bladder infection. It may also occur in patients with suprapontine lesions and in some patients with bladder outlet obstruction.

An important consideration in spinal cord injury patients with lesions above T5, and in some patients with lesions between T5 and T8, is that they may develop autonomic dysreflexia. In such patients there is a danger of cerebral hemorrhage; they should be treated with anticholinergic drugs (9). If the precipitous bladder contraction is catheter induced, however, and does not occur at other times, there is no need to treat the patient. This is a significant consideration, since anticholinergic drugs cause constipation, already a problem with spinal cord injury patients. In addition, it may be impossible to do a radiological voiding cystourethrogram or urodynamic studies in these patients because the catheter is vigorously ejected by the precipitous bladder contraction (9).

We have made the diagnosis of catheter-induced precipitous bladder contractions by doing a sonographic voiding cystourethrogram with the catheter on one day (Fig. 9.13**A**) and repeating the examination without a catheter on another day (Fig. 9.13**B**). In patients in whom the precipitous bladder contraction was catheter induced, we have found no precipitous contraction later, without the catheter; in fact,

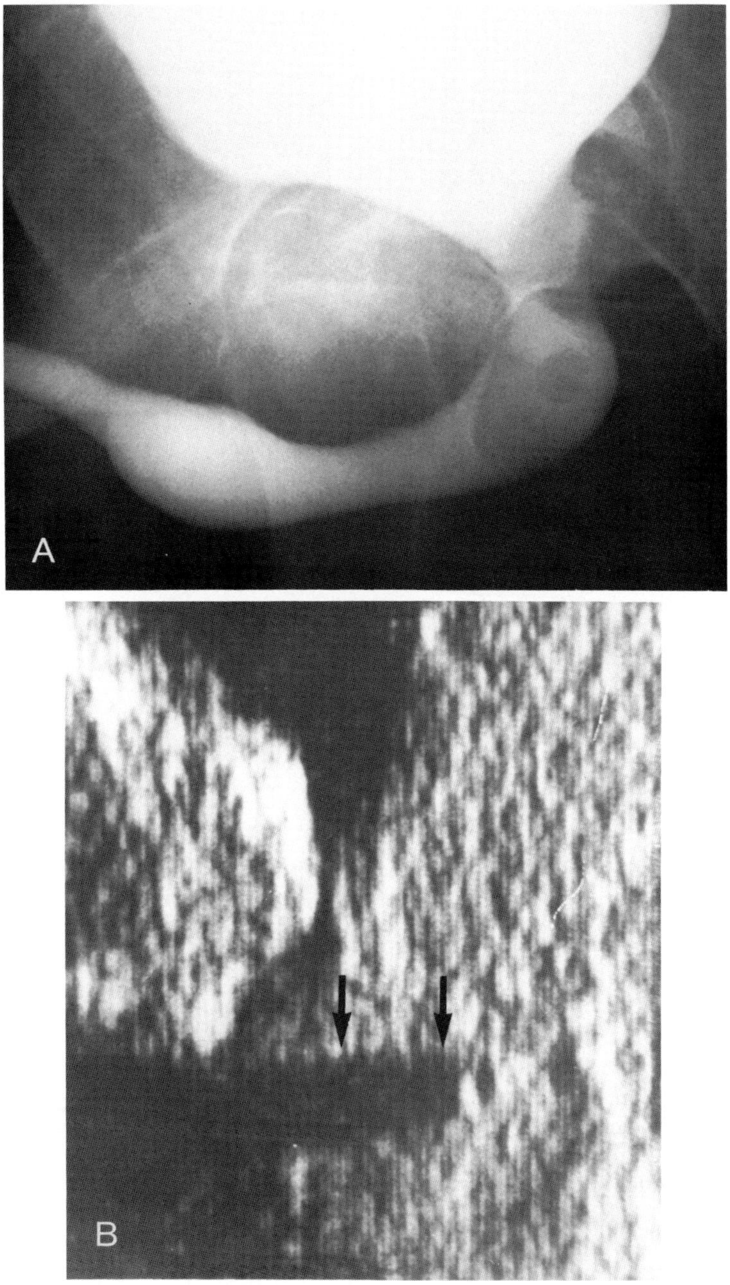

Figure 9.12. False passage in posterior urethra. A radiological voiding cystourethrogram (**A**) appears normal. The sonographic study (**B**) demonstrates the false passage (*arrows*). (Reproduced with permission from Perkash I, Friedland GW. Ultrasonographic detection of false passages arising from the posterior urethra in spinal cord injury patients. J Urol 1987;137:701. Copyright by Williams & Wilkins, 1987.)

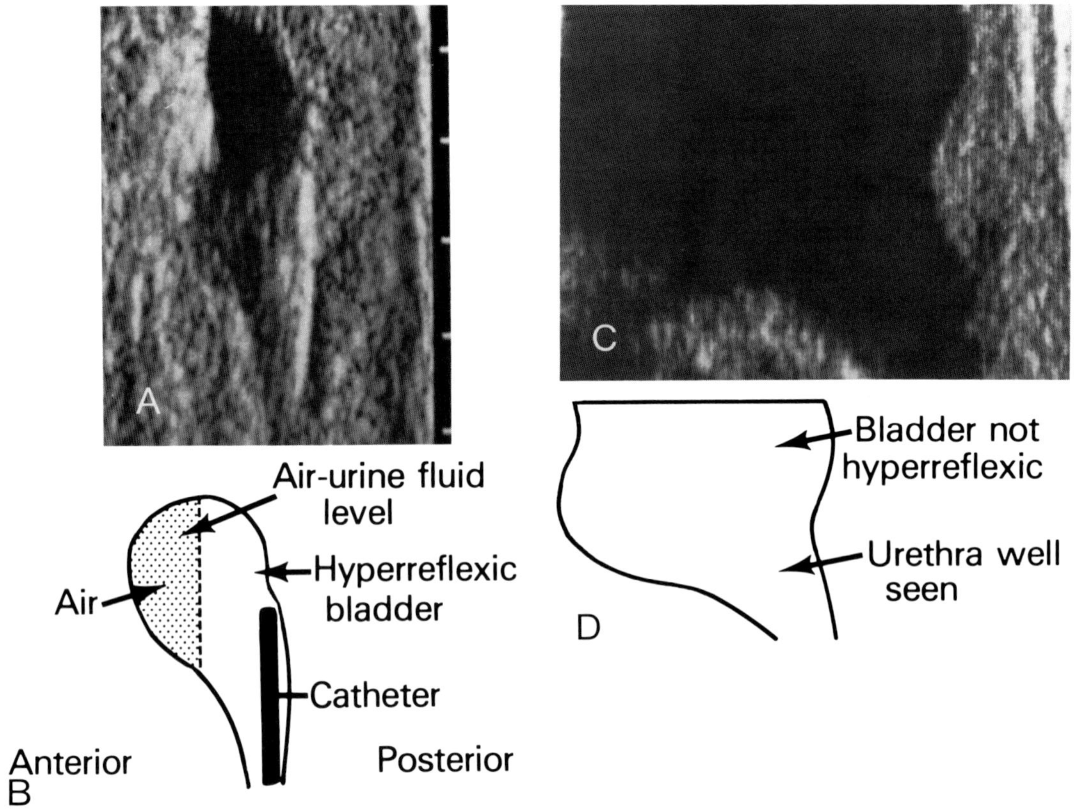

Figure 9.13. Catheter-induced precipitous bladder contractions. **A** and **B,** Precipitous contractions with catheter in bladder. **C** and **D,** Repeat study on another day without a catheter shows reflex bladder without precipitous contractions. (Reproduced with permission from Perkash I, Friedland GW. Catheter-induced hyperreflexia in spinal cord injury patients. Diagnosis by sonographic voiding cystourethrography. Radiology 1986;159:453.)

we have found that about 50% of all precipitous bladder contractions are catheter induced (9).

We found that, using real-time sonographic control to introduce the catheter into the bladder, we could prevent catheter-induced precipitous bladder contractions. There is always some residual urine in the bladder in spinal cord injury patients; but stopping the advance of the catheter just before reaching the bladder wall stopped precipitous bladder contractions (9).

We recently found a second cause of catheter-induced precipitous bladder contractions. A patient with incomplete spinal cord lesions can be very sensitive to touch at the bladder neck posteriorly, perhaps because this is the main sensory area of the bladder. When the tip of the catheter touches this area, patients often complain immediately of discomfort; further, touching this area in these patients can result in a precipitous bladder contraction.

It would not have been possible to make any of the above-mentioned observations without transrectal sonography.

USE OF SONOGRAPHY TO TRAIN SPINAL CORD INJURY PATIENTS TO VOID

If patients with an upper motor neuron lesion do the Credé maneuver to open the bladder neck, the bladder neck may actually close (Fig. 9.2**A** and **B**); thus those very efforts can increase bladder pressure very significantly, even to the point of causing reflux.

If the patient performs suprapubic tapping, as described above, however, there is little elevation in bladder pressure and no danger of reflux. The urethra opens widely (Fig. 9.2**C** and **D**) and the bladder is emptied more completely than with the Credé maneuver.

When these patients tap their bladders on

their own, however, we have found that they do not know how much or how often to tap, leading at times to significant postvoid residuals, even after surgery.

To overcome this problem, we have been teaching patients to perform tapping during transrectal sonography, allowing them to watch the monitor to see how effective the tapping is (13). This has proved very successful and is now part of the routine training of these patients at our institution.

USE OF TRANSRECTAL SONOGRAPHY AFTER TRANSURETHRAL SPHINCTEROTOMY

Patients who have transurethral sphincterotomies for posterior ledges or for detrusor–bladder neck or detrusor-sphincter dyssynergia must be observed to check the success of the surgery. Traditionally, this has been done using urodynamic studies and a radiological voiding cystourethrogram, but we have found that transrectal sonography is a quick, simple, and inexpensive follow-up examination. If the bladder neck and urethra are widely patent and if the bladder empties completely and rapidly, transrectal sonography alone provides a sufficient check (Fig. 9.14).

We have also been able to reduce the number of intravenous urograms these patients need. The normal routine is one intravenous urogram a year, but we have found that if the bladder neck and urethra are widely patent and if there are no signs and symptoms, there is no need to do an intravenous urogram.

CONCLUSIONS

Transrectal sonography is now a routine part of the dynamic evaluation of the lower urinary tract at our institution. We recently compared the number of radiological voiding cystourethrograms done before the advent of transrectal sonography with the present and found that we now do 95% fewer radiological examinations than before.

This is an important consideration, especially in the younger patient, who formerly received much greater radiation dosages to the gonads through repeated radiological voiding cystourethrograms. It was once said that the examination was necessary despite the radia-

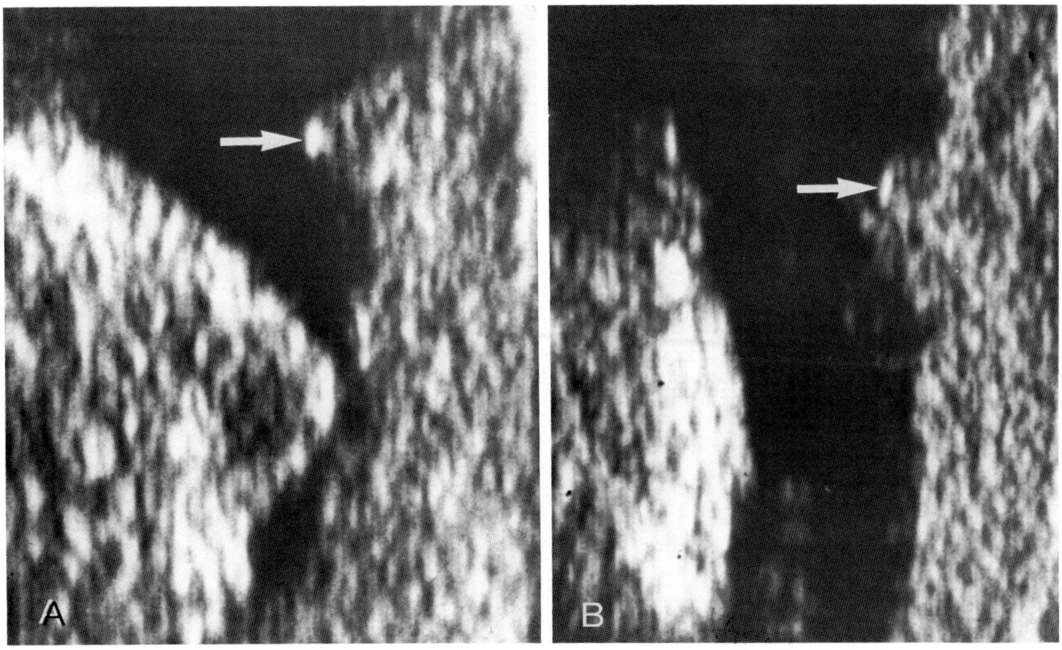

Figure 9.14. Value of transrectal sonography for follow-up of patients after surgery. **A,** Before transurethral sphincterotomy, there is a prominent posterior ledge (*arrow*) and detrusor-sphincter dyssynergia. **B,** After transurethral sphincterotomy, the bladder neck and urethra are widely patent. (Reproduced with permission from Perkash I, Friedland GW. Posterior ledge of the bladder neck: the crucial diagnostic role of ultrasonography. Urol Radiol 1986;8:175.)

tion and that it caused no harm to the patient. We now recognize that, though this may be true, there could possibly be genetic changes in future generations. Until recently this also was not a consideration, as it was not expected that patients with neuromuscular dysfunction would father children, but as a number of these patients are young, are married, or may marry, and may wish to father children, it is now a very real consideration.

Transrectal sonography is a simple, quick, and cost-effective means of investigating many patients. It is easy to perform and causes minimal discomfort in neurologically intact patients.

Transrectal sonography cannot tell us whether a patient has vesicoureteral reflux. If the urologist considers it essential to the management of the patient to know whether reflux is present, a radiological or scintigraphic voiding cystourethrogram will still have to be done. Transrectal sonography cannot produce images of the pendulous urethra; but for the majority of patients with functional disorders, that information is of little or no significance.

References

1. Perkash I. Neuromuscular diseases of the bladder. In: Friedland GW, Filly R, Goris ML, et al., eds. Uroradiology: an integrated approach. New York: Churchill Livingstone, 1983:1291.
2. Shapeero G, Friedland GW, Perkash I. Transrectal sonographic voiding cystourethrography. Studies in neuromuscular dysfunction. AJR 1983;141:83.
3. Friedland GW, Perkash I. Neuromuscular dysfunction of the bladder and urethra. Semin Roentgenol 1983;18:255.
4. Resnick M, Yalla SV. Management of urinary incontinence in the elderly. N Engl J Med 1985;131:800.
5. Brazda JF. Washington report. The Nation's Health 1983;13:3.
6. Hald T, Bates P, Bradley WE. The standardization of terminology of lower urinary tract function. Glasgow: International Continence Society, 1984:1–34.
7. Resnick NM, Yalla SV. Detrusor hyperactivity with impaired contractile function. JAMA 1987; 257:3076.
8. Perkash I, Friedland GW. Principles of modern urodynamic studies. Invest Radiol 1987;22:279.
9. Perkash I, Friedland GW. Catheter-induced hyperreflexia in spinal cord injury patients. Diagnosis by sonographic voiding cystourethrography. Radiology 1986;159:453.
10. Perkash I, Friedland GW. Posterior ledge of the bladder neck: the crucial diagnostic role of ultrasonography. Urol Radiol 1986;8:175.
11. Perkash I, Friedland GW. Transrectal ultrasonography of the lower urinary tract: evaluation of bladder neck problems. Neurourol Urodynam 1986;5:299.
12. Perkash I, Friedland GW. Ultrasonographic detection of false passages arising from the posterior urethra in spinal cord injury patients. J Urol 1987;137:701.
13. Perkash I, Friedland GW. Using transrectal sonography to teach patients with spinal cord injury to retrain their bladders. Radiology 1984; 152:228.
14. Perkash I, Friedland GW. Real-time gray-scale transrectal linear array ultrasonography in urodynamic evaluation. Semin Urol 1985;3:49.
15. Porena M, Vespaspiani G, Vergili G, Lombi R, Mearini E, Rosi P, Micali F. Real-time transrectal sonographic voiding cystourethrography. Urology 1987;30:171.
16. Shabsigh R, Fishman TJ, Krebs M. The use of transrectal longitudinal real-time ultrasonography in urodynamics. J Urol 1987;138:1416.
17. McNeal J. The prostate gland: morphology and pathobiology. Monogr Urol 1983;4:3.
18. Yalla SV, Sharma GVRK, Barsamian EM. Micturitional static urethral pressure profile during voiding and implications. J Urol 1980;124:649.
19. Blaivas JG, Norlen LJ. Primary bladder neck obstruction. World J Urol 1984;1:191.
20. Manolin RA. Voiding cystourethrography with synchronous measurements of pressures and flow in the diagnosis of subvesical obstruction in men: radiological view. J Urol 1987;137:1196.
21. Blaivas J. Multichannel urodynamic studies. Urology 1984;23:421.
22. Hinman F. Nonneurogenic neurogenic bladders (the Hinman Syndrome): 15 years later. J Urol 1986;136:769.
23. Raz S, Smith RB. External sphincter spasticity syndrome in female patients. J Urol 1976; 115:443.
24. Perley MJ, Guz SB. Hysteria: the stability and usefulness of clinical criteria. N Engl J Med 1962;266:421.
25. Korzets I, Garb R, Lewis S, Bernheim JL. Reversible renal failure due to psychogenic urinary retention. Postgrad Med J 1985;61:465.

CHAPTER 10

Ultrasonography of the Prostate

MATTHEW D. RIFKIN, M.D.
MARTIN I. RESNICK, M.D.

Prostate cancer is the most prevalent cancer in men and the most commonly diagnosed malignancy in the American male population. It is also the second most lethal tumor in men in the United States (Fig. 10.1). It has been estimated, based on both autopsy and prostatectomy specimens from patients from bladder cancer, that over 40% of men over 60 years of age harbor prostate malignancy (1–3). While many (if not most) of these cancers may not be clinically significant, prostate cancer is the second most common cause of cancer deaths in the American male population, and 30,000 men will die each year from the disease process (4). There are over 100,000 newly diagnosed prostate cancers each year in the United States (4). However, as yet, we have not always been able to determine which of these cancers will become a clinically significant disease process and which will not cause morbidity and mortality (Fig. 10.2).

Until the advent of advanced diagnostic imaging studies, the only means to detect prostate cancer was by the digital rectal examination or serendipitously during pathological evaluation of a surgical specimen (from a transurethral resection of the prostate [TURP] for benign disease). These clinical diagnostic techniques, however, often limited the diagnosis of prostate cancer to relatively advanced stages. Thus, early detection, with potentially better survival rate, eluded the clinicians.

For these reasons, other modalities for detection and early diagnosis of prostate cancer are essential. In addition to the development of certain serum markers—i.e., prostate specific antigen (PSA) and prostatic acid phosphatase (PAP)—a variety of diagnostic imaging modalities, including computed tomography (CT), magnetic resonance imaging (MRI), and radionuclide studies, have been used in an attempt to diagnose early cancer. To date, none have showed satisfactory results.

Ultrasound was developed with crude equipment in the 1950s and 1960s. With the development of sophisticated equipment and technology for endorectal ultrasound in the late 1980s and early 1990s, cancers as small as a few millimeters that are not detectable by any other means are now being routinely diagnosed.

However, while imaging can be used for detection and diagnosis of disease, it also plays an important part in staging of a diagnosed cancer. Prostate ultrasonography is of value in the assessment of nonmalignant disorders of the prostate as well.

This chapter discusses the role of sonography in the evaluation of the prostate.

PROSTATE ANATOMY

The understanding of prostate anatomy on both the gross and the microscopic levels has changed during the past few decades. An understanding of both is essential in using newer cross-sectional imaging techniques.

The prostate in the normal postpubescent male, prior to the onset of benign enlargement, is an ovoid-conical structure, usually no larger than a walnut. It measures approximately 3.5 cm in transverse width, 3.5 to 4.0 cm cephalocaudad length, and 2.5 to 3.0 cm in anterior-posterior dimension. The apex or inferior margin of the gland is conical and is adjacent to the urogenital diaphragm. The superior, most cephalad margin of the prostate is broader and is termed the base of the gland. It is adjacent to the inferior margin, also termed the base, of the bladder (Fig. 10.3).

Adjacent to the anterior portion of the prostate is a collection of veins termed Santorini's plexus embedded in a collection of fat and fascia. The lateral margins of the prostate include draining veins and periprostatic fat, and in the posterolateral margins are another bilaterally paired collection of vessels and nerves, termed the lateral venous plexi or neurovascular bundles. Posteriorly, the prostate is separated from

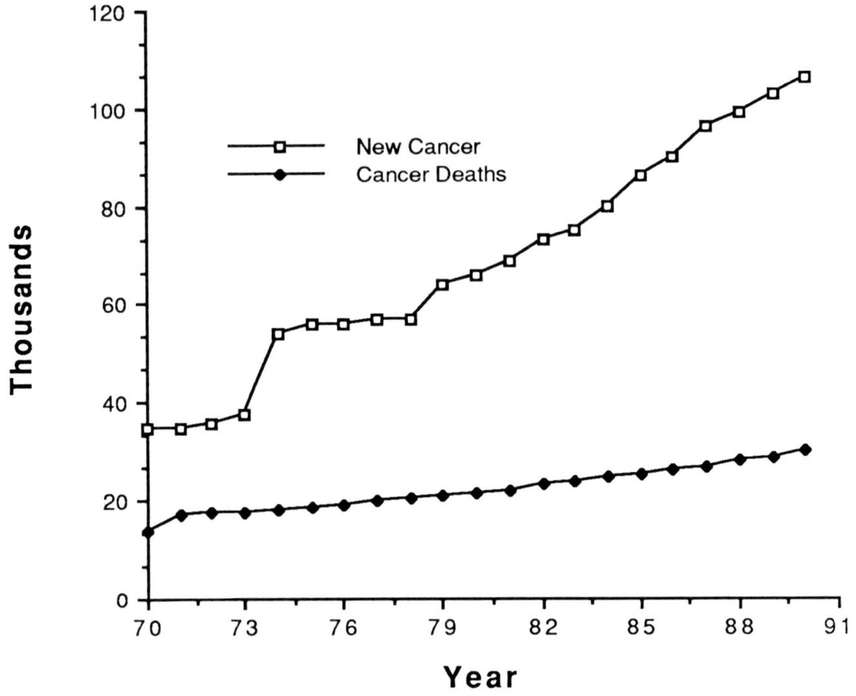

Figure 10.1 A graph obtained from statistics from the American Cancer Society demonstrates that the number of new cases diagnosed per year is increasing more rapidly than the number of deaths per cancer.

the rectum by periprostatic fat and a thin fascial membrane, Denonvillier's fascia.

There is a thin fibrous capsule surrounding the prostate, predominantly identified in the lateral and posterior margins. There is interruption of capsule at the base, where the internal sphincter enters, and at the apex, where the external sphincter exits.

Superior to the prostate, posteriorly positioned between the urinary bladder anteriorly and the rectum posteriorly are the two paired seminal vesicles. These symmetrically shaped, variably sized structures are composed of fluid-filled tubules. The vas deferens (continuations of the epididymis and the scrotum) insert and join the medial aspect of the seminal vesicles, forming the bilaterally paired ejaculatory ducts.

Within the prostate, the description and understanding of the intrinsic anatomy of the prostate gland have changed dramatically during the past few decades.

For example, classic prostate anatomy, termed Lowsley's lobar concept of anatomy, has been used to identify the prostate and prostatic pathology since the early 1900s (5). In this description, the prostate is divided into five major lobes. The first lobe, in the anterior portion of the prostate, is termed the anterior lobe. It is situated from the anterior margin of the gland to the level of the prostatic (also termed the posterior) urethra posteriorly. The middle or median lobe is a smaller area between the superior prostatic urethra (as its anterior margin) and the ejaculatory ducts (as the median lobe's posterior margin). This lobe extends from the base (the cephalad margin of the prostate) caudad to the midportion of the prostate, to the level of the verumontanum (where the ejaculatory ducts insert into the prostatic urethra). The posterior lobe encompasses the posterior portion of the prostate and is situated posterior to the ejaculatory ducts and the inferior intraprostatic urethra. The posterior lobe extends to the posterior margins of the gland (Fig. 10.3). The two large lateral lobes (the fourth and fifth lobes) extend from the lateral margin of the prostate bilaterally to the middle part of the gland. Despite these distinct anterior-posterior "boundaries," none of the lobes have clearly defined medial margins. Additionally, Lowsley's concept of anatomy did not take into con-

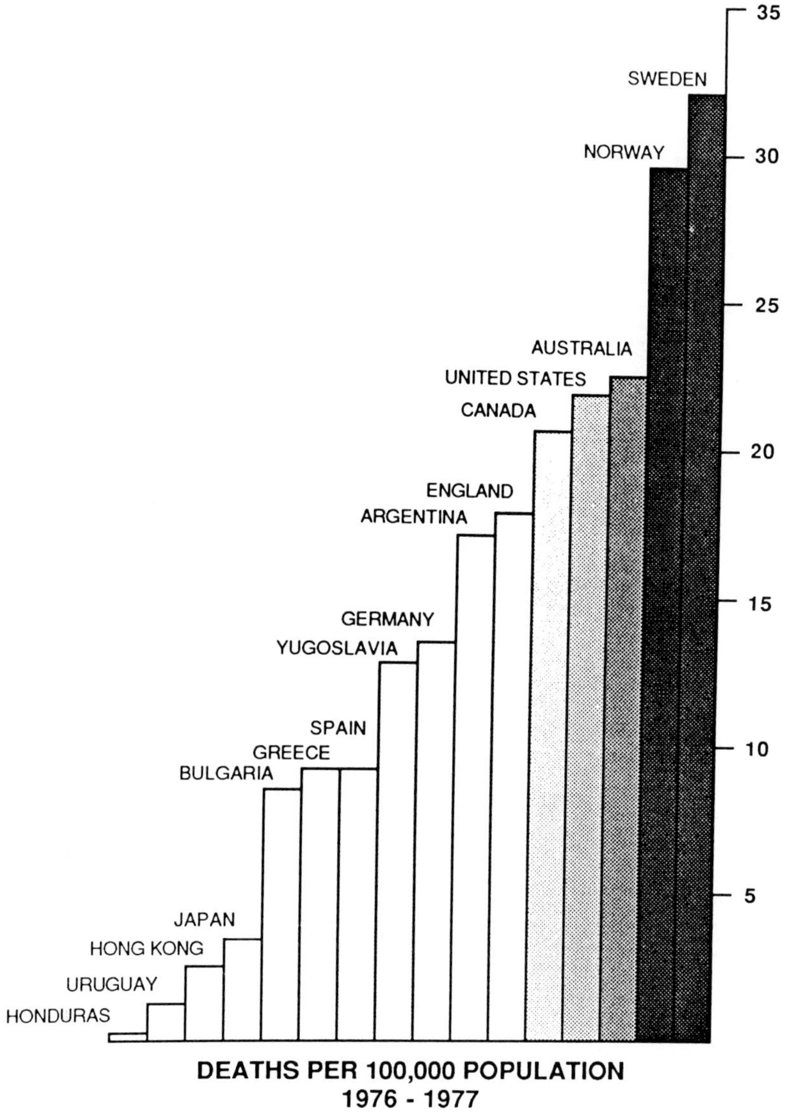

Figure 10.2. Mortality rates from 1976 to 1977 differ from country to country, whereas the prevalence (the number of cases within the generalized population) is similar. (Reprinted with permission from Rifkin MD. Ultrasound of the prostate. New York: Raven Press, 1987.)

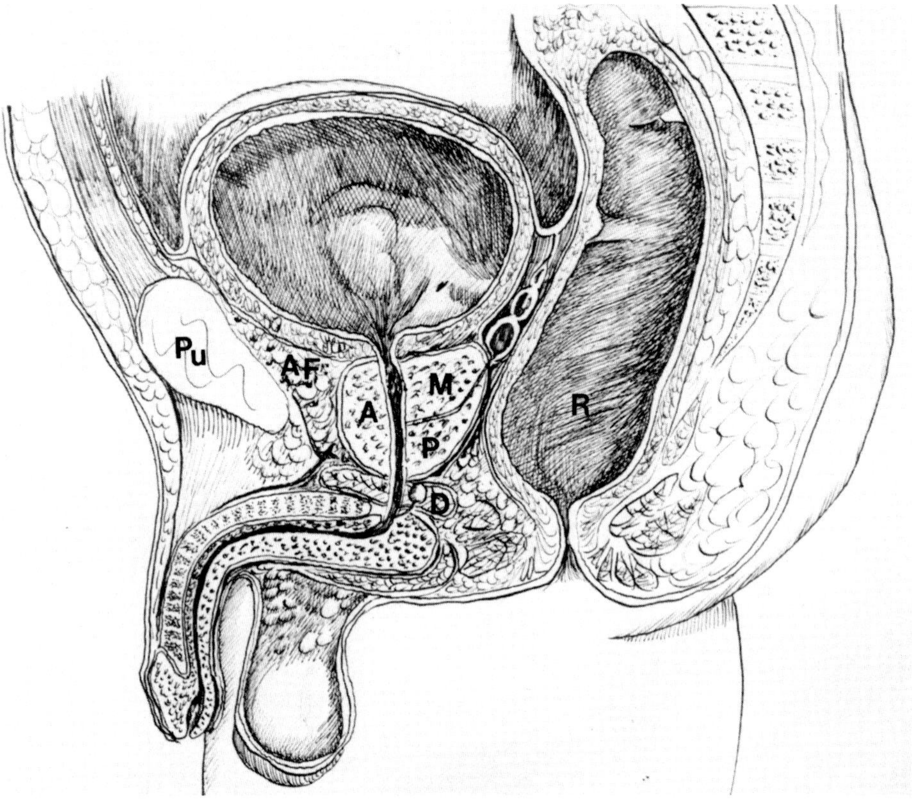

Figure 10.3. The prostate is divided into five lobes. The anterior lobe (*A*) is situated anterior to the prostatic urethra. The median lobe (*M*) is situated between the urethra and the ejaculatory ducts. The posterior lobe (*P*) is situated in the posterior portion of the prostate. The prostate is situated between the pubic bones (*Pu*) and anterior prostatic fat and fascia (*AF*) and posteriorly, the rectum (*R*). The base of the urinary bladder (*B*) abuts the superior portion of the prostate, the base of the gland, and the inferior or apical portion of the prostate is adjacent to the urogenital diaphragm (*D*).

sideration the different histologic components of the prostate but is based purely on anatomical position of the tissue as defined in the embryonic and fetal gland (5).

Since the 1960s, a "zonal" concept of anatomy, initially developed by Dr. John McNeal (6), has evolved. It has been modified over the past 25 years (7–13). This anatomical orientation defines the prostate in terms of its cellular components. It divides the gland into three major areas: the anterior portion of the prostate, the central or inner gland, and the peripheral or outer gland (Fig. 10.4). This terminology can be modified slightly to correlate with cross-sectional imaging.

1. Anterior Prostate—The anterior portion of the gland is fibromuscular stroma, which is quite thick anteriorly and is nonglandular tissue. The thin, fibrous prostate capsule, laterally and posteriorly, is an extension of the thick anterior fibromuscular stroma. The anterior prostate encompasses about one-third of the volume by the normally nonenlarged gland.
2. Central or Inner Gland—The central or inner gland is the central (inner) area of the prostate and includes a number of different structures: the proximal urethra (and its lining), the transition zone, and the smooth muscle of the internal sphincter. The thin lining of the proximal urethra (the periurethral glandular tissue) extends from the base (the superior portion of the prostate) cephalad to the level of the verumontanum. The smooth muscle fibers of the internal sphincter are extensions of the base of the urinary bladder. The transition zone is a small bilobed structure situated just cephalad to the verumontanum. The transition

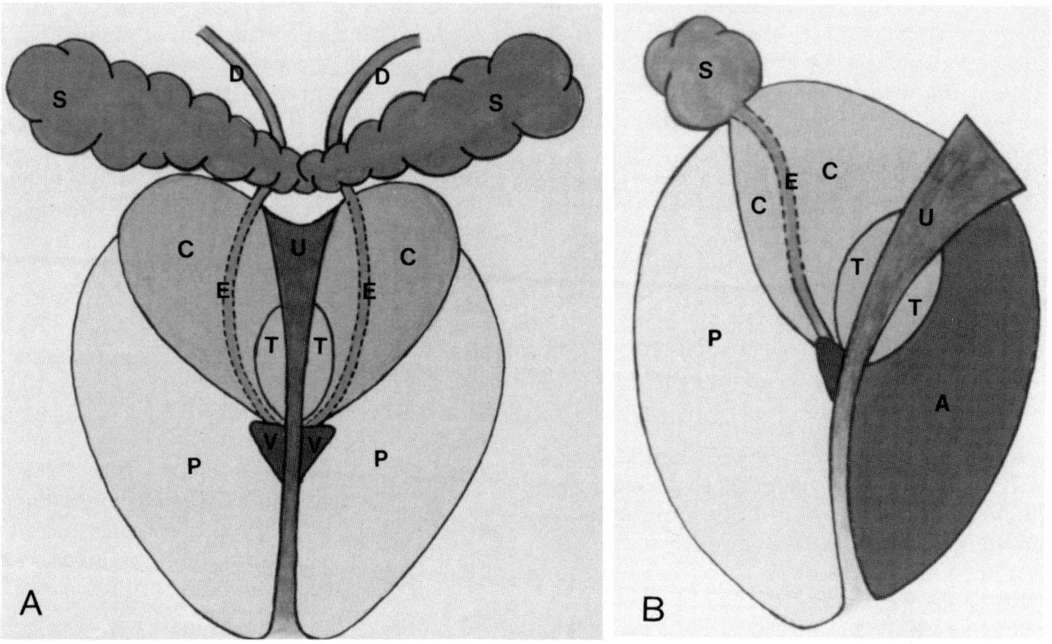

Figure 10.4. Zonal anatomy. Line diagrams demonstrates the prostate in coronal (**A**) and midline sagittal (**B**) orientations. *D,* vas deferens; *S,* seminal vesicles, *E,* ejaculatory ducts; *U,* urethra and urethral ducts; *T,* transition zone; *V,* verumontanum; *C,* central zone; *P,* peripheral zone; *A,* anterior prostatic fat and fascia.

zone is acinar tissue and along with the periurethral glandular tissue is the only acinar tissue not part of the peripheral gland. The central gland encompasses about 5% of the volume of the glandular prostate in the young male.

3. Peripheral or Outer Gland—The peripheral or outer gland is composed exclusively of prostatic acinar tissue. It is divided into central and peripheral zones. The central zone should not be confused with the central (inner) gland. It is situated posterior to the bladder neck or internal sphincter and is distinctly separate from the central gland. It extends posteriorly from the central gland to surround the bilaterally paired ejaculatory ducts. Similar to the central gland, the central zone extends inferiorly to the level of the verumontanum. The peripheral zone comprises the posterior, the apical (inferior), and the lateral, posterolateral, and anterolateral portions of the prostate (Fig. 10.5). It is the largest portion of the gland, approximately 70% of the volume of the normal postpubescent prostate and about 95% of the volume of the glandular prostate.

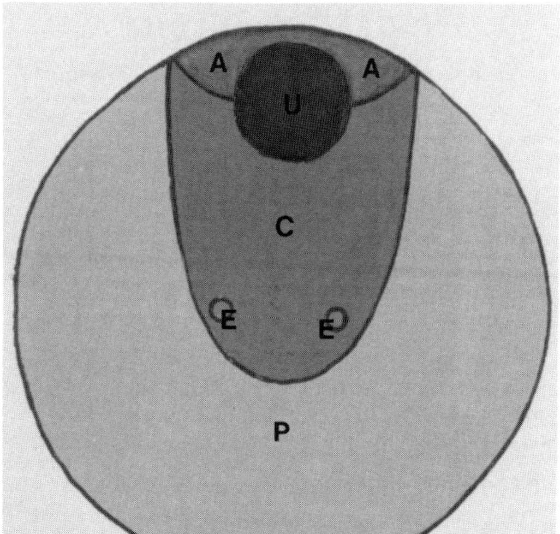

Figure 10.5. Zonal anatomy, axial orientation. A large portion of the peripheral (*P*) and central (*C*) zones are situated anteriorly. *A,* anterior prostatic fat and fascia; *E,* ejaculatory ducts; *U,* urethra and urethral tissues.

A comparison of Lowsley's lobar and McNeal's zonal concepts of anatomy is possible and important because of the need to compare clinical findings (clinicians may still refer to lobar anatomy) to imaging studies (which should employ zonal anatomy):

1. The anterior lobe correlates with the anterior fibromuscular stroma;
2. The median lobe and central zone are similar, but the latter is larger, extending slightly more posteriorly;
3. The sum of the posterior and two lateral lobes correlates to a large extent with the peripheral zone.

Initially, McNeal's concept of zonal anatomy had little utility in the clinical sphere or in diagnostic imaging. However, with the development of cross-sectional imaging studies, in particular endorectal prostate ultrasound and MRI, the zonal concept of anatomy became a useful technique to apply to imaging because it is able to define the different areas. Both ultrasound and MRI can differentiate the normal central gland from the normal peripheral gland. In the hyperplastic prostate, they differentiate benign hyperplastic areas from the normal tissue. The zonal concept of anatomy is also used because it also incorporates a clearer understanding of the pathogenesis of disease.

PATHOGENESIS OF DISEASE

The development of prostatic pathology was poorly understood and impossible to correlate accurately with areas of the prostate using Lowsley's concepts of lobar anatomy. It was previously thought, for example, that cancers would only arise in the posterior lobe and benign prostatic hyperplasia would develop predominantly in the lateral and, to a lesser degree, the median lobes. These concepts were based on the clinical presentation of pathology, not on the actual position of the tumors or on a cellular basis. They are inaccurate.

It is now understood that prostate cancer develops in the acinar tissue, predominantly the peripheral or outer prostate (11–13). While the peripheral zone is three times larger in volume than the central zone (in the normal-sized gland), prostate cancer develops seven times more frequently in the peripheral zone (11–13). Approximately 70% of all cancers develop in the peripheral zone and 10% in the central zone. An additional 20% develop from the transition zone of the central gland. There are portions of the peripheral gland that are situated in the anterior half of the prostate. It has been shown that about 50% of cancer arises in the anterior half of the prostate, including all cancers from the transition zone (20% of the total) and the central zone (10%), and cancers from the anteriorly situated portions of the peripheral zone (20% of the total) (7) (Table 10.1).

Benign prostatic hyperplasia (BPH), in contrast, develops exclusively from the central gland, approximately 95% from the transition zone and 5% from the periurethral glandular tissue (Table 10.2). However, not all benign pathologic processes develop in the central gland.

Prostatitis, or inflammation of the prostate, develops exclusively in the acinar prostate. This distribution is similar to prostate cancer, since it develops predominantly in the peripheral gland.

ULTRASOUND IMAGING TECHNIQUES

There are a number of imaging approaches using ultrasound that can be used to evaluate the prostate. These include (*a*) the transabdominal approach, (*b*) the transperineal approach, (*c*) the endourethral approach, and (*d*) the endorectal approach.

Transabdominal Approach—The transabdominal approach uses conventional ultrasound equipment. It requires the urinary bladder to be distended with fluid prior to the examination. The transducer (usually 3.5 to 5 MHz) is placed just superior to the symphysis pubis and is angled caudad to visualize the

Table 10.1.
Origins of Prostate Cancer

Peripheral (outer) gland	80%
Peripheral zone	70%
Central zone	10%
Central (inner) gland	
Transition zone	20%

Table 10.2.
Origins of Benign Prostate Hyperplasia

Central (inner) gland	100%
Transition zone	95%
Periurethral glandular tissue	5%

prostate. Longitudinal and transverse images must be obtained. The major benefit of this technique is to evaluate prostate size (Fig. 10.6). Most internal texture changes will not be identified. A transurethral resection of the prostate (TURP) defect may be identified as an anechoic, fluid-filled defect in the base of the gland. Occasionally in patients with prostatic hyperplasia causing bladder outlet obstruction, the bladder wall may be identified as being thickened. Additionally, postvoid residua can be obtained.

Transperineal Approach—The transperineal approach uses conventional ultrasound imaging equipment identical with that used in the transabdominal approach. The transducer is placed on the perineum and angled cephalad. The prostate may be defined, but internal texture changes are no better identified than the transabdominal approach. Slight distention of the urinary bladder will occasionally help delineate the gland.

Transurethral Approach—The transurethral approach requires specialized transducers that are placed into the urethra. These were initially developed to evaluate the urinary bladder wall but can also be used to evaluate the prostate as they are withdrawn slowly (14, 15). They can delineate the prostate by using a 7.5- to 10-MHz transducer but have limited penetration. Additionally, the study is invasive and usually no more diagnostic than the clinically more accepted endorectal approach.

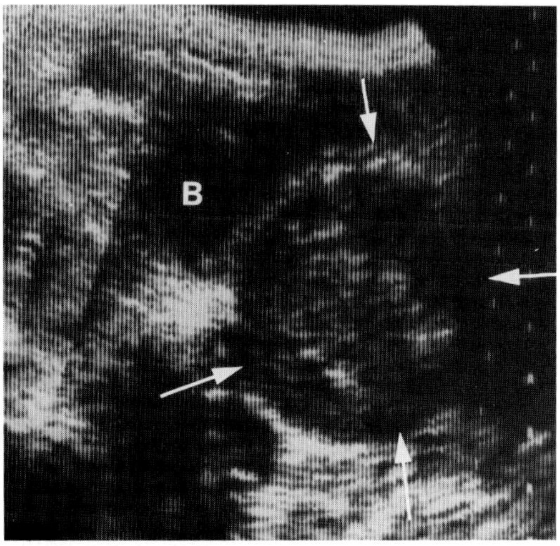

Figure 10.6. Abdominal ultrasound. Longitudinal scan demonstrates an enlarged prostate (*arrows*) with poor determination of the internal prostate texture. *B*, bladder.

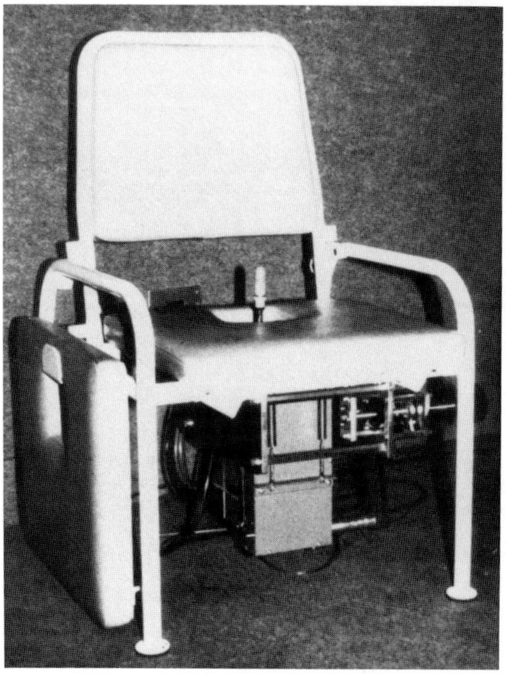

Figure 10.7. Rotating chair. One of the first endorectal scanners used a chair with the transducer placed in the seat. (Reprinted with permission from Rifkin MD. Ultrasound of the prostate. New York: Raven Press, 1988.)

Endorectal Ultrasound—Endorectal ultrasound is a relatively old technique developed initially in the 1950s to evaluate the rectal wall. However, with improvement of equipment, this has become the most accepted technique to evaluate internal tissue changes of the prostate.

When prostate ultrasound was first developed using endorectal probes, a single orientation was available. The early probes used a rotating crystal and was termed "radial" scanning (Fig. 10.7). In the late 1970s and early 1980s, a second type of equipment, a longitudinally oriented, flat, linear array transducer was developed to image the prostate in a longitudinal orientation. More recently, mechanical and phased-array sector scanners have been used (15–19).

In the mid 1980s, further refinement was made so that "biplane" probes were developed (Fig. 10.8). These instruments used a variety of techniques to image the prostate in multiple orientations. The true biplane probe evaluates

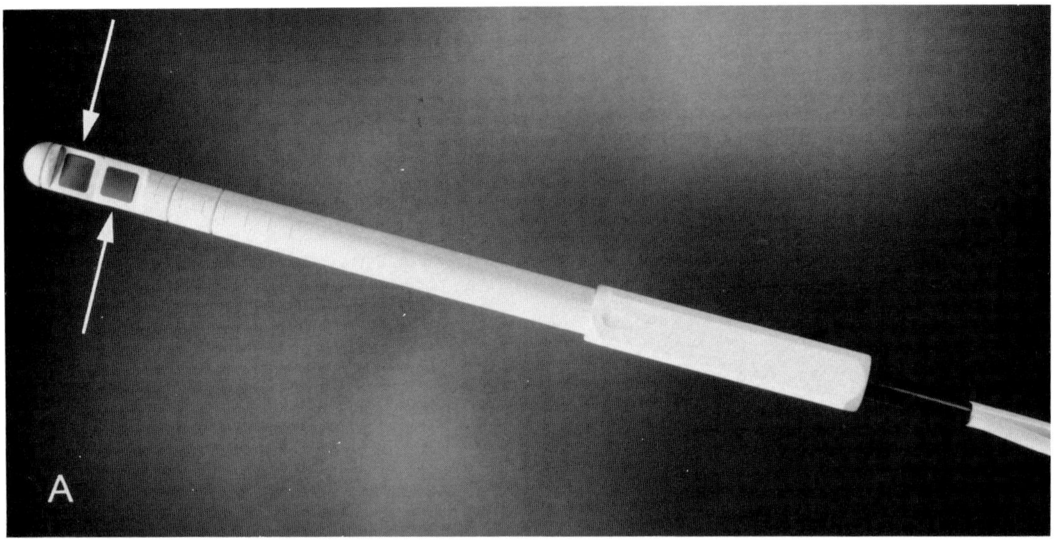

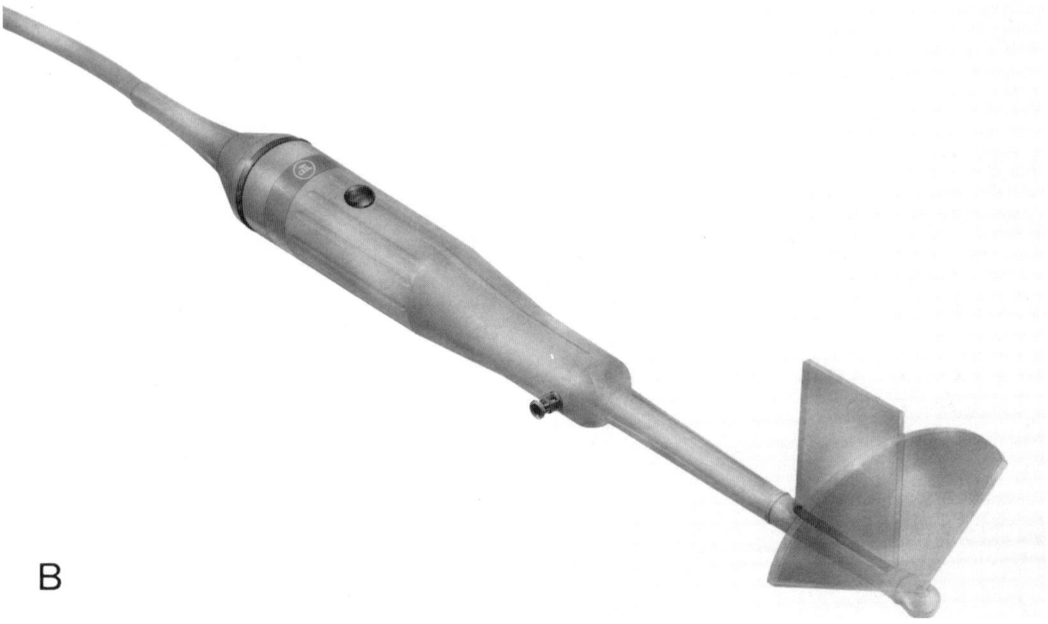

Figure 10.8. Biplane probes. One type of biplane instrument (**A**) demonstrates two different transducer crystals (*arrows*) placed at the tip. This will give perpendicularly oriented images (**B**).

the prostate in axial and longitudinal orientations, and the most common technology incorporated two distinctly separate transducers into a single endorectal probe. Other technology includes incorporation of a single crystal that can be rotated in a variety of positions. This has been termed an "omnidirectional" transducer. A single crystal placed at the end of the probe, an "end-fire" orientation, can also be used. This, however, requires manipulation and manual rotation of the probe during scanning. This equipment can view the prostate in an oblique coronal orientation (15, 20).

While early equipment used 3.5-MHz transducers, the more sophisticated modern technology has used higher-resolution, higher-frequency transducers with more sharply focused near fields that permit better evaluation of the posterior portion of the prostate and delineation of smaller areas of abnormality.

The use of a variety of imaging planes (at least two) allows prostatic visualization in three dimensions, thus permitting more accurate localization of abnormalities and extent of disease. Multiple images can be obtained by a variety of techniques, including multiple single-phase transducers, incorporation of two fixed transducers into a single probe (biplane probes), and multi- and omnidirectional imaging, in which a single transducer rotates within the probe or a single oblique or end-fire transducer is rotated to allow omnidirectional imaging.

Regardless of the type or types of transducers used, there are three major planes that should be understood prior to beginning an ultrasound study: the axial, the sagittal, and the "oblique" coronal-axial orientations. All orientations view the cross-sectional anatomy in slightly different presentations, although axial and "oblique" coronal-axial planes may appear similar. The true axial plane permits rapid assessment of the size, shape, and symmetry of the prostate. Scans obtained in the most cephalad position will visualize the seminal vesicles as symmetrically paired structures.

PATIENT PREPARATION

In many instances, no patient preparation is required for a diagnostic endorectal sonographic examination. However, in certain instances, when extensive fecal material is noted on the pre-ultrasound digital rectal examination, a cleansing enema may be required.

PATIENT POSITION

Patients may be examined in a variety of positions, including the decubitus, lithotomy, and knee-chest positions. All are appropriate, and the preferences of the patient and examiner should be the guides to the position used.

NORMAL ENDORECTAL SONOGRAM

The normal endorectal ultrasound (which is usually seen only in men under the age of 40) will have sonographic appearances different from pathologically riddled glands. However, an understanding of the normal is essential to understand the abnormal.

The normal inner prostate is generally low level in echogenicity (hypoechoic) compared to the outer gland. This is well seen on all views.

When scanning the prostate using the axial orientation, the transducer is usually placed deep within the rectum, just cephalad to the seminal vesicles (Fig. 10.9). The initial scans will demonstrate the vas deferens either just superior to the seminal vesicle or at the level of the seminal vesicles, just anterior to the two paired seminal vesicles. The vas deferens and seminal vesicles have similar low-level acoustic reflectivity, suggesting a predominant fluid component (Fig. 10.10). As the transducer is withdrawn slightly to the level of the base of the gland, a hypoechoic area (the inner gland) will be identified anteriorly placed and in the midline (Fig. 10.11). The central and peripheral zones have similar sonographic appearances. As the probe is withdrawn progressively caudad, another subtle anterior hypoechoic area may be identified, the anterior fibromuscular stroma. The remainder of the gland has relatively homogeneous, moderately high acoustic reflectivity. On the axial orientation, the apex of the prostate is occasionally poorly identified, although the surrounding musculature will be seen (Fig. 10.12).

When scanning in the longitudinal orientation with a side-viewing transducer, the probe is placed into the rectum to the level of the prostate (Fig. 10.13). At that point, a midline image will be obtained. In the midline, the hypoechoic central or inner prostate will be identified (Fig. 10.14). A small amount of fluid within the urinary bladder helps delineate the base of the prostate more accurately. The hypoechoic area extends to the level of the verumontanum, where the central zone and the central (inner) prostate terminate. The peripheral prostate is relatively homogeneous in echogenicity. The seminal vesicles are seen in cross section and appear as rounded or oblique rounded, slightly less echogenic areas than the normal prostate. They are situated in the superior aspect of the prostate, just anterior to the rectum. To evaluate the lateral portions of the gland on the longitudinal orientation, the probe is rotated slightly clockwise or counterclock-

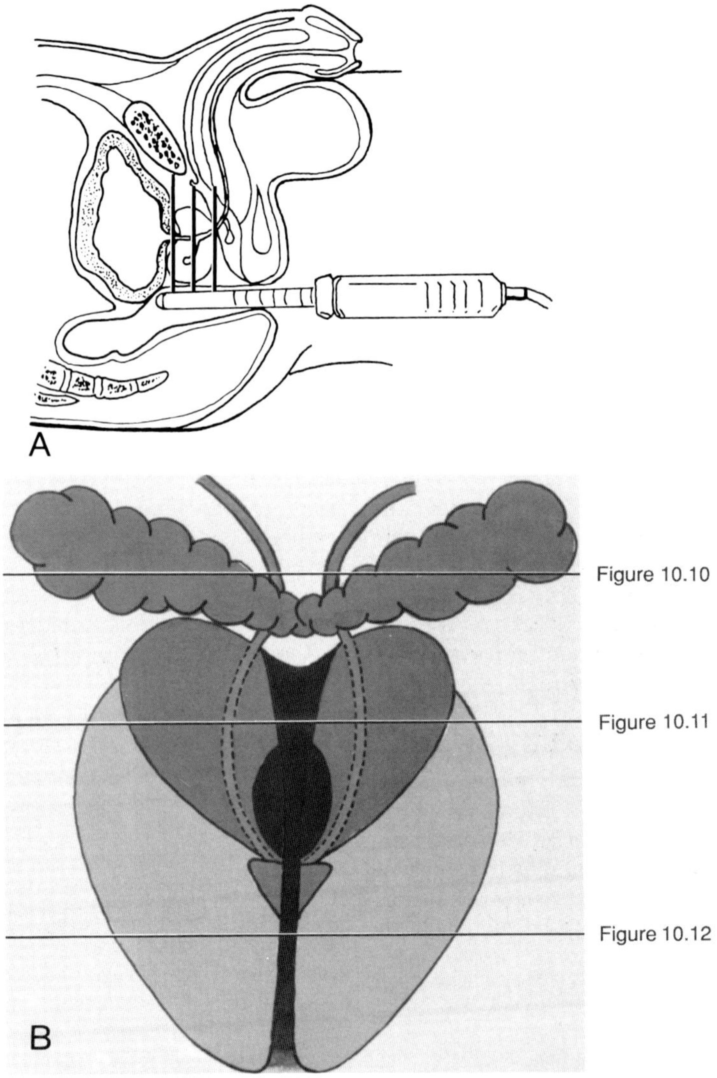

Figure 10.9. Axial scan technique. Line diagram (**A**) demonstrates various axial section (*lines*) of the prostate. These will image the prostate at different sections of the gland (**B**).

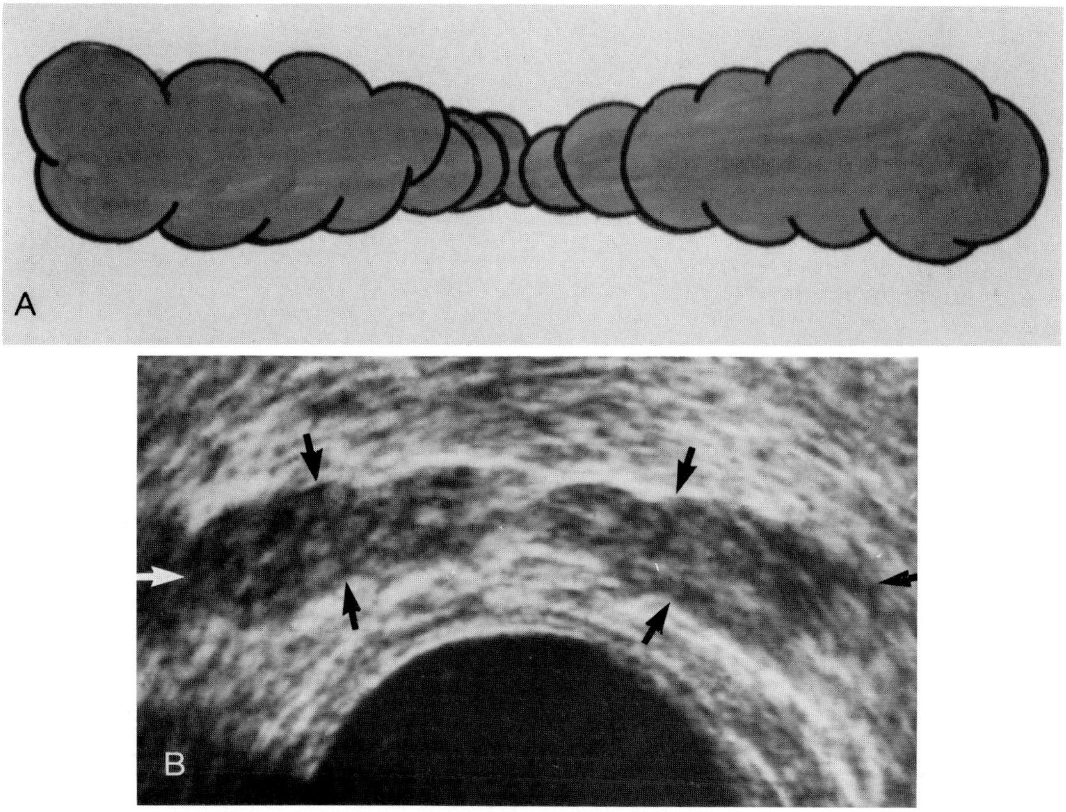

Figure 10.10. Seminal vesicles. Axially oriented views of the seminal vesicles (*arrows*) will demonstrate the structures to be symmetrical in size, shape, and echogenicity.

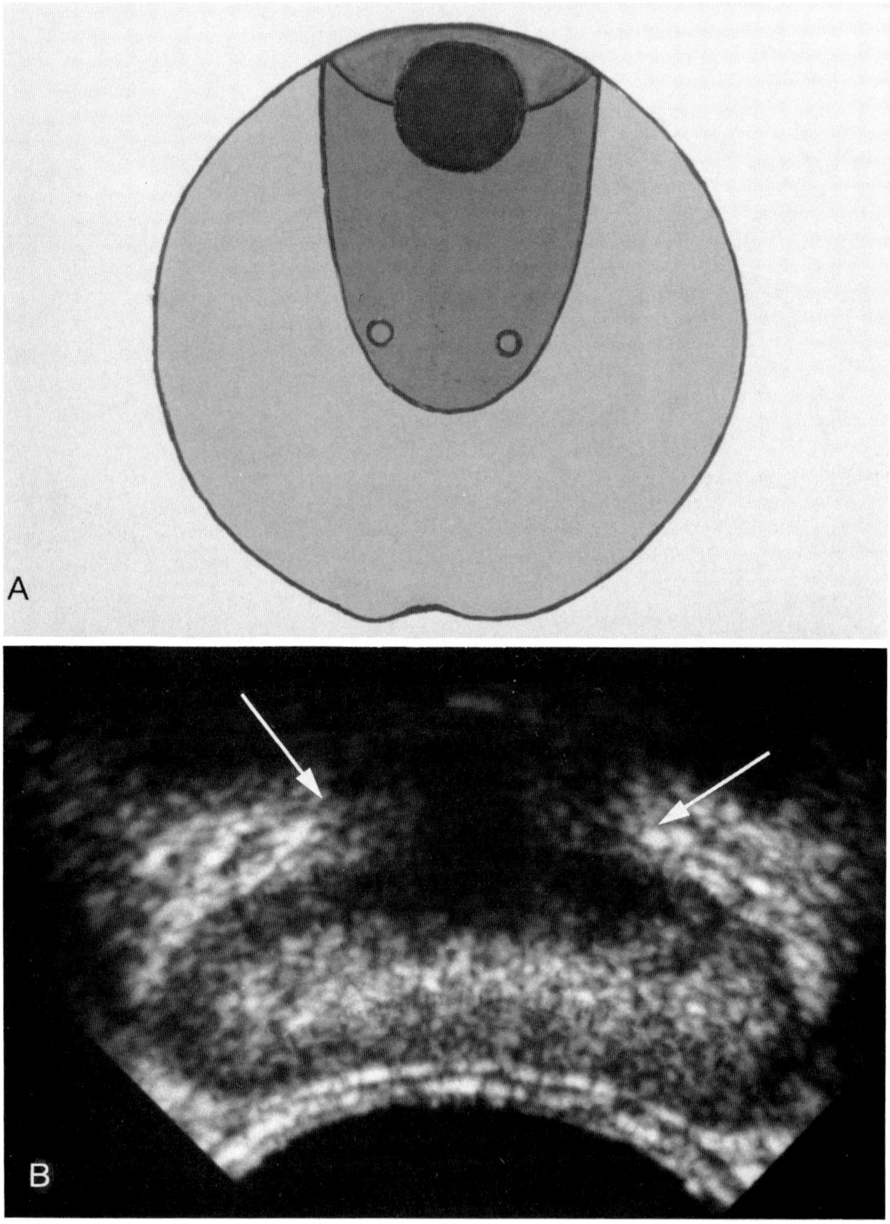

Figure 10.11. Base of the prostate. At the base of the prostate, a hypoechoic area (*arrows*) will differentiate the central or inner prostate from the outer gland. The hypoechoic area is composed of the smooth muscle of the internal sphincter and portions of the periurethral tissues.

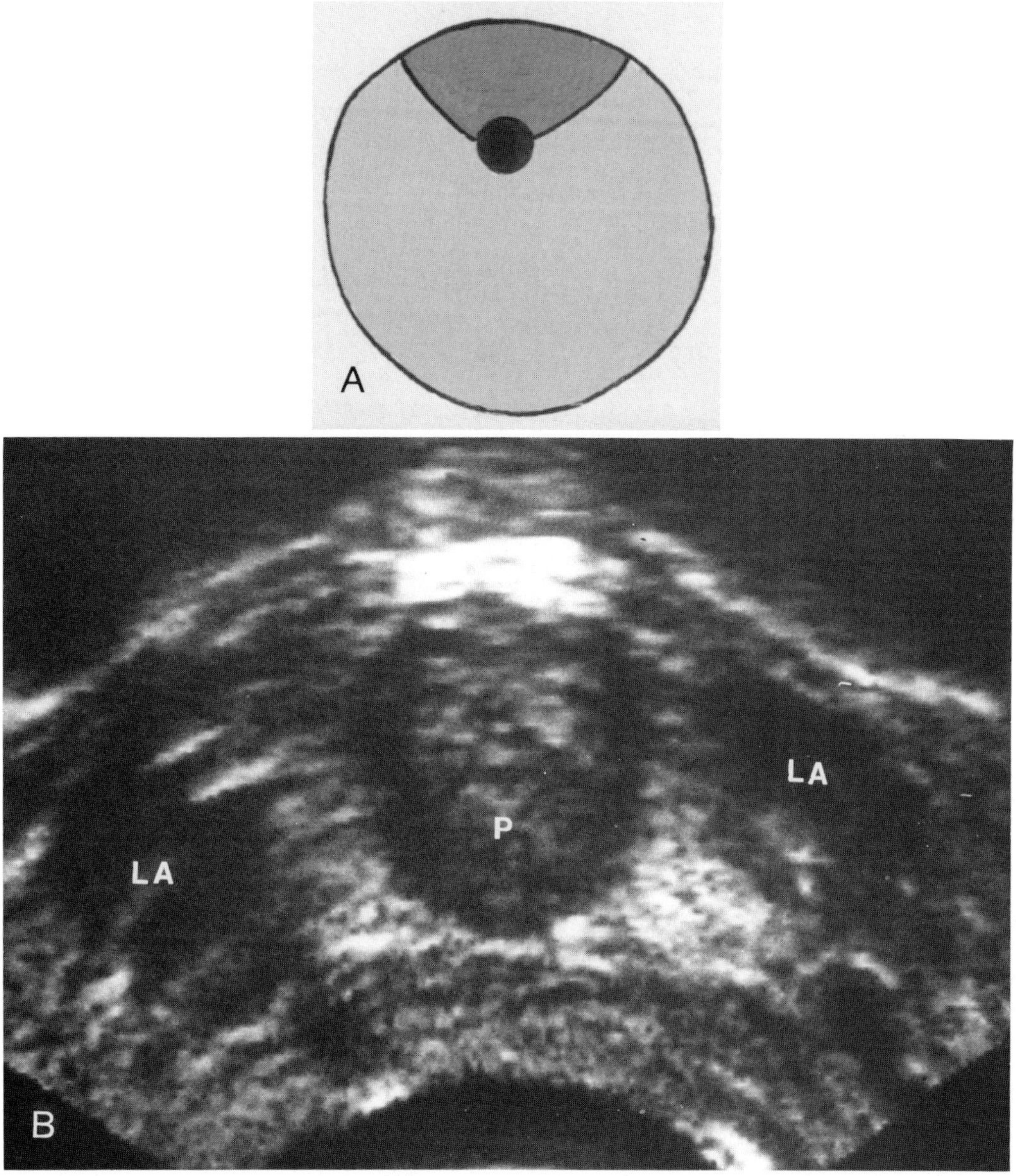

Figure 10.12. Apex of the prostate. Axial scans of the apex of the prostate (*P*) will demonstrate the gland to be homogeneous without delineation of the structures situated at the base. The prostate is smaller and is surrounded by the levator ani (*LA*) muscles laterally.

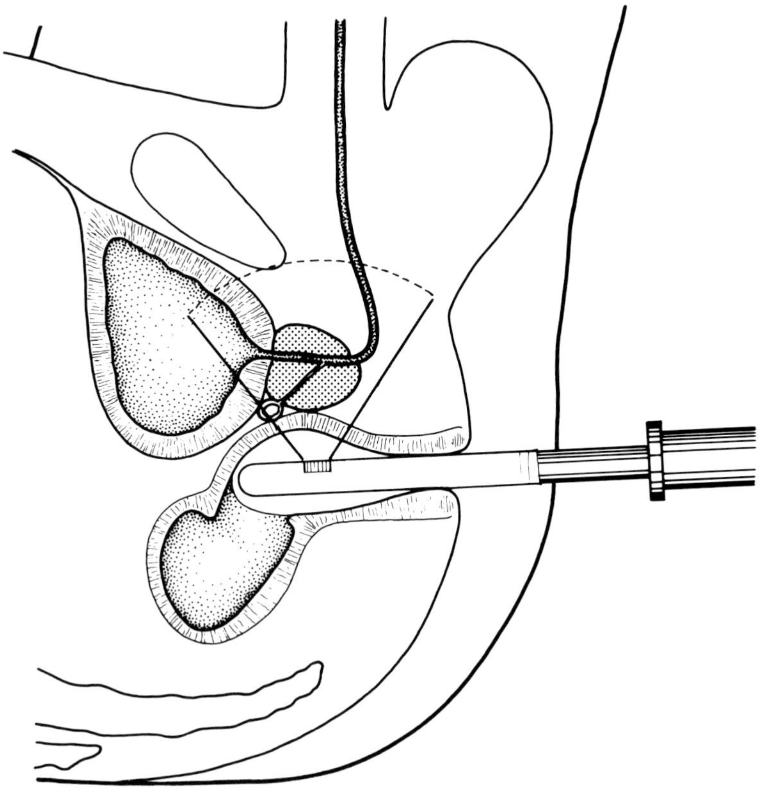

Figure 10.13. Longitudinal scanning is performed by placing a transducer within the rectum and identifying the entire prostate on a single image. (Reprinted with permission from Rifkin MD. Ultrasound of the prostate. New York: Raven Press, 1988.)

wise (Fig. 10.15). As the probe is rotated, the hypoechoic central structures (inner prostate) and the urethra are no longer seen (Fig. 10.16). The prostate then appears relatively homogeneously echogenic with a surrounding highly echogenic margin, the periprostatic fat. The periprostatic fat is seen surrounding the prostate, except at the apex of the prostate, where the external sphincter is present and at the superior midline portion of the gland at the base of the prostate.

The so-called coronal images are not truly coronal. They are obliquely oriented axial or obliquely oriented coronal images (Fig. 10.17). To obtain these, a transducer with an end- or oblique-fire orientation is necessary. The probe is placed in the rectum and angled toward the urinary bladder. This will evaluate the base of the prostate; when the probe is angled less steeply, toward the anterior abdomen, an oblique axial orientation of the body and apex of the gland is obtained. These images are very similar in appearance to the true axial scans but have an elongated appearance (Fig. 10.18).

On both the coronal and axial images, the prostate is surrounded by the highly echogenic periprostatic fat. This may be normally disrupted in the posterolateral margins of the prostate, where the neurovascular bundles are situated bilaterally. Symmetry should be preserved.

Anterior to the prostate in all orientations, tubular fluid-filled structures, the vessels of Santorini's plexus, may be identified.

SONOGRAPHIC CRITERIA FOR DIAGNOSIS

There are certain sonographic characteristics that are essential to understand prior to examining patients with suspected prostate pa-

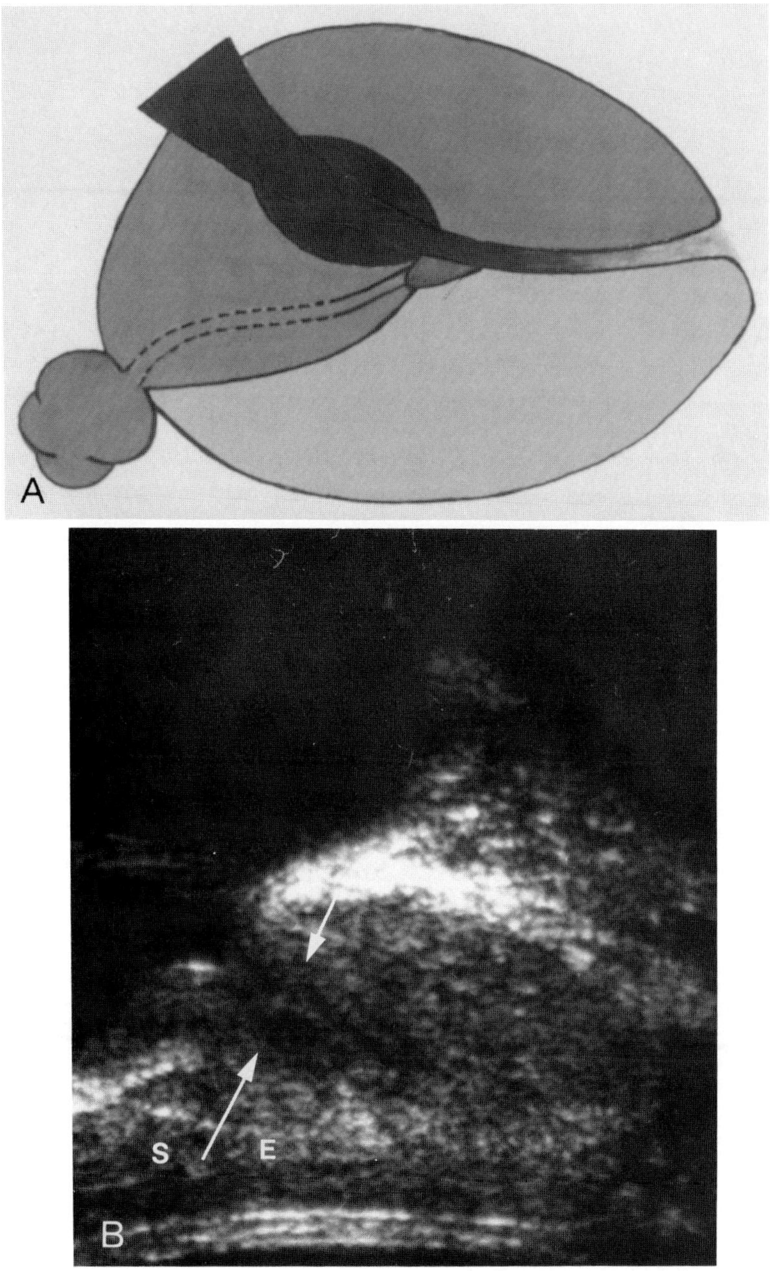

Figure 10.14. Midline longitudinal orientation will demonstrate a small hypoechoic area (*arrows*) corresponding to the inner prostate. The peripheral prostate has similar sonographic characteristics. The seminal vesicle (*S*) is identified as a more rounded structure at it is seen in cross section, and the ejaculatory duct (*E*) may be identified segmentally as a thin, hypoechoic structure surrounded by two slightly echogenic lines, the walls of the ejaculatory duct.

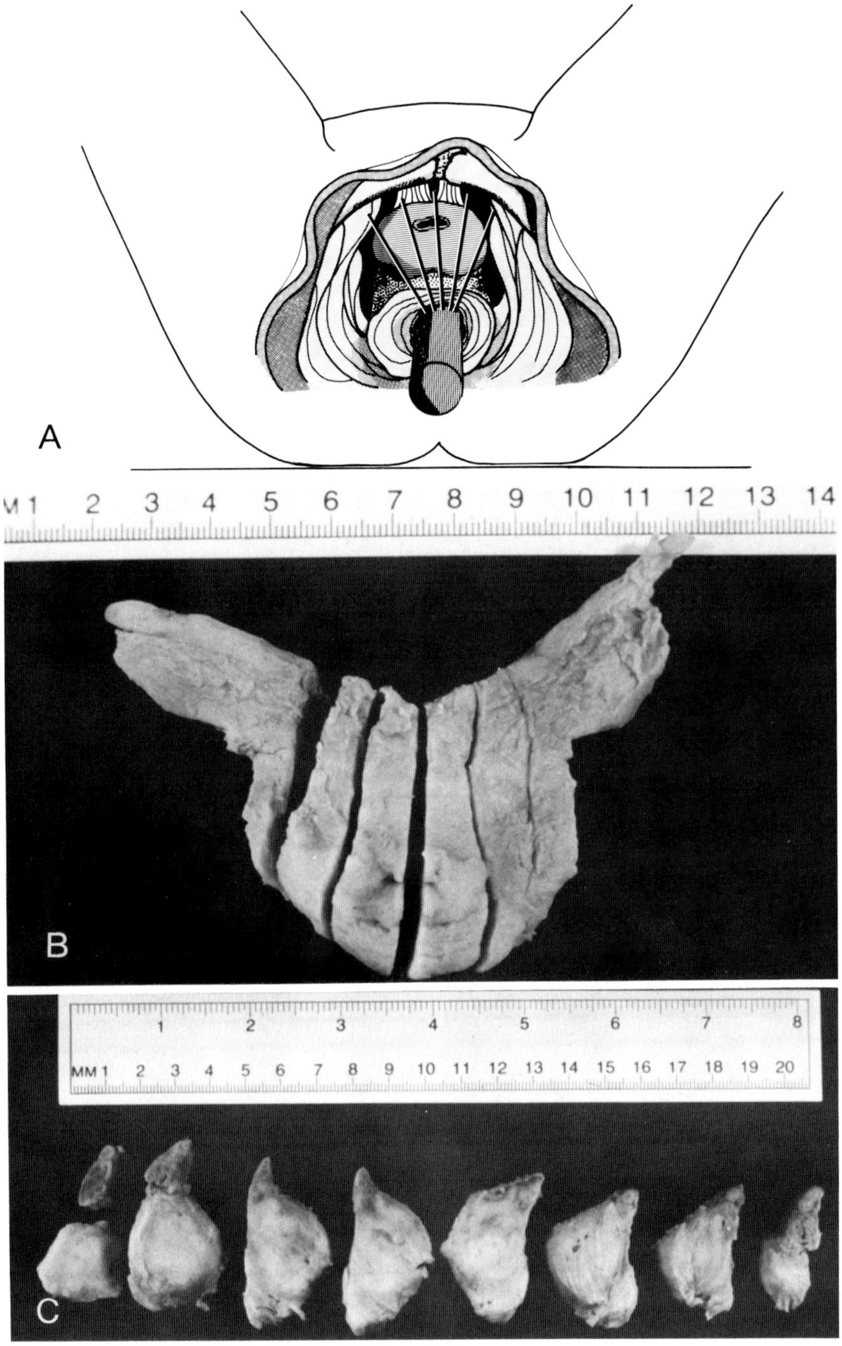

Figure 10.15. Lateral images, longitudinal orientation. To obtain lateral views of the prostate in a longitudinal orientation, the probe, when placed in the rectum, is rotated clockwise and counterclockwise (**A**). This will demonstrate pie-shaped sections of the prostate (**B** and **C**), with larger portions of the prostate in seen the midline and smaller portions laterally. The seminal vesicles will be cut in cross section and appear rounded or oblique. (Reprinted with permission from Rifkin MD. Ultrasound of the prostate. New York: Raven Press, 1988.)

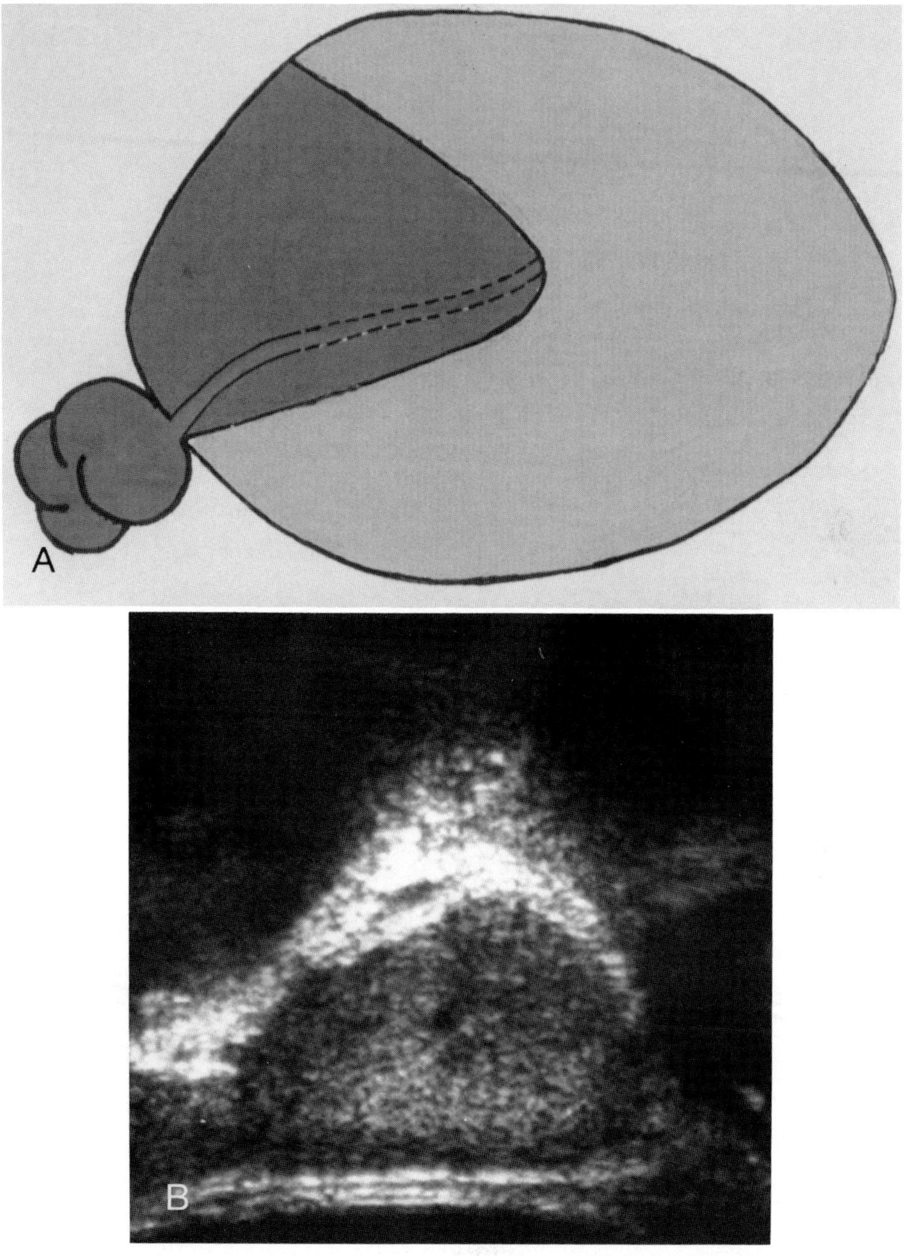

Figure 10.16. Lateral aspect of the prostate. When longitudinally oriented lateral aspects of the prostate are identified, a hypoechoic central or inner prostate is no longer seen, since this area is not positioned laterally. The gland will then appear relatively homogeneous, without differences in echogenicity in the central and peripheral zones.

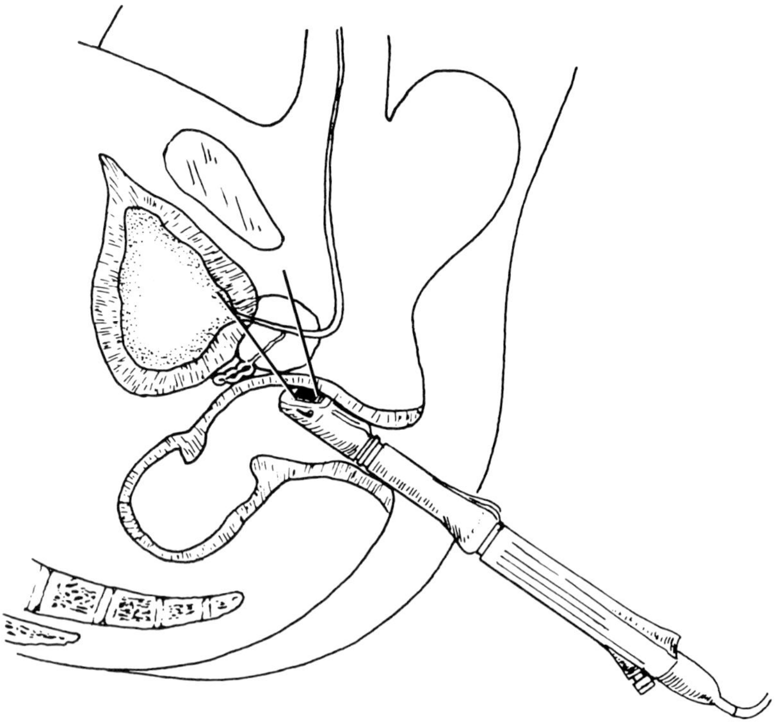

Figure 10.17. Oblique coronal-axial orientation. With an end- or oblique-fire transducer placed in the prostate, by angling the transducer slightly toward the base or apex of the gland, oblique images of the prostate will be obtained.

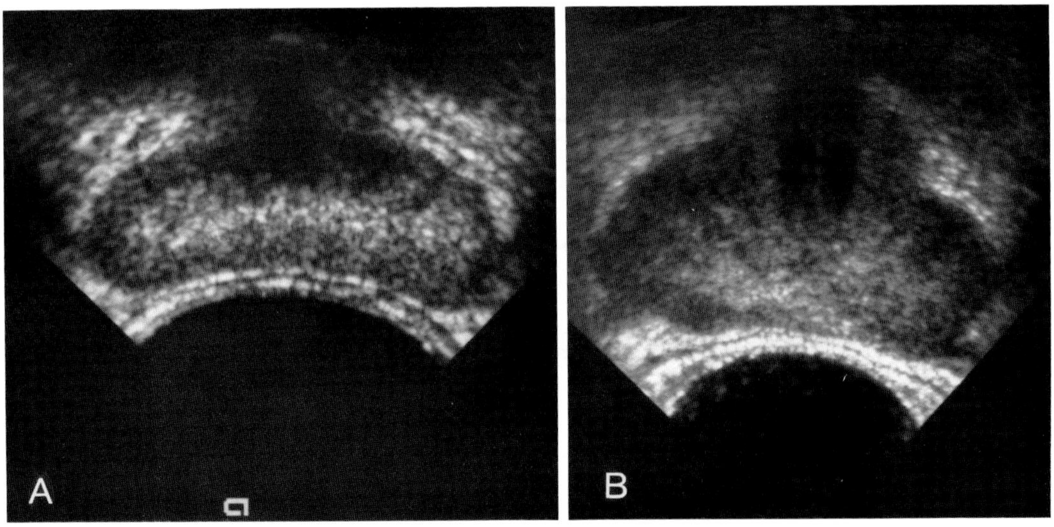

Figure 10.18. Oblique images of the prostate. True axial image (**A**) is compared to an oblique coronal-axial image (**B**) demonstrating elongation of the prostate.

thology. The prostate must be examined carefully. This includes the entire gland, the margins of the prostate, and intrinsic areas within the prostate. A suggested approach includes evaluation of the prostate (Table 10.3), foal lesions within the gland (Table 10.4), and the periprostatic tissues (Table 10.5) (15).

BENIGN HYPERPLASIA

Benign changes of the gland can include a variety of findings. Most commonly, benign prostatic hyperplasia (BPH) occurs. This develops from the transition zone and the periurethral glandular tissues and is frequently seen as a relatively well-differentiated mass that involves the periurethral area.

This area will occur in the normally hypoechoic internal sphincter–transition zone–periurethral glandular (inner prostate) area. It is frequently well demarcated (both on the sonogram and pathologically) from the uninvolved acinar tissues (Fig. 10.19). On occasion, BPH may be so large it causes compression of the central zone (so that it is essentially no longer seen) and may also compress the peripheral zone, which may appear to be only a few millimeters in thickness. Changes from BPH may also compress the lateral margins of the gland, causing capsular bulge and distortion. Benign change should never infiltrate or disrupt the capsule of the gland or infiltrate into the periprostatic fat (20).

Table 10.3.
Evaluation of Prostate

- Margins of prostate
  - Smooth
  - Irregular
- Capsule (pericapsular fat)
  - Intact
  - Disrupted
- Peripheral zone
  - Identified
    - Yes
    - No
  - Normal
    - Yes
    - No
- Central gland
  - Normal
  - Abnormal
    - Diffuse
    - Focal
- Architecture
  - Symmetrical
  - Asymmetrical
- Focal abnormality
  - Yes
  - No
- Urethra
  - Normal position
  - Abnormal position

Table 10.4.
Evaluation of Focal Lesions of the Prostate

- Are focal lesions present?
  - Yes
  - No
- How many?
- Where are they found?
  - Peripheral zone
  - Central gland
- Margins of focus
  - Well defined
  - Poorly defined
- Echogenicity of focus
  - Anechoic
  - Hypoechoic
  - Isoechoic
  - Hyperechoic
  - Mixed echogenicity
- Is there a halo sign present?
- Are there any calculi present?
  - Yes
  - No
  - Where?
- Secondary sonograpic characteristics
  - Shadowing (attenuation)
  - Enhancement

Table 10.5.
Evaluation of Periprostatic Tissues

- Capsule (pericapsular fat)
  - Normal
  - Bulged but intact
  - Eroded
  - Invaded
- Lymph nodes
  - Absent
  - Present
- Seminal vesicles
  - Symmetrical
  - Asymmetrical
- Seminal vesicle—prostate "nipple"
  - Normal
  - Abnormal
- Seminal vesicle—prostate "angle"
  - Normal
  - Abnormal

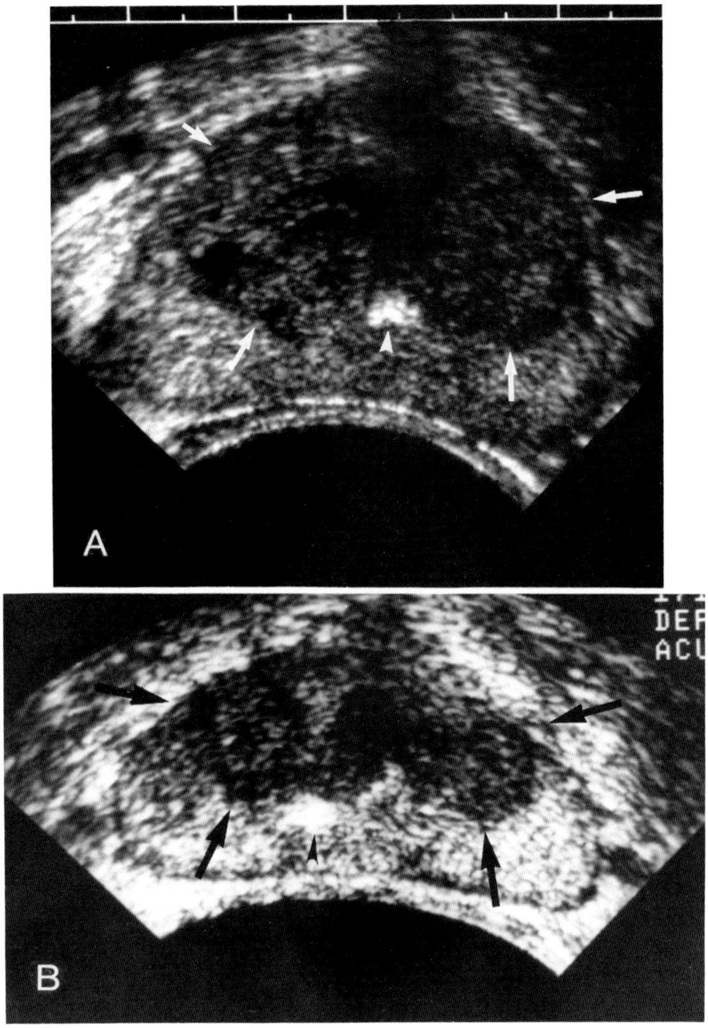

Figure 10.19. Benign prostatic hyperplasia. Classically, benign prostatic hyperplasia will be seen as enlargement of the central or inner prostate (*arrows*), causing compression and distortion of the peripheral prostate. There can be a variety of echogenic areas within the hyperplastic tissue corresponding to the combination of epithelial, muscular, and nodular components. Calcifications (*arrowheads*) may be seen within the areas separating the hyperplastic central or inner prostate and a compressed outer gland.

PROSTATITIS

Prostatitis is an inflammatory condition of the prostate that can affect men of all ages. It may preferentially involve the peripheral zone but can also involve the central tissues of the gland. A classic finding in acute prostatitis is a hypoechoic rim surrounding either the periurethral tissues or involving the acinar tissue. This hypoechoic area has been suggested to be edema. It is usually well demarcated.

Most commonly, prostatitis is not imaged until it is diagnosed in the later subacute or chronic stage. At this time, there is no distinctly abnormal sonographic appearance that is diagnostic of the disease process. Diffuse or focal abnormalities of the prostate may be seen, including architectural disruption or even focal hypoechoic areas within the central or peripheral portions of the prostate.

Prostatic abscesses may develop secondary to prostatitis or surgical manipulation; i.e., transurethral resection of the prostate, cystoscopy, etc. While most cases of prostatitis involve the peripheral prostate (and thus abscesses also develop in the outer gland), after manipulation, abscesses can develop centrally. Abscesses will generally be anechoic or relatively hypoechoic areas with good margins and relatively good through transmission, suggesting the predominantly fluid (although in many cases complicated fluid) nature of the collection (Fig. 10.20). Abscesses may also, as elsewhere in the body (when seen by ultrasound), have relatively thick walls. The diagnosis on ultrasound is not

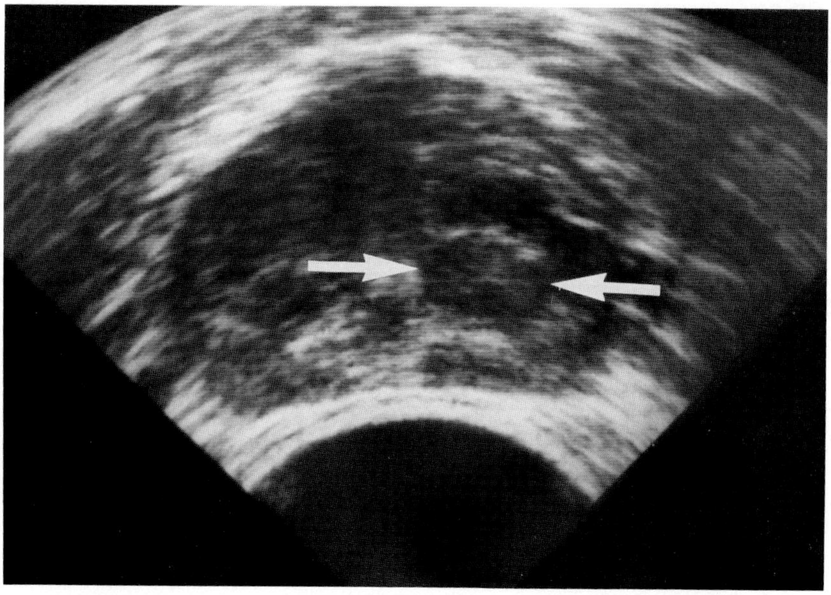

Figure 10.20. Prostatic abscess. Axial orientation demonstrates a relatively hypoechoic area (*arrows*) within the central gland. This corresponded to a prostatic abscess that developed following cystoscopy.

pathognomonic, and clinical correlation is often necessary (15).

CALCULI

Calculi may form as a secondary process to inflammation (i.e., chronic prostatitis), or may be a de novo dystrophic process. They usually develop from corpora amylacea, a proteinaceous material that is indigenous to the prostate. In general, the calculi form along the urethra (i.e., periurethral), however, in cases of benign prostatic hyperplasia, they may be seen along the periphery of the hyperplastic nodule, the area known as the surgical capsule.

Calculi, as seen on ultrasound, are usually brightly echogenic (Fig. 10.21). They are more echogenic than any other structures within the prostatic or periprostatic tissues. They may cause acoustic shadowing, particularly when large. Even the smaller calculi, a millimeter or two in size, will cause acoustic shadowing if a properly focused transducer with a narrow beam width is used. Careful scanning techniques may be necessary to demonstrate sonographic attenuation.

Calculi should never be confused with malignant change of the prostate. Prostatic calculi may occur in an area of malignancy. However, they are not due to the cancer.

MISCELLANEOUS BENIGN CONDITIONS

There are a variety of other conditions that may involve the prostate. Many of these can affect the outer gland and mimic malignancy. These include smooth muscle (particularly that surrounding the ejaculatory ducts), inflamed tissue, atrophy, and infarction, among others.

PROSTATE CANCER

Prostate cancer is a pervasive disease in the American male population. Sonographically, it may have a variety of appearances (21). A classic finding, particularly in the small cancer, is a hypoechoic (i.e., less echogenic than normal surrounding prostatic tissue) lesion in the peripheral prostate, particularly the peripheral zone (15, 21). These areas may range from having no internal echoes to having some subtle areas of (increased) echogenicity (Figs. 10.22 to 10.25). While cancers are well seen because of their contrast differences, they are usually irregular with poorly defined margins. They are frequently situated adjacent to the prostatic capsule. Bulging and erosion may be seen, a sign indicative of an invasive process. These lesions can be seen when they are as small as a few millimeters. As these hypoechoic lesions enlarge, they can spread along the capsule and

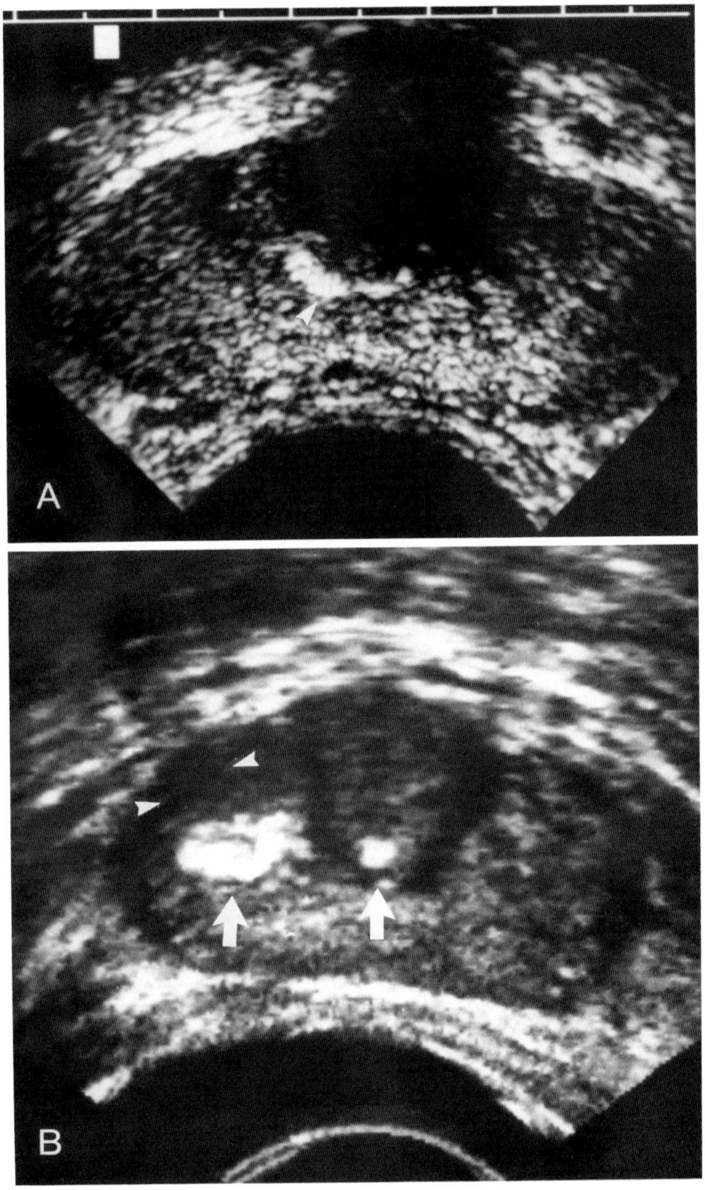

Figure 10.21. Calcifications. Calculi within the prostate will appear brightly echogenic (*arrows*). Depending on their size and the technique used during scanning, the calcifications may not shadow (**A**) or may demonstrate subtle acoustic shadowing (*arrowheads* in **B**).

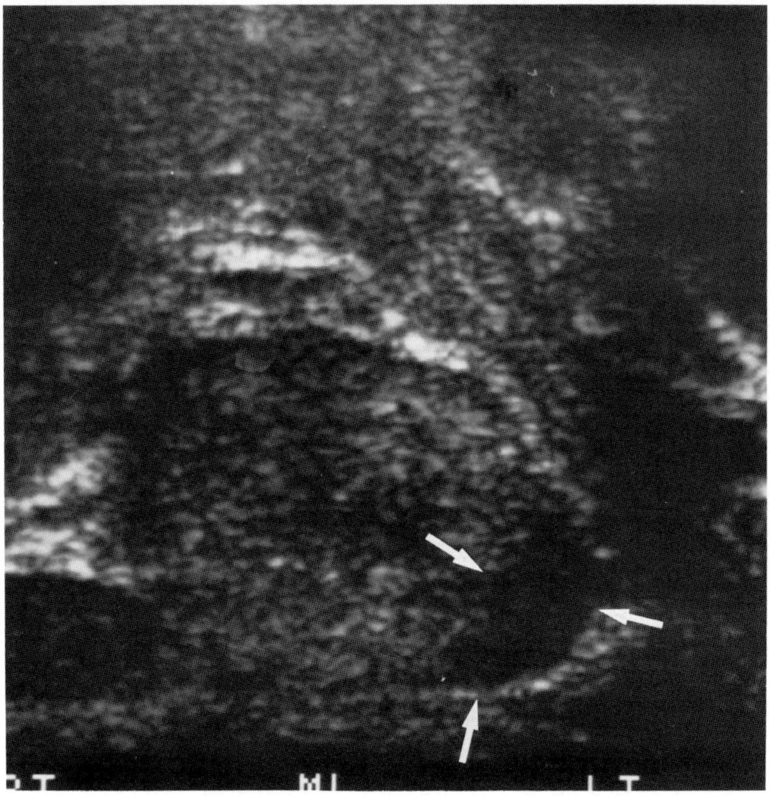

Figure 10.22. Prostate cancer. Longitudinal orientation demonstrates an essentially anechoic lesion (*arrows*) in the apex of the prostate. This is not a fluid-filled collection, there are no sharp walls, and no good through transmission is identified.

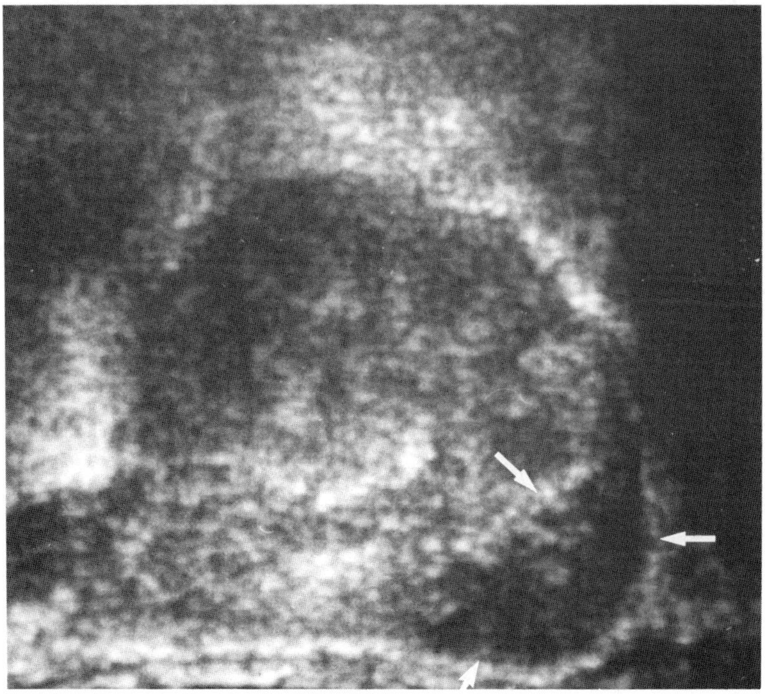

Figure 10.23. Prostate cancer situated in the apex of the prostate (*arrows*) is seen on this longitudinal scan. While the lesion is hypoechoic, there are subtle scattered acoustic reflectors within the tumor.

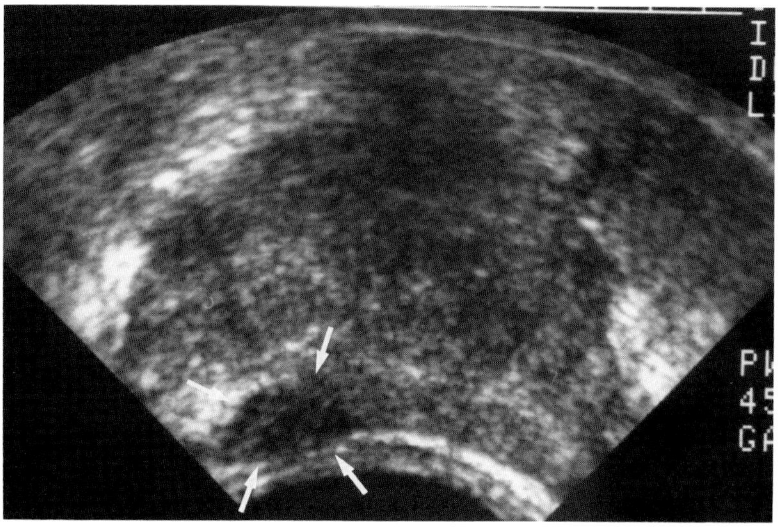

Figure 10.24. Prostate cancer. Axial orientation demonstrates asymmetric focus in the right posterior portion of the prostate (*arrows*) corresponding to the cancer. There are subtle acoustic reflectors within this hypoechoic lesion.

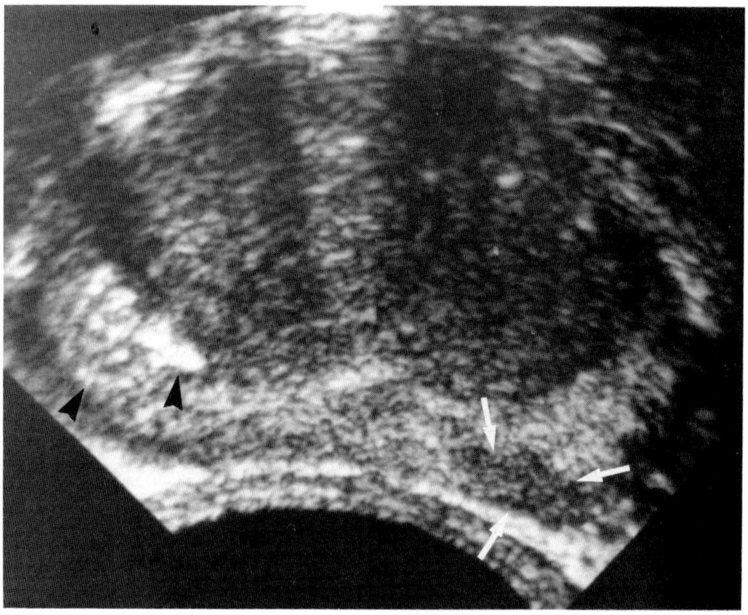

Figure 10.25. Prostate cancer. In the left posterolateral aspect of the prostate (*arrows*) a cancer is seen as a hypoechoic, poorly marginated lesion disrupting the normally hyperechoic peripheral prostate. Note calcifications (*arrowheads*) in the right lateral aspect of the prostate. These are unrelated to cancer.

appear elongated, infiltrate through the capsule, or actually extend into the inner prostatic tissues. Lesions as they enlarge may also appear to be slightly more echogenic than the smaller tumors and have been called (depending on the researcher) slightly more echogenic (or hypoechoic) compared to normal prostatic tissue, or to have mixed echogenic appearances (21–25) (Figs. 10.26 to 10.29). There is much confusion regarding these types of lesions. The areas of increased echogenicity are quite subtle and generally are not indicative of prostate calculi, but are more likely due to infiltration of normal or benign prostatic tissues. These lesions are poorly marginated and may be seen in larger lesions.

An isoechoic lesion is one that cannot be differentiated from normal prostatic tissue sonographically by echogenic characteristics. However, they may cause capsular bulge.

The exact cause of changes in echogenicity has not been clearly differentiated but it has been suggested to be due to changes in cellular differentiation, tumor size, fibrous reaction, or other causes (11, 15, 20, 21, 23). A study demonstrated that the well-differentiated tumors are in general more hypoechoic than normal tissue, the more isoechoic lesions are moderately differentiated, and the more anaplastic lesions have mixed or hyperechoic characteristics (11). Another study has suggested that 25% of cancers are not seen by ultrasound (and are thus isoechoic) (24). A further study has suggested that increasing echogenicity may be related not only to cellular differentiation but also to the amount of fibrosis present within the tumor (21).

Regardless of the reason or cause for echogenic changes, the following characteristics are suggested that will help differentiate a normal from an abnormal area.

1. A distinctly abnormal echogenic focus within the peripheral zone.

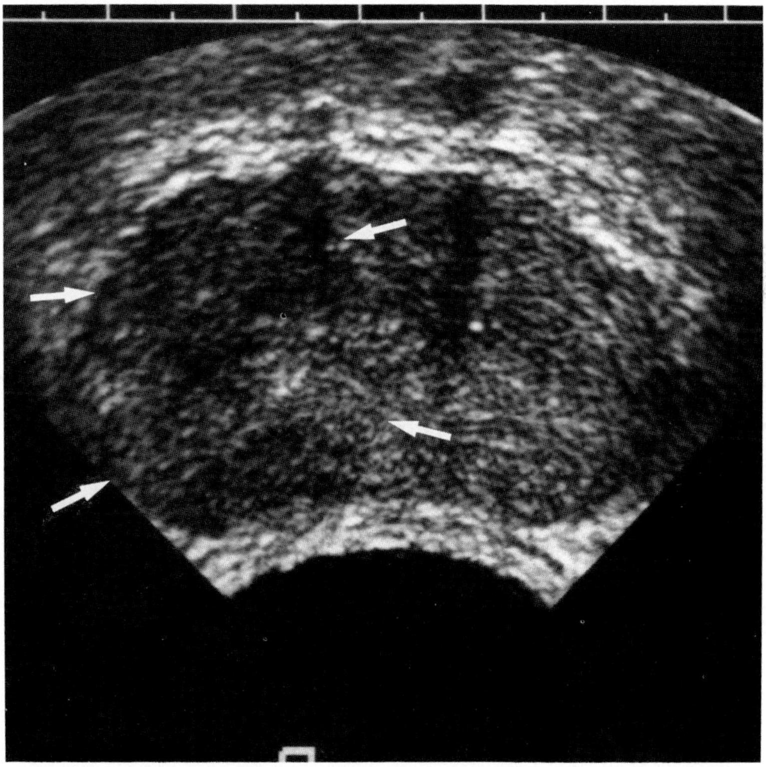

Figure 10.26. Prostate cancer. Prostate cancer is seen infiltrating the entire posterior and right lateral aspects of the prostate (*arrows*). The tissue is not clearly defined, although there are subtle hypoechoic areas.

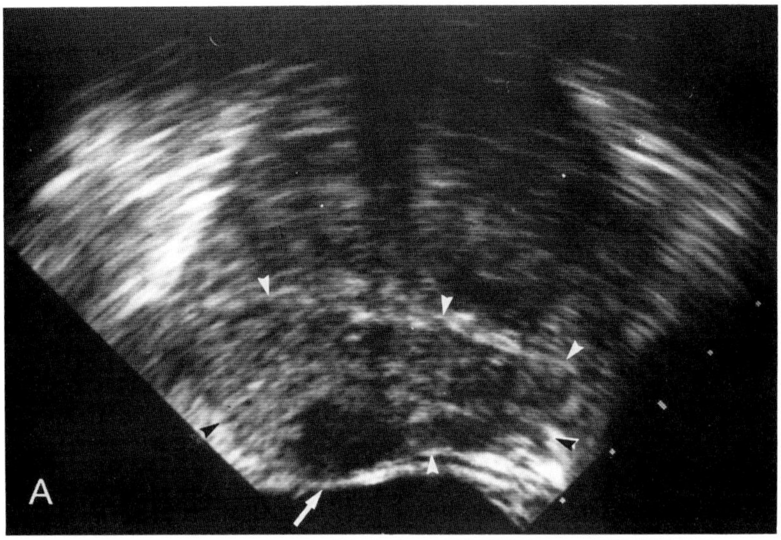

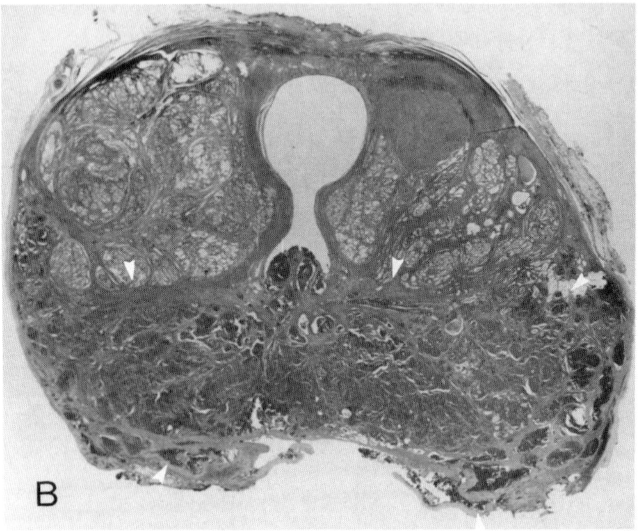

Figure 10.27. Prostate cancer. A small hypoechoic focus (*arrow*) is seen in the posterior portion of the prostate. However, the entire posterior prostate as defined by the ultrasound (**A**) and radical prostatectomy section (**B**) is involved by cancer (*arrowheads*).

2. Asymmetry in echogenic characteristics of the prostate, particularly the peripheral zone.
3. Asymmetry in size or shape of the prostate, particularly in the peripheral zone.
4. Capsular distortion.
5. Capsular disruption.
6. Loss of normal differentiation between the central tissues and the peripheral zone.

Specificity of Prostate Cancer

Unfortunately, while the sonogram may differentiate many abnormal areas on the sonogram, regardless of the echogenic characteristics, it is not a pathognomonic diagnosis for a specific process. Thus, sonographically guided biopsies must be undertaken (which are described below). It has been shown that the positive predictive value of a peripherally oriented hypoechoic lesion has ranged from 0 to 50% (Table 10.6) (26–31). Overall, the average positive predictive value of peripherally oriented hypoechoic lesions being malignant is approximately 25 to 30%. Lesions that are palpable or have an elevated prostate-specific antigen (PSA) level are more likely malignant than

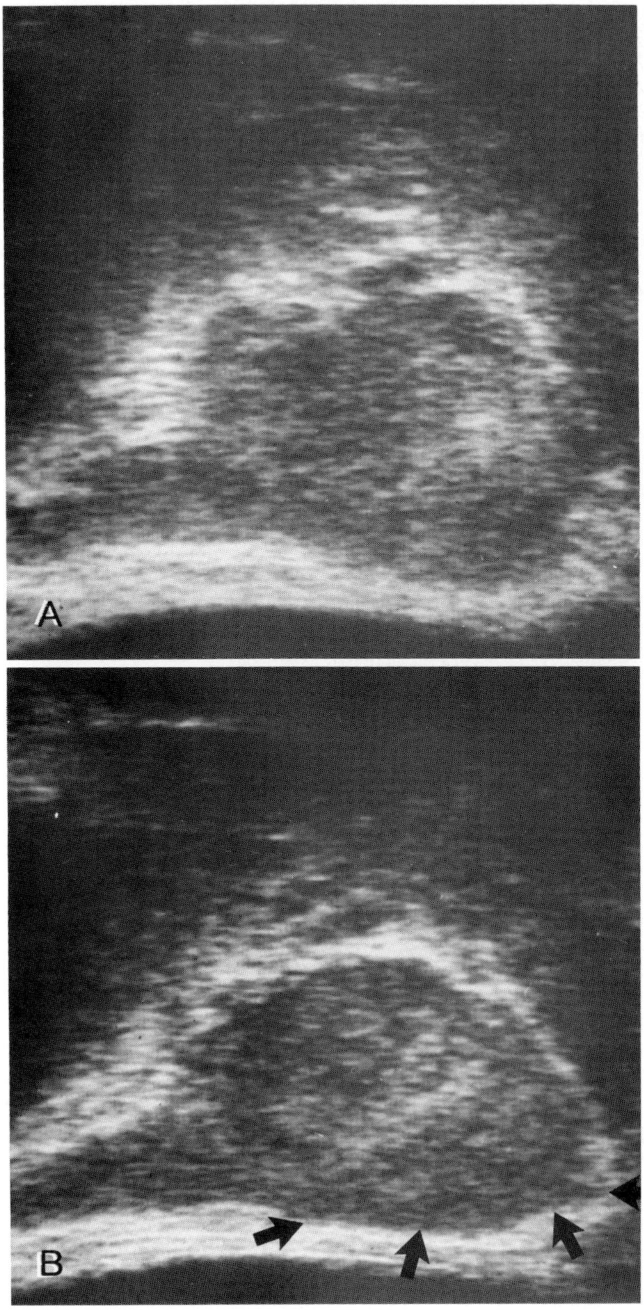

Figure 10.28. Prostate cancer. Two longitudinally oriented scans, one on the patient's right (**A**) and the other on the patient's left (**B**), demonstrate no differences in acoustic reflectivity. However, there is capsular bulge on the left (*arrows*), capsular infiltration that are suggestive of an isoechoic but obvious cancer if secondary sonographic characteristics are identified. (Reprinted with permission from Rifkin MD. Ultrasound of the prostate. New York: Raven Press, 1988.)

those that are nonpalpable or have a normal PSA level (32).

Prostate Biopsy

While it may not be necessary to biopsy all palpable prostatic lesions with ultrasound guidance, it is a very valuable tool, particularly for subtle or nonpalpable lesions (33–35). A number of techniques can be used for sonographically guided prostate biopsy. All are relatively equally accurate and have their major advantages and disadvantages (15). The most frequently used and easiest approaches include endorectal sonographically guided transperineal (36–39) and transrectal biopsies (15, 20, 40). The transperineal biopsy requires that the patient be in the lithotomy position, and local anesthesia must be used. The transrectal

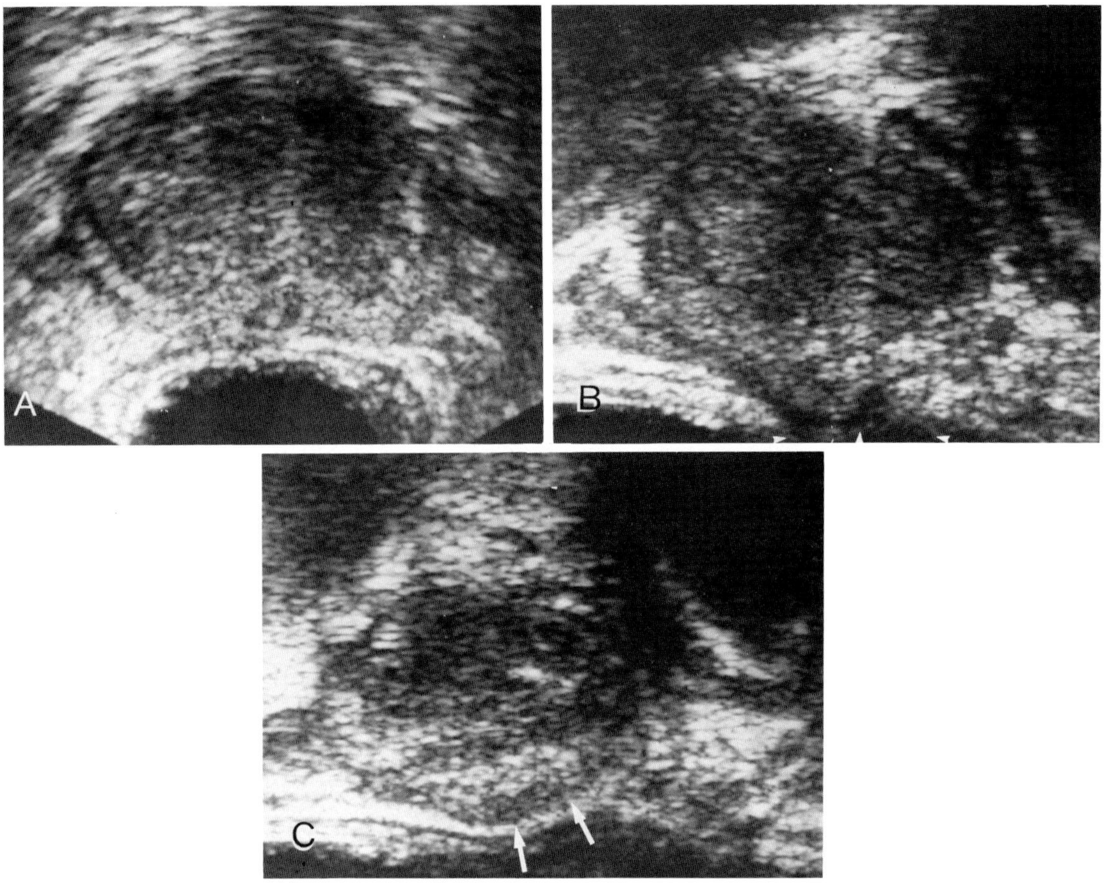

Figure 10.29. Prostate cancer. An isoechoic prostate cancer seen on the axial image (**A**). There is disruption of the peripheral prostatic fat by tumor. This is better appreciated on the longitudinally oriented linear array scans, which demonstrate clear destruction of the periprostatic on the right fat (**B**) compared to the left (**C**). (Reprinted with permission from Rifkin MD. Ultrasound of the prostate. New York: Raven Press, 1988.)

biopsy can be performed with the patient in the decubitus position and does not require the use of anesthesia.

The use of an automatic trigger device has greatly simplified the biopsy, increased the rapidity of the biopsy, and eliminated most of the discomfort. It is essential when using these automatic trigger devices, regardless of the approach used, that the needle be placed in front of the lesion so that the excursion of the needle will obtain tissue at the level of the tumor.

TRANSPERINEAL BIOPSY

The longitudinally oriented linear array or sector scanner can be used for guidance for the transperineal biopsy. To perform this biopsy, the patient is placed in the lithotomy position (Fig. 10.30). Both cytology and core biopsies can be used. To perform the biopsy, following a diagnostic ultrasound, the perineum should be cleansed with an antimicrobial solution. Extensive 1% xylocaine should be given. A skin "wheal" should be raised in the area to be biopsied, i.e., right, midline, or left side, then deeper subcutaneous tissue anaesthesia should be given. Then, using ultrasound for guidance, a longer needle should be placed into the deeper subcutaneous tissues and the pericapsular region of the prostate. Local anesthesia should then be given to these areas. While initially the patient may experience some burning, if an appropriate interval of time (approximately 15 to 30 seconds) is allowed between injections of local anesthesia, the patient should experience

Table 10.6.
Positive Predictive Value (PPV) of the Hypoechoic Peripheral Lesion Diagnosed by Ultrasound-Guided Biopsy

	No. of Lesions	No. of Cancers	PPV	Reference
			%	
	80	17	21.7	26
	353	89	25	27
	109	20	18	28
	149	77	52	29
	43	0	0	30
	138	50	36	31
Total	872	255	29	

little, if any, discomfort. Overall, about 15 to 20 ml of 1% xylocaine should be administered.

Following administration of local anesthesia, the probe is placed in the rectum and rotated to the lesion to be biopsied. A guide should be attached prior to probe insertion, and the needle placed in the appropriate groove, into the subcutaneous tissues of the perineum, and advanced to the lesion to be biopsied. Cytology or core biopsies can be performed with direct visualization of the needle entering the lesion.

Complications are quite unusual with a transperineal biopsy and include at most minor hematuria. Because sterile technique is used, no antibiotic treatment is usually required and no patient preparation is usually needed.

TRANSRECTAL BIOPSY

The transrectal biopsy uses a slightly different technique. The patient is placed in the decubitus position with the knees toward the patient's chest. Prior to biopsy, a cleansing enema should be given and antibiotic treatment administered prophylactically. The longitudinal or oblique longitudinally oriented images can be used, although an end-fire transducer permits immediate changing between the axial and longitudinal orientations (Fig. 10.31). Once the probe is placed into the rectum with the appropriate guide attached, the lesion is localized, the needle guide line of sight placed on the screen, and the biopsy needle advanced. The tip of the needle is seen compressing upon the rectal tissues, and the biopsy can be performed with either core biopsy or aspiration technique. Because of the rapidity of the procedure and the lack of nerve fibers within the rectal wall (but not the anal sphincter, which is highly sensitive to needle puncture), the biopsy is usually simple, accurate, and essentially pain free. Complications, however, are not uncommon, although they are usually not clinically significant. The most frequent include hematuria, hematospermia, and hematochezia. The risk of urosepsis is approximately 1%.

COMPARISON OF TRANSRECTAL AND TRANSPERINEAL BIOPSIES

Both approaches are highly accurate for diagnosing prostatic pathology. The rectal biopsy can be used with great accuracy for almost all lesions. However, theoretically, if fluid-filled lesions or abscesses are suspected, the use of the transrectal biopsy may "superinfect" the lesion. Thus, it may be prudent to use the transperineal approach for these areas. Additionally, when using a transrectal approach, the needle may perforate the anterior venous plexus when biopsying a very anterior prostate lesion. It may be advisable in these circumstances to use the transperineal approach, where the vessels can be more easily avoided.

Table 10.7.
Staging of Prostate Cancer

Stage A and stage B cancers are clinically felt to be confined to the prostate without extension into the periprostatic fat or pelvic lymph nodes and beyond.
- Stage A1 tumors—lesions that are histologically well differentiated and are present in only a few "chips" or pieces of the specimen
- Stage A2 tumors—lesions that are histologically anaplastic or, if histologically well differentiated, present in a large amount of the specimen

Stage B tumors are clinically palpable. These can be subdivided into:
- Stage B1 tumors—those that are confined to one portion of the gland
  - Stage B1N—tumors that are confined to one side of the gland and measure less than 1.5 cm in diameter
- Stage B2 tumors—tumors that are multifocal or are large, i.e., present on both sides of the prostate.

Stage C and D tumors have extended beyond the confines of the prostate.
- Stage C1 tumors—those that have extended beyond the confines of the prostate into the periprostatic fat
- Stage C2 tumors—those that involve the seminal vesicle(s).
- Stage D tumors—those that have extended into the pelvic lymphs or beyond

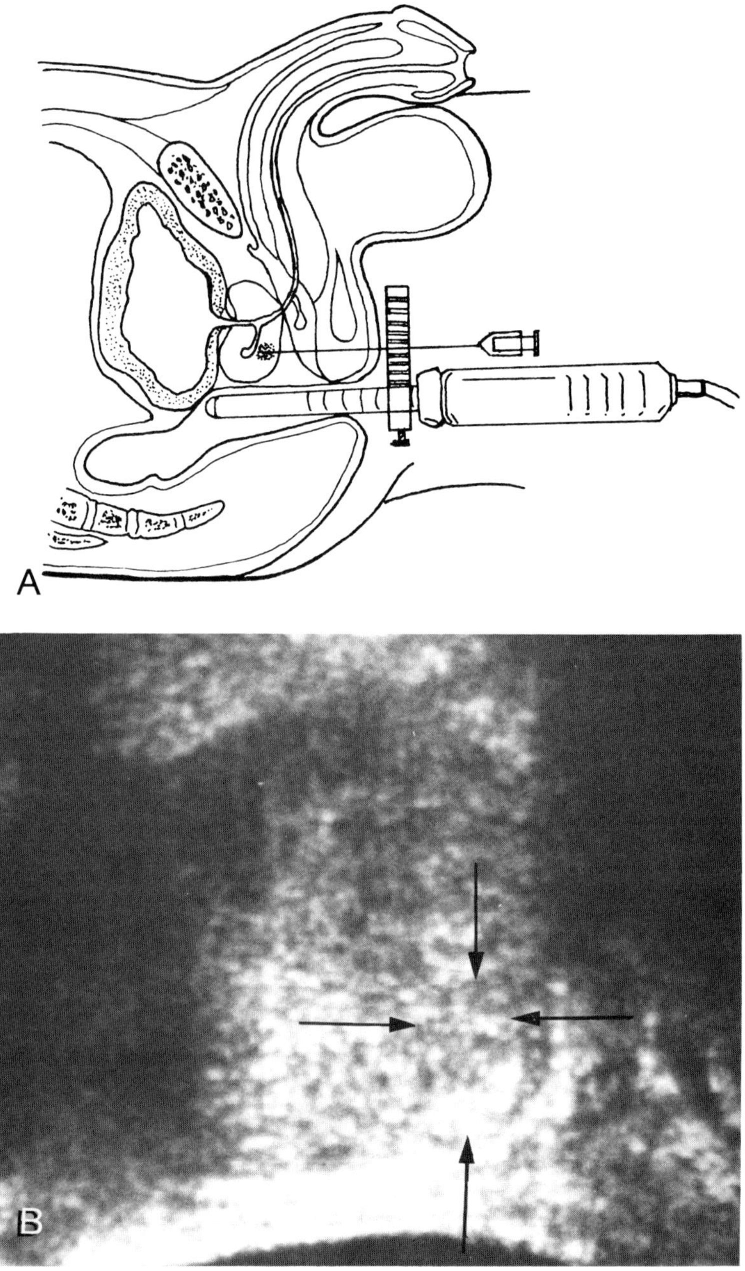

Figure 10.30. Transperineal oriented biopsy. **A,** The technique of longitudinally oriented transperineal biopsy. **B,** Preliminary scan demonstrates a hypoechoic area of disruption (*arrows*). **C, D, E,** Line of sight is placed on the screen and the needle (*arrowheads*) is sequentially advanced until the biopsy is performed.

COMPLICATIONS

Complications for each approach are usually clinically insignificant. However, hematuria, hematospermia, and blood in the fecal material are more common (although not necessarily clinically significant) with the transrectal biopsy.

Theoretically, the risk of sepsis developing is increased (even with administration of pro-

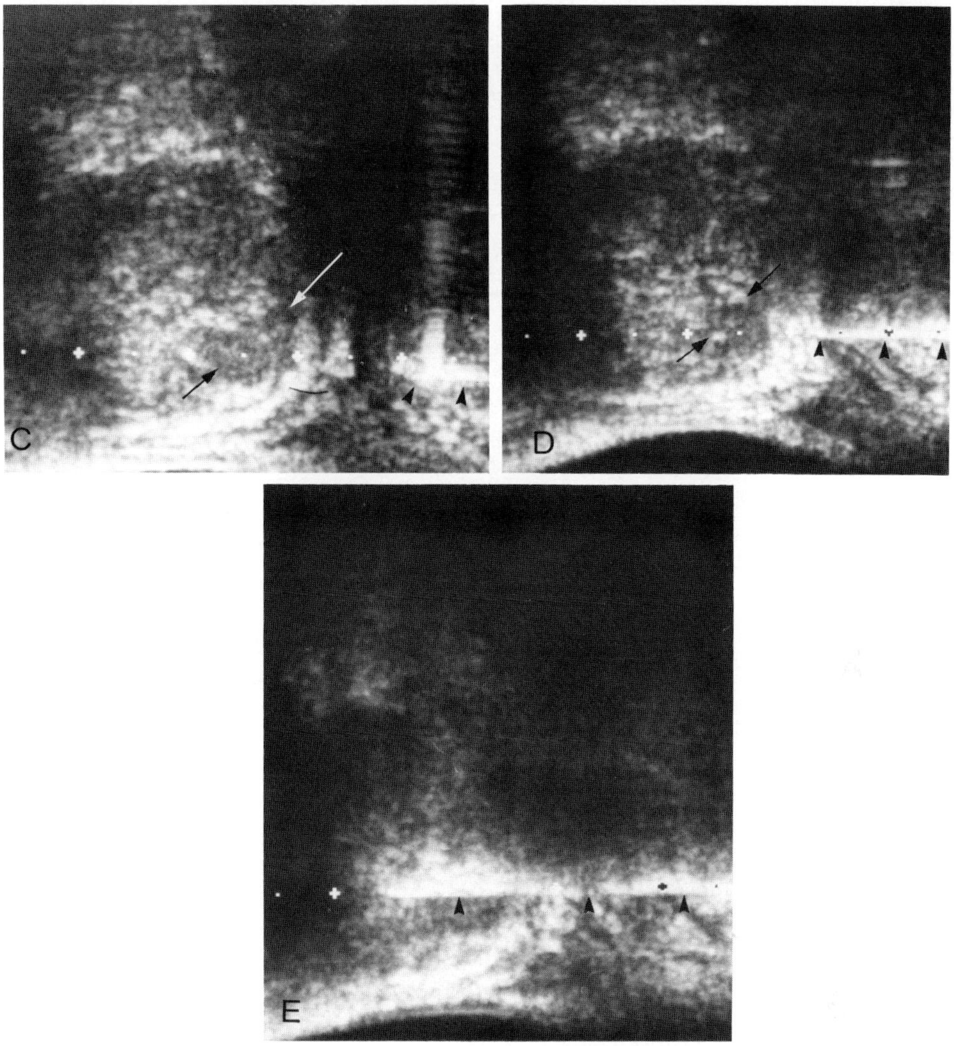

Figure 10.30. C, D, and **E.**

phylactic antibiotics) with the transrectal approach. However, this complication is still unusual.

Not all prostatic lesions should necessarily be biopsied by endorectal sonographic guidance. There are many prostate cancers that are palpable but may not be identified clearly by prostate ultrasound because of their isoechoic characteristics. In these cases, it is recommended that conventional digitally guided biopsy be performed first for a digitally palpated lesion. Only when the biopsy is negative and the clinical suspicion is still high should sonographically guided biopsy be undertaken. However, for subtly palpable or the nonpalpable lesions, ultrasound-guided biopsy is the only accurate technique for obtaining a diagnosis.

Staging

Diagnosis of prostate cancer is only one aspect of imaging. Staging or evaluation of the extent of disease is also essential when performing imaging. It is necessary to evaluate the extent of tumor, since treatment may vary, depending on the localization or extent of spread of cancer at the time of diagnosis. While a number of systems are used in the United States, the modified Whitmore-Jewett system is most frequently used. This categorizes the extent of prostate cancer into a number of

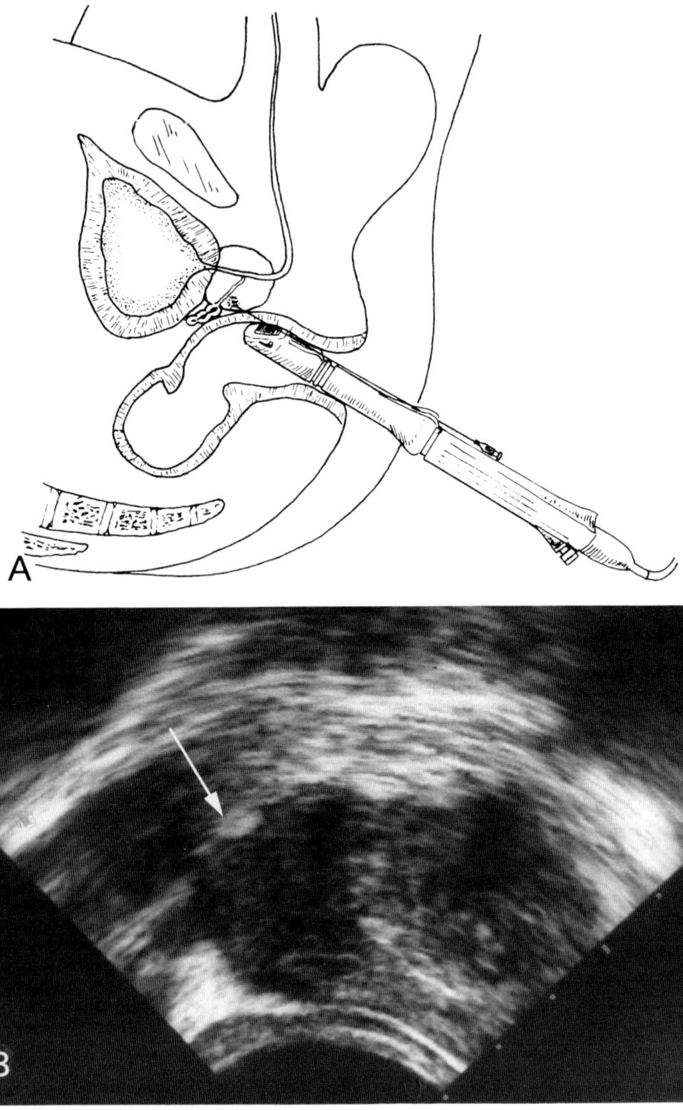

Figure 10.31. Transrectal biopsy. **A,** Line diagram demonstrates the theory and technique of transrectal biopsy. **B,** A preliminary axially oriented scan demonstrates a hypoechoic area (*arrow*) of abnormality in the right lateral aspect of the prostate. **C,** The lesion is seen with longitudinally oriented sector scan technique. **D,** Biopsy is performed showing the needle (*arrowheads*) within the lesion during biopsy.

groups, i.e., clinically suspected versus non-suspected, size, local disease versus spread of cancer, and pelvic lymph node involvement (Table 10.7). Staging is quite important, since advanced disease (stage C and D cancers) are treated differently from more localized (stage A and B) tumors. A variety of imaging modalities can be used for staging prostate cancer. These include computed tomography (CT) and magnetic resonance imaging (MRI) in addition to ultrasound. CT and MRI both detect lymphadenopathy. CT has little success in detecting focal disease of the prostate or subtle extension into periprostatic fat. MRI can detect intrinsic disease of the gland as well as capsular infiltration.

Prostate ultrasound using an endorectal approach is limited to the evaluation of intrinsic disease. Both capsular infiltration and seminal vesicle involvement can be detected by endorectal ultrasound.

Capsular infiltration is defined and detected as capsular bulge and asymmetry of the gland with irregularity of the periprostatic fat (the

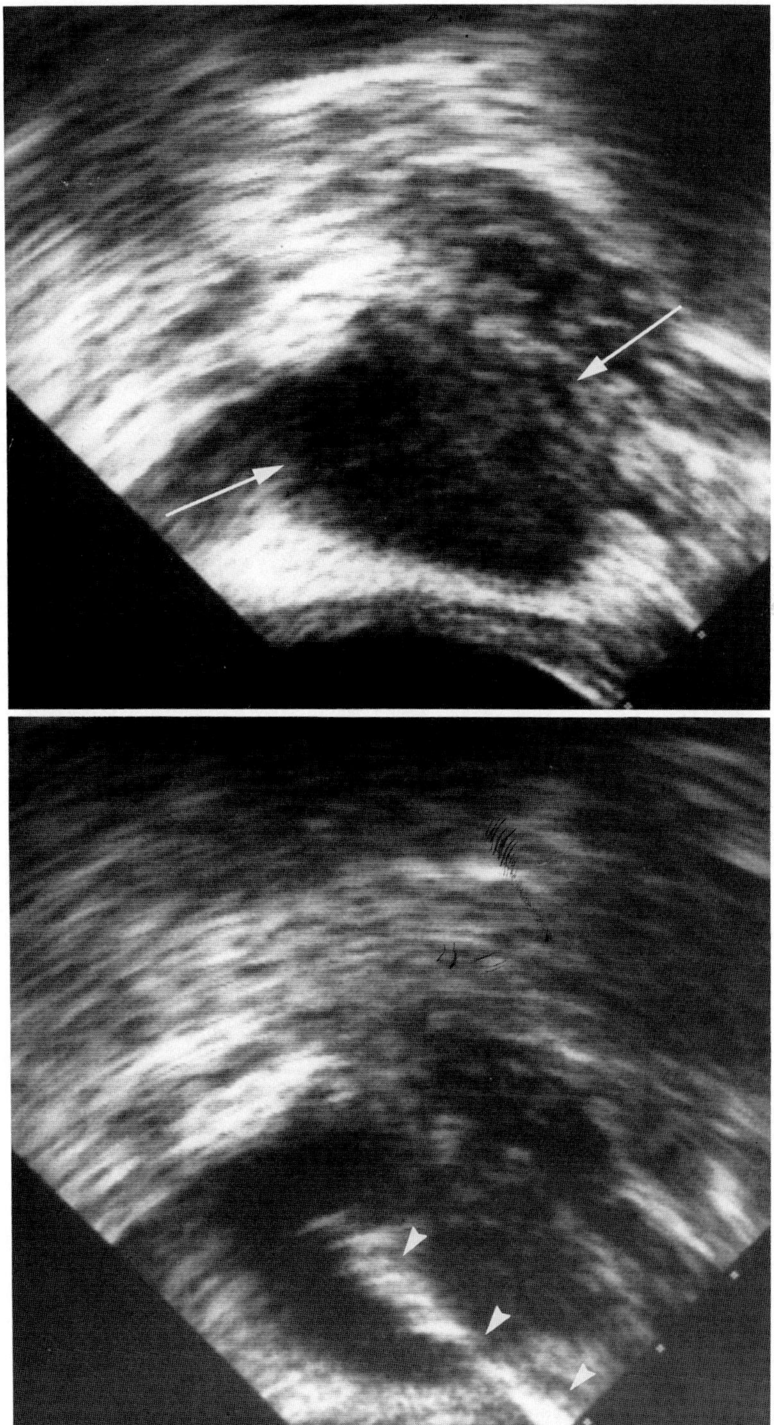

Figure 10.31 C and **D.**

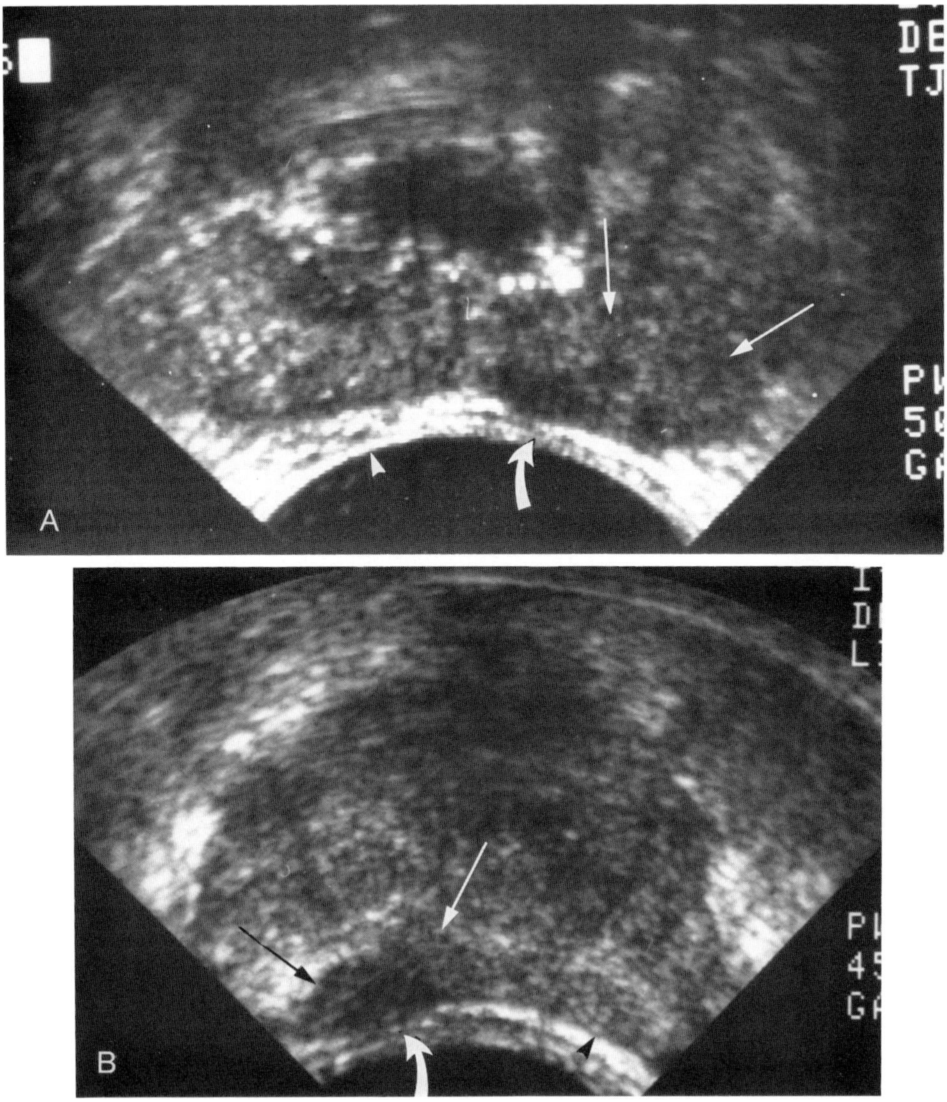

Figure 10.32. Fat infiltration. Two different patients demonstrate poorly defined **(A)** and well-defined **(B)** cancers (*arrows*). Note that the bright echogenic fat, which is normally identified in the uninvolved areas (*arrowheads*) is disrupted (*curved arrows*) at the site of pericapsular fat infiltration.

hyperechoic area surrounding the prostate) (Fig. 10.32). Direct extension of tumor may also be identified. Seminal vesicle involvement is usually detected by asymmetry of the seminal vesicles in size and echogenicity (Fig. 10.33).

The accuracy of ultrasound has not been adequately determined, although the ability to differentiate between localized and invasive cancer appears to range between 60 and 80% accuracy (41–44). Endorectal ultrasound is most accurate when cancer has spread beyond the confines of the prostate, having accuracy reports between 70 and 90%. This accuracy improves when the clinical suspicion is increased (accuracies approaching 80 to 90%) and is significantly reduced when the clinical suspicion is confined cancer, yet there is pathologic evidence of tumor invasion into the pericapsular fat (in these cases, accuracy ranges between 50 to 70%). Endorectal ultrasound cannot define pelvic lymph node involvement.

Radiation Seed Implantation

Preliminary results have suggested that percutaneous implantation of radioactive seeds may be a useful technique for treatment of cer-

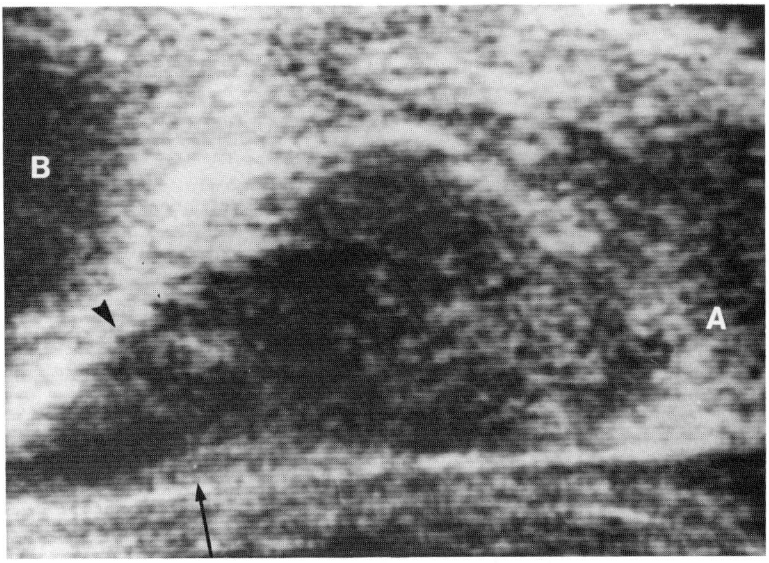

Figure 10.33. Seminal vesicle involvement. Longitudinal orientation demonstrates seminal vesicle involvement best. The entire prostate is disrupted by hypoechoic areas. There is also direct infiltration of the seminal vesicles anteriorly (*arrowhead*) and posteriorly (*arrow*), consistent with seminal vesicle infiltration. *A,* apex; *B,* bladder.

tain prostatic cancers (45–47). Using an approach modified from the ultrasound-guided biopsy technique, placement of radioactive seeds into the prostate and periprostatic bed can be performed using endorectal sonographic guidance. This is a simple technique, but it does require approximately 30 to 60 minutes time, and thus sedation or anesthesia may be required. Transperineal approaches are used and seeds can be placed with great accuracy into the prostate. Complications include the possibility of bleeding, loss of seeds through urination, and possible sepsis. The efficacy of this modality in eradicating prostate cancer is currently unknown in that there are no long-term results in patients treated in this manner.

Applications in Screening

Should screening be used to detect early prostate cancer and, if so, should ultrasound be the modality employed? The statistics suggest that yes, prostate cancer may require large-scale screening for earlier detection and treatment, but the dilemma regarding the growth pattern of prostate cancer complicates the answer. For example, prostate cancer is the most prevalent and frequently diagnosed cancer in the American male population (4). However, while the mortality of the disease is significant (the second most common), more men will die with unsuspected and clinically undiagnosed prostate cancer than from malignancy that has been detected and treated (4). Why the discrepancy? Autopsy studies have shown that over 30% (and up to 50%) of men over 50 years of age who have died from a cause other than prostate cancer have cancer on serially sectioned prostates. While many of these are microscopic and probably insignificant, some may be quite large (2). An additional study of men undergoing cystoprostatectomy for bladder cancer (but no suspected prostate cancer) has shown that 47% harbored clinically unsuspected prostate cancer, confirming the results of the autopsy studies (3).

An important consideration—yet to be fully evaluated—is what constitutes an important clinically significant cancer. McNeal has suggested that prostate cancer becomes both more anaplastic and more invasive as it enlarges (11). He has also shown that the metastatic potential of the tumor is essentially nil before the tumor reaches 1 cm^3 in volume but increases dramatically above that volume (11). While treatment options have been defined (but not universally accepted) for prostate cancer (e.g., that confined malignancy be treated by radical surgery and invasive disease by "palliative" therapy), new approaches may have to be defined (48, 49). For example, should all nonpalpable cancer (many being detected by ultrasound screening) be treated? If so, with what type of therapy? Will the morbidity of treatment be more significant than the potential morbidity of an untreated small cancer?

Assuming screening is necessary, another important consideration is the efficacy and comparative accuracy of screening with ultrasound compared to conventional techniques such as the digital rectal examination. Preliminary studies have suggested that ultrasound is more accurate and sensitive in detecting prostate cancer than the digital rectal examination (50–52). However, these studies were constructed to prove the benefit of ultrasound. Either the results of the physical examination were ignored or the expertise of the examiner was not necessarily as great as those performing and interpreting the ultrasound. Additionally, these studies were statistically biased to show great accuracy of ultrasound. Both assumed that if the ultrasound did not show an abnormality, no cancer existed! This is obviously fallacious. A prospective study, examining over 200 men with prostate cancer, all of whom underwent radical prostatectomy (because of clinical stage A or B disease) has shown that endorectal ultrasound using "state-of-art" equipment could not detect 40% of cancers greater than 5 mm in size (41). These "large" tumors (not the microscopic lesions) are those that need to be detected if a technique is to be used appropriately for screening.

Is prostate ultrasound a screening tool? No, not today, but it may be in the future. Cancer can be detected, but the data are not available to show the following: (*a*) the sensitivity and specificity of the technique applied to the appropriate patient population: (*b*) the accuracy of ultrasound compared to other modalities; (*c*) improvement in patient prognosis by detecting and treating the cancers that would be identified by an early screening program.

SUMMARY

There are a number of indications for which prostate ultrasound is essential. These include the following (20):

1. A mass identified on digital rectal examination. Ultrasound can be used to identify the mass and determine its suspiciousness for cancer or a possible benign process such as cyst or calcification mimicking malignancy (Figs. 10.34 and 10.35).
2. Asymmetry of the gland in size on digital rectal examination.
3. Induration without distinct mass of the prostate on digital rectal examination. Endorectal ultrasound can determine if induration may represent malignant infiltration.
4. Mass on digital rectal examination and negative conventional biopsy. Studies have shown that over 50% of masses felt by digital rectal examination that have had con-

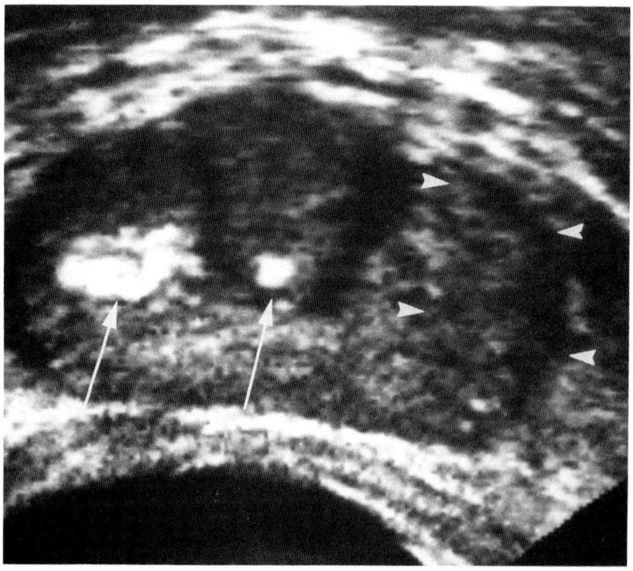

Figure 10.34. Calcification mimicking carcinoma. The digital rectal examination suggests a mass or nodularity in the right portion of the prostate. Endorectal ultrasound demonstrates calculi (*arrows*) in the right side, not secondary to cancer. However, a hypoechoic focus (*arrowheads*) on the left side is identified that was not palpable, but was biopsied and proven to be carcinoma.

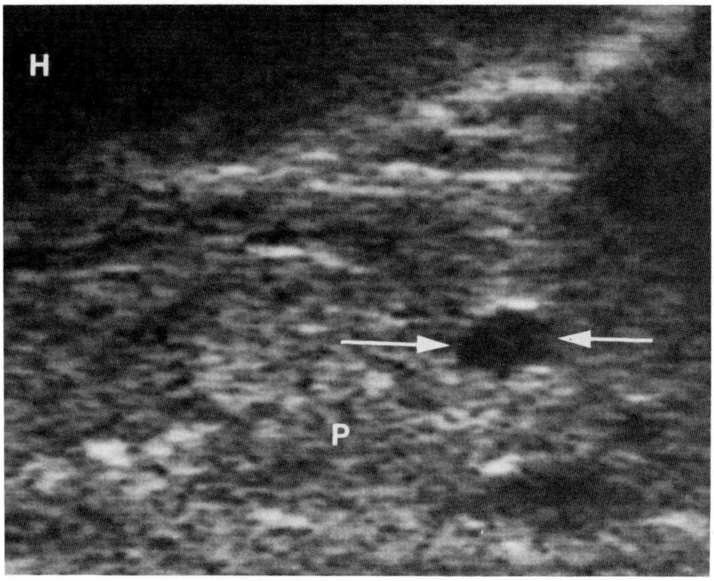

Figure 10.35. Prostate cyst. Longitudinal orientation of the prostate demonstrates a palpable abnormality secondary to cyst. The cyst is identified as an anechoic area (*arrows*) with good back wall and enhanced sound through transmission suggestive of a simple cyst. *P*, prostate; *H*, toward patient's head.

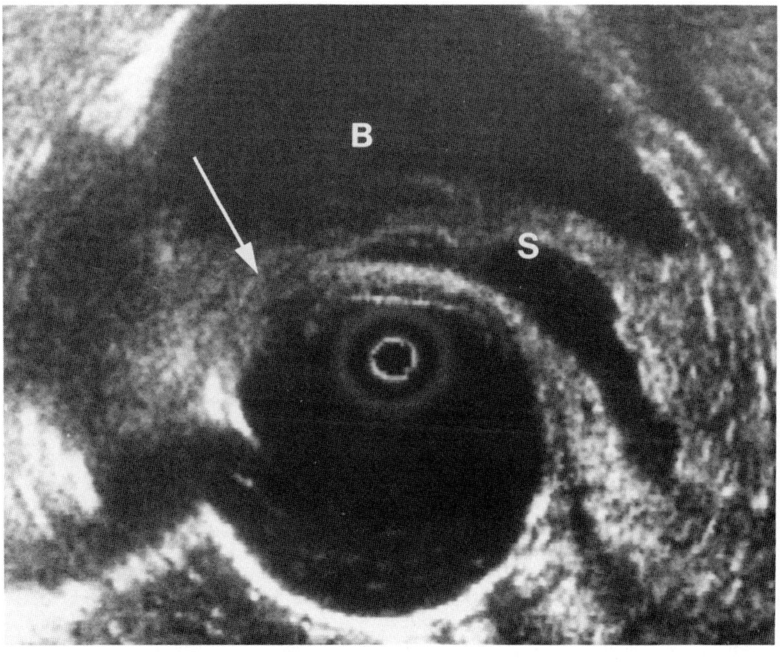

Figure 10.36. Agenesis of seminal vesicles. Axially oriented scan demonstrates a normal-appearing left seminal vesicle (*S*). There is no seminal vesicle seen on the right side (*arrow*) consistent with agenesis. Urinary bladder (*B*) is identified.

ventional biopsy that have showed no evidence of cancer, when biopsied by prostate ultrasound guidance, will demonstrate malignancy (8).

5. Staging of cancer on a patient diagnosed on a TURP with a normal digital rectal examination. These men may have large cancers not detected by digital rectal examination.

A TURP may detect cancer in the pathology specimen, but ultrasound may define the extent of the lesion.

6. Staging of prostate cancer. Prostate ultrasound may determine capsular infiltration or seminal vesicle invasion, which may change the therapeutic approach.
7. Elevated biochemical markers. Patients with normal digital rectal examinations may have elevated prostate-specific antigen (PSA), prostatic acid phosphatase levels, or other serum studies that may suggest the presence or extension of prostate cancer. Prostate ultrasound may delineate and determine the extent of cancer in these individuals.
8. Biopsy guidance.
9. Radioactive seed implantation. This technique is an extension of prostate biopsy guidance. Some studies have shown that by placing radioactive seeds percutaneously through the perineum into the prostate, an adequate therapeutic approach is possible (15, 16). This negates the need for external beam radiation (possibly minimizing some of the complications of radiotherapy). Further work must be performed regarding this technique to determine its exact placement in the therapeutic approach to prostate cancer.
10. Monitoring of prostate cancer. Endorectal ultrasound may determine further extension of prostate cancer in patients undergoing treatment of the disease.
11. Infertility, inflammation, or congenital abnormalities. Ultrasound may determine some congenital abnormalities or anomalies such as absence of the seminal vesicles (Fig. 10.36), ejaculatory duct obstructions, or others. These may, in certain individuals, be clinically important abnormalities that can be evaluated by prostate ultrasound.
12. Screening. As stated, prostate ultrasound has not yet been shown to be an effective tool for screening for prostate cancer. Further work must be performed to elucidate its exact place in detecting unexpected cancer.

References

1. Franks LM. Latent carcinoma of the prostate. J Pathol Bacteriol 1954; 68:603–616.
2. Scott R Jr, Mutchnik D, Laskowski TZ, Schmalhorst WR. Carcinoma of the prostate in elderly men: incidence, growth characteristics and clinical significance. J Urol 1969; 101:602–607.
3. Montie JE, Wood DP Jr, Pontes JE, Boyett J, Levin HS. Adenocarcinoma of the prostate cystoprostatectomy specimens removed for bladder cancer. Cancer 1989; 63:381–385.
4. Silverberg E, Boring CC, Squires TS. Cancer statistics, 1990. CA 1990; 40:9–26.
5. Lowsley OS. Embryology, anatomy, and surgery of the prostate gland. Am J Surg 1930; 8:526–541.
6. McNeal JE. Morphogenesis of prostatic carcinoma. Cancer 1965; 18:1659–1666.
7. McNeal JE. Regional morphology and pathology of the prostate. Am J Clin Pathol 1968; 49:347–357.
8. McNeal JE. Origin and development of carcinoma in the prostate. Cancer 1969; 23:24–34.
9. McNeal JE. Anatomy of the prostate: an historical survey of divergent views. Prostate 1980; 1:3–13.
10. McNeal JE. The prostate gland. 1983 Monographs in Urology 1983; 4:3–33.
11. McNeal JE, Kindrachuk RA, Freiha FS, Bostwick DG, Redwine EA, Stamey TA. Patterns of progression in prostate cancer. Lancet 1986, 1:60–63.
12. McNeal JE. Normal anatomy of the prostate and changes in benign prostatic hypertrophy and carcinoma. Seminars in US, CT, MRI 1988; 9(5):329–334.
13. McNeal JE. The prostate gland. Mongr Urol 1988; 9:36–54.
14. Resnick MI, Willard JW, Boyce WH. Recent progress in ultrasonography of the bladder and prostate. J Urol 1977; 117:444–446.
15. Rifkin MD. Ultrasound of the prostate. New York: Raven Press, 1988.
16. Watanabe H, Kaiho H, Tanaka M, Terasawa Y. Diagnostic application of ultrasonotomography of the prostate. Invest Urol 1971; 8:548–559.
17. Resnick MI, Willard JW, Boyce WH. Ultrasonic evaluation of the prostatic nodule. J Urol 1978; 120:86–89.
18. Rifkin MD, Kurtz AB, Choi HY, Goldberg BB. Endoscopic ultrasonic evaluation of the prostate using a transrectal probe: prospective evaluation and acoustic characterization. Radiology 1983; 149:265–271.
19. Rifkin MD, Friedland GW, Shortliffe L. Prostatic evaluation by transrectal endosonography: detection of carcinoma. Radiology 1986; 158:85–90.
20. Rifkin MD, Dahnert W, Kurtz AB. Progress in radiology. State of the art. Endorectal sonography of the prostate gland. AJR 1990; 154:691–700.
21. Rifkin MD, McGlynn ET, Choi H. Echogenicity of prostate cancer correlated with histologic grade and stromal fibrosis: endorectal US studies. Radiology 1989; 170:549–552.
22. Rifkin MD, Gatsonis C, Zerhouni E, et al. Endorectal US and MR imaging: accuracy of staging prostate cancer. Presented at the 7th Scientific Assembly and Annual Meeting of the Radiological Society of North America, Chicago, November 1989.

23. Hamper UM, Sheth S, Walsh PC, Epstein JI. Bright echogenic foci in early prostatic carcinoma: sonographic and pathologic correlation. Radiology 1990; 176:339–343.
24. Dahnert WF, Hamper UM, Eggleston JC, Walsh PC, Sanders RC. Prostatic evaluation by transrectal sonography with histopathologic correlation: the echopenic appearance of early carcinoma. Radiology 1986; 158:97–102.
25. Salo JO, Rannikko S, Makinen J, Lehtonen T. Echogenic structure of prostatic cancer imaged on radical prostatectomy specimens. Prostate 1987; 10:1–9.
26. Rifkin MD, Choi H. Endorectal prostate ultrasound: implications of the small peripherally place hypoechoic lesion. Radiology 1988; 166: 619–622.
27. Rifkin MD. Unpublished data.
28. MacIntyre RC, Peron SE, Madrazo B, Cerny JC. Ultrasound guided needle biopsy of the prostate gland. J Urol 1987; 137(4 Part 2); 242A.
29. Lee F, Littrup PJ, Kumasaka GH, Borlaza GS, McLeary RD. Use of transrectal ultrasound in the diagnosis, guided biopsy, staging and screening of prostate cancer. Radiographics 1987; 7:617.
30. Chancellor MB, McHugh TA, Dorr RP, VanAppledorn CA. Transrectal prostate ultrasonography before transurethral prostatectomy, its value in screening for stage A cancer. J Urol 1987; 137(4 Part 2): 242A.
31. Ragde H, Bagley CM Jr, Aldape HC, Blasko JC. Prostate cancer screening with high resolution transrectal ultrasound. J Endourology 1989; 3(2):115–123.
32. Lee F, Torp-Pedersen S, Littrup PJ, et al. Hypoechoic lesions of the prostate: clinical relevance of tumor size, digital rectal examination and prostate-specific antigen. Radiology 1989; 170:29–32.
33. Resnick MI. Transrectal ultrasound guided versus digitally directed prostatic biopsy: a comparative study. J Urol 1988; 139:754–757.
34. Ajzen SA, Goldenberg SL, Allen GJ, Cooperberg PL, Chan NH, Jones EC. Palpable prostatic nodules: comparison of US and digital guidance for fine-needle aspiration biopsy. Radiology 1989; 171:521–523.
35. Rifkin MD, Dahnert W, Pisarchik J, Matteucci T. Ultrasound guided biopsy of the prostate. A necessary tool (even for palpable nodules) Presented to the 34th Annual Convention of the American Institute of Ultrasound in Medicine, March 4–7, 1990, New Orleans.
36. Rifkin MD, Kurtz AB, Goldberg BB. Prostate biopsy utilizing transrectal ultrasound guidance: diagnosis of nonpalpable cancers. J Ultrasound Med 1983; 2:165–167.
37. Rifkin MD, Kurtz AB, Goldberg BB. Sonographically guided transperineal prostatic biopsy: preliminary experience with a longitudinal linear array transducer. AJR 1983; 139:745–747.
38. Fornage BD, Touche DH, Deglaire M, Faroux MJC, Simatos A. Real-time ultrasound-guided prostatic biopsy using a new transrectal linear array transducer. Radiology 1983; 146:547–548.
39. Holm HH, Gammelgaard J. Ultrasonically guided precise needle placement in the prostate and the seminal vesicles. J Urol 1981; 125:385–387.
40. Torp-Pedersen ST, Lee F, Littrup PJ, Siders DB, Kumasaka GH, Solomon MH, McLeary RD. Transrectal biopsy of the prostate guided by transrectal ultrasound: experience with longitudinal and multiplanar scanning. Radiology 1988; 170:23–27.
41. Rifkin MD, Zerhouni EA, Gatsonis CA, et al. Comparison of MRI and US in staging early prostate cancer: results of a multi-institutional cooperative trial. N Engl J Med, 1990; 323:621–626.
42. Andriole GL, Kavoussi LR, Torrence RJ, Lepor H, Catalona WJ. Transrectal ultrasonography in the diagnosis and staging of carcinoma of the prostate. J Urol 1988; 140:758–760.
43. Perrapato SD, Carothers GG, Maatman TJ, Soechtig CE. Comparing clinical staging plus transrectal ultrasound with surgical-pathologic staging of prostate cancer. Urology 1989; 33:103–105.
44. Scardino PT, Shinohara K, Wheeler TM, St. C. Carter S. Staging of prostate cancer: value of ultrasonography. Urol Clin North Am 1989; 16(4):713–734.
45. Holm HH, Juul N, Pedersen JF, Hansen H, Stroyer I. Transperineal 125-iodine seed implantation in prostatic cancer guided by transrectal ultrasonography. J Urol 1983; 130:283–286.
46. Lee F, Meiselman L, Torp-Pedersen S. The development of ultrasound guided iodine-125 therapy, the Copenhagen-Ann Arbor experience. Presented at the Second International Symposium on Transrectal Ultrasound in Diagnosis and Management of Prostate Cancer, Detroit, September 21–22, 1987.
47. Blasko J, Ragde H. Seattle experience with transperineal percutaneous radioisotope implantation for prostatic carcinoma utilizing transrectal ultrasound and template guidance. Presented at the Second International Symposium on Transrectal Ultrasound in the Diagnosis and Management of Prostate Cancer, Detroit, September 21–22, 1987.
48. McNeal JE, Price HM, Redwine EA, Freiha FS, Stamey TA. Stage A versus Stage B adenocarcinoma of the prostate: morphological comparison and biological significance. J Urol 1988; 139:61–65.
49. Adolfsson J, Fahraeus B. The natural course of prostatic carcinoma in relation to initial cytological grade. J Urol 1988; 140:1452–1454.
50. Lee F, Littrup PJ, Torp-Pedersen ST, et al. Prostate cancer: comparison of transrectal US and digital rectal examination for screening. Radiology 1988; 168:389–394.
51. Ragde H, Bagley CM Jr, Aldape HC, Blasko JC. Prostate cancer screening with high resolution transrectal ultrasound. J Endourology 1989; 3:115–123.
52. Cooner WH, Mosley BR, Rutherford CL Jr, et al. Prostate cancer detection in a clinical urologic practice by ultrasonography, digital rectal examination and prostate specific antigen. J Urol, 1990; 143:1146–1154.

CHAPTER 11

Ultrasonography of the Penis

TOM F. LUE, M.D.
HEDVIG HRICAK, M.D.

Recent advances in ultrasonography and in our understanding of the physiology of erection have resulted in improved noninvasive diagnosis of pathologic conditions of the penis. This chapter reviews the use of high-resolution ultrasonography in the evaluation of penile anatomy, Peyronie's disease, trauma, urethral strictures, and vasculogenic impotence.

HIGH-RESOLUTION ULTRASOUND

Technique

To evaluate the penis, real-time equipment with high-frequency transducers (preferably 10 MHz) is needed (1). The penile shaft is scanned by placing the probe directly on the penile body; the penile bulb is scanned through the perineum. Transverse and longitudinal sections are routinely obtained, with coronal sections also if the region of interest warrants them (1). The anatomy can be demonstrated with the penis in the flaccid state, but the corpora are better displayed during erection. The penile urethra will be better seen if it is distended by intraurethral injection of sterile gel or saline (2).

Normal Anatomy

The penile body comprises three intimately attached erectile structures that can be differentiated from each other by their anatomical position: the two lateral penile corpora cavernosa and the ventral and medial corpus spongiosum (Fig. 11.1) (3). The thick tunica albuginea, which is composed of collagen tissue, appears as an echogenic rim surrounding the cavernous bodies (1); however, it cannot be distinguished sonographically from Buck's fascia, the fibrous tube-like structure enveloping it.

In the flaccid state, the corpora cavernosa demonstrate a hypoechoic pattern interrupted by central echogenic dots representing the deep (cavernous) artery. During erection, the corpora increase in size and echogenicity: the pattern can be uniform throughout or a relatively hypoechoic area may be seen in the periarterial region (1). When flaccid, the three corporeal bodies exhibit a similar echogenicity; during erection the corpora cavernosa often have a higher echogenicity. Within the shaft of the penis the corpus spongiosum emits a uniformly low to medium echogenicity, with the urethra appearing as an echogenic focus.

The transperineal approach is necessary to scan the bulbous portion of the corpus spongiosum. In the sagittal plane, the urethra appears as an echogenic line. When distended with either saline or gel, the lumen can be evaluated. This is especially helpful for urethral strictures (2). The attachment of the crura to the ischium can be seen, as can the ischiocavernosus muscle covering its medial aspect. The entrance of the deep artery to the corpus cavernosum at the hilum can be appreciated, and the deep dorsal vein and dorsal artery are seen between the tunica albuginea and Buck's fascia on the dorsum of the penis. The superficial dorsal vein outside Buck's fascia is only occasionally visible.

The portion of the tunica albuginea that is interposed between the paired corpora cavernosa forms an incomplete septum and appears as an echogenic line in both the transverse and coronal planes.

Pathologic States

CONGENITAL ANOMALIES

Diphallus is demonstrable on ultrasound. However, as a rule congenital anomalies are better evaluated by magnetic resonance imaging (4), as their complexity renders precise assessment difficult on the small field of view provided by sonography.

PEYRONIE'S DISEASE

Peyronie's disease is a thickening of the tunica albuginea that extends to varying degrees

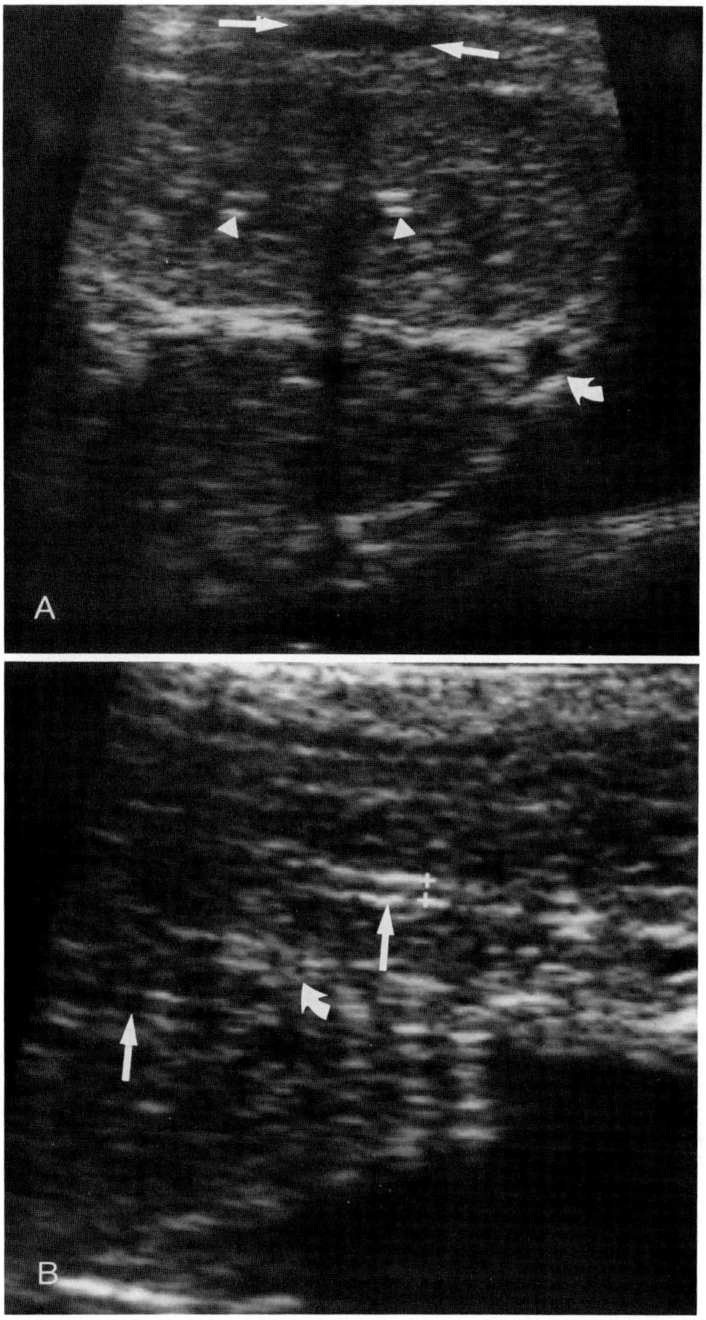

Figure 11.1. Normal penile anatomy. **A,** Transverse view. *Straight arrows,* deep dorsal vein; *arrowheads,* cavernous arteries; *curved arrow,* urethral vein. **B,** Longitudinal view. *Straight arrows,* cavernous arteries; *curved arrow,* septum.

into the corpora cavernosa. Often physical examination is sufficient; however, ultrasound can evaluate the size and thickness of the plaque (5, 6) and the possibility of compromise of the cavernous arteries and dorsal arteries and veins. The plaque appears as a localized thickening of the tunica albuginea with an echo pattern that varies with age (6): in the earlier stages, it is hypoechoic, but it becomes increasingly hyperechoic until its end stage, when calcification is apparent as dense, hyperechoic lesions with acoustical shadowing. The possibility of differentiating mature calcified plaques from more recent ones is helpful in determining the correct medical or surgical treatment (6). If the latter is chosen, the distance between the plaque and the cavernous artery should be measured. Ultrasound can also be used for follow-up.

FIBROSIS OF THE PENIS

Penile fibrosis is a known complication of prolonged priapism (7) and a recently recognized complication of intracavernous injection of vasoactive agents. The penis must be scanned in both the flaccid and erect states. During erection, extensive fibrosis will be seen as a nonhomogeneous echo pattern with a patchy, asymmetrical area of decreased signal intensity. As yet, no large studies comparing the sensitivities of ultrasound and penile biopsy have been reported.

PENILE TRAUMA

A peripenile hematoma consequent to acute rupture of the penis appears as an echo-poor mass adjacent to the corpora cavernosa (8). Tunical disruption is demonstrable as well. However, magnetic resonance imaging, with its larger field of view and better contrast between the corpora and tunica, is preferable (4). Ultrasound can be used to evaluate a posttraumatic intracavernous hematoma (9) or detect an intrapenile foreign body (10, 11).

URETHRAL STRICTURE

Urethral strictures secondary to trauma or inflammatory disease require surgical intervention, for which the length and thickness of the scar are important considerations. Voiding cystourethrography and retrograde urethrography demonstrate length but offer no information about thickness or the status of the corpus spongiosum. For these purposes, penile ultrasound has been advocated (2, 12, 13). In a study by McAninch et al. (2) ultrasound more accurately assessed stricture length than did retrograde urethrography when compared with the "gold standard" of open urethroplasty.

Distention of the urethra with gel or saline allows classification of the degree of spongiofibrosis (Fig. 11.2). However, ultrasonography is limited to the penile urethra and cannot assess the prostatic urethra.

DUPLEX ULTRASOUND

Histologic studies in penile tissues fixed in the flaccid and erect states clearly show tremendous arterial and arteriolar dilation during the erectile process (14). This phenomenon occurs regardless of the mode of experimental induction: viz. electrical stimulation or injection of vasodilators such as papaverine (15) or

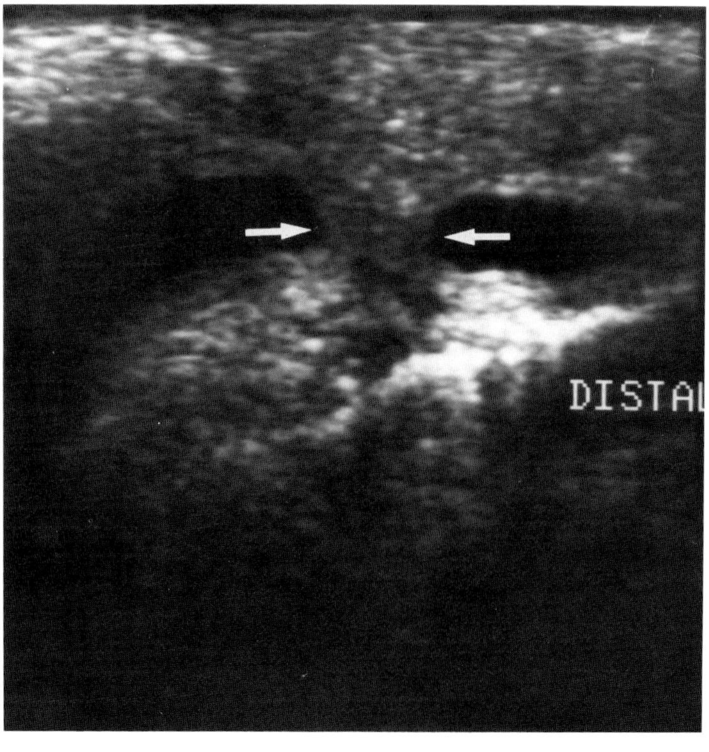

Figure 11.2. Sonourethrogram demonstrates a severe focal noncompressive stricture (*arrows*). Note that the normal segment of the urethra is distensible during saline filling and easily compresses the spongiosum. (Reprinted from McAninch JW, Laing FC, Jeffrey RB Jr. Sonourethrography in the evaluation of urethral strictures: a preliminary report. J Urol 1988;139: 294–297.)

prostaglandin E_1 (16). In our search for an accurate functional test of the penile arteries, we began using duplex ultrasound in 1983 (1). Over the past 5½ years, we have performed this test in more than 1200 patients and can recommend it as reliable and reproducible.

Indications: One can argue that this test may be indicated in almost all impotent patients because of its minimal invasiveness and the ability to assess the penile arteries accurately. However, at the present time, we perform duplex ultrasonography only if a patient responds poorly to intracavernous injections and the treatment strategy requires more accurate evaluation of the penile arteries.

Contraindications: Duplex ultrasonography itself carries no contraindications. However, we do not recommend intracavernous injection of papaverine in patients with sickle cell anemia, severe bleeding diatheses, or severe liver disease.

Technique

A real-time mechanical-sector duplex scanner with an imaging frequency of 10 MHz is used (1, 17). The duplex probe contains two piezoelectric transducers positioned in a geometric configuration that allows simultaneous imaging and Doppler flow studies (the latter performed with the pulsed, range-gated Doppler subsystem operating at a fundamental frequency of 4.5 MHz). Blood flow velocity is quantified with the system's real-time gray-scale spectrum analyzer with Fast Fourier Transform (FFT) analysis (50 FFTs/sec with a frequency resolution of 50 Hz). The simultaneous display of the anatomic image during Doppler analysis allows accurate placement of the Doppler sample volume into the small vessels of the penis for conversion of frequency data into angle-independent velocity data. The length of the sample volume can be varied from 0.6 to 10.0 mm; most often, 1.3 mm is used. The Doppler beam and sample volume are positioned in the vessel, and the angle cursor can be aligned manually in parallel. The system's computer automatically measures the Doppler angle (displayed at the top of the image) and converts frequency to velocity. Peak flow velocity at peak systole is measured by moving the cursor, located below the time baseline, to the point (FFT bin) in the cardiac cycle where the flow velocity is highest. The peak and average velocities are automatically calculated and displayed above the velocity histogram.

Initially, the ultrasound study is performed on the entire penis in the flaccid state to evaluate penile anatomy, including the size and shape of the corpora and the diameters of the arteries (measured by electronic calipers). Measurements are taken in the transverse and longitudinal planes near the base of the penis. A rubber band is then placed at the penile base and 60 mg of papaverine or 10 μg of prostaglandin E_1 is injected into either corpus cavernosum with a 25-gauge needle. Digital pressure is applied to the injection site for 2 to 3 min, and the rubber band is cut. Gray-scale imaging and pulsed Doppler analysis are again performed at the base of the penis.

The routine duplex examination consists of measuring vessel diameter in both the systolic and diastolic phases, blood flow velocity at peak systole in the cavernous artery, and blood flow alone in the dorsal artery. This is usually done 5 and 15 min after the injection. The diameter and flow of the deep dorsal vein can also be measured if venous leakage is suspected.

Serious complications include priapism and hypotension. To prevent priapism, one should observe the patient for 1 hr after the injection. If erection persists, one should aspirate the penis or inject diluted epinephrine (10 to 20 μg/ml saline) or phenylephrine hydrochloride (Neo-Synephrine) (100 to 200 μg/ml) every 5 min until detumescence. With this approach, only four cases of priapism of more than 6 hours' duration have been seen in our more than 1200 patients over the past 5 years.

Ultrasound Findings During Erection

TRANSVERSE VIEW

In patients with a good erection after intracavernous injection of a vasodilator, the echo pattern is usually homogeneous and the cavernous arteries are easily recognizable for their greater echogenicity and striking pulsation (Fig. 11.3). Two patterns of pulsation can be appreciated: concentric, in which the diameter of the artery is appreciably larger in the systolic phase and smaller in the diastolic (in healthy young men); nonconcentric, in which the diameter shows no appreciable change but the artery moves from side to side (healthy men of middle age or older). In patients with a poor arterial response after injection (Fig. 11.4) or in those with cavernous fibrosis, the echo pattern is irregular and the cavernous arteries are dif-

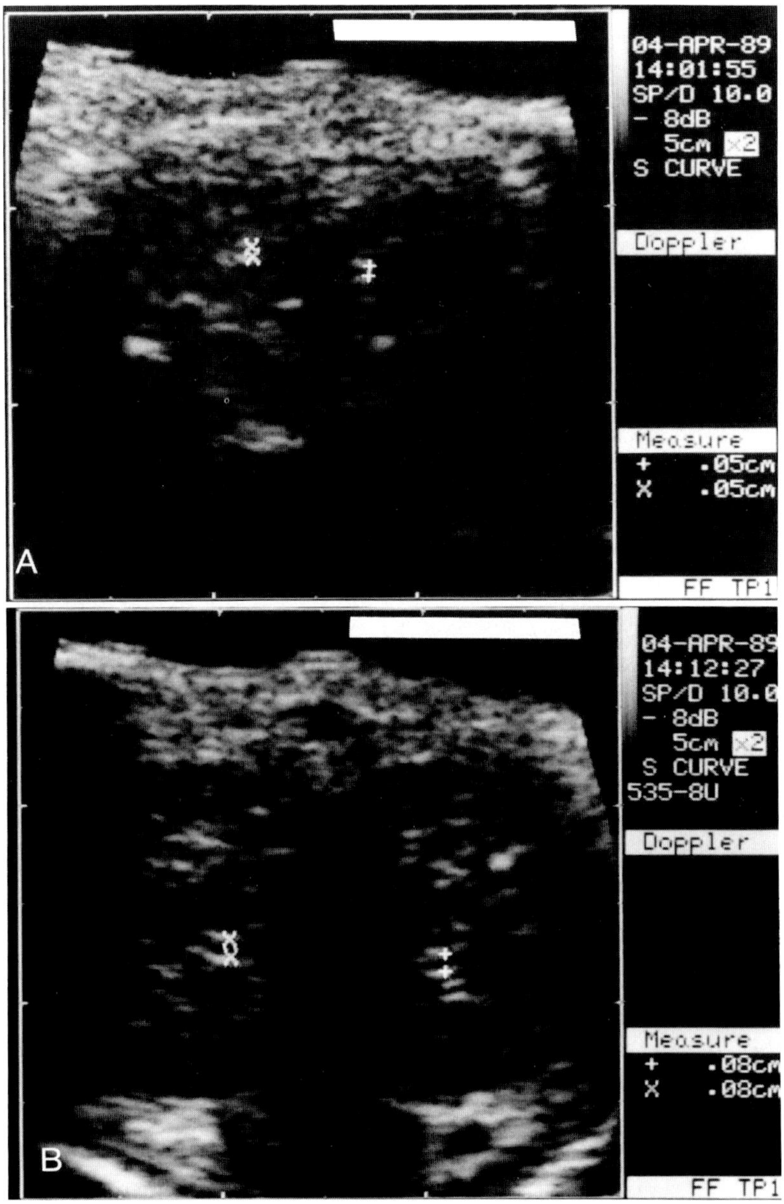

Figure 11.3. Good arterial response to papaverine. **A,** Before injection, transverse view. The cavernous arteries measure 0.05 cm bilaterally. **B** and **C,** Transverse and longitudinal views after injection show dilation of both cavernous arteries (diameter, 0.08 cm). **D** and **E,** Pulsed Doppler study. Monitoring gray-scale sonogram at the left upper corner displays the placement of the cursor on the cavernous artery. At the right upper corner, the velocity histogram shows the peak (33 cm/sec, right; 45 cm/sec, left) and average (19 cm/sec, right; 29 cm/sec, left) velocities. Below is the gray-scale velocity waveform. **F,** The deep dorsal vein measures 0.2 cm in diameter.

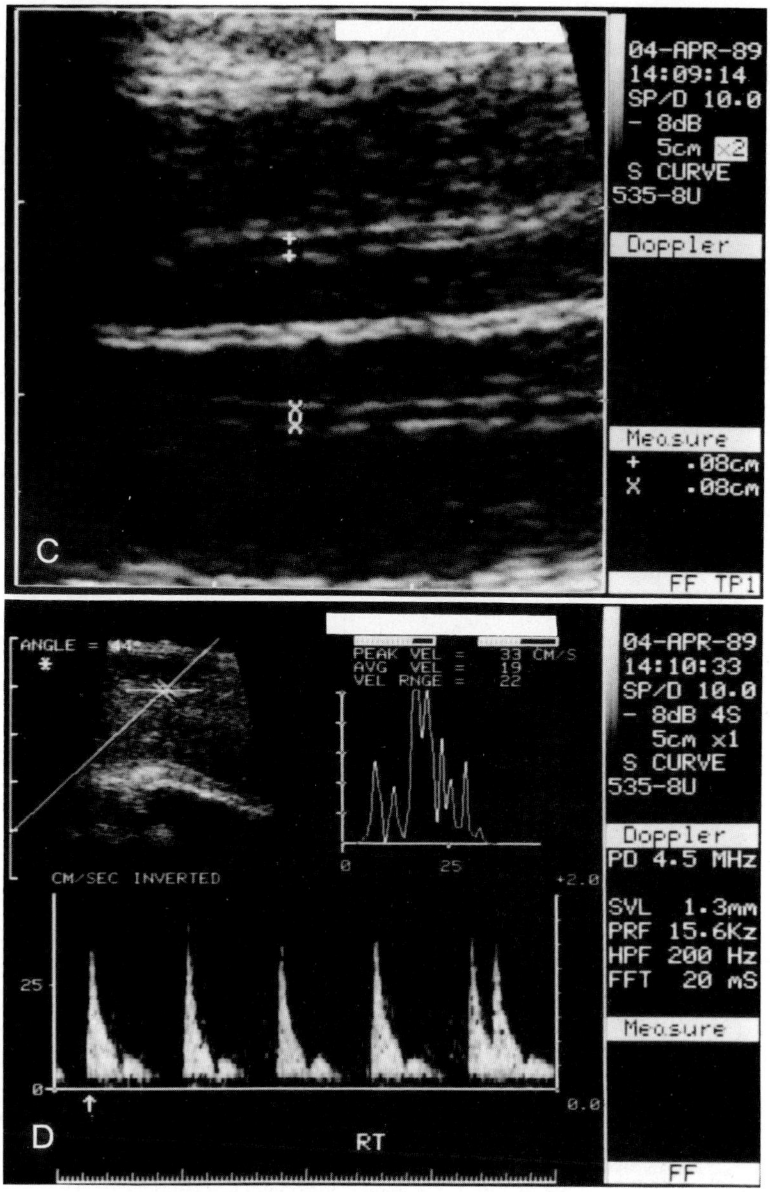

Figure 11.3. C and **D.**

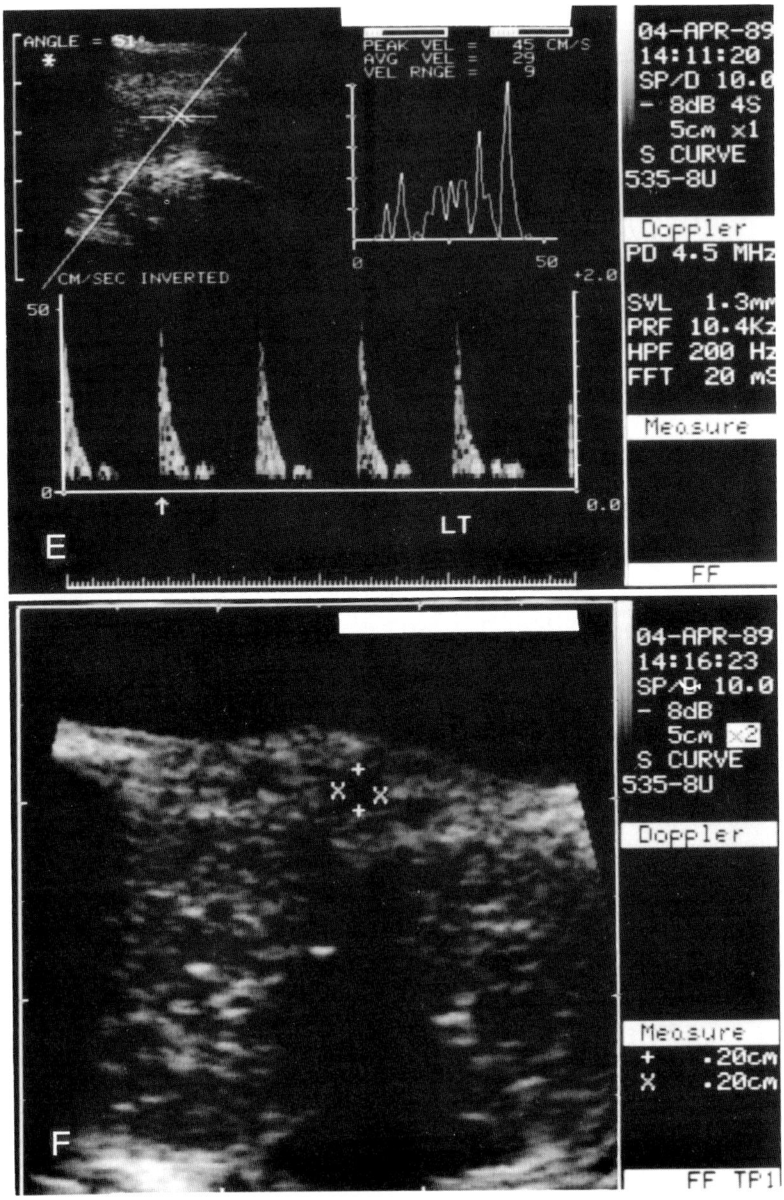

Figure 11.3. E and F.

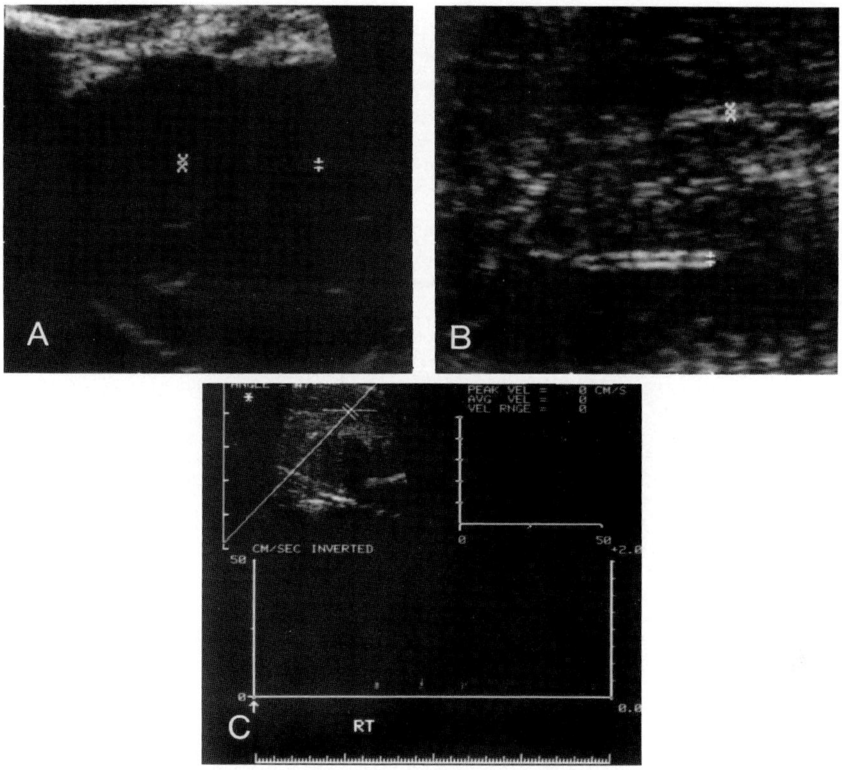

Figure 11.4. Severe arterial insufficiency. **A,** Before injection, transverse view. The diameters of the cavernous arteries are 0.04 and 0.05 cm. **B,** After injection, longitudinal view. The diameters are unchanged. **C,** Flow in the deep right artery is not measurable.

ficult to identify (even if distinguishable, the pulsations may not be recognizable). The thickened tunica albuginea is demonstrated as an echogenic rim surrounding the cavernous bodies.

LONGITUDINAL VIEW

Positioning the probe on the lateral aspect of the penis provides a better assessment of arterial health: both corpora cavernosa, their arteries, and the septum can be seen in the same field. In the flaccid state, the cavernous arteries appear as interrupted segments because they are constricted and assume a zig-zag course in the corpora cavernosa. In nervous patients and those with cavernous fibrosis (Fig. 11.5), they cannot be easily differentiated from the erectile tissue. After intracavernous injection of a vasodilator, the cavernous artery will exhibit vigorous concentric pulsations in healthy young men; the lumen will be large and the arterial wall thin (Fig. 11.3). Doppler study will reveal an excellent peak flow of more than 30 cm/sec with sharp waveforms. Diastolic flow is large in the latent phase of erection but disappears with full erection. In older potent men, the arterial wall usually appears thicker, although they may still achieve adequate flow and erection after intracavernous injection. In patients with severe atherosclerosis, the arterial wall appears thickened and irregular with a small lumen and poor flow (Fig. 11.4). Branches of one cavernous artery passing through the septum to supplement the opposite corpus are frequently seen when the contralateral artery is absent or has undergone occlusion or stenosis (Fig. 11.6).

CLINICAL FINDINGS AND CONSIDERATIONS

In normal patients, the most consistently useful values for assessing arterial function are postinjection diameter and peak flow velocity. Because individual penile size and the amount

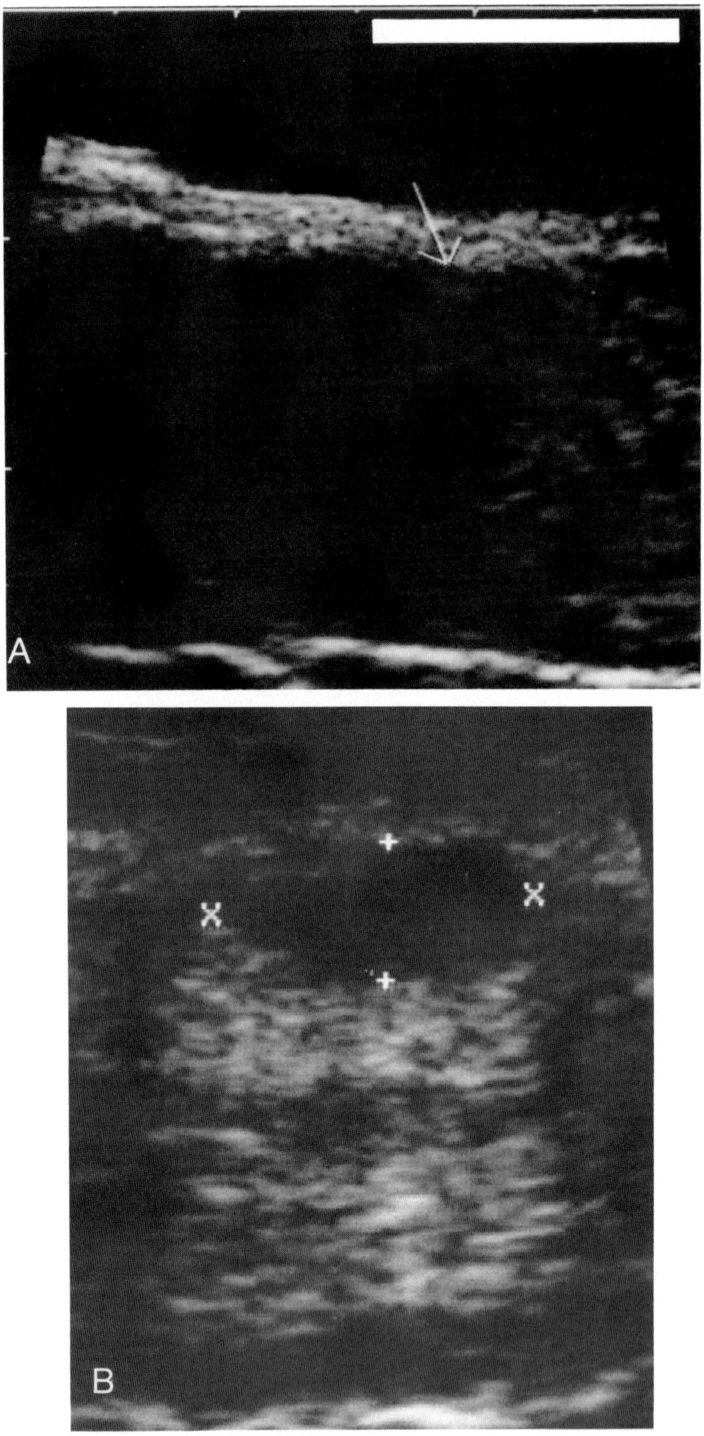

Figure 11.5. **A,** Longitudinal view of the penis shows increased echogenicity (fibrosis) in the distal third secondary to cavernosography 6 months previously. **B,** This longitudinal view shows a localized fibrotic area secondary to intracavernous papaverine therapy.

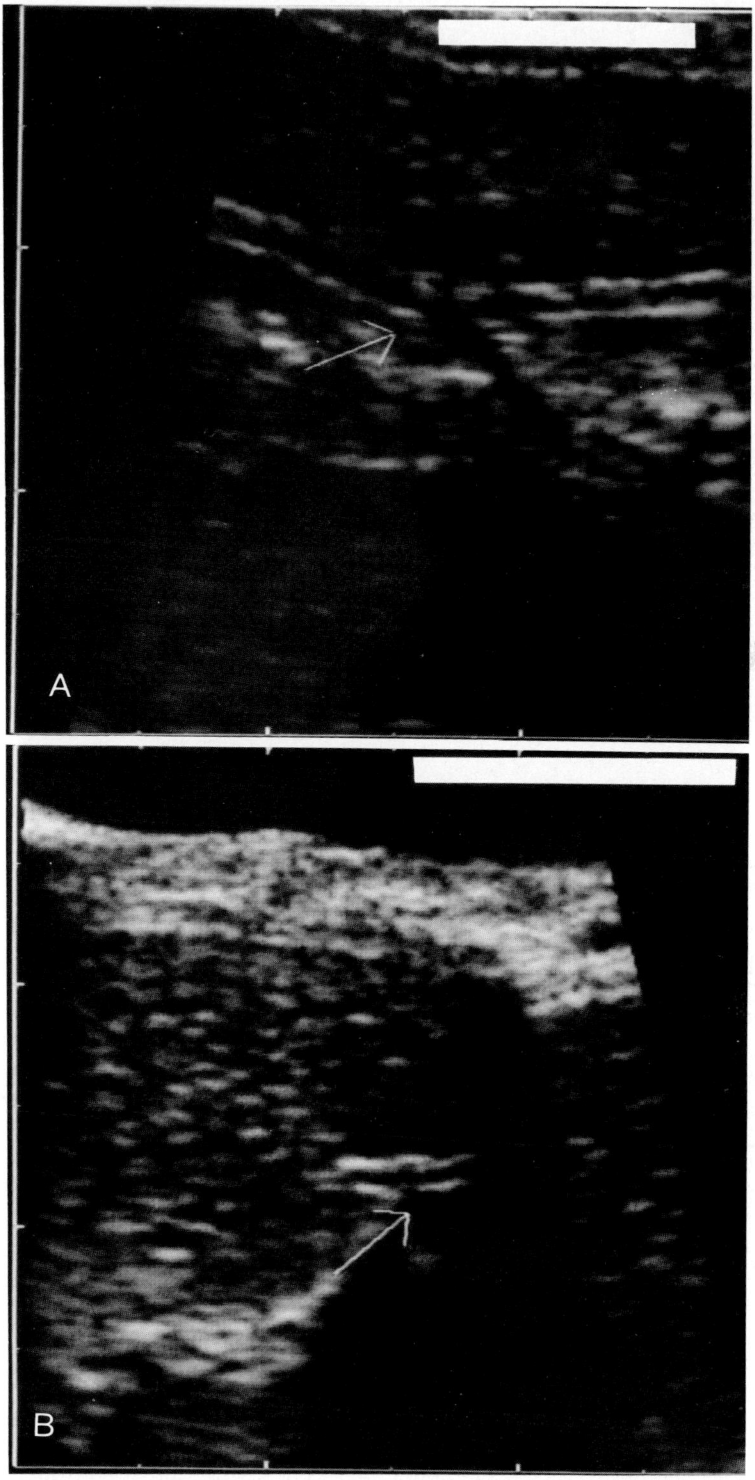

Figure 11.6. Branching of the cavernous artery with occlusion of the contralateral cavernous artery. **A,** Longitudinal view. **B,** Transverse view. In **C** is shown an anastomosis between the dorsal and cavernous arteries.

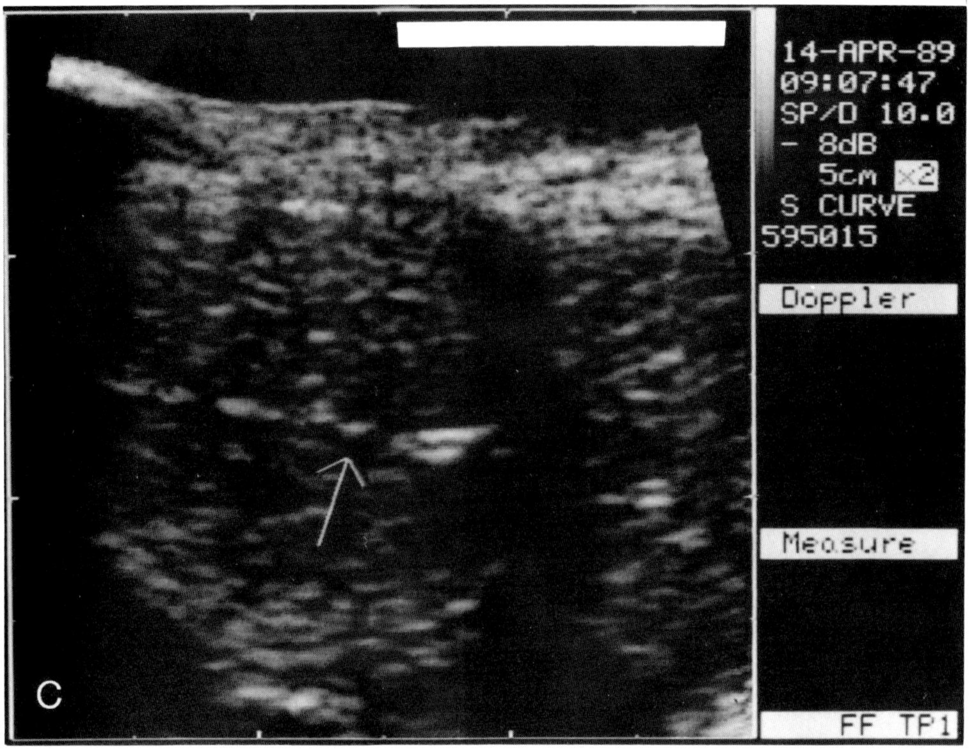

Figure 11.6. C.

of venous drainage vary widely, a "normal" value for arterial flow cannot be determined. In addition, intracavernous injection is not a physiologic event, and the flow increase is not as rapid as in sexually stimulated erection. Therefore, ±2 standard deviations from the mean is assigned as an adequate arterial response (mean postinjection diameter >0.07 cm, mean peak flow velocity >25 cm/sec [the low limit of the 95% confidence level derived from 18 control subjects]) (Table 11.1). In addition, the pulse waveform, pulsation pattern, and thickness of the arterial wall are considered useful accessory values.

In our first 657 patients (Table 11.2), 75% were found to have some degree of penile arterial insufficiency (not surprising in that the majority of our patients were over 50 years old). Patients under 40 had a significantly better arterial response than did those over 60 ($p < 0.05$). Diabetes mellitus and coronary artery disease were statistically significant factors in determining the diameter and peak flow velocity before and after injection of papaverine. The complications were relatively minor (Table 11.3).

The analysis of human results is based on our initial laboratory work. Electrostimulation of the cavernous nerve in dogs and monkeys caused an immediate increase of arterial flow in both the systolic and diastolic phases and a drop in pressure in the internal pudendal artery, denoting decreased peripheral resistance and vasodilation. With increasing intracavernous pressure, the blood flow through the internal pudendal artery gradually decreased owing to filling of the sinusoidal spaces and increasing resistance until, during full erection, it was only slightly above the prestimulation level. Timing is important in assessing penile arterial flow: during the latent and tumescent phases, the flow will be more than in the fully erect phase.

In larger arteries, increased peak flow velocity may indicate segmental stenosis; in a small vessel such as the cavernous artery, however, it indicates a good response to intracavernous injection. In addition, according to Laplace's law, a twofold increase in diameter can effect a 16-fold increase in flow. Thus, the diameter increase may in fact be the most important diagnostic indicator. We believe that only patients

Table 11.1.
Peak Flow Velocity and Inner Diameter of the Deep Arteries after Papaverine Injection in 18 Normal Men

	Diameter			
Age	Before	After	Increase	Peak Velocity
	cm	*cm*	*%*	*cm/sec*
45.8	0.51±0.09[a]	0.89±0.11	78.28±25.69	34.80±5.02
95% Confidence limits	0.33–0.69	0.67–1.11	26.9–129.66	24.76–44.84

[a] Mean ± S.D.

Table 11.2.
Differential Diagnosis of Impotence in 657 Patients

Neurogenic	28
Psychogenic	20
Predominantly venogenic	97
Predominantly arteriogenic	210
Mixed (arteriogenic + venogenic)	282
Others	20

Table 11.3.
Complications of Papaverine Injection for Ultrasonography in 657 Patients

Complication	No. of Patients
Moderate to severe hematoma	56
Dizziness and facial flushing	16
Hypotension	4
Prolonged erection (>1 hr)	61
Priapism (>6 hr)[a]	3

[a] Resolved by aspiration or injection of diluted phenylephrine hydrochloride.

with an adequate postinjection diameter and peak flow velocity can be considered as having an adequate arterial response.

Because the diameter and flow velocity measurements taken during full erection are different from those obtained during the latent phase, this study is not useful in patients who develop full erection after intracavernous injection unless it is performed before full erection occurs. We now routinely measure flow velocity and diameter increase 3 to 5 min after injection to avoid this problem. After relaxation of the smooth muscles of the arterioles and the cavernous tissues with injection, the erection becomes a function of the interplay between the arterial and venous flow. The critical level of arterial flow reduction that will render the patient impotent may vary from person to person owing to variations in penile volume and venous drainage.

Our tests involve high-resolution, small-part sonography, which can magnify the arterial vessels for accurate measurement of the inner diameter of the individual arteries (measurement error ± 0.01 cm). Although conventional continuous-wave Doppler analysis is accurate, it is less than ideal here, as it detects a mixture of signals from all the blood vessels in the path of the sound beam. The pulsed Doppler technique can scan the individual deep and dorsal arteries separately to identify specific pathologic conditions.

Except in very anxious patients, erection induced by intracavernous injection is not subject to psychologic inhibition. When the erectile response is considered together with the arterial status, the magnitude of venous drainage can be estimated. Duplex ultrasonography can be performed in the office, and the results are easily reproducible. It is more accurate than penile angiography for evaluating the cavernous arteries and avoids the risks associated with angiography and arterial catheterization in patients with atherosclerosis.

References

1. Lue TF, Hricak H, Marich KW, Tanagho EA. Vasculogenic impotence evaluated by high-resolution ultrasonography and pulsed Doppler spectrum analysis. Radiology 1985;155:777–781.
2. McAninch JW, Laing FC, Jeffrey RB Jr. Sonourethrography in the evaluation of urethral strictures: a preliminary report. J Urol 1988; 139:294–297.
3. Tanagho EA. Anatomy of the genitourinary tract. In: Tanagho EA, McAninch, eds. Smith's general urology. San Mateo, CA: Appleton & Lange, 1988:1–15.
4. Hricak H, Marotti M, Gilbert TJ, et al. Normal penile anatomy and abnormal penile conditions: evaluation with MR imaging. Radiology 1988; 169:683–690.
5. Hamm B, Friedrich M, Kelami A. Ultrasound imaging in Peyronie disease. Urology 1986; 28:540–545.
6. Balconi G, Angeli E, Nessi R, de Flaviis L. Ultrasonographic evaluation of Peyronie's disease. Urol Radiol 1988;10:85.

7. Hamm B, Friedrich M, Kelami A. Ultrasound imaging of the corpora cavernosa after priapism. Eur Urol 1985;11:210–211.
8. Oesterling JE, Bromberg WD, Albertson PC. Xeroradiography and ultrasonography in the evaluation of a penile injury. J Urol 1986;135: 791–793.
9. Sasso F, Vacilotto D, Controneo A, Destito A, Alcini E. Posttraumatic intracavernous haematoma: diagnostic and therapeutic perspectives. Int Urol Nephrol 1987;19:429–432.
10. Niedrach WL, Lerner RM, Linke CA. Penile abscess involving the corpus cavernosum: a case report. J Urol 1989;141:374–375.
11. Suarez G, Baum N. Ultrasonography in evaluation of mechanical problems of inflatable penile prosthesis. Urology 1987;30:388–389.
12. Dierks PR, Hawkins H. Sonography and penile trauma. J Ultrasound Med 1983;2:417–419.
13. Gluck DC, Bundy AL, Fine C, Loughlin KR, Richie JP. Sonographic rethrogram: comparison to roentgenographic techniques in 22 patients. J Urol 1988;140:1404–1408.
14. Lue TF, Tanagho EA. Functional anatomy and mechanism of penile erection. In: Tanagho EA, Lue TF, McClure RD, eds. Contemporary management of impotence and infertility. Baltimore: Williams & Wilkins, 1988:39–50.
15. Virag R, Frydman D, Legman M, Virag H. Intracavernous injection of papaverine as a diagnostic and therapeutic method in erectile failure. Angiology 1984;35:79–87.
16. Stackl W, Hasun R, Marberger M. Intracavernous injection of prostaglandin E_1 in impotent men. J Urol 1988;140:66–68.
17. Wetzner SM, Tutunjian J, Marich KW. Duplex scanning: a vascular diagnostic technology. Am Rev Diagnostics 1983;1:31.

CHAPTER 12

Ultrasound in Pediatric Urology

THOMAS E. SUMNER, M.D.

The pediatric patient is ideally suited for ultrasound. Small size and relative lack of body fat facilitate scanning since ultrasound imaging is based on the acoustic impedance of normal and pathological tissue. The fact that it is painless and does not employ irradiation further enhances the appeal of ultrasonography. Recent technical advances have resulted in high-resolution real-time scanners, and Doppler capability has further expanded diagnostic applications. In addition to initial diagnostic evaluation, follow-up pediatric urologic assessment with ultrasound has become popular due to its relatively low cost and efficiency.

Accurate renal ultrasonography is particularly valuable in children, since 55% of abdominal masses in infants and children are renal in origin (1). Differentiation between solid (echoic, echogenic) and cystic (anechoic) lesions is diagnostically reliable. Mixed echogenicity (solid and cystic patterns) may be seen with renal tumors. Current clinical indications to be discussed in addition to abdominal mass evaluation include infiltration, obstructive lesions, intrinsic renal disease (congenital and acquired), and imaging workup of infection.

NORMAL NEONATAL RENAL ULTRASOUND

The normal infant kidney differs sonographically from the adult kidney. Its cortical echogenicity is equal to or greater than adjacent normal liver (Fig. 12.1**A**). Infant medullary pyramids are larger relative to the remainder of the kidney, resulting in their prominent appearance (Fig. 12.1**B**). This appearance mimics multiple cysts, but the characteristic radial arrangement of pyramids around the central echo complex usually differentiates this condition. Increased neonatal renal cortical echogenicity (Fig. 12.1**C**) may be related to several factors: glomeruli occupying greater volume (19% in infants versus 9% in adults), thinner glomerular basement membrane in adults, and infant glomeruli being surrounded by a cuboid epithelium, which regresses with time; also, the neonatal cortex contains 20% of the loops of Henle (2). This "neonatal" cortical sonographic appearance changes to the "adult" pattern (renal cortex less echogenic than adjacent normal liver) between 2 and 3 months of age, with 90% simulating the adult appearance by 4 months. In addition to increased cortical echogenicity, decreased medullary echogenicity is typical in neonatal kidneys. This condition may be due to relative cortical hyperechogenicity or related to less echogenicity of the renal sinus due to less peripelvic fat in infants (3).

NEONATAL ABDOMINAL MASSES

Accurate diagnostic imaging is important for distinguishing the origin, content, and nature of abdominal masses. Since approximately 85% of abdominal masses in children, especially neonates, involves the kidneys or retroperitoneal structures, combined imaging of these structures is essential. Following palpation of an abdominal mass, a plain radiograph is usually obtained to attempt better definition of a suspected mass or to detect calcifications. The excretory urogram has largely been replaced by "screening" ultrasonography in both equivocal and highly suspect pediatric patients. The site of origin and type of content are usually established by abdominal sonography, with the exception of exophytic or large border lesions that blend with adjacent viscera. The latter situations are often further evaluated by computed tomography (CT) or magnetic resonance imaging (MRI). Assessing renal function is usually best achieved with radionuclide imaging.

The most common nonobstructing mass of the newborn period is the multicystic dysplastic kidney (MCDK). Two forms of multicystic kidneys are encountered: hydronephrotic and pelvoinfundibular. Ureteropelvic atresia during the metanephric stage of intrauterine development is the generally accepted etiology of

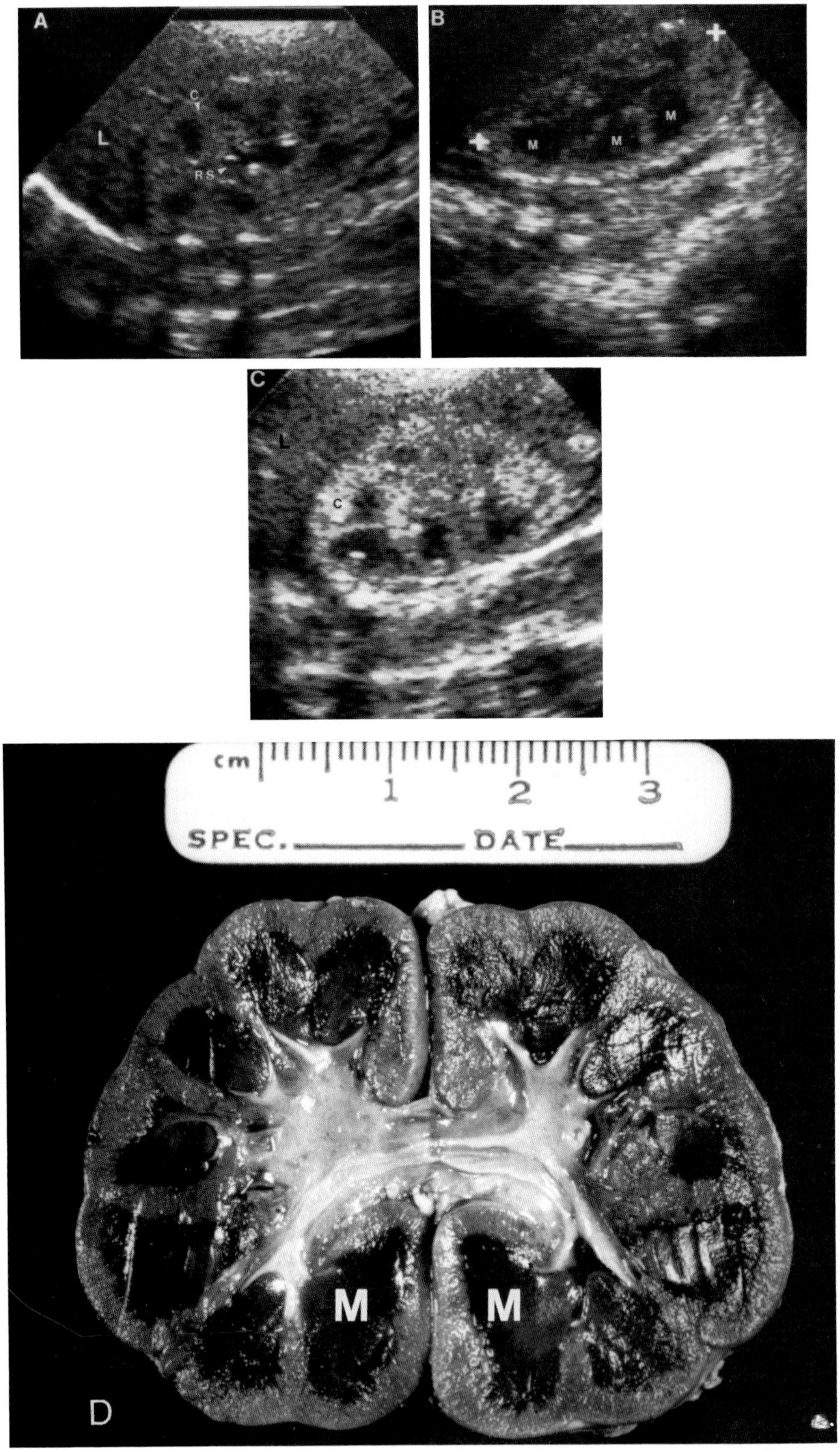

Figure 12.1. Normal infant kidney. Longitudinal supine view of right kidney. **A,** The renal cortex (*C*) is equal in echogenicity to the adjacent liver (*L*). The renal sinus (*RS*) is less echogenic than in adult patients. **B,** The renal medullary pyramids (*M*) in the infant are larger relative to the rest of the kidney and appear prominent. **C,** The renal cortex (*C*) is more echogenic than the adjacent liver (*L*). **D,** Gross specimen; note the prominent medullary pyramids (*M*).

MCDK. If only the ureter is atretic, the rare hydronephrotic form results, with multiple cysts replacing the pelvicaliceal system (4); if both the ureter and renal pelvis are atretic, the common pelvoinfundibular form results with multiple cysts of various sizes arranged in a disordered manner without reniform tissues or shape (5). Usually large and unilateral, a MCDK grossly has a grapelike appearance due to multiple smooth-walled, noncommunicating cysts (Fig. 12.2**A**). Microscopically, dysplastic renal parenchyma is seen, with varying amounts of connective tissue and cartilage (Fig. 12.2**B**); however, 5 to 20% of patients have relatively well differentiated renal tissue (6). Contralateral abnormalities such as vesicoureteral (VU) reflux, ureteropelvic junction (UPJ) obstruction, or crossed ectopia occurs in 20% of MCDK cases; only 20% are found in children beyond the age of 2 years, as most are detected in the neonatal period.

The diagnosis of MCDK can usually be made

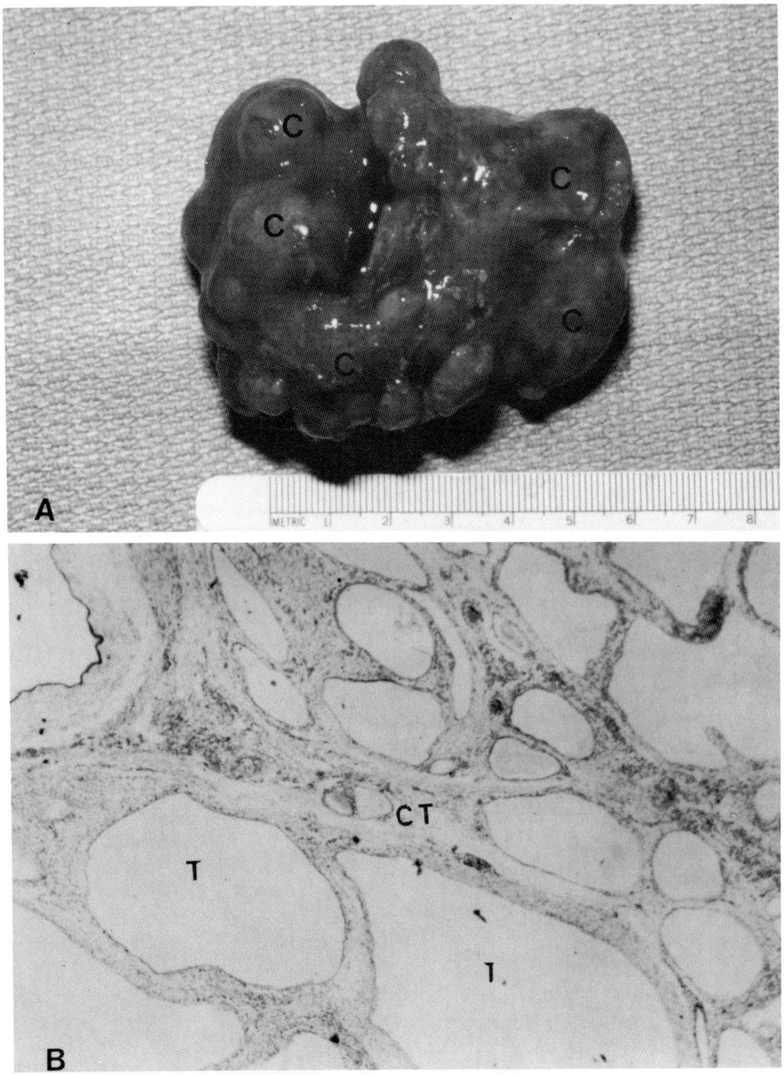

Figure 12.2. Multicystic dysplastic kidney. **A,** Gross specimen demonstrating cysts (*C*) of various sizes in dysplastic kidney. (From Sumner TE et al. Neonatal abdominal real-time sonography. RadioGraphics 1981;1(3):29–40.) **B,** Microscopic appearance with complete absence of normal parenchyma; numerous thick-walled collecting tubule cysts (*T*) are found; loose connective tissue (*CT*) fills space between cysts. (From Sumner TE et al. Real-time sonography of congenital cystic kidney disease. Urology 1982;20(1):97–101.)

with sonography. Typical sonograms show a multiloculated cystic mass with internal linear echoes representing curvilinear septa dividing it into cysts of various sizes (Fig. 12.3**A**). Its lobulated outline and disorderly arrangement of cysts usually distinguished MCDK from a severely hydronephrotic kidney; the latter usually appears reniform with symmetrically arranged dilated calices surrounding a medial hydropelvis (Fig. 12.3**B**). Difficulty arises in the rare case of a unilocular multicystic kidney resembling a severe UPJ obstruction (Fig. 12.3**C**). However, sonographic differentiation can usually be made by identifying the dilated extrarenal pelvis with its medial tapering, typical of UPJ obstruction (7). Doppler sonography may prove helpful in that the vascular pedicle is often absent in MCDK, so lack of renal arterial flow may be diagnostic.

Nonvisualization during excretory urography or radionuclide imaging is characteristic of MCDK. Occasionally, multiple cysts may be

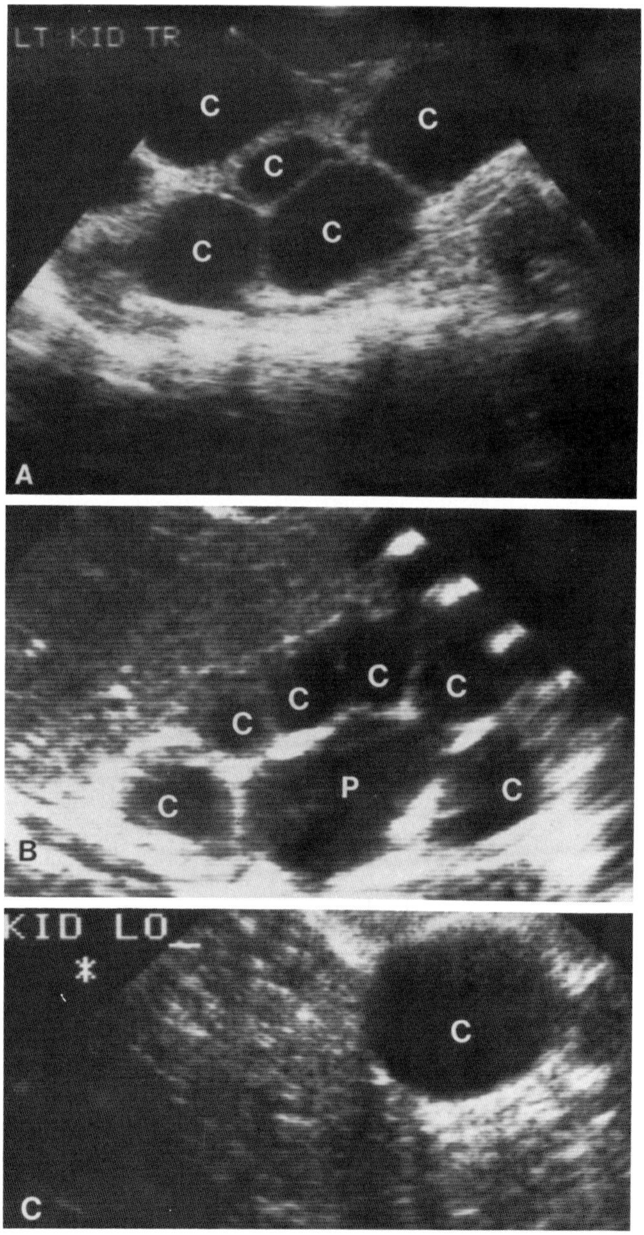

Figure 12.3. Multicystic dysplastic kidney. **A,** Supine longitudinal renal sonography demonstrates multiple anechoic areas separated by echogenic septations representing cysts (*C*). **B,** Typical longitudinal supine sonogram of hydronephrosis. *P,* pelvis; *C,* calices. **C,** Longitudinal renal sonogram of "unilocular" multicystic kidney (*C*). (From Sumner TE: Evaluation of the nonvisualizing or poorly visualized kidney. In: McCullough DL, ed. Difficult diagnoses in urology. New York: Churchill Livingstone, 1988: 3–21. Used by permission.)

demonstrable during early phases of excretory urography, with nonfunction at 30 min to 1 hr; 24- to 48-hr delay films in these cases may show puddling within the cysts, depending on the amount of functioning renal parenchyma (8). Other imaging modalities, such as percutaneous puncture and cystography, may be confirmatory. Percutaneous puncture under ultrasound guidance may distinguish between MCDK and severe unilateral hydronephrosis if no renal pelvis is identified or opacification of renal tubules occurs (9) (Fig. 12.4). Cystography is helpful if reflux occurs into a hypoplastic ureter (Fig. 12.5).

Other masses of the neonatal period include renal vein thrombosis, polycystic kidney disease, mesoblastic nephroma, and nephromegaly. All of these lesions are echogenic on ultrasonography and may be unilateral or bilateral. Renal vein thrombosis (RVT) in the neonate is often a complication of dehydration or sepsis, frequently with a maternal history of diabetes. Gross hematuria and flank mass is the usual presentation. Nonvisualization of the kidney during excretory urography is characteristic, although there may be faint visualization or a dense and persistent nephrogram; nuclear renal scans demonstrate either nonfunction or diminished and prolonged isotope uptake. Renal sonography excludes hydronephrosis or MCDK as the cause of a nonfunctioning, enlarged kidney. Typical sonographic features of RVT include nephromegaly with distorted architecture with varying degrees of cortical echogenicity (Fig. 12.6). RVT may be acute or chronic. Acutely, decreased echogenicity related to edema and hemorrhage is seen; later, echogenicity increases owing to cellular infiltration and fibrosis (10). This sonographic sequence occurs relatively quickly in the neonate (by 8 days) compared with adults (11). The primary thrombosis begins in the small intrarenal branches, then extends into larger veins and eventually into the inferior vena cava. Doppler ultrasonography may establish the diagnosis of RVT by demonstrating diminished or absent venous flow. Nonsurgical treatment is recommended since the involved kidney or kidneys revert to normal or become small and atrophic (12). Calcification occurs within the intrarenal veins in 30% of affected kidneys (13).

A neonate with bilateral renal masses usually has polycystic kidney disease (PCKD).

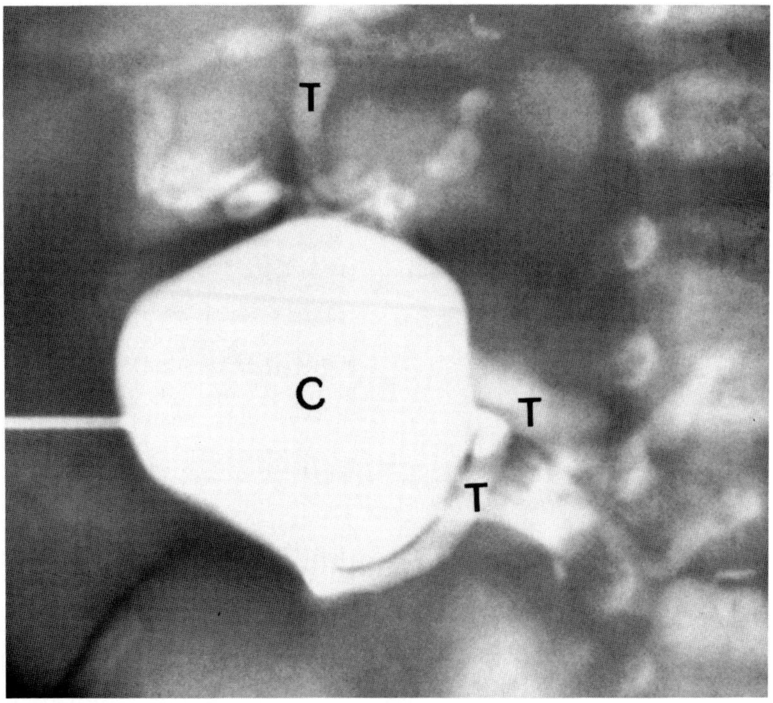

Figure 12.4. Multicystic dysplastic kidney. Percutaneous opacification of huge cyst (*C*) and ectatic collecting tubules (*T*).

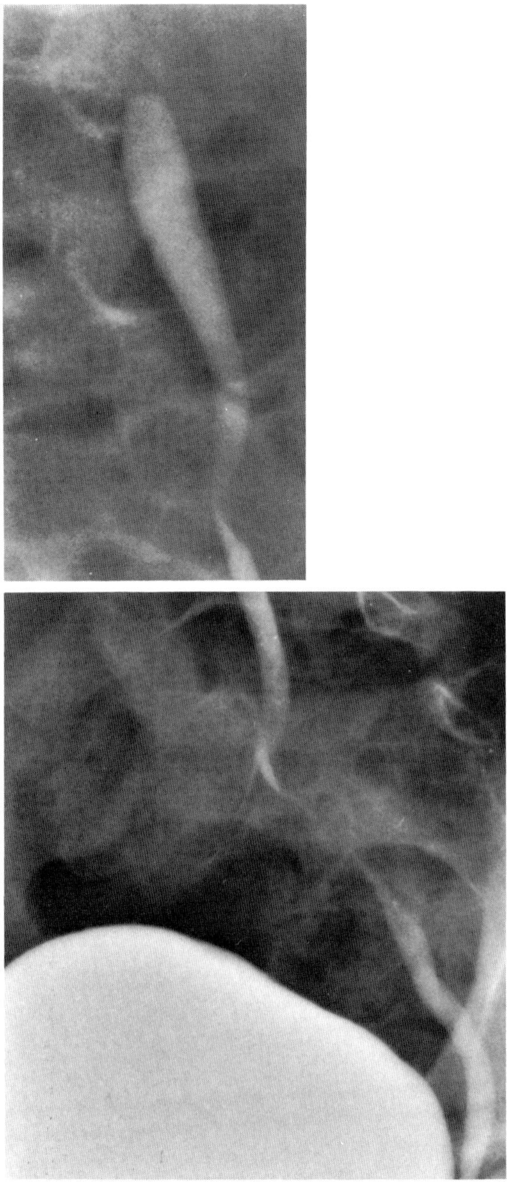

Figure 12.5. Multicystic dysplastic kidney. Cystogram demonstrating reflux into hypoplastic ureter.

Both the recessive (infantile) and dominant (adult) types occur in the newborn period. "Polycystic" is a misnomer in that neither of these conditions is necessarily cystic, although small or large cysts can be found in either (14). Infantile PCKD usually has ectatic collecting tubules simulating microscopic cysts. Sonography typically reveals echogenic kidneys with a "salt and pepper" pattern (Fig. 12.7); excretory urography (Fig. 12.8**A**) or CT (Fig. 12.8**B**) demonstrates a striated nephrogram. Childhood

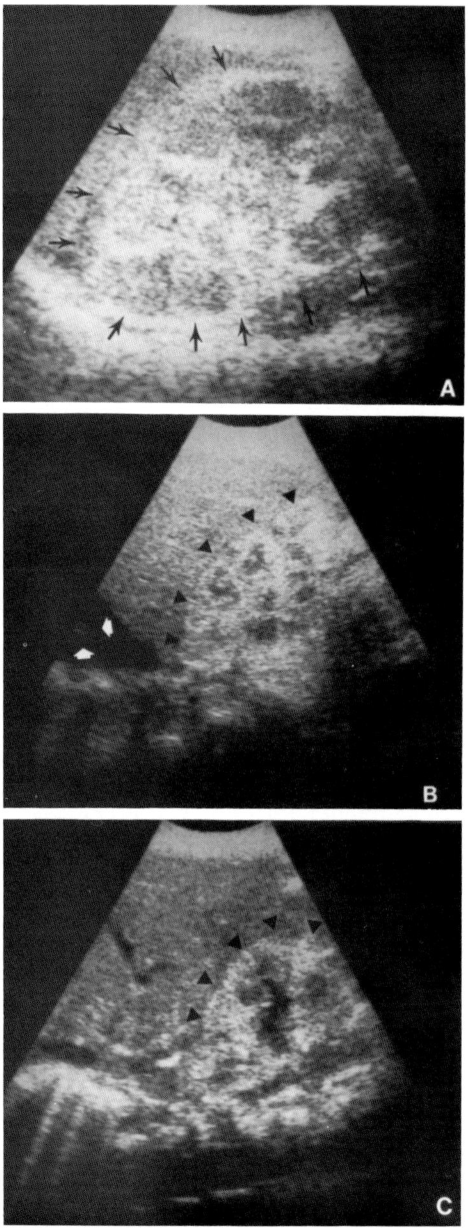

Figure 12.6. Renal vein thrombosis in a newborn with hematuria. **A,** Initial renal longitudinal sonogram demonstrating slightly enlarged kidney with poorly visualized pyramids. *Arrows* delineate renal borders. **B** and **C,** Serial subsequent renal sonograms demonstrating decreasing renal size with increased echogenicity. Note clot (*white arrowheads*) in the inferior vena cava in **B.** *Black arrowheads* delineate renal borders in **B** and **C.** (From Sumner TE, Volberg FM. Evaluation of the nonvisualizing or poorly visualized kidney. In: McCullough DL, ed. Difficult diagnoses in urology. New York: Churchill Livingstone, 1988: 3–21. Used by permission.)

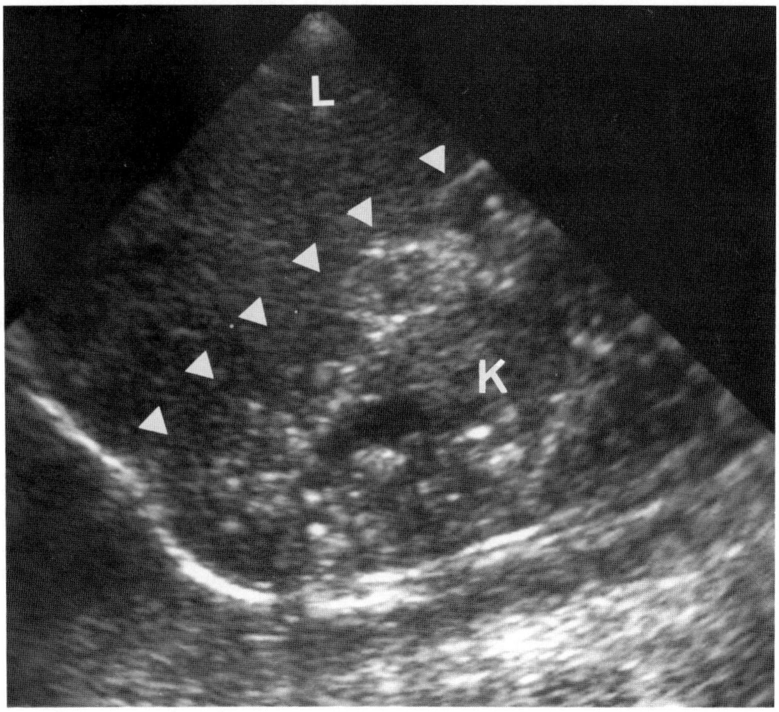

Figure 12.7. Infantile polycystic kidney disease. Longitudinal renal ultrasound demonstrates "salt and pepper" appearance. *L,* liver; *K,* kidney. *Arrows* delineate renal borders.

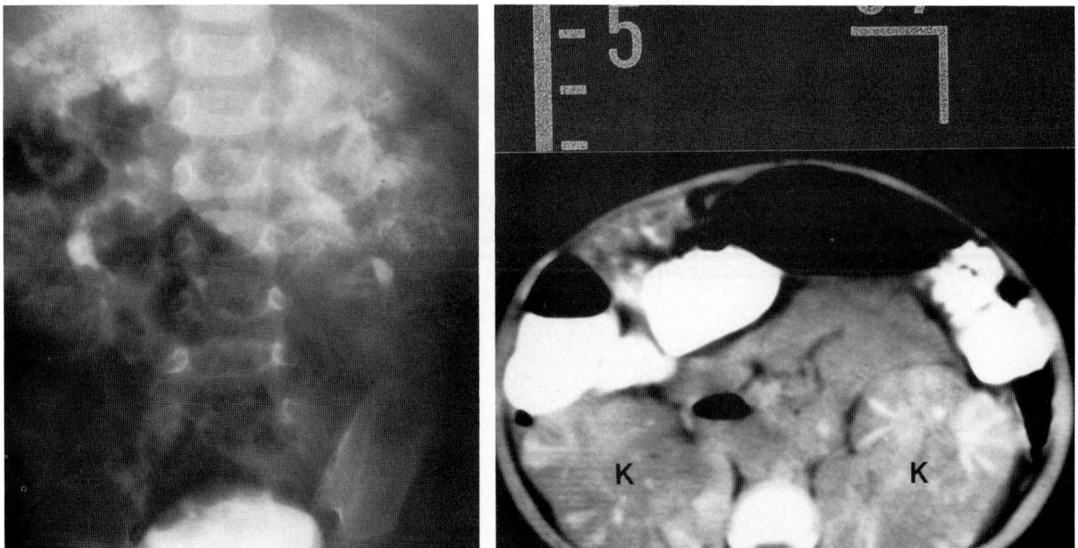

Figure 12.8. Infantile polycystic kidney disease. **A,** Intravenous urogram demonstrates striated nephrogram. **B,** CT after infusion demonstrates striated nephrogram. *K,* kidney.

PCKD represents a spectrum between the infantile and juvenile forms. The infantile form has more severe renal involvement, less hepatic fibrosis, and a poorer prognosis. The juvenile form has less renal involvement with a better prognosis; these patients may present with complications of hepatic disease. Renal ultrasonography in older children with recessive polycystic disease may demonstrate a cortical rim of normal echogenicity with the remainder of the kidney echogenic (14). Adult PCKD, an autosomal dominant condition, usually presents in the third and fourth decades but has been reported in young children and has also been identified in fetuses and infants (15). Sonography demonstrates large kidneys bilaterally with increased echogenicity due to interfaces of small cysts; scattered larger cysts can be seen (Fig. 12.9). Although diffuse and bilateral, markedly asymmetric involvement occurs in 8% of individuals with adult PCKD, sometimes stimulating a mass (16), sonographic screening of siblings and parents of the pediatric patient with suspected adult PCKD often established the diagnosis (Fig. 12.10). Liver involvement in the neonate is quite rare, but hepatic cysts reportedly occur in at least 60% of patients.

Mesoblastic nephroma is the most common solid renal tumor encountered in the neonatal period (up to 3 months of age). The most frequently used synonym is fetal renal hamartoma; other synonyms include leiomyomatous hamartoma, mesenchymal hamartoma of infancy, benign congenital Wilms' tumor, fibroma, fibromyoma, fibrosarcoma, and congenital fibrosarcoma (17). It usually appears as a neonatal abdominal mass without race or sex predilection. Mesoblastic nephroma is a benign tumor without distant metastases expected, but histologic examination is necessary to distinguish it from the rare neonatal Wilms' tumor. Radiologic findings resemble Wilms' tumor. Excretory urography reveals an intrarenal mass with collecting system distortion (Fig. 12.11). Hydronephrosis is minimal or absent, but there may be nonvisualization of one or more calices (17). Sonography reveals varying degrees of echogenicity, likely due to varying amounts of cystic change within these tumors (Fig. 12.12); in addition, hemorrhage and necrosis may result in relatively hypoechoic or anechoic areas (17). Computed tomographic examination may demonstrate a heterogeneous mass with areas of contrast enhancement (18). Hartman et al. described reduced CT density

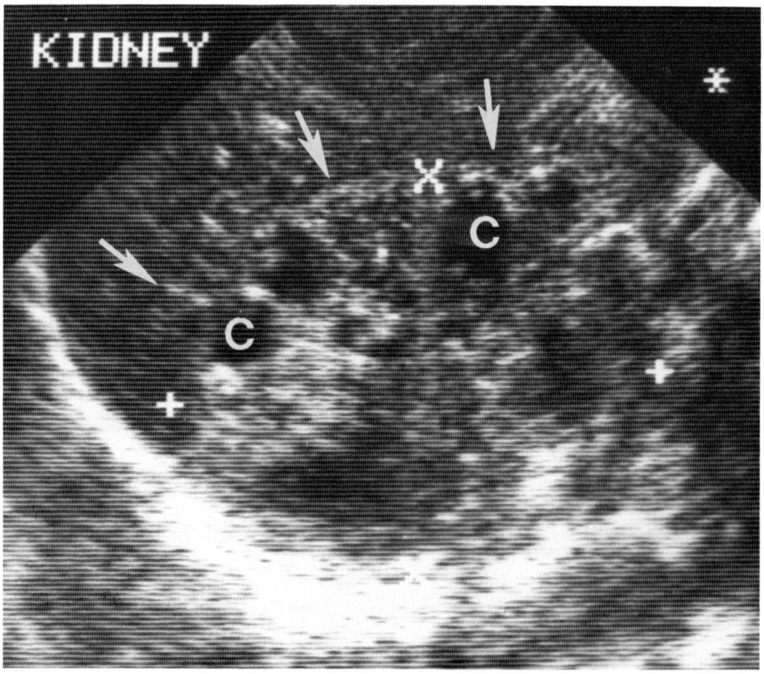

Figure 12.9. Adult polycystic kidney disease. Eight-month-old with sonographic demonstration of variously sized cysts (*C*). *Arrows* and + delineate renal borders.

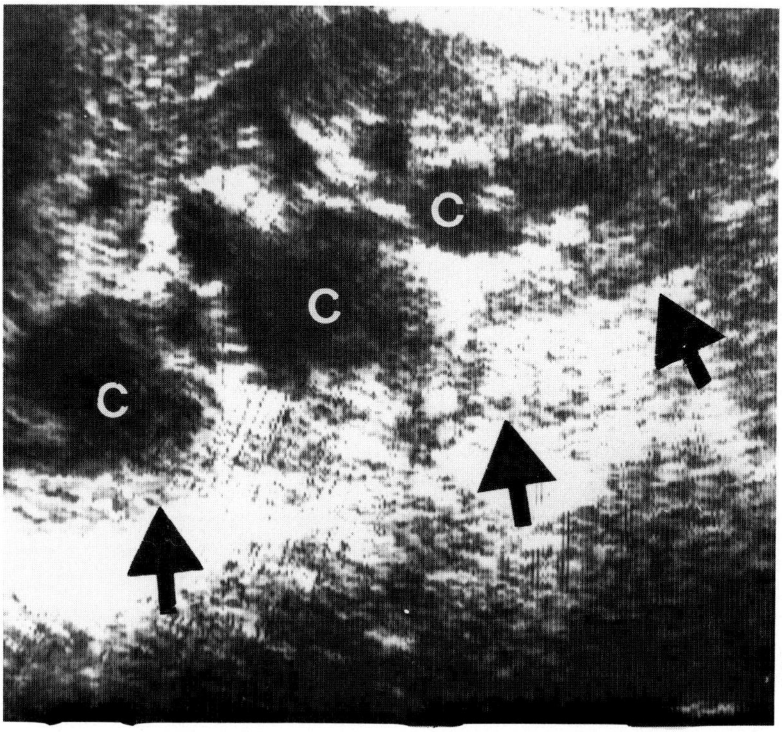

Figure 12.10. Adult polycystic kidney disease. Mother of pediatric patient illustrated in Fig. 12.9; longitudinal renal ultrasound demonstrates multiple cysts (*C*). *Arrows* delineate renal borders.

and minimal contrast enhancement corresponding to ultrasonographic anechoic areas (Fig. 12.13) (17). Angiography is nonspecific with irregular neovascularity (Fig. 12.14) and is recommended only if outlining vascular anatomy is important in surgical planning. Treatment is local resection.

The last group of neonatal renal masses is nephromegaly. Nephromegaly implies enlarged kidneys with normal sonographic architecture. Infants with congenital nephrosis and those with the Beckwith-Wiedemann syndrome (Fig. 12.15) should be considered in this group. Patients with Beckwith-Wiedemann syndrome have an increased incidence of nephroblastomatosis, so tumor screening is recommended during the first 4 to 6 years of life.

CHILDHOOD RENAL MASSES

Beyond the neonatal period, cystic renal masses to be considered include MCDK, PCKD, simple cysts, and hydronephrosis. MCDK and PCKD are discussed in the preceding section on neonatal renal masses, and hydronephrosis is discussed in the following section on obtrusive lesions. Simple renal cysts are seldom found in children and rarely cause symptoms. An abdominal mass is the most frequent presenting feature with occasional hematuria, proteinuria, or hypertension. Multiple bilateral cysts are suggestive of polycystic disease in that multiple simple cysts in childhood are exceptionally rare (19, 20). Children with tuberous sclerosis may have macroscopic cysts indistinguishable from adult PCKD; the renal disease may precede cutaneous or neurologic manifestations. Renal cysts have also been described with Zellweger's (cerebrohepatorenal) syndrome (21); macroscopic cysts may occur in infants born to mothers who have abused cocaine.

Solid renal masses to be considered include Wilms' tumor, multilocular cystic nephroma, nephroblastomatosis, renal cell carcinoma, renal lymphoma and leukemia, and angiomyolipoma. Mesoblastic nephroma is discussed with neonatal renal masses, as most occur be-

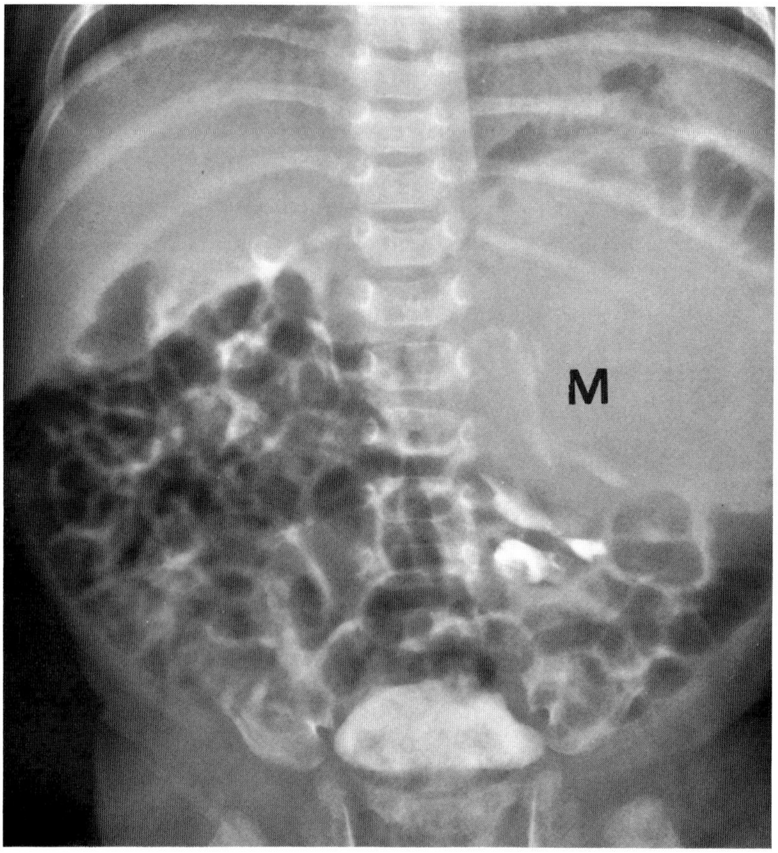

Figure 12.11. Mesoblastic nephroma. Excretory urography reveals left intrarenal mass (*M*) distorting collecting system.

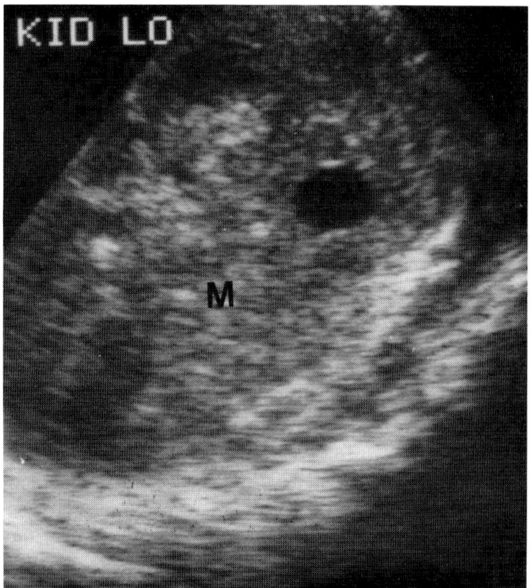

Figure 12.12. Mesoblastic nephroma. Longitudinal sonogram shows echogenic intrarenal mass (*M*).

fore age 3 months; only three of 20 children were age 2 years or older in the review series of Hartman et al. (17). Wilms' tumor (WT) is the most common renal neoplasm of childhood. WT has a medium age at presentation of 3 to 4 years, with 80% diagnosed by age 6 years. Bilaterality incidence is 5%, Most children are asymptomatic until abdominal distension or mass is discovered. Fifty percent of patients have hypertension. Uncommon signs are pain, hematuria, and fever. Associated anomalies include cryptorchidism, hemihypertrophy, hair and nail abnormalities, hypospadias, and cardiovascular abnormalities; aniridia occurs in a small percentage of WT patients.

Radiographic evaluation of WT has changed in the past decade. A plain abdominal radiograph is usually obtained for detection of a renal mass or tumor calcification. Previously diagnosed by excretory urography and venography, Wilms' tumor is now diagnosed by ultrasound and computed tomography. WT on ultrasound is an echogenic intrarenal mass

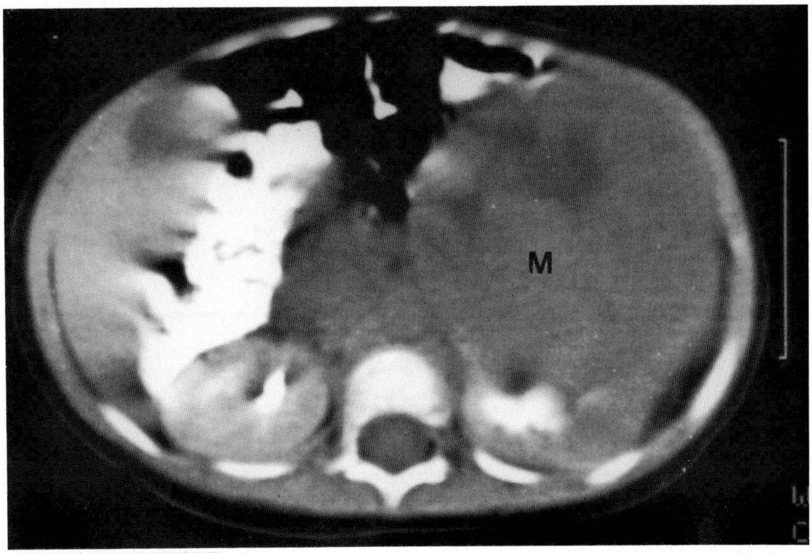

Figure 12.13. Mesoblastic nephroma. Computed tomographic study demonstrates heterogeneous left renal mass (*M*). (Courtesy of Dr. Marilyn J. Seigel, Mallinckrodt Institute of Radiology, St. Louis, MO.)

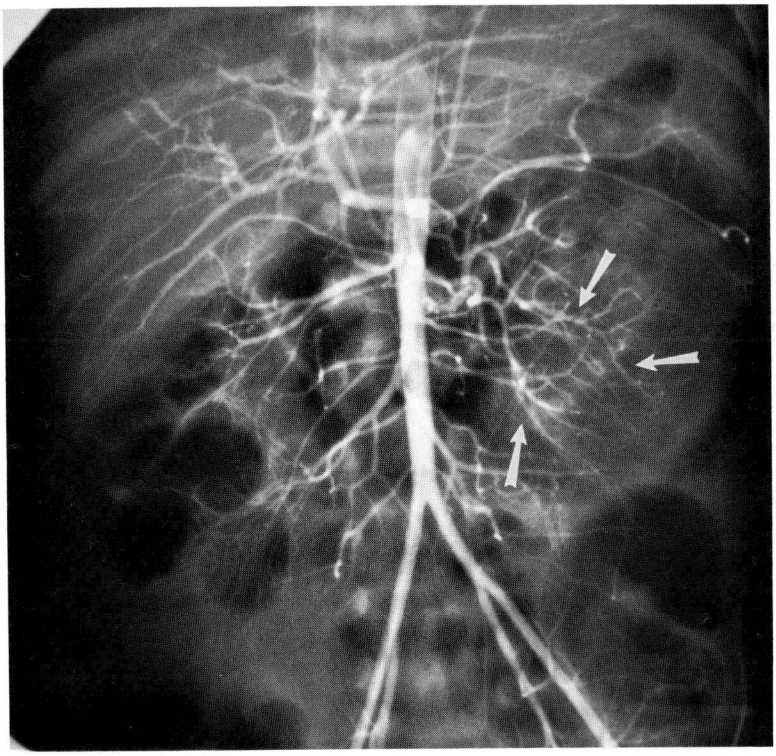

Figure 12.14. Mesoblastic nephroma. Aortogram reveals left renal neovascularity (*arrows*).

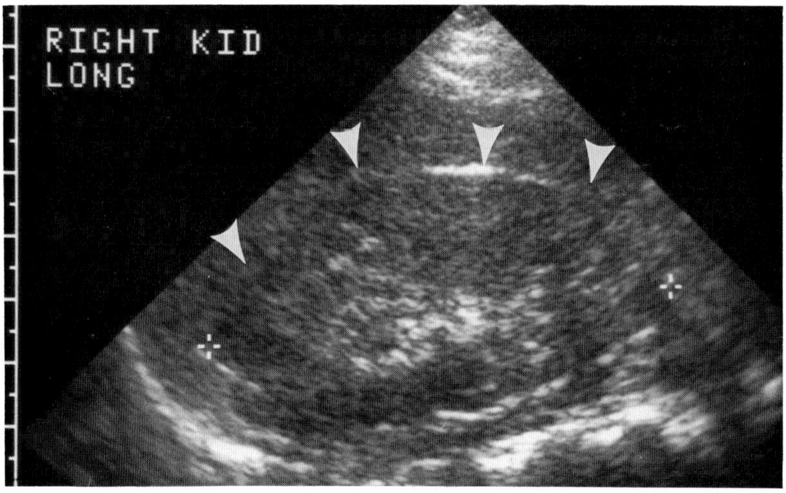

Figure 12.15. Beckwith-Wiedemann syndrome. Longitudinal sonogram shows nephromegaly with normal sonographic architecture. *Arrowheads* and + delineate renal borders.

(Fig. 12.16). Hypoechoic or anechoic areas are related to cystic areas in the tumor or tumor necrosis; obstructed calices may produce cystic areas within the mass. Sonography of the contralateral kidney may reveal other tumors (Fig. 12.17) or nephroblastomatosis. Regional lymph nodes and the liver should be scanned for metastases and the inferior vena cava, renal vein, and right atrium assessed for possible tumor thrombus (Fig. 12.18). Duplex Doppler sonography facilitates the evaluation of vessels prone to tumor thrombus and the confirmation of vascular encasement and displacement. Ultrasound can be limited by bowel gas, and mod-

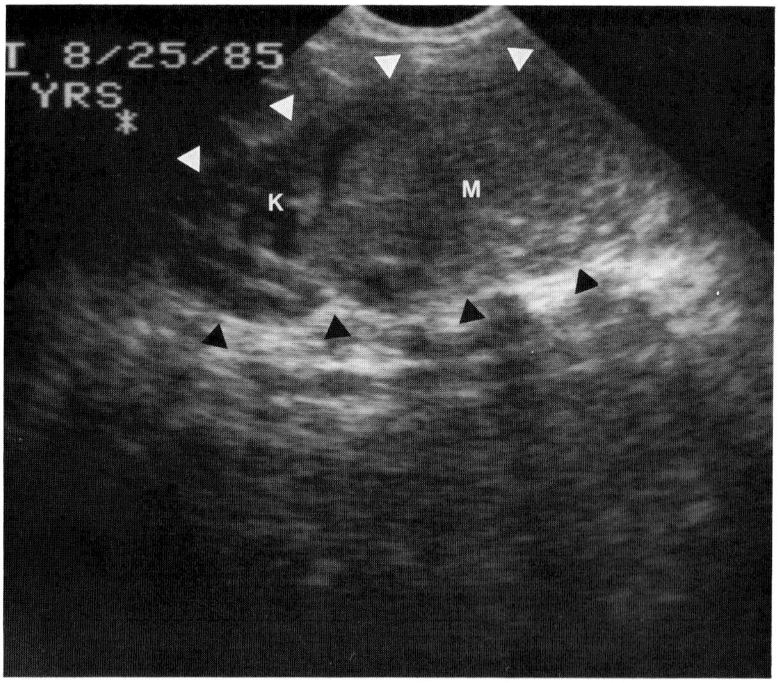

Figure 12.16. Wilms' tumor. Longitudinal ultrasound showing an echogenic mass (*M*) arising from the lower pole of the kidney (*K*). *Arrowheads* delineate renal borders.

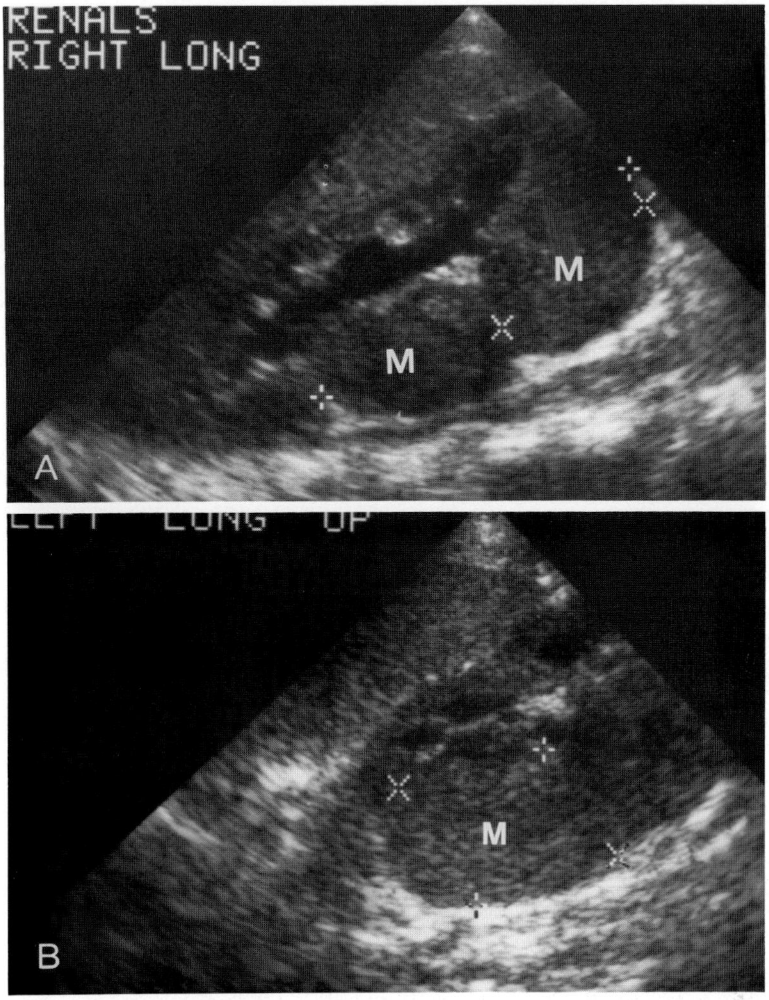

Figure 12.17. Bilateral Wilms' tumor. Longitudinal right (**A**) and left (**B**) renal sonograms revealing variously sized echogenic masses (*M*).

ern real-time ultrasound sector scanning cannot produce an entire abdominal cross section. For these reasons CT is usually done if the ultrasound is positive or suspicious for a tumor. CT is excellent for demonstrating the primary tumor; local or distant abdominal spread to nodes, vessels, or liver; and pulmonary metastases. The primary tumor appears as an intrarenal mass, especially well seen after contrast enhancement (Fig. 12.19). Tumor in the inferior vena cava is seen after bolus contrast injection, although false positives have been reported for caval involvement by tumor (22). Preliminary studies with magnetic resonance imaging (Fig. 12.20) suggest it is equal to CT for the evaluation of WT and is particularly well suited for the detection of caval involvement (23).

Multilocular cystic nephroma is an uncommon benign renal neoplasm mainly affecting boys in childhood and women in adulthood. Plain radiographs may reveal curvilinear calcification. A predominately cystic multilocular mass is the typical sonographic appearance, although an echogenic mass without cysts has been reported. On CT, the cysts appear as low-density round masses that do not communicate with the collecting system and are not enhanced with contrast infusion (24).

Nephroblastomatosis refers to persistence of primitive renal parenchymal tissue postnatally. Nephromegaly is typical with varying

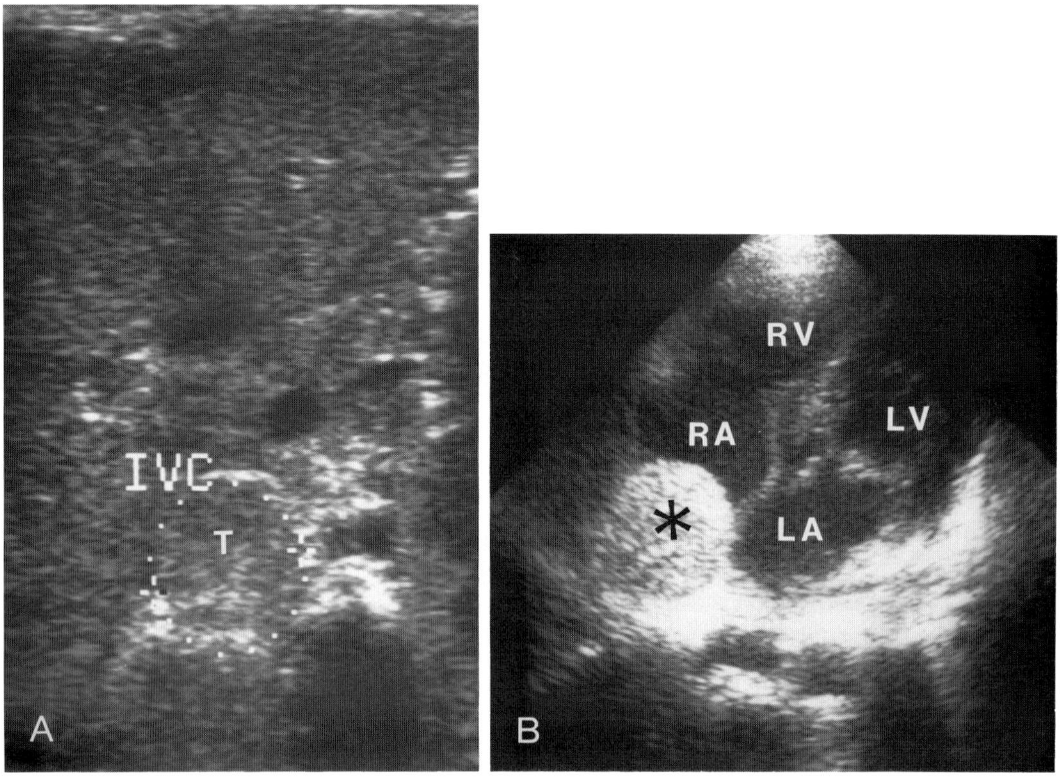

Figure 12.18. Wilms' tumor. **A,** Transverse sonogram showing tumor thrombus (*T*) in inferior vena cava (*IVC*). **B,** Cardiac ultrasound shows thrombus in right atrium (*). (*RA*), right atrium; *LA,* left atrium; *RV,* right ventricle; *LV,* left ventricle.

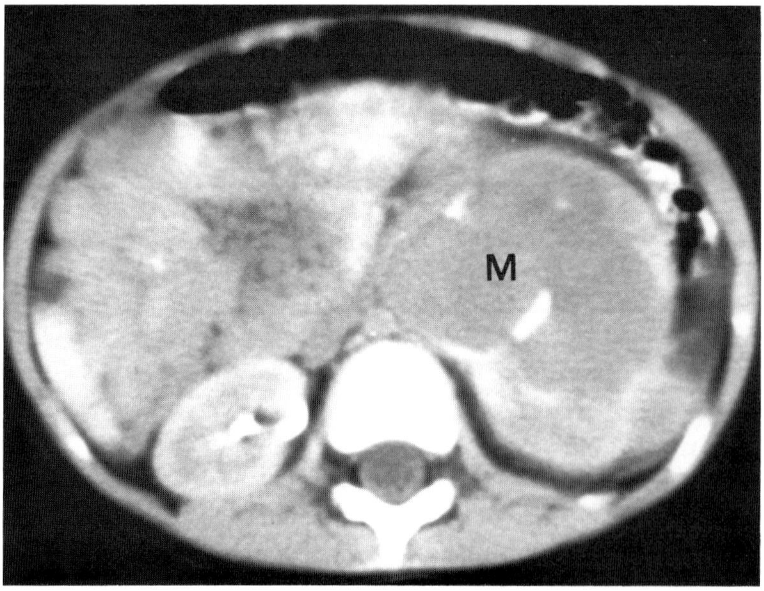

Figure 12.19. Wilms' tumor. Computed tomography showing intrarenal mass (*M*).

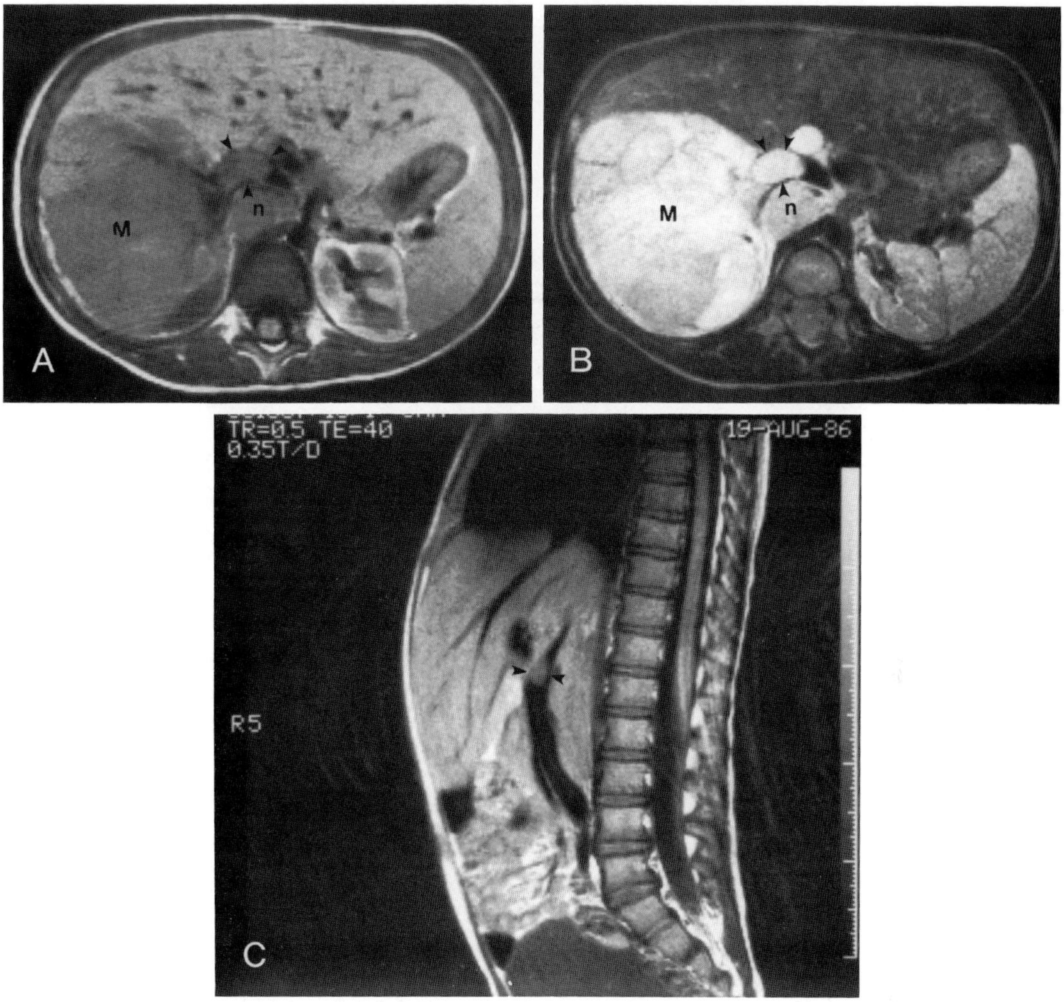

Figure 12.20. Magnetic resonance imaging of Wilms' tumor. **A** and **B,** T1- and T2-weighted cross-sectional scans with tumor (*M*) in right kidney and renal vein and inferior vena cava (*arrows*) lymph node (*n*) containing tumor. **C,** Sagittal scan showing inferior vena cava containing tumor (*arrows*). (Courtesy of Jerald P. Kuhn, M.D., Childrens' Hospital of Buffalo, Buffalo, NY.)

degrees of renal parenchymal dysfunction. A higher incidence of renal tumors in children with nephroblastomatosis is reported, although the level of risk for development of Wilms' tumor is not known (25). Sonography reveals an enlarged kidney and subtle peripheral hyperechoic or hypoechoic cortical masses. Excretory urography may show some caliceal distortion, CT is more sensitive than ultrasound or excretory urography for detection of rests of nephroblastomatosis. These lesions appear as nonenhancing cortical plaques of tissue well demarcated from normal renal parenchyma (26).

Renal cell carcinoma (RCC) occurs rarely in the first 2 decades of life. In an extensive review of more than 1500 patients, less than 0.5% presented before age 20 years. The almost equal sex incidence contrasts with male preponderance in adults. In comparison to WT, RCC in childhood and adolescence usually presents with a smaller abdominal mass that is frequently not palpable or visible on plain abdominal radiographs. Ultrasound and CT findings resemble Wilms' tumor (Fig. 12.21). However, this rare neoplasm should be considered in the older child with hematuria and renal calcification on plain films (27). Recently a 2½ month

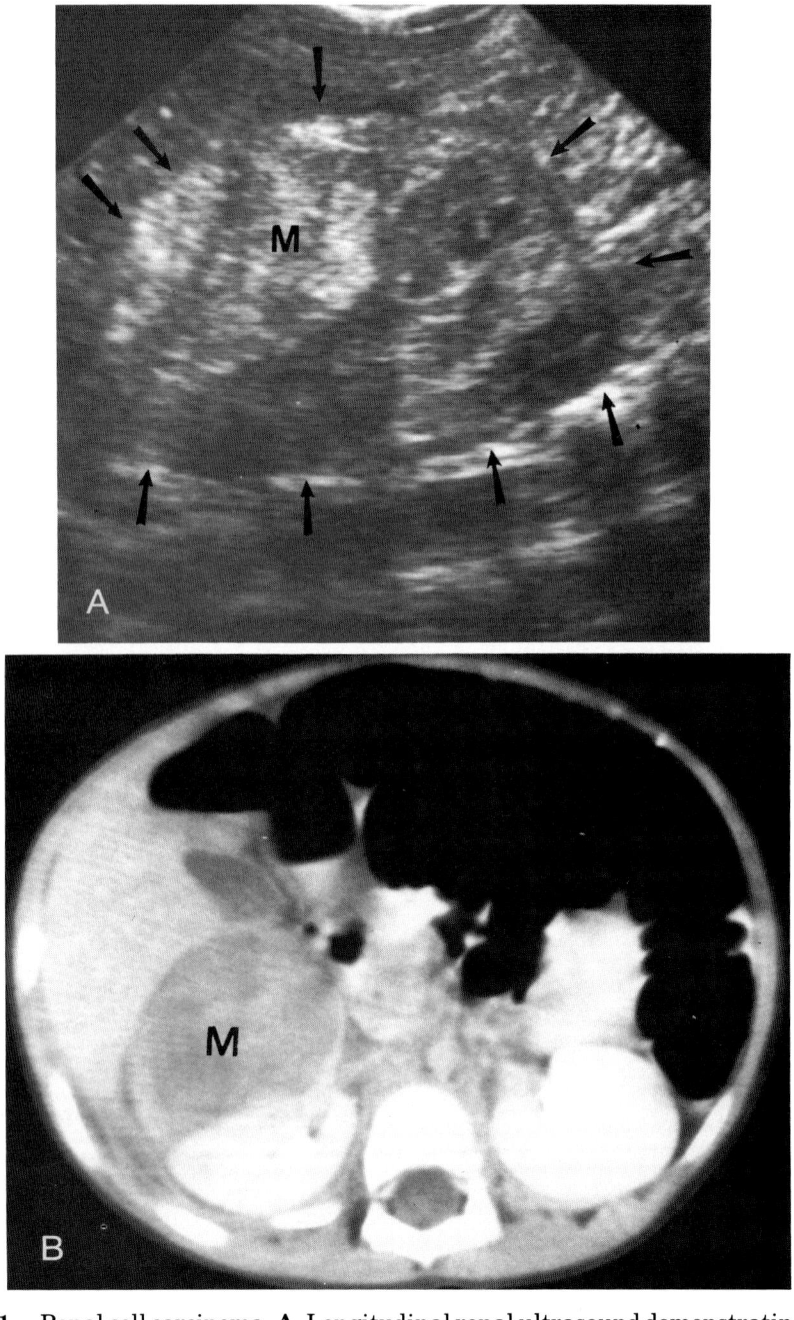

Figure 12.21. Renal cell carcinoma. **A,** Longitudinal renal ultrasound demonstrating echogenic mass (*M*). *Arrows* delineate renal border. **B,** Abdominal CT revealing intrarenal mass (*M*).

old child has been reported with undifferentiated renal cell carcinoma (28). Prognosis depends on the stage of disease at presentation; RCC is less responsive to multimodal therapy than is Wilms' tumor.

Renal lymphoma typically produces either smooth nephromegaly or lobulated parenchymal masses. Primary lymphoma is rare because the kidney does not have lymphoid tissue; however, the kidney represents one of the most common extranodal sites of metastatic lymphoma. Non-Hodgkin's lymphoma more commonly involves kidneys than does Hodgkin's disease. Large cell American Burkitt lymphoma in children commonly has renal involvement (29). Ultrasound usually reveals hypoechoic renal parenchymal masses (Fig. 12.22), with similar findings on excretory urography or CT. Leukemic infiltration is rarely demonstrable radiographically, although the incidence of detection at autopsy is 50%. Diffuse infiltration is the rule, with a focal renal mass rarely found. Sonography usually reveals highly echogenic and enlarged kidneys (Fig. 12.23), and CT shows diffuse enlargement (30).

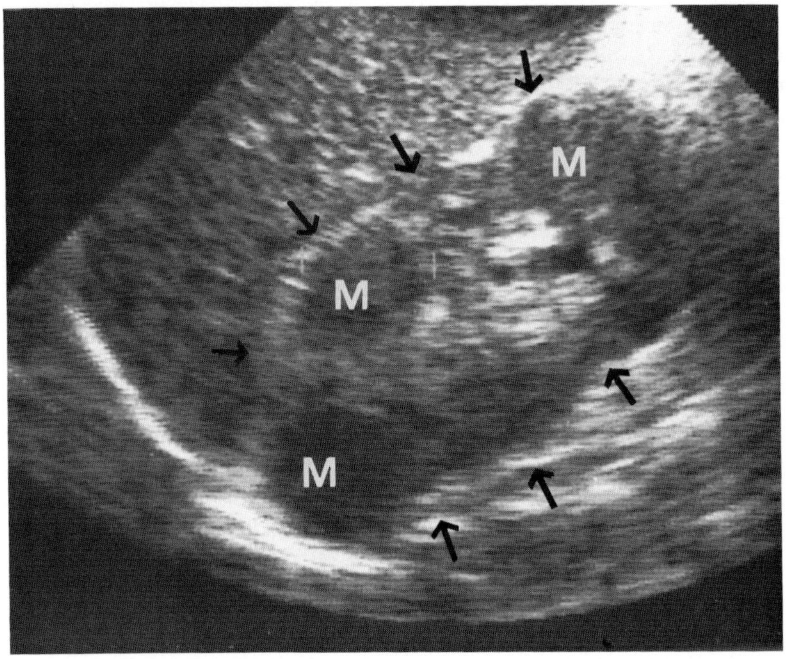

Figure 12.22. Lymphoma. Longitudinal renal ultrasound showing hypoechoic renal masses (*M*). *Arrows* delineate renal borders.

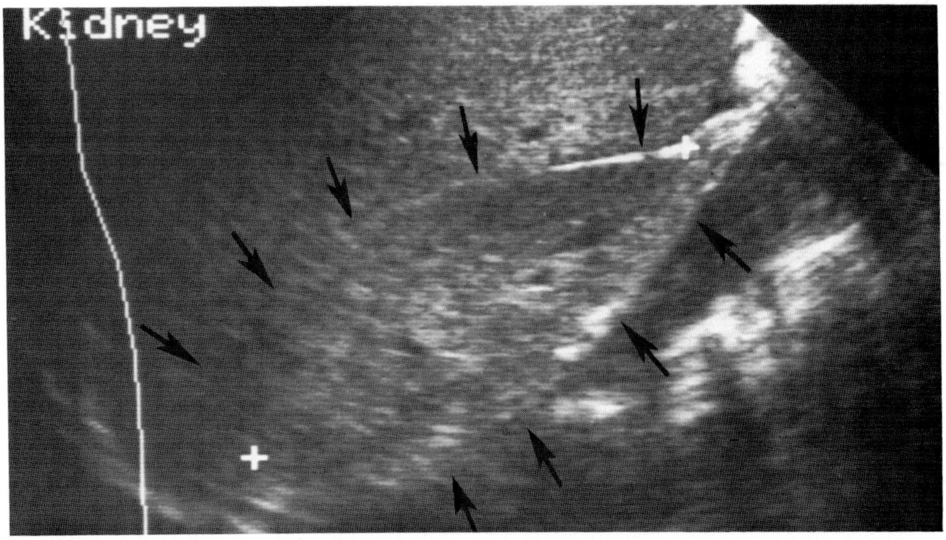

Figure 12.23. Leukemia. Nephromegaly with increased echogenicity on ultrasound. *Arrows* and + delineate renal borders.

Angiomyolipoma occurs in up to 50% of tuberous sclerosis patients (31). Of 23 tuberous sclerosis patients reported by Narla et al., the earliest detection of angiomyolipoma was at 5 years, although renal cysts in association with tuberous sclerosis were found in the newborn period (32). Renal lesions were found more frequently with increasing age. Sonography is recommended for screening for renal lesions. Angiomyolipomas are typically extremely echodense due to fat content. Large lesions are easily confirmed by CT, whereas detection of fat by ultrasound is easier. Ultrasound should also detect associated renal tumors such as Wilms' tumor or renal cell carcinoma.

OBSTRUCTIVE LESIONS

Ureteropelvic junction (UPJ) obstruction is the most common congenital obstruction of the urinary tract. Possible etiologies include congenital bands, aberrant blood vessels, intrinsic muscle fiber abnormalities in the pelvis, and fibrosis due to collagen deposition. One-third of all intrinsic lesions are associated with an extrinsic factor, such as bands or vessels. Most UPJ obstructions are on the left, with a 10 to 25% bilaterality incidence and association with contralateral multicystic dysplastic kidney (MCDK). The most common cause of hydronephrosis in the pediatric age group is UPJ obstruction; it is common in the neonate and very common in children older than 5 years. Most neonates with UPJ obstruction present with a prenatal ultrasonographic diagnosis and abdominal mass, or a urinary tract infection. Older children have their hydronephrosis detected as an asymptomatic mass or during an incidental abdominal radiograph; occasionally hematuria, especially after trauma, is the presenting finding. Pain or a urinary tract infection evaluation may also reveal hydronephrosis. Due to nonvisualization or poor visualization during excretory urography (Fig. 12.24**A**), delayed films may be helpful by revealing a dilated renal pelvis without filling of the distal ureter (Fig. 12.24**B**), indicating UPJ obstruction. Ultrasonography, which does not rely on renal function, shows pyelectasis and caliectasis without ureterectasis (Fig. 12.24**C**); if ureteral dilatation is detected, vesicoureteral reflux or distal ureteral obstructions must be excluded. A radionuclide diuretic study may be required to document UPJ obstruction and assess the degree of obstruction. This test is performed using [^{99m}Tc]DTPA (Fig. 12.25**A–C**); after 20 min 1 to 2 mg/kg furosemide (Lasix) is given intravenously, and background-corrected time-activity histogram curves are generated for each kidney and sections of their respective ureter (Fig. 12.25**D** and **E**). Each kidney is individually evaluated, since computer programs permit quantitative split glomerular filtration rate (GFR) assessment. However, in cases of extremely poor renal function with extremely low GFR or severely dilated collecting systems, the Lasix renogram may be falsely positive or negative. In these situations, a percutaneous ureteral perfusion study (Whitaker test) may be the only reliable means of establishing UPJ obstruction (33, 34). Diuretic renography may also be used pre- and postoperatively to correlate surgical results and to diagnose intermittent UPJ obstruction. If renography reveals hydroureteronephrosis, a cystogram is necessary to detect vesicoureteral (VU) reflux or distal ureteral obstruction. Infection, bladder distention, and VU reflux can cause urinary tract dilatation without obstruction. Accurate diagnosis of VU reflux by ultrasonography has been reported and may decrease the need for repetitive cystograms (35). Distal ureteral obstruction may be due to congenital or acquired ureterovesical junction (UVJ) obstruction. Congenital etiologies include primary megaureter (obstructive and nonobstructive), primary megaureter with coexisting bladder saccule, simple ureterocele, ectopic ureterocele, and ectopic ureter. Acquired causes include distal ureteral stricture following ureteral reimplantation, neurogenic bladder, edema, and inflammation. Neurogenic bladder patients may develop urinary tract dilatation secondary to incomplete emptying, urinary tract infection, or reflux; serial ultrasonography has proved useful in evaluating dilatation, bladder emptying, and reflux and in detecting renal scarring, thereby obviating repeated radiographic or radionuclide examinations.

MEGAURETERS

Primary megaureters can be obstructive or nonobstructive. Primary obstructive megaureter (megaloureter), usually discovered in infants and young children, frequently involves the left ureter but is bilateral in 20%. Obstruction is due to a narrowed aperistaltic juxtavesicular ureteral segment ranging from 0.5 to 4 cm in length. It is postulated that congenital absence of spiral musculature with second-

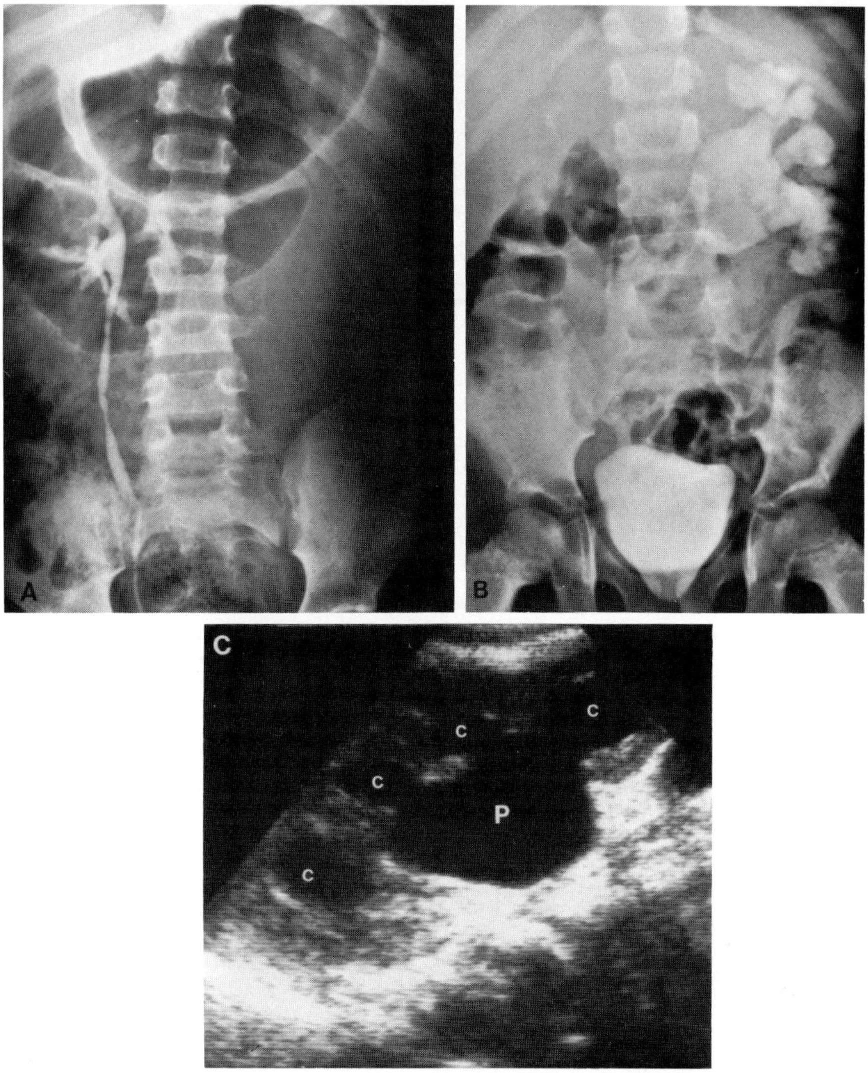

Figure 12.24. Left ureteropelvic junction obstruction. **A,** Nonvisualization during excretory urography. **B,** Dilated renal pelvis without ureteral opacification on delayed films. **C,** Renal sonography reveals pelvicaliectasis without ureterectasis. *P,* pelvis; *C,* calices. (From Sumner TE, Volberg FM. Evaluation of the nonvisualizing or poorly visualized kidney. In: McCullough DL, ed. Difficult diagnoses in urology. New York: Churchill Livingstone, 1988: 3–21. Used by permission.)

ary local muscular hypertrophy produces the obstruction. Associated fibrosis of the involved ureteral segment further limits the expansion and peristalsis. Excretory urography typically shows ureteral dilatation above a distal narrowed segment (Fig. 12.26**A** and **B**). At fluoroscopy, lack of peristalsis of the involved segment produces bulbous ureteral dilatation proximal to the narrow juxtavesical ureter. Voiding cystourethrography should be performed to exclude VU reflux or bladder outlet obstruction (36). Finding reflux suggests refluxing rather than primary obstructive megaureter, but the two conditions are not mutually exclusive. Reflux may coexist with distal ureteral obstruction, in which case reflux may obscure the obstructive component. Percutaneous studies can assess the degree of obstruction in an unoperated dilated system and evaluate the results of interventional techniques, such as balloon dilatation (Fig. 12.26**C**) (37). Primary obstructive (idiopathic) megaureter is rare, and

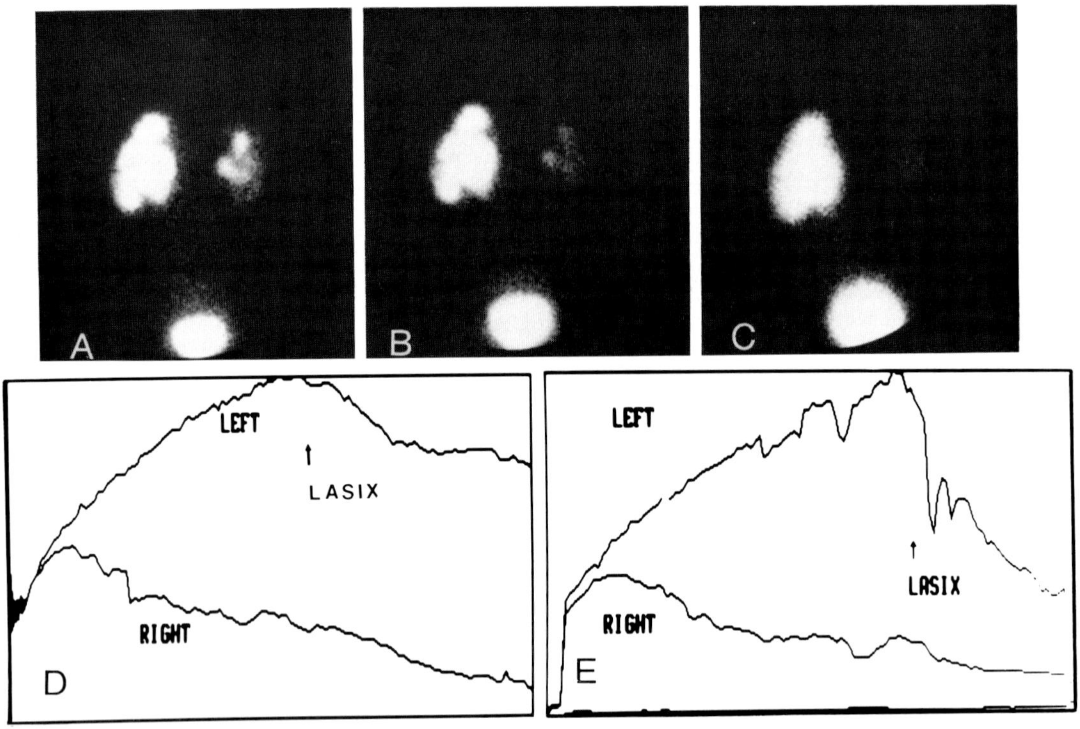

Figure 12.25. Diuretic radionuclide urography. **A, B, C,** [^{99m}Tc]DTPA sequential posterior images after Lasix administration consistent with left UPJ obstruction. **D,** Renogram curve on the right is normal. The obstructive pattern on the left with flattened response to Lasix is consistent with left UPJ obstruction. **E,** Postoperative diuretic renogram demonstrating improved response to Lasix. (From Sumner TE, Volberg FM. Evaluation of the nonvisualizing or poorly visualized kidney. In: McCullough DL, ed. Difficult diagnoses in urology. New York: Churchill Livingstone, 1988: 3–21. Used by permission.)

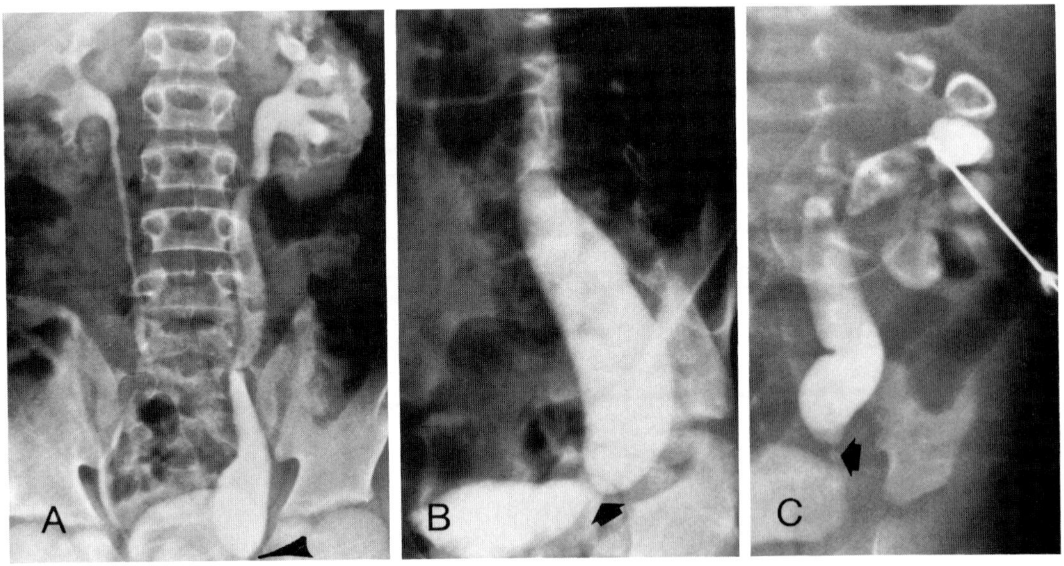

Figure 12.26. Primary obstructive megaureter (megaloureter). **A,** Intravenous urogram demonstrating fusiform distal ureteral dilatation (*arrowhead*) in primary megaureter. **B,** A narrowed distal ureteral segment at the juxtavesical level (*arrowhead*) is demonstrated on oblique view during intravenous urography. **C,** Percutaneous nephrostogram demonstrating distal ureteral narrowing (*arrowhead*) in primary obstructive megaureter. (From Sumner TE, Volberg FM. Evaluation of the nonvisualizing or poorly visualized kidney. In: McCullough DL, ed. Difficult diagnoses in urology. New York: Churchill Livingstone, 1988: 3–21. Used by permission.)

no definite etiology other than "embryonic widening" is implicated. Flow studies are normal (Fig. 12.27).

Acquired megaureters are usually diagnosed after ureteral reimplantation for ureterovesical (UV) reflux. If distal ureteral obstruction persists after the usual 6-week postoperative edema stage, acquired distal ureteral obstruction should be suspected. Documentation of distal ureteral obstruction in equivocal cases can be provided by Lasix excretory urography or [^{99m}Tc]DTPA "diuretic scans." Bladder wall thickening associated with neurogenic bladders may produce distal ureteral obstruction.

Other obstructing lesions to be considered include simple and ectopic ureteroceles, ectopic

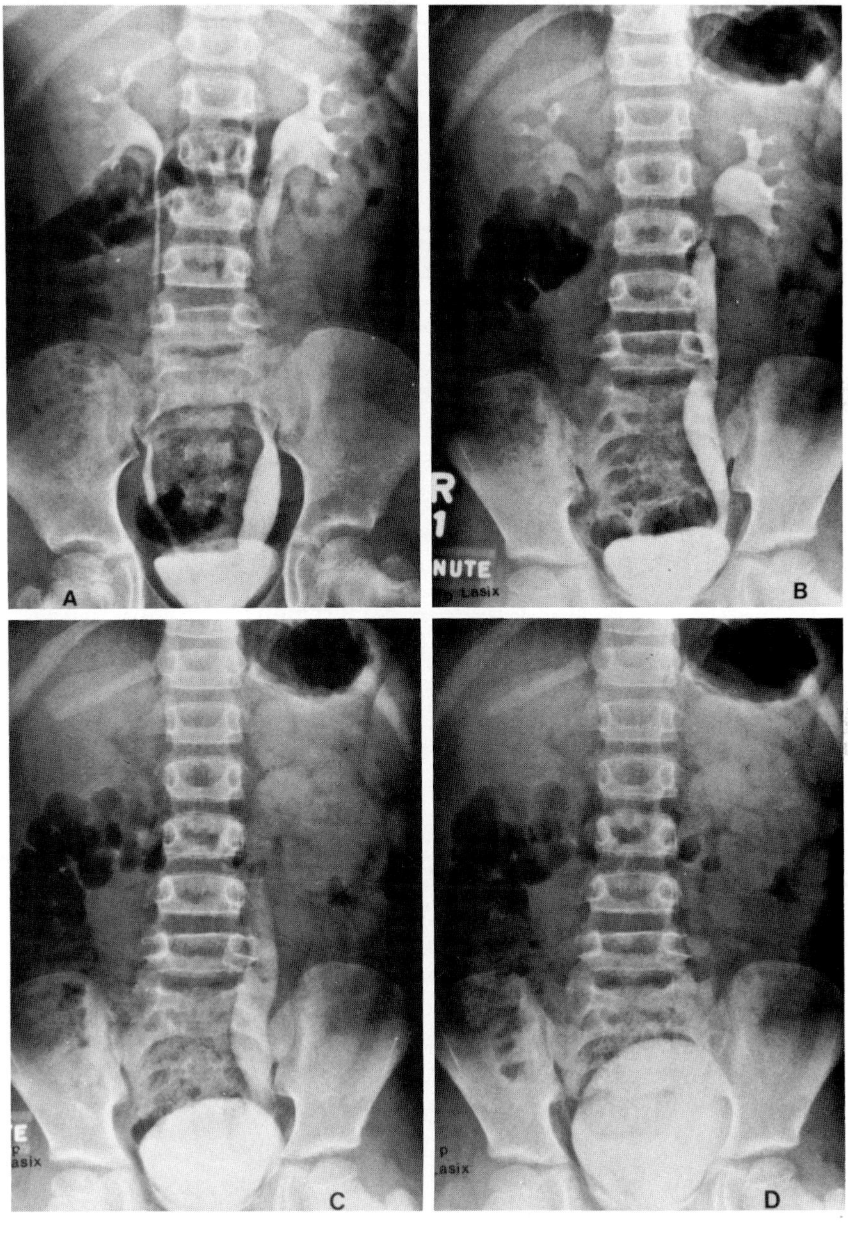

Figure 12.27. Primary nonobstructive (idiopathic) megaureter. **A,** Intravenous urogram demonstrating left megaureter with mild pelvicaliectasis. **B, C,** and **D,** Sequential films at 1, 5, and 10 min after Lasix administration demonstrating complete "washout." (From Sumner TE, Volberg FM. Evaluation of the nonvisualizing or poorly visualized kidney. In: McCullough DL, ed. Difficult diagnoses in urology. New York: Churchill Livingstone, 1988: 3–21. Used by permission.)

ureter, and posterior urethral valves. Simple ureteroceles are rarely seen in children and seldom produce obstruction beyond the neonatal period. Neonates may present with a flank mass and nonvisualization of an obstructed kidney due to UV junction (UVJ) obstruction by a simple ureterocele (Fig. 12.28**A** to **C**). Bladder sonography may demonstrate the ure-

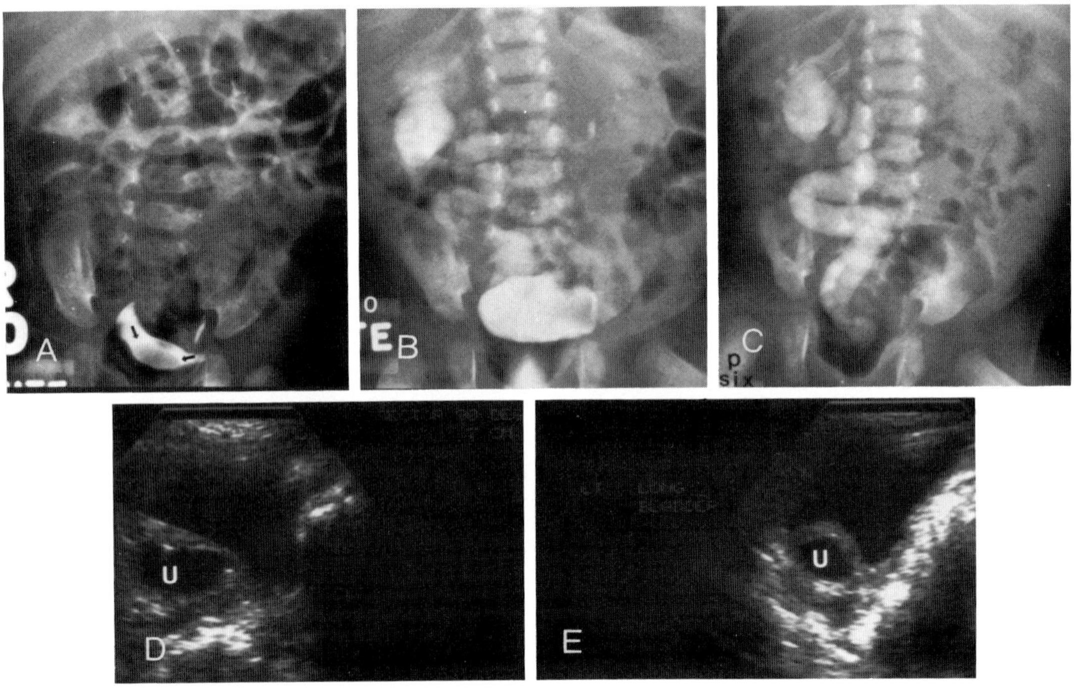

Figure 12.28. Obstructing simple ureterocele. **A,** Faint right renal visualization at 10 min; note ureterocele defect (*arrows*). **B,** Moderate right ureteropyelocaliectasis at 60 min during intravenous urography. **C,** Confirmation of right UVJ obstruction on 10-min film after Lasix administration. **D** and **E,** Transverse and longitudinal supine bladder sonograms demonstrating ureterocele (*U*). (From Sumner TE, Volberg FM. Evaluation of the nonvisualizing or poorly visualized kidney. In: McCullough DL, ed. Difficult diagnoses in urology. New York: Churchill Livingstone, 1988: 3–21. Used by permission.)

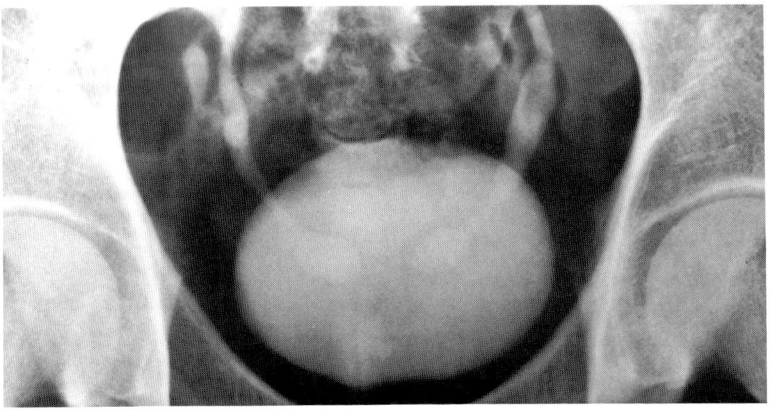

Figure 12.29. Simple ureterocele. Bilateral "cobra head" appearance during excretory urography. (From Sumner TE, Volberg FM. Evaluation of the nonvisualizing or poorly visualized kidney. In: McCullough DL, ed. Difficult diagnoses in urology. New York: Churchill Livingstone, 1988: 3–21. Used by permission.)

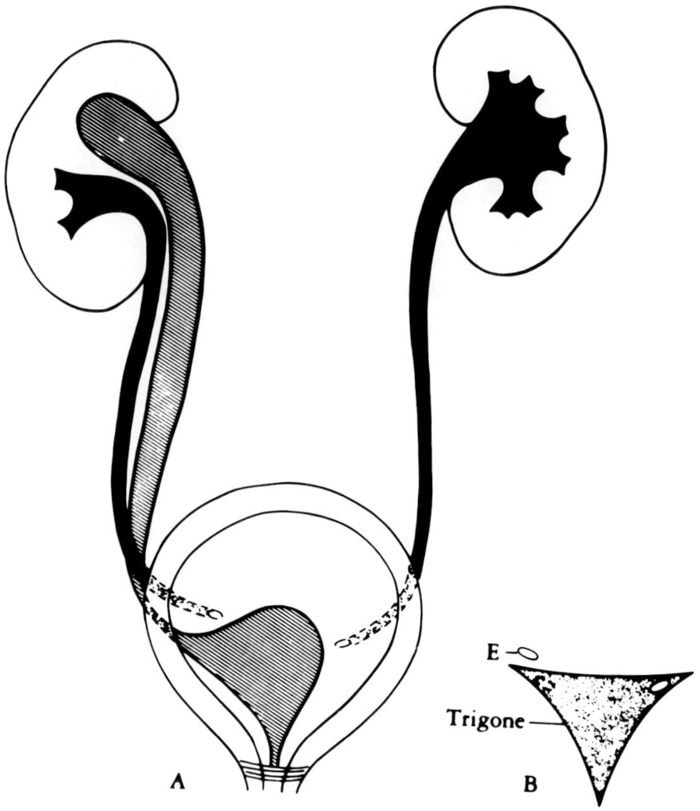

Figure 12.30. Weigert-Meyer rule. **A,** Typical features of ectopic ureterocele. There is usually duplication of the upper urinary tract. Flattening of the lower-pole calices produces a "drooping lily" appearance. The ureter of the lower-pole moiety is displaced laterally on the side of the ureterocele. The mass in the bladder is due to a ureterocele of the distal ureter of the upper-pole moiety. The Weigert-Meyer rule states that the ectopic ureteral orifice of the upper-pole moiety is medial and causal to its normal location. **B,** Frequently, the ureteral orifice for the lower-pole moiety is slightly ectopic (*E*). It lies lateral and cephalad to its normal location. There may be vesicoureteral reflux into the ureter draining the lower-pole moiety. (From Sumner TE, Volberg FM. Evaluation of the nonvisualizing or poorly visualized kidney. In: McCullough DL, ed. Difficult diagnoses in urology. New York: Churchill Livingstone, 1988: 3–21. Used by permission.)

terocele (Fig. 12.28**D** to **E**); reflux is uncommon with this type of ureterocele. In adults, simple ureteroceles typically produce a "cobra head" appearance in the bladder during excretory urography (Fig. 12.29).

Ectopic ureteroceles are frequently seen in children and represent cystic dilatation of ectopic ureter(s) beneath the bladder mucosa. In boys this condition usually occurs without ureteral duplication and is occasionally associated with posterior urethral valves. In girls it is usually associated with the upper moiety of a duplex kidney whose ureter inserts distal to the orifice of the lower-pole ureter (Fig. 12.30). The obstructed upper moiety frequently cannot be seen on early films of excretory urography, and the upper-pole hydronephrosis may cause a horizontal splayed lower-pole appearance stimulating a "drooping lily" (Fig. 12.31**A**). A typical lucent filling defect in the bladder may be seen during excretory urography (Fig. 12.31**A**) or cystography (Fig. 12.31**B**). The upper moiety may eventually opacify on delayed excretory urography films (Fig. 12.31**C**). Cystourethrography should be performed in these patients, since approximately 50% demonstrate VU reflux. Renal and bladder sonography are diagnostic (Fig. 12.32). Occasionally an ectopic ureterocele can resemble a bladder diverticulum due to bulging through the bladder wall during voiding (Fig. 12.33). Rarely, the ectopic ureterocele may be inadvertently cathe-

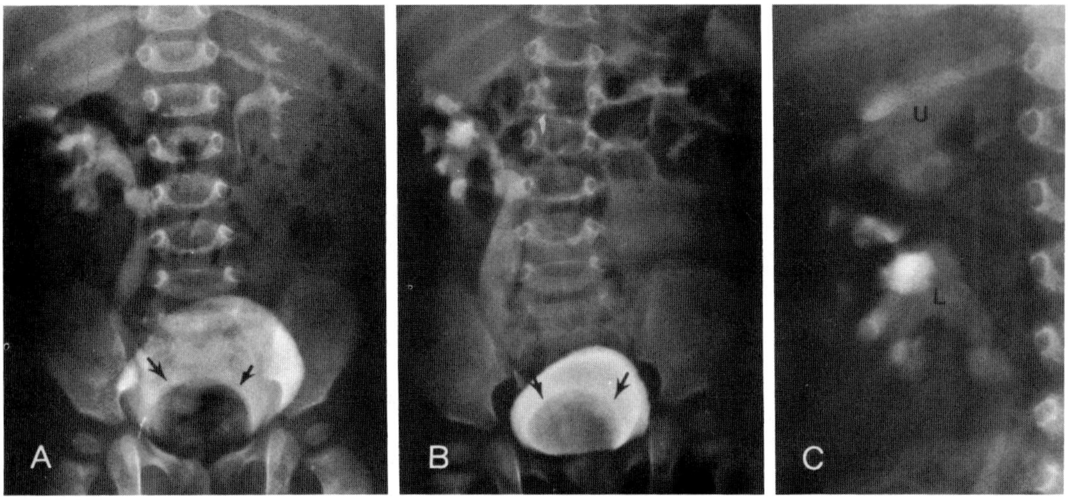

Figure 12.31. Ectopic ureterocele. **A,** Early film during excretory urography demonstrating nonvisualization of upper pole and bladder filling defect (*arrows*). **B,** Voiding cystogram demonstrating reflux into lower moiety and bladder filling defect (*arrows*). **C,** Delayed excretory urogram film demonstrating upper-pole (*U*) and lower-pole (*L*) hydronephrosis. (From Sumner TE, Volberg FM. Evaluation of the nonvisualizing or poorly visualized kidney. In: McCullough DL, ed. Difficult diagnoses in urology. New York: Churchill Livingstone, 1988: 3–21. Used by permission.)

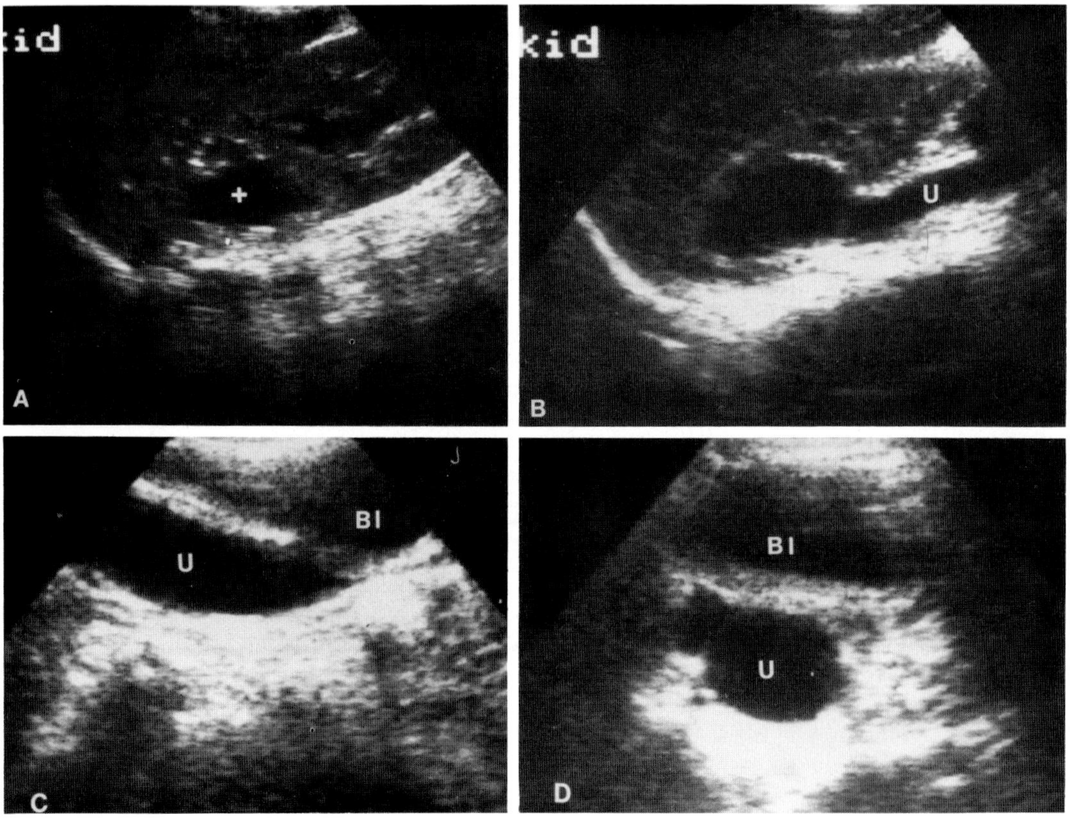

Figure 12.32. Ectopic ureterocele sonography. **A, B,** and **C,** Sequential longitudinal renal sonograms demonstrating the subtended upper moiety (+ in **A**), its dilated ureter (*U*) in ***B,*** and distal upper-moiety ureteral (*U*) dilatation to the level of the bladder (*Bl*) in ***C. D,*** Transverse bladder sonography demonstrating the right ectopic ureterocele (*U*) in the bladder (*Bl*). (From Sumner TE, Volberg FM. Evaluation of the nonvisualizing or poorly visualized kidney. In: McCullough DL, ed. Difficult diagnoses in urology. New York: Churchill Livingstone, 1988: 3–21. Used by permission.)

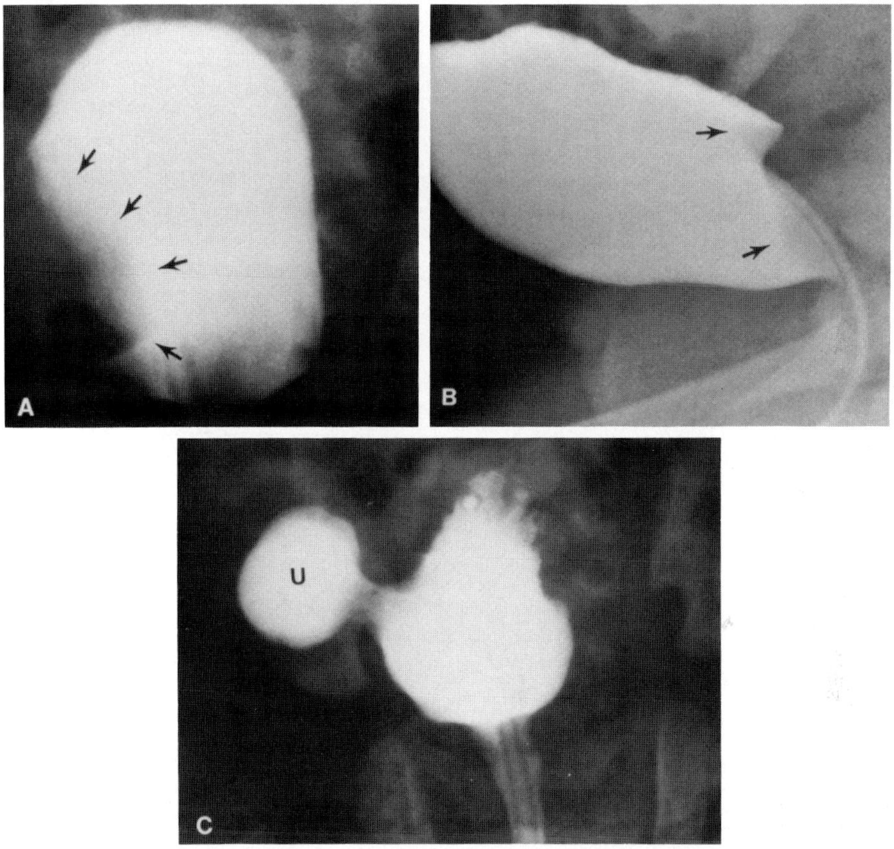

Figure 12.33. Ectopic ureterocele. AP (**A**) and lateral (**B**) films during bladder filling demonstrating lucent-filling defect (*arrows*) due to utereocele. **C,** Ectopic ureterocele (*U*) bulging through the bladder wall during voiding. (From Sumner TE, Volberg FM. Evaluation of the nonvisualizing or poorly visualized kidney. In: McCullough DL, ed. Difficult diagnoses in urology. New York: Churchill Livingstone, 1988: 3–21. Used by permission.)

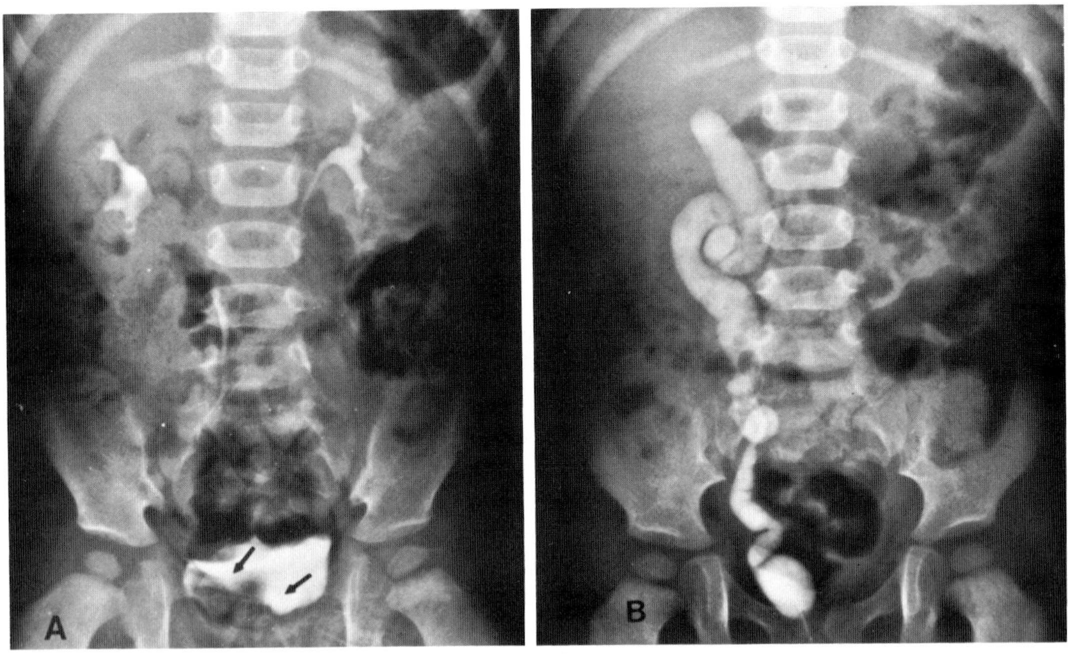

Figure 12.34. Ectopic ureterocele. **A,** Intravenous urogram demonstrating "drooping lily" appearance on right with nonvisualization of upper moiety; bladder filling defect (*arrows*) due to utereocele. **B,** Catheterization of a right ectopic ureterocele during voiding cystourethrography, with opacification of its subtended ureter to the upper moiety. (From Sumner TE, Volberg FM. Evaluation of the nonvisualizing or poorly visualized kidney. In: McCullough DL, ed. Difficult diagnoses in urology. New York: Churchill Livingstone, 1988: 3–21. Used by permission.)

terized during a voiding cystourethrogram (Fig. 12.34).

Ectopic ureters are usually single and often obstructed, resulting in nonvisualization during excretory urography. Ectopic sites of insertion are the seminal vesicles and posterior urethra (Fig. 12.35) in males and along the urethra in females. Rarely, ectopic insertion occurs with a duplex kidney, and voiding cystourethrography may reveal the ectopic insertion (Fig. 12.36).

POSTERIOR URETHRAL VALVES

The most common cause of severe urinary tract obstruction in the male infant is posterior urethral valves. Fifty percent are discovered during the first 3 months of life, but occasionally older children and adults are discovered to have hydronephrosis secondary to posterior urethral valves. Ultrasonography in these patients reveals hydroureteronephrosis (usually bilateral) and an abnormally thickened bladder wall due to muscular hypertrophy (Fig. 12.37). Similar bladder wall thickening with associated hydroureteronephrosis may occur in patients with neurogenic bladders. Differentiating this condition from posterior urethral valves requires urethral imaging. Angled sonographic views of the bladder base may demonstrate posterior urethral dilatation proximal to valves, but the sensitivity and specificity of this method are unknown (38). A voiding cystourethrogram is usually performed to confirm the diagnosis (Fig. 12.38). Vesicoureteral reflux occurs in 45% of these patients, but a hypertrophied trigone may prevent reflux. Antegrade pyelography will demonstrate hydroureteronephrosis with ureterovesical obstruction due to bladder hypertrophy (Fig. 12.39).

Unexplained ascites in the newborn male should be considered to be due to posterior urethral valves until proven otherwise. The obstructed renal collecting system decompresses by rupturing the area of least resistance—the caliceal fornix—with extravasation of urine into the perirenal space (urinoma) (Fig. 12.40) or decompression into the peritoneal cavity (urinary ascites) (39). Therefore, sonographic detection of ascites should suggest the etiology of urine extravasation and be followed by uri-

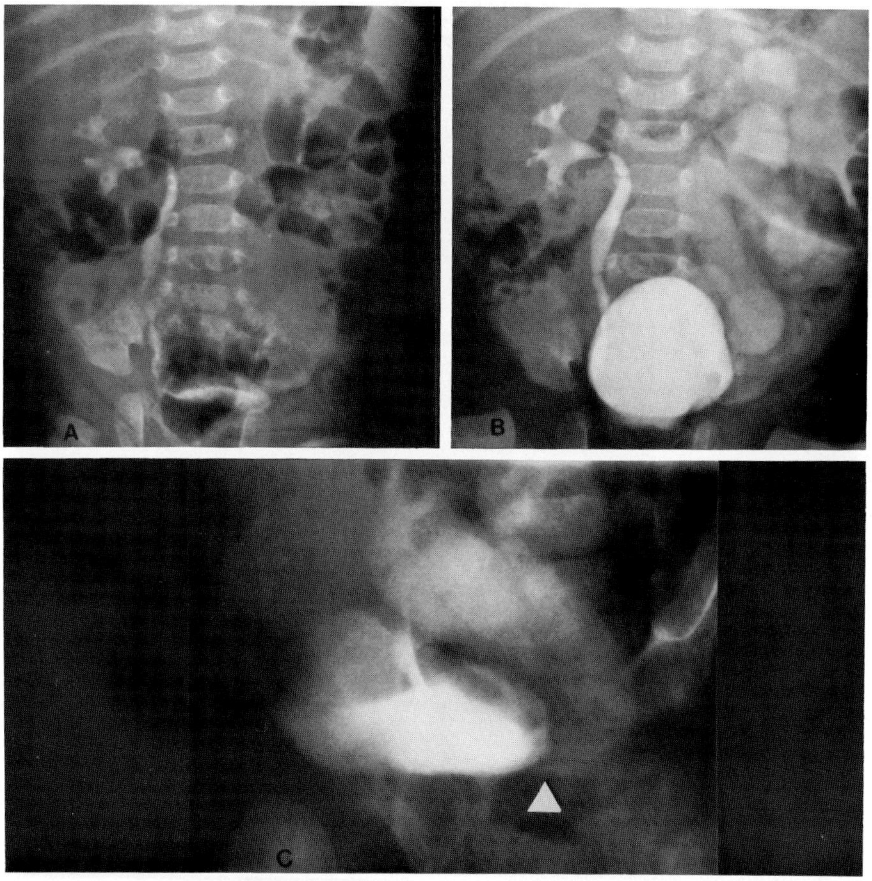

Figure 12.35. Ectopic ureter. Male infant with left flank mass. **A,** Nonvisualization of the left kidney during early intravenous urogram film. **B,** Delayed intravenous urogram film demonstrating marked left pelvicaliecstasis and ureterectasis. **C,** Oblique intravenous urogram film demonstrating ectopic insertion of the left ureter into the posterior urethra (*arrowhead*). (From Sumner TE, Volberg FM. Evaluation of the nonvisualizing or poorly visualized kidney. In: McCullough DL, ed. Difficult diagnoses in urology. New York: Churchill Livingstone, 1988: 3–21. Used by permission.)

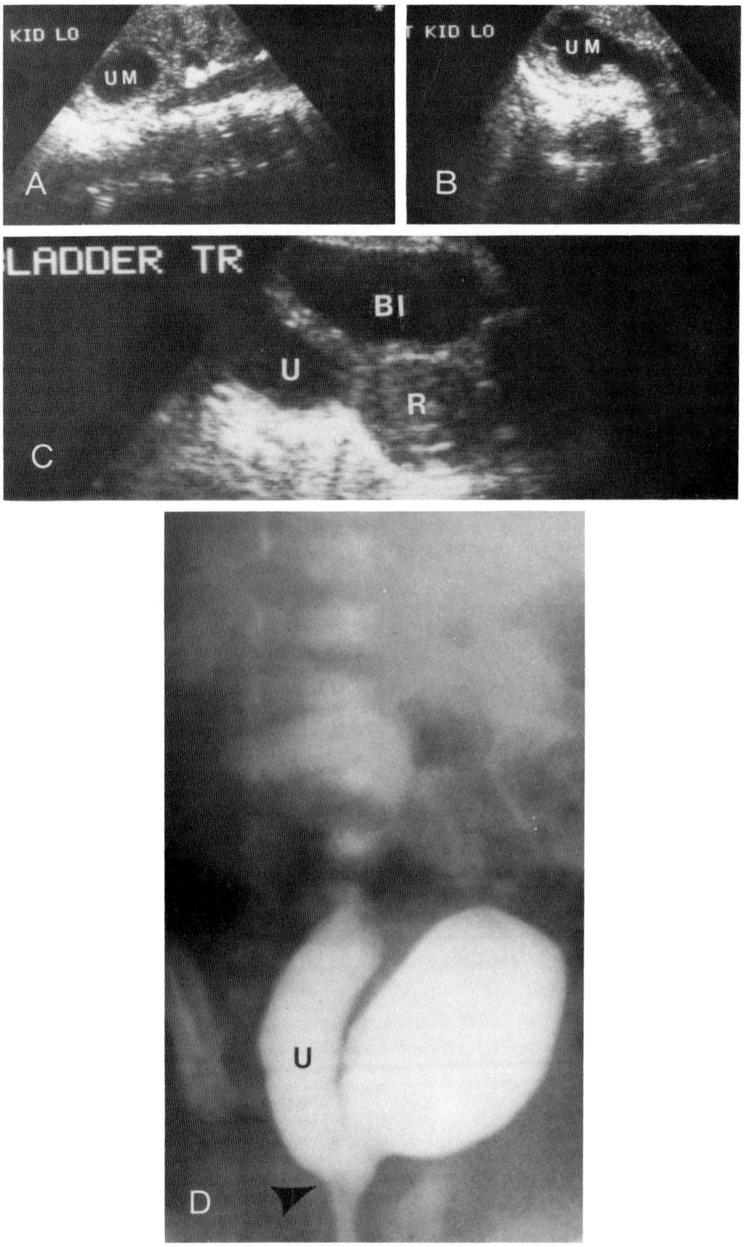

Figure 12.36. Ectopic ureter. Female infant with right flank mass. **A** and **B,** Serial longitudinal supine right renal sonograms demonstrating obstructive upper moiety (*UM*) of duplex kidney. **C,** Transverse bladder sonography demonstrating ectopic insertion of right upper-moiety ureter (*U*). *Bl,* bladder; *R,* rectum. D, Voiding cystourethrogram demonstrating right upper-moiety ureter (*U*) ectopically inserting into urethra (*arrowhead*). From Sumner TE, Volberg FM. Evaluation of the nonvisualizing or poorly visualized kidney. In: McCullough DL, ed. Difficult diagnoses in urology. New York: Churchill Livingstone, 1988: 3–21. Used by permission.)

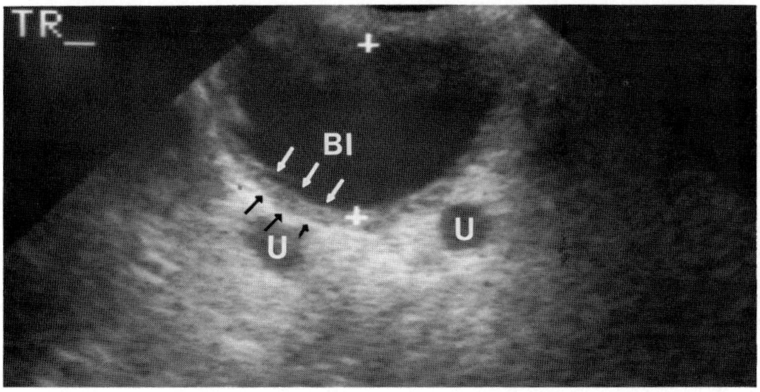

Figure 12.37. Posterior urethral valves. Bladder (*Bl*) sonogram reveals an abnormally thick wall (*arrows*) due to muscular hypertrophy. *U,* ureter.

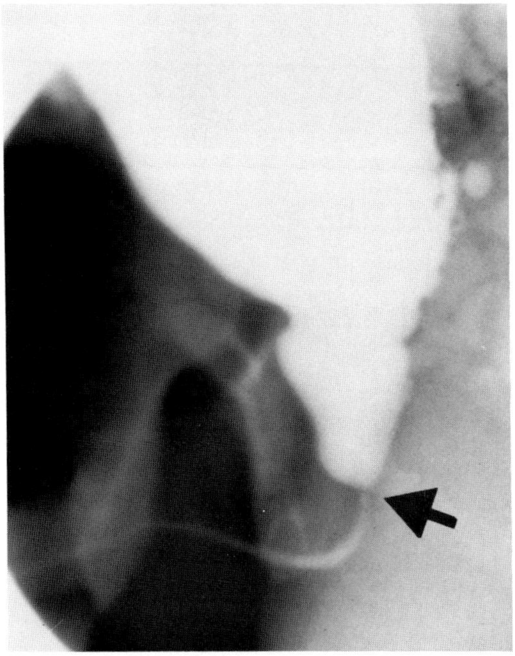

Figure 12.38. Posterior urethral valves. Voiding cystourethrogram demonstrates posterior urethral valves (*arrow*).

nary tract evaluation for detection of hydroureteronephrosis or urinoma formation. Rarely, an obstructed bladder ruptures into the peritoneum (40).

Hydroureteronephrosis may also be caused by extrinsic pressure on the urinary system. Extrinsic abnormalities include imperforate anus, intersex anomalies, and tumor. Syndromatic causes of dilatation include the megacystis-microcolon-intestinal hypoperistalsis (M-M-IH) syndrome or the Eagle-Barrett ("prune belly") syndrome. Ultrasonography can be of diagnostic and prognostic value in these conditions in evaluation of hydroureteronephrosis.

INTRINSIC RENAL DISEASE (CONGENITAL AND ACQUIRED)

Congenital intrinsic renal diseases include renal tubular acidosis (RTA), congenital nephrotic syndrome, and renal dysplasia. The sonographic appearance of RTA is unremarkable unless nephrocalcinosis occurs (Fig. 12.41). Ultrasonography of renal dysplasia may demonstrate hyperechogenicity with or without normal corticomedullary differentiation (Fig. 12.42). Acquired intrinsic disease conditions include renal ischemia and renal artery thrombosis. Renal ischemia is usually manifested by renal tubular and cortical nec-

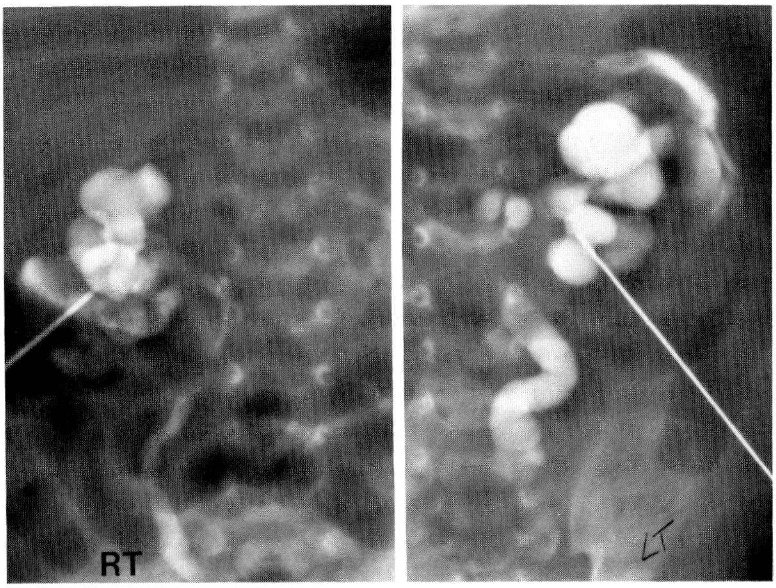

Figure 12.39. Posterior urethral valves. Antegrade pyelography demonstrating marked bilateral hydroureteronephrosis with ureterovesical obstruction to bladder hypertrophy.

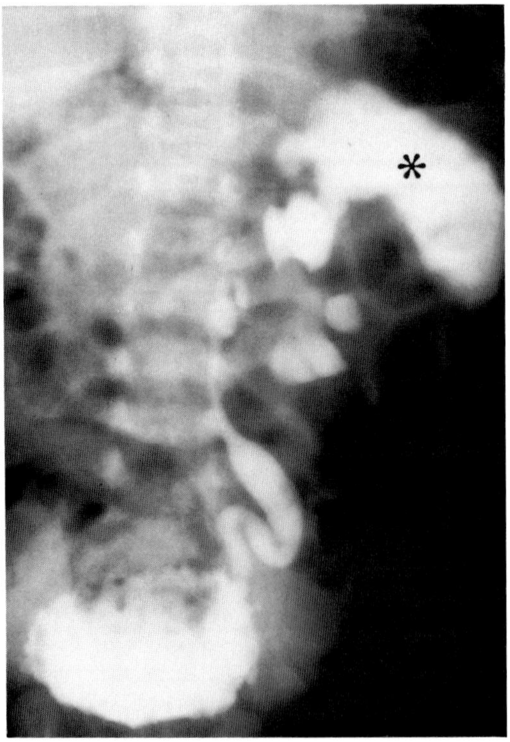

Figure 12.40. Urinoma due to posterior urethral valves. Voiding cystourethrogram reveals urinoma (*) due to rupture of an obstructed renal collecting system.

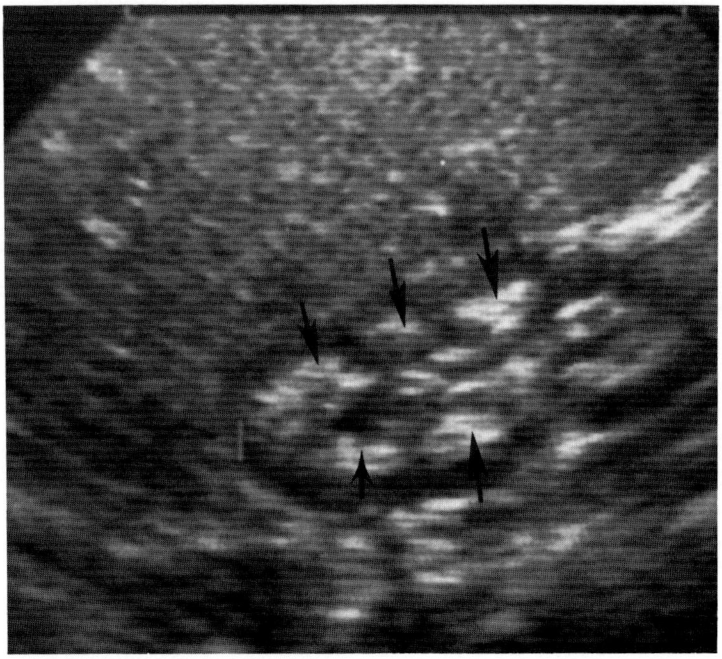

Figure 12.41. Nephrocalcinosis. Longitudinal renal sonogram showing focal areas of increased echogenicity (*arrows*) due to nephrocalcinosis.

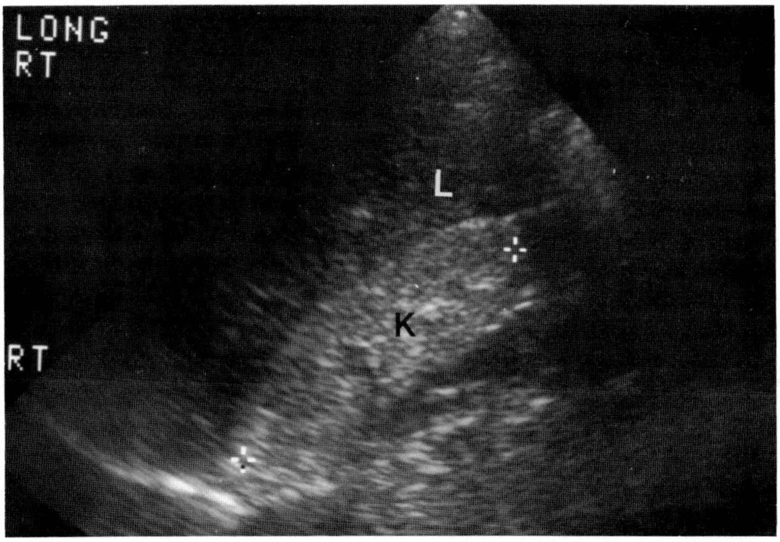

Figure 12.42. Renal dysplasia. Longitudinal renal sonogram revealing a tiny echogenic kidney (*K*). *L,* liver. + delineates renal borders.

rosis, whereas renal artery thrombosis produces hypertension. Ultrasonography may help differentiate these conditions by demonstrating alterations of cortical or medullary echogenicity and changes in renal architecture. Renal ischemia usually has increased cortical echogenicity with normal corticomedullary differentiation (41) (Fig. 12.43). Renal artery thrombosis has a normal sonographic appearance, so Doppler ultrasound may prove diagnostic if no renal artery flow is detected. Confirming no renal arterial flow may require

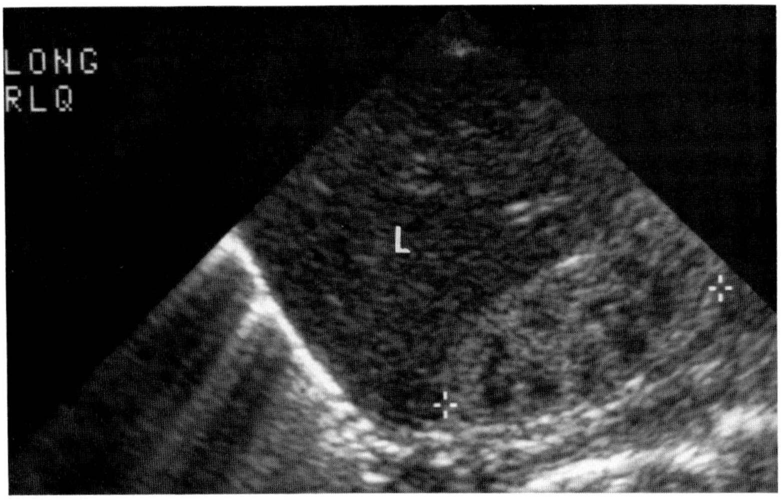

Figure 12.43. Acute tubular necrosis. Longitudinal renal sonogram demonstrates diffuse increased echogenicity. *L,* liver. + delineates renal borders.

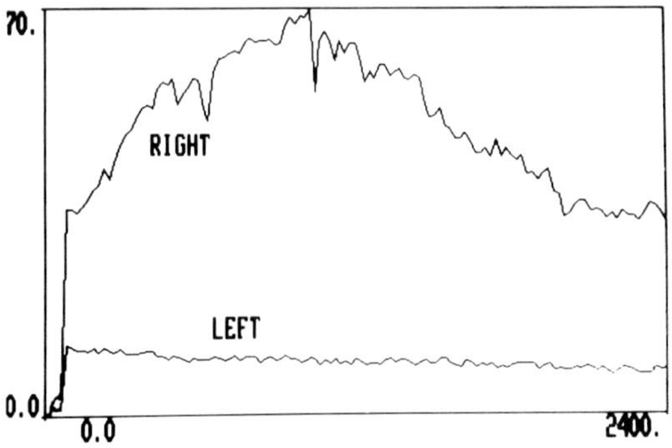

Figure 12.44. Renal ischemia. Renal isotopic study confirming no arterial flow on left.

an isotopic renal flow study (Fig. 12.44). If aortic sonography reveals intraluminal echoes (Fig. 12.45**A**), aortography will confirm aortic or renal arterial thrombosis (Fig. 12.45**B**).

RENAL INFECTIONS

Ultrasound has become increasingly popular in the evaluation of children with urinary tract infection. During acute pyelonephritis, both excretory urography and ultrasonography may be normal. Positive ultrasound findings include increased renal size with diffuse increased renal parenchymal echogenicity due to edema or inflammation (Fig. 12.46). Unilateral nephromegaly is the usual finding, but bilateral renal enlargement is much less specific (42). Focal renal changes may be detected during excretory urography and ultrasonography in patients with focal pyelonephritis or lobar nephronia. This condition represents a localized bacterial renal infection without major suppuration. Sonographically, a localized renal mass, hypoechoic or hyperechoic, will disrupt the corticomedullary definition. Similar disruption of renal architecture may be produced by a normal variant (pseudotumor)—a column of Bertin (Fig. 12.47). Confirmation of the latter may necessitate excretory urography (Fig. 12.48) or a [^{99m}Tc]glucoheptonate renogram. The column of Bertin will have normal uptake, whereas focal inflammation will have decreased radioisotope uptake (43). However, a tumor would resemble focal inflammation on the renogram, so sequential ultrasound examination during medical treatment may be warranted; rapid change with resolution of the "mass" would be expected in response to antibiotic therapy in cases of lobar nephronia. Sonography is also useful for detecting perinephric fluid collections and abscess; these conditions are frequently difficult to identify during excretory urography or scintigraphy. Ultrasound can also be used for percutaneous drainage and abscess aspiration (44). Chronic pyelonephritis often produces small kidneys indicative of endstage renal disease. Sonography reveals hyperechoic kidneys with irregular borders due to scarring (Fig. 12.49). However, these findings are not pathognomonic in that similar sono-

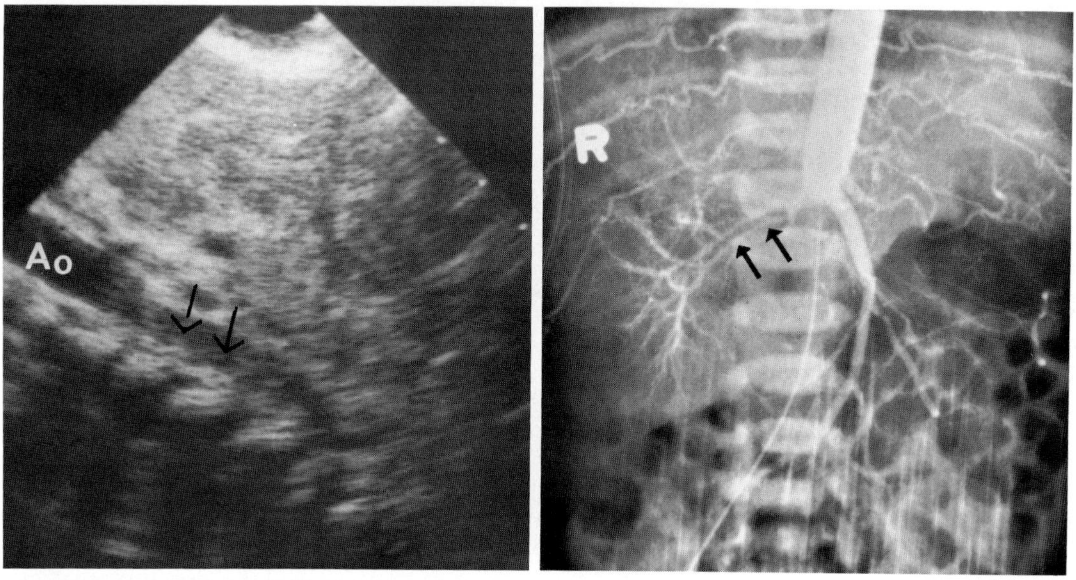

Figure 12.45. **A,** Longitudinal aortic sonogram demonstrates echoes (*arrows*) in the distal abdominal aorta (*Ao*). **B,** Aortogram reveals complete occlusion of the left renal artery and minimal right renal arterial flow (*arrows*).

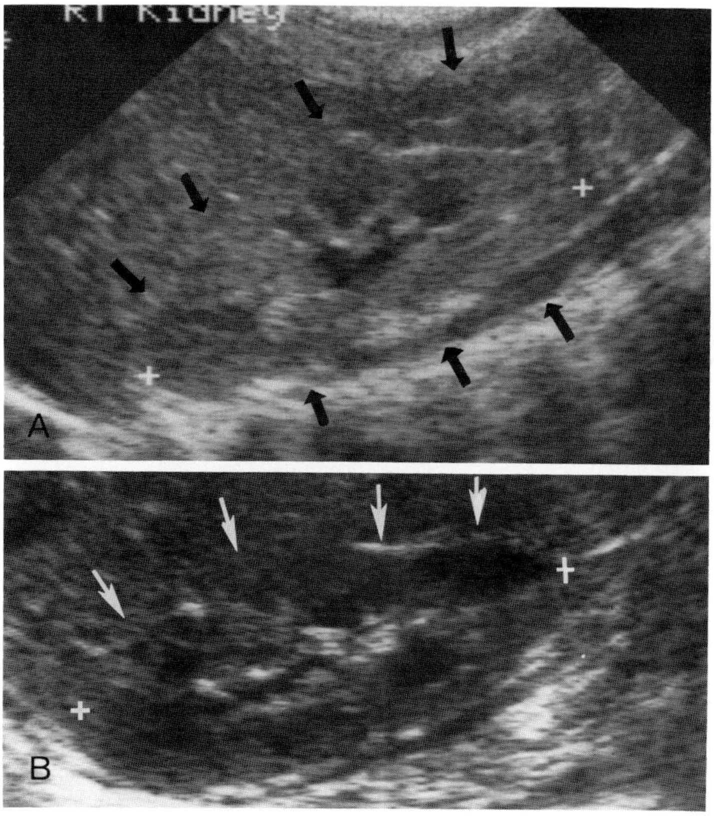

Figure 12.46. Acute pyelonephritis. A, Initial longitudinal renal sonogram demonstrates nephromegaly with increased echogenicity. **B,** Follow-up longitudinal sonogram demonstrates normal renal size and echogenicity. *Arrows* and + delineate renal borders.

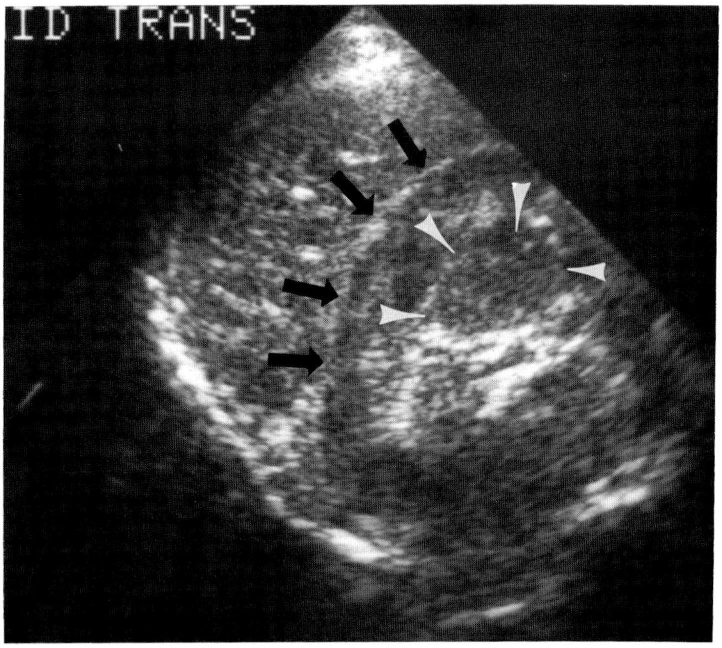

Figure 12.47. Renal pseudotumor. Transverse renal sonogram reveals localized echoic area (*white arrowheads*) with echogenicity similar to surrounding renal parenchyma. *Black arrows* delineate renal border.

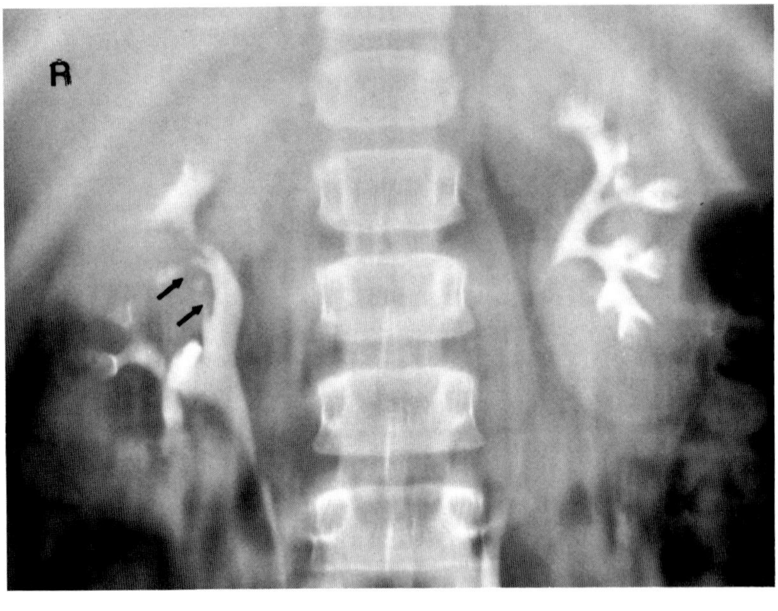

Figure 12.48. Renal pseudotumor. Excretory urography shows slight right upper-pole caliceal displacement (*arrows*).

grams can be seen in chronic glomerulonephritis and hypertensive or ischemic disease.

All children with urinary tract infection require imaging evaluation to identify those having or being at risk for renal parenchymal damage. Since most urinary tract infections are ascending infections from the bladder (except in neonates, in whom they are hematogenous), bladder evaluation and detection of vesicoureteral reflux is an appropriate initial procedure. Voiding cystourethrography (VCUG), fluoroscopic or isotopic, should be performed.

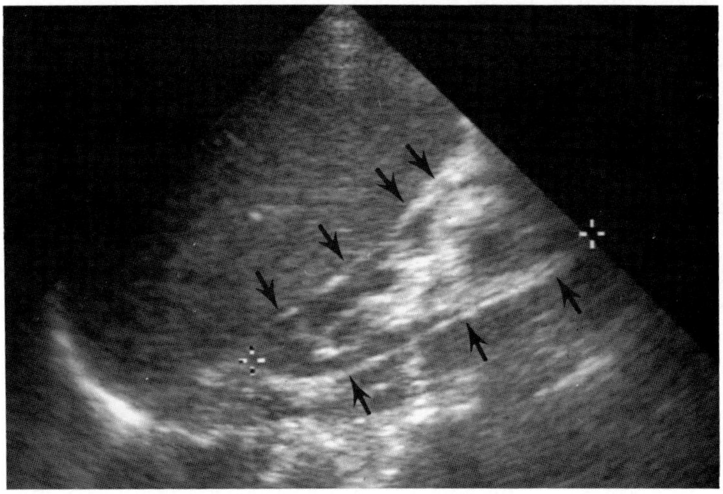

Figure 12.49. Chronic pyelonephritis. Renal sonography reveals small, scarred, hyperechoic kidney. *Arrows* and + delineate renal borders.

Fluoroscopic VCUG is necessary in boys to evaluate anatomic abnormalities of the urethra. Isotopic VCUG, although lacking anatomic specificity, significantly reduces radiation exposure. In girls, the ovarian dose is 1% of that from a fluoroscopic VCUG (45). Therefore many institutions recommend initial fluoroscopic VCUG in males and nuclear VCUG in females. Radionuclide VCUG, by permitting continuous visualization, is theoretically a more sensitive indicator of reflux; however, it cannot delineate intravesical pathology such as ureterocele or stone or a duplex system. We prefer radionuclide VCUG for all follow-up examinations in both boys and girls. Ultrasonography has been advocated in screening for vesicoureteral reflux but it is both time consuming and inefficient; therefore, ultrasound is not widely used to appraise reflux (46).

In the nonrefluxing child, renal sonography is appropriate and quite sensitive for detecting obstruction or congenital anomalies in addition to approximating renal size. Uncomplicated duplex collecting systems and small cortical scars may be missed with ultrasound. Scarring may occur without reflux, but 90% of scarred kidneys are drained by refluxing ureters. Furthermore, increasing grades of reflux are associated with increasing incidence of cortical scars. With Internal Grades I and II reflux, some physicians feel sonography is sufficient, since small parenchymal scars are not significant. However, Huland and Busch reported appreciable renal scarring with Grade II reflux (47). Since renal cortical scans using glucoheptonate or disodium monomethanearsonate (DMSA) are probably the most sensitive way to detect scarring, radioisotope studies are recommended for Grades II through V reflux. The excretory urogram can be valuable in refluxers, but because of overlying bowel gas, it is not as sensitive as the renogram. Also, renal function may be compromised with Grades IV and V reflux, so a radionuclide renal function scan may be of particular value in these situations.

The above described imaging workup is followed with patients responding well to antibiotic therapy. VCUG (fluoroscopic or isotopic) may be developed for up to 6 weeks; some physicians prefer to continue antibiotic coverage until the VCUG is performed. If the patient is not responding to antibiotic therapy, ultrasonography is recommended to detect congenital anomalies or surgically correctable lesions. As mentioned, renal sonography may be normal during acute pyelonephritis, and further evaluation with [^{99m}Tc]glucoheptonate may be warranted to detect focal lesions. Occasionally CT scanning may be necessary to exclude perirenal inflammation undetected during ultrasonography due to obscuration by bowel gas. In patients with fever of unknown origin and normal urine culture, additional imaging with [^{67}Ga]gallium citrate or ^{111}In-tagged leukocytes has been recommended to demonstrate an extrarenal or unsuspected intrarenal site of infection (48). Magnetic resonance imaging will soon be widely available and may also be used for investigating urinary tract infections in the pediatric patient.

References

1. Griscom NT. The roentgenology of neonatal abdominal masses AJR 1965;93:447–463.
2. Haller JO, Berdon WE, Friedman AP. Increased renal cortical echogenicity: a normal finding in neonates and infants. Radiology 1982;142:173–174.
3. Behan M, Kezam E. The echogenic characteristics of fatty tissues and tumors. Radiology 1978;129:143–151.
4. Felson B, Cussen LJ. The hydronephrotic type of unilateral congenital multicystic disease of the kidney. Semin Roentgenol 1975;10:113–123.
5. Griscom NT, Vawter GF, Fellers FX. Pelvoinfundibular atresia: the usual form of multicystic kidney; 44 unilateral and two bilateral cases. Semin Roentgenol 1975;10:125–131.
6. Kirks DR, Merten DF, Grossman H, Bowie JD. Diagnostic imaging of pediatric abdominal masses: an overview. Radiol Clin North Am 1981;19:(3)527–545.
7. Young LW, Wood BP, Spohr CH, Panner B. Delayed excretory urographic opacification—a puddling effect, in multicystic renal dysplasia. Ann Radiol (Paris) 1974;17:391–396.
8. Bearman SB, Hine PL, Sanders RC. Multicystic kidney: a sonographic pattern. Radiology 1976;118:685–688.
9. Saxton HM, Golding SJ, Chantler C, Haycock GD. Diagnostic puncture in renal cystic dysplasia (multicystic kidney). Evidence on the aetiology of the cysts. Br J Radiol 1981;54:555–561.
10. Rosenfield AT, Zeman RK, Cronan JJ, Taylor KJW. Ultrasound in experimental and clinical renal vein thrombosis. Radiology 1980;137:735–741.
11. Rosenberg ER, Trought WS, Kirks DR, et al. Ultrasonic diagnosis of renal vein thrombosis in neonates. AJR 1980;134:35–38.
12. Belman AB, King LR. The pathology and treatment of renal vein thrombosis in the newborn. J Urol 1972;107:852–855.
13. Sutton TJ, LeBlanc A, Gauthier N, Hassan M. Radiologic manifestations of neonatal renal vein thrombosis on follow-up examinations. Radiology 1977;122:435–438.
14. Melson GL, Shackelford GD, Cole BR, McClennan BL. The spectrum of sonographic findings in infantile polycystic kidney disease with urographic and clinical correlations. J Clin Ultrasound 1985;13:113–119.
15. Pretorius DH, Lee ME, Manco-Johnson ML, et al. Diagnosis of autosomal dominant polycystic kidney disease in utero and in the young infant. J Ultrasound Med 1987;6:249–255.
16. Porch P, Noe NHN, Stapleton FB. Unilateral presentation of adult-type polycystic kidney disease in children. J Urol 1986;135:744–746.
17. Hartman DS, Lesar MSL, Madewell JE, et al. Mesoblastic nephroma: radiologic-pathologic correlation of 20 cases. AJR 1981;136:69–74.
18. Bitter JJ, Harrison DA, Kaplan J, et al. Mesoblastic nephroma. J Comput Assist Tomogr 1982;6:180–183.
19. Gordon RL, Pollack HM, Popky GL, et al. Simple serous cysts of the kidney in children. Radiology 1979;131:357–361.
20. Siegel MJ, McAlister WH. Simple cysts of the kidney in children. J Urol 1980;123:75–78.
21. Weese-Mayer DE, Smith KM, Reddy JK, et al. Computerized tomography and ultrasound in the diagnosis of cerebro-hepato-renal syndrome of Zellweger. Pediatr Radiol 1987;17:170–172.
22. Glazer GM, Callen PW, Parker JJ. CT diagnosis of tumor thrombus in the inferior vena cava: avoiding the false positive diagnosis. AJR 1981;137:1265–1267.
23. Dietrich RB, Kangarloo H. Kidneys in infants and children: evaluation with MR. Radiology 1986;159:215–221.
24. Madewell JE, Goldman SM, Davis CJ Jr, et al. Multilocular cystic nephroma: a radiographic-pathologic correlation of 58 patients. Radiology 1983;146:309–321.
25. Gonzales-Crussi F. Wilms' tumor (nephroblastoma) and related renal neoplasms of childhood. Boca Raton, FL: CRC Press, 1984.
26. Fernbach SK, Feinstein KA, Donaldson JS, et al. Nephroblastomatosis: comparison of CT with US and urography. Radiology 1988;166:153–156.
27. Chan HSL, Daneman A, Gribbin M, Martin DJ. Renal cell carcinoma in the first two decades of life. Pediatr Radiol 1983;13:324–328.
28. Senga Y, Taguchi H, Asao T, Misugi K. Undifferentiated renal cell carcinoma in infancy: report of a case and review of literature. Pediatr Pathol 1986;5:157–165.
29. Hartman DS, Davis CJ Jr, Goldman SM, et al. Renal lymphoma: radiologic-pathologic correlation of 21 cases. Radiology 1982;144:759–766.
30. Araki T. Leukemic involvement of the kidney in children: CT features. J Comput Assist Tomogr 1982;6:781–784.
31. Price EB Jr, Mostofi FK. Symptomatic angiomyolipoma of the kidney. Cancer 1965;18:761–774.
32. Narla LD, Solvis TL, Watts FB, Nigro M. The renal lesions of tuberosclerosis (cysts and angiomyolipoma)—screening with sonography and computerized tomography. Pediatr Radiol 1988;18:205–209.
33. Whitaker RH. Percutaneous upper urinary tract dynamics in equivocal obstruction. Urol Radiol 1981;2:187–189.
34. Senac MO Jr, Miller JH, Stanley P. Evaluation of obstructive uropathy in children: radionuclide renography vs. the Whitaker test. AJR 1984;143:11–15.
35. Kessler RM, Altman DH. Real-time sonographic detection of vesicoureteral reflux in children. AJR 1982;138:1033–1036.
36. Friedland GW. Hydronephrosis in infants and children. Part 2. Curr Probl Diagn Radiol 1978;7:(9)3–14.
37. Glanz S, Gordon DH, Butt K, et al. Percutaneous transrenal balloon dilatation of the ureter. Radiology 1983;149:101–104.
38. Gilsanz V, Miller JH, Reid BS. Ultrasonic characteristics of posterior urethral valves. Radiology 1982;145:143–145.
39. MacPherson RI, Leithiser RE, Gordon L, et al. Posterior urethral valves: an update and review. Radiographics 1986;6:753.
40. Trulock TS, Finnerty DP, Woodard JR. Neonatal

bladder rupture: case report and review of literature. J Urol 1985;133:271–273.
41. Slovis TL. Pediatric renal anomalies and infections. Neonatal and pediatric ultrasonography. Clin Diagn Ultrasound 1989;24:170–174.
42. Johnson CE, DeBax BP, Shurin PA, DeBartolomeo R. Renal ultrasound evaluation of urinary tract infections in children. Pediatrics 1986;78:871–878.
43. Traisman ES, Conway JJ, Traisman HS, et al. The localization of urinary tract infection with ^{99m}Tc glucoheptonate scintigraphy. Pediatr Radiol 1986;16:403–406.
44. Towbin RB, Ball WS. Pediatric interventional radiology. Radiol Clin North Am 1988;26(2): 419–440.
45. Taylor A, Eshima D, Fritzberg AR, et al. Comparison of iodine-131 OIH and technetium-99m Mag^3 renal imaging in volunteers. J Nucl Med 1986;27:795–803.
46. Schneider K, Jablonski C, Weissner M, et al. Screening for vesicoureteral reflux in children using real-time sonography. Pediatr Radiol 1984;14:400–403.
47. Huland H, Busch R. Pyelonephritic scarring in 213 patients with upper and lower urinary tract infection: long term follow-up. J Urol 1984; 132:936–939.
48. Reid BS, Bender TM. Radiographic evaluation of children with urinary tract infections. Recent advances in practical pediatric radiology. Radiol Clin North Am 1988;26(2):393–407.

CHAPTER 13

Scrotum and Contents

ELLEN M. O'MARA, D.O.
MATTHEW D. RIFKIN, M.D.

A scrotal mass or enlargement of the scrotum is usually first detected by the patient on self-examination or by the physician during the course of a routine medical checkup. The diagnosis of scrotal disease often rests primarily on careful palpation of the testis since the clinical symptoms are nonspecific, variable, and frequently misleading (1). A discrete scrotal mass or diffuse enlargement of the scrotum may result from a broad spectrum of conditions, including primary and metastatic tumors of the testis or epididymis, cysts, varicoceles, fluid collections (hydroceles or hematoceles), torsion, trauma, and inflammatory and postinflammatory processes. Current imaging modalities for evaluation of the scrotum in addition to ultrasound include nuclear medicine, computed tomography, magnetic resonance imaging, and, to a lesser extent, venous angiography.

Ultrasound has become the primary imaging modality for analysis of the scrotum and its contents (2). When the clinical diagnosis of a scrotal abnormality requires confirmation, sonography may be useful for (*a*) differentiating intratesticular from extratesticular origin as the cause of scrotal enlargement or mass; (*b*) assessing testicular size; (*c*) demonstrating the presence of occult neoplasm; (*d*) differentiating the causes of acute scrotum; (*e*) evaluating the integrity of the testicle in cases of trauma or infection; (*f*) following up after unilateral orchiectomy for testicular carcinoma for the possibility of recurrence in the contralateral testis; (*g*) determining the presence or absence of a varicocele in an infertility workup; and (*h*) locating an undescended testis (3–10). In some cases, however, ultrasound remains a complementary procedure to one of the previously mentioned modalities for the diagnosis of intrascrotal pathology (e.g., torsion).

The aim of this chapter is to discuss the variety of scrotal abnormalities and pathologies with attention to the role of ultrasound in imaging and diagnosis. Where relevant, the role of the clinical evaluation as well as other imaging modalities including nuclear medicine, computed tomography, magnetic resonance imaging, and venography will be evaluated and correlated with the clinical history and physical examination of the scrotum.

TECHNIQUE

Sonographic imaging of the testes is optimally performed using a short-focused, high-resolution, real-time 7.5- or 10-MHz transducer. The latter can theoretically resolve areas as small as 0.5 mm. Direct contact scanning may be preferable to using a water path; however, a water path may be beneficial in some instances. Synthetic water delay systems in the form of a gel mattress are readily available for this purpose (11–15). Large amounts of acoustic gel should be used to reduce hair artifacts.

To prepare for imaging, the penis is retracted over the patient's lower abdomen. The scrotum can then be supported by a towel draped beneath it or, alternatively, it may be cradled in the examiner's gloved hand (Fig. 13.1). In the latter instance, the examiner's finger can be identified as an echogenic band in the appropriate relationship to the palpable abnormality on the images obtained (Fig. 13.2). Correlation of palpatory with ultrasonographic findings is mandatory. Images are obtained in sagittal and transverse planes with oblique projections as needed. The time-gain-compensation (TGC) curve and over-gain settings are adjusted to provide uniform echogenicity of the testicle (3, 11).

EMBRYOLOGY

Embryologically, the testes begin to develop during the fifth week of fetal life as a proliferation of cells of the celomic epithelium, underlying mesenchyme, and primordial germ cells. The germinal epithelium and mesenchyme

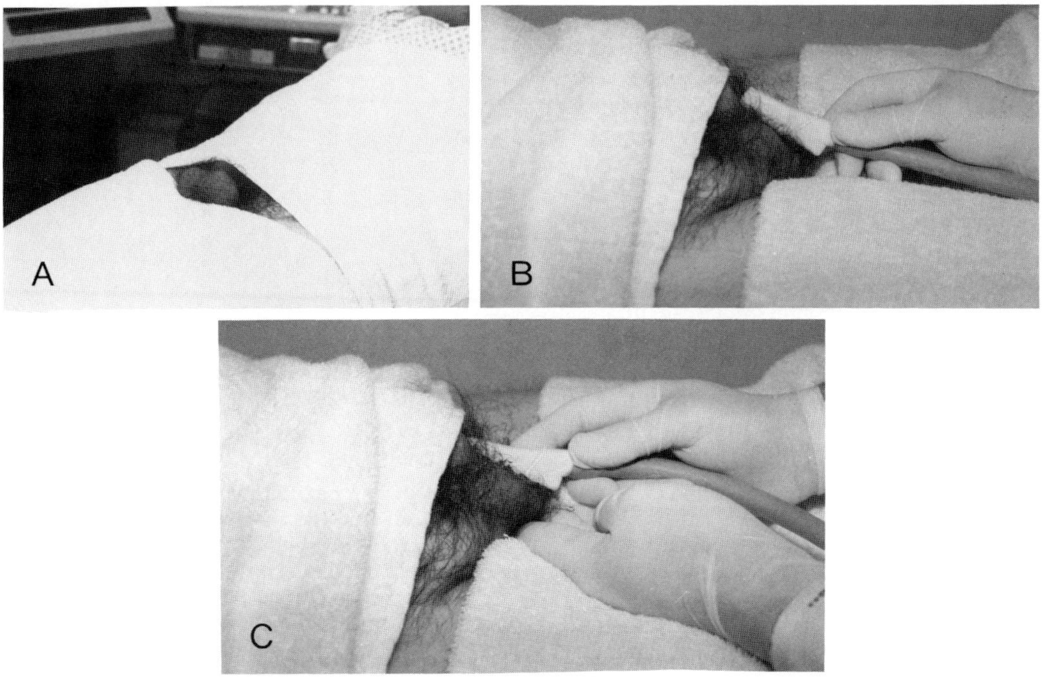

Figure 13.1. Scrotal ultrasound technique. The patient is placed in a supine position and the scrotum is supported by the use of a towel draped beneath it. The penis is retracted over the lower abdomen and covered by a second towel (**A**). Copious amounts of acoustic gel should be used and placed on both the scrotal skin and the transducer. The transducer is then placed on the anterior aspect of the scrotum, which can be supported by the towel alone (**B**). Alternatively, the scrotum can be cradled by the examiner's gloved hand (**C**).

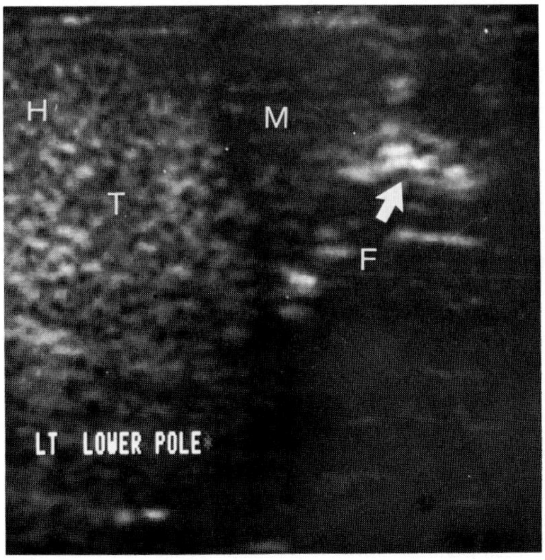

Figure 13.2. Finger localization of scrotal mass. The examiner's finger (*F*) can be identified as an echogenic band in contact with an extratesticular mass (*M*) adjacent to the lower pole of the left testis (*T*) on this sagittal image. *H*, toward patient's head.

produce a bulge on the medial side of each mesonephros called the gonadal ridge. Finger-like epithelial cords grow into the mesenchyme, forming an outer cortex and an inner medulla. The cortex regresses and the medulla differentiates into a testis. During the sixth week of fetal life, the primordial germ cells migrate into the mesenchyme and are incorporated into the primary sex cords. The primary sex cords condense and extend into the medulla of the gonad to form the rete testis. The prominent sex cords, called the seminiferous cords, lose their connection with the germinal epithelium because of the development of a thick fibrous capsule, the tunica albuginea. The enlarging testis separates from the degenerating mesonephros and becomes suspended by the mesorchium. The seminiferous cords develop into the seminiferous tubules, which are made up of two cell types, the sustentacular cells of Sertoli (derived from the germinal epithelium) and the spermatogonia (derived by the primordial germ cells). The fetal testes produce hormones that stimulate adjacent mesonephric tissue to be transformed into efferent ductules, which develop into the epididymis. Beyond the epididymis, the mesonephric duct acquires smooth muscle and becomes the ductus deferens (11, 16).

As the mesonephros degenerates, a ligament, the gubernaculum, descends on either side of the abdomen from the lower pole of the gonads, passing through the abdominal wall and attaching to a labial scrotal swelling. Later, a sac of peritoneum called the processus vaginalis forms ventral to the gubernaculum and herniates through the lower abdominal wall along the path of the gubernaculum. The processus vaginalis carries layers of the abdominal wall and thereby forms the inguinal canal. By 28 weeks, the testes have descended from the dorsal abdominal wall to the inguinal rings. The gubernaculum does not grow as rapidly as the body wall and therefore allows the testes to descend through the inguinal canal. By about 32 weeks, the testes have entered the scrotum. Ninety-seven percent of all term newborns have normally descended testicles. During the first 3 months after birth, some undescended testicles may descend into the scrotum. The process of descent is controlled by gonadotropins and androgens. Maternal gonadotropins have disappeared by the fourth week of neonatal life (11, 16).

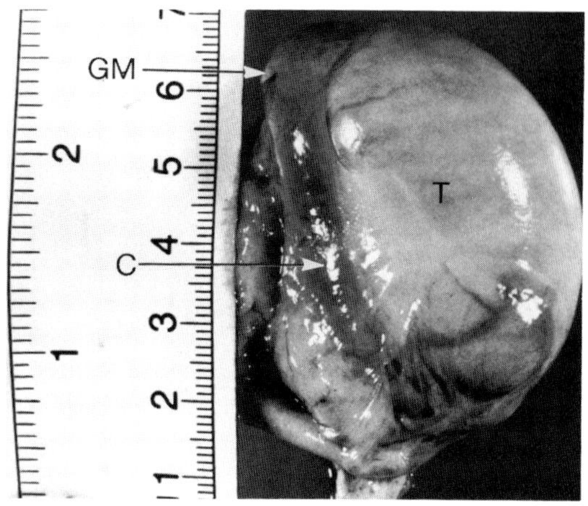

Figure 13.3. Pathologic specimen of a normal testis and epididymis. The epididymal head, also termed the globus major (*GM*), and epididymal body or corpus (*C*) course along the dorsolateral aspect of the testis (*T*).

NORMAL ANATOMY

The normal, mature testicle is ovoid in configuration, measuring approximately 4.0 × 3.5 × 2.5 cm (Fig. 13.3) (2). It may on occasion have a more rounded appearance, especially during later life. The testis is composed of more than 250 separate lobules, which contain the seminiferous tubules, the site of spermatogenesis. (Fig. 13.4). The lobuli testis are separated from each other by fibrous septae that join at the mediastinum testis. The mediastinum represents the invagination of the fibrous capsule that envelopes the testis, otherwise known as the tunica albuginea. The septula testis, which form the margins of the lobuli testis, are located between the mediastinum and the tunica albuginea. The testicular vessels course through the mediastinum (3, 10, 17). The appendix testis is situated at the superior pole and is present in up to 93% of men (18). It represents a remnant of the müllerian duct. Other appendages have been infrequently identified and are rarely seen with ultrasound. These include the paradidymis (organ of Giraldes) and the superior and inferior vas aberrans of Haller (18).

The epididymis lies along the superoposterolateral aspect of the testis (Fig. 13.3). Its overall size is 6 to 7 cm, and it contains more than 6 m of coiled tubule. The epididymal head, also termed the globus major or caput epididymis, is round or triangular and measures approximately 6 to 15 mm in width. It is connected to the testis via the vasa efferentia and represents the confluence of approximately 10 efferent ducts from the rete testis into a single duct, the ductus epididymis. The latter forms the body (corpus) of the epididymis, measuring approximately 2 to 4 mm in diameter. It courses caudally along the dorsolateral aspect of the testis to the inferior pole to form the tail or globus minor. The globus minor measures approximately 2 to 4 mm in diameter. From this point, the ductus epididymis ascends medially and cephalad, acquiring a muscular coat to become the ductus deferens (2, 3, 10). A small protuberance may arise from the epididymal head, known as the appendix of the epididymis. This is present in approximately 33% of all males (3).

The scrotum is composed of many different tissue layers (Fig. 13.5). During the process of descent, the testes become invested with layers of tissue corresponding to the many layers of abdominal wall musculature. The testes, invested by the tunica albuginea, come to rest in

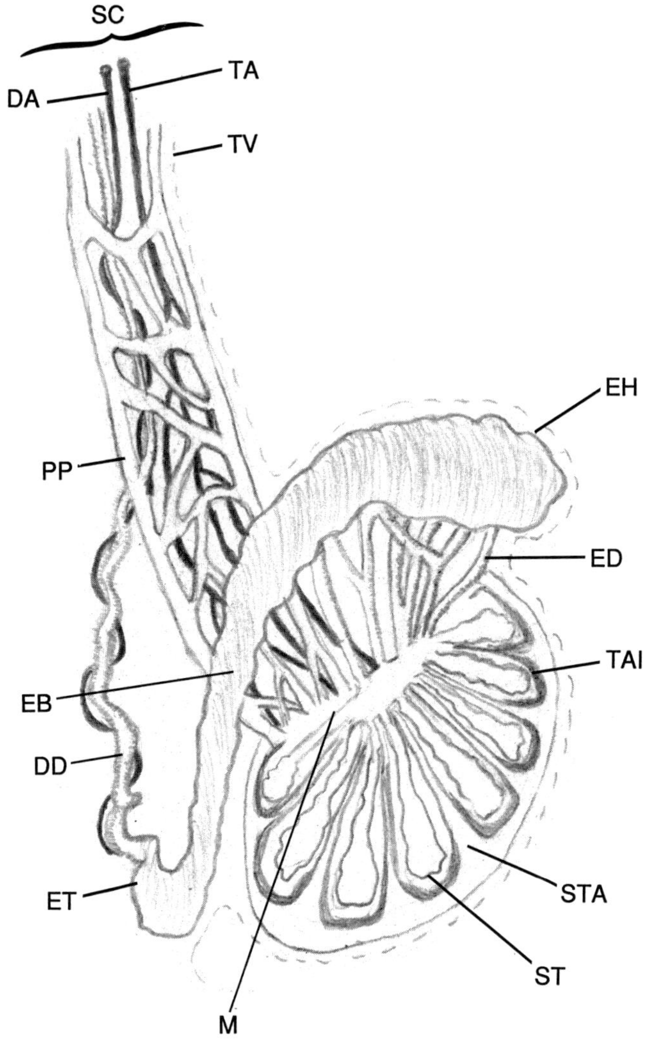

Figure 13.4. Anatomy of the testicle and epididymis. *SC,* spermatic cord; *TA,* testicular artery; *TV,* tunica vaginalis; *EH,* epididymal head; *ED,* efferent ductules; *ST,* seminiferous tubules; *TAI,* tunica albuginea; *STA,* septa of tunica albuginea; *M,* mediastinum; *ET,* epididymal tail; *EB,* epididymal body; *DD,* ductus deferens; *PP,* pampiniform plexus; *DA,* deferential artery.

a pouch formed by the skin and tunica dartos. During its descent, the testis is accompanied by the processus vaginalis, which originates from peritoneum. The processus vaginalis eventually envelopes the testis and forms attachment to the posterior scrotal wall above, below, medial, and lateral to the testis, leaving the posterior aspect of the testis uncovered. The lateral aspect of the epididymis is also attached to the posterior scrotal wall in this process. This investing layer is then called the tunica vaginalis and is located between the tunica dartos and the tunica albuginea (3). It is composed of two layers of tissue, visceral and parietal. The visceral layer, a serous membrane, produces secretions and the parietal layer contains lymphatics, important for absorption (18). A potential space exists between these two layers into which bowel can herniate and in which fluid can collect and form a hydrocele or hematocele, etc.

Normal Sonographic Anatomy

The normal testicle demonstrates a homogeneous, low to medium level of echogenicity, similar to that of the thyroid (Fig. 13.6). Except in the presence of a hydrocele, the tunica albuginea and the appendix testis are not routinely visualized (Fig. 13.7). The mediastinum testis is seen as a brightly echogenic thick band that parallels the epididymis (Fig. 13.8). The septula testis may be visualized as echogenic or hypoechogenic linear structures. The individual lobuli are not routinely defined. The var-

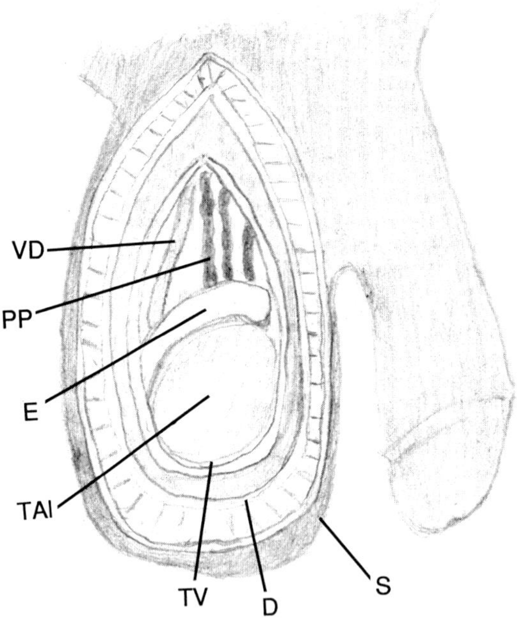

Figure 13.5. Anatomy of the scrotum. *PP*, pampiniform plexus; *E*, epididymis; *S*, skin; *D*, dartos; *TV*, tunica vaginalis; *TAI*, tunica albuginea; *VD*, vas deferens.

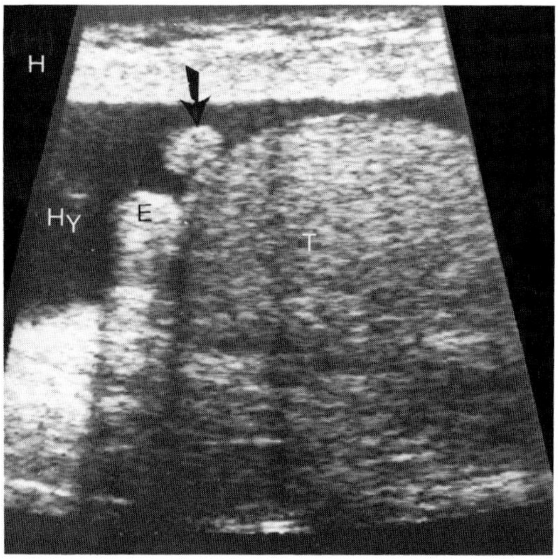

Figure 13.7. Appendix of the testicle. The appendix of the testis (*arrow*) is visualized because of the presence of a small hydrocele (*Hy*). The normal epididymis (*E*) is located just posterior to this structure on the longitudinal image. Note the normal testicular echogenicity (*T*). *H*, toward patient's head.

ious scrotal layers are indistinguishable, appearing as a highly echogenic stripe (3).

The echogenicity of the epididymal head is equivalent to or slightly greater than that of the testis (Fig. 13.9). The echogenicity of the body may be slightly less than or equal to that of the testis (Fig. 13.10). The differences are due to the greater number of tubules in the epididymal head. Frequently, the tail may not be clearly visualized on sonography (11).

The spermatic cord is connected to the testis at the mediastinum (Fig. 13.11). It is composed of the pampiniform plexus of veins, testicular and deferential arteries, lymphatics, nerves (genital branch of the genitofemoral nerve and

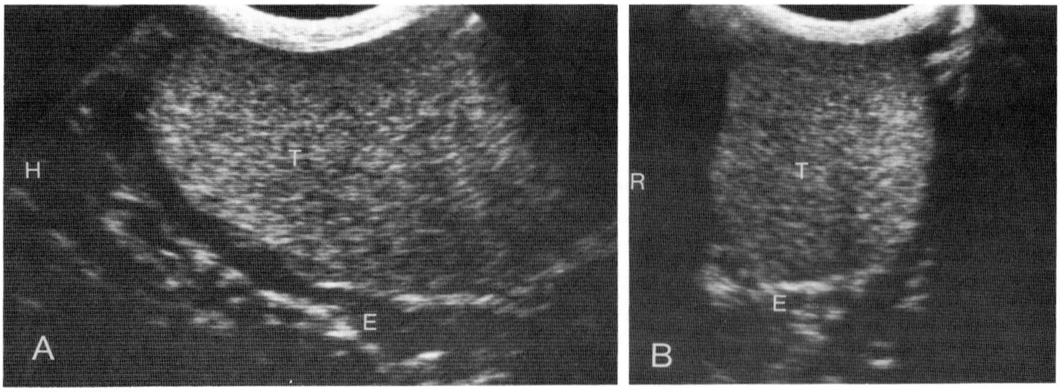

Figure 13.6. Normal scrotal ultrasound. Real-time images of the normal scrotum in longitudinal (**A**) and transverse (**B**) orientations demonstrating the normal low to medium homogeneous echotexture of the ovoid-shaped testis (*T*). The normal epididymis (*E*) lies posterior to the testis. *H*, toward patient's head; *R*, patient's right side.

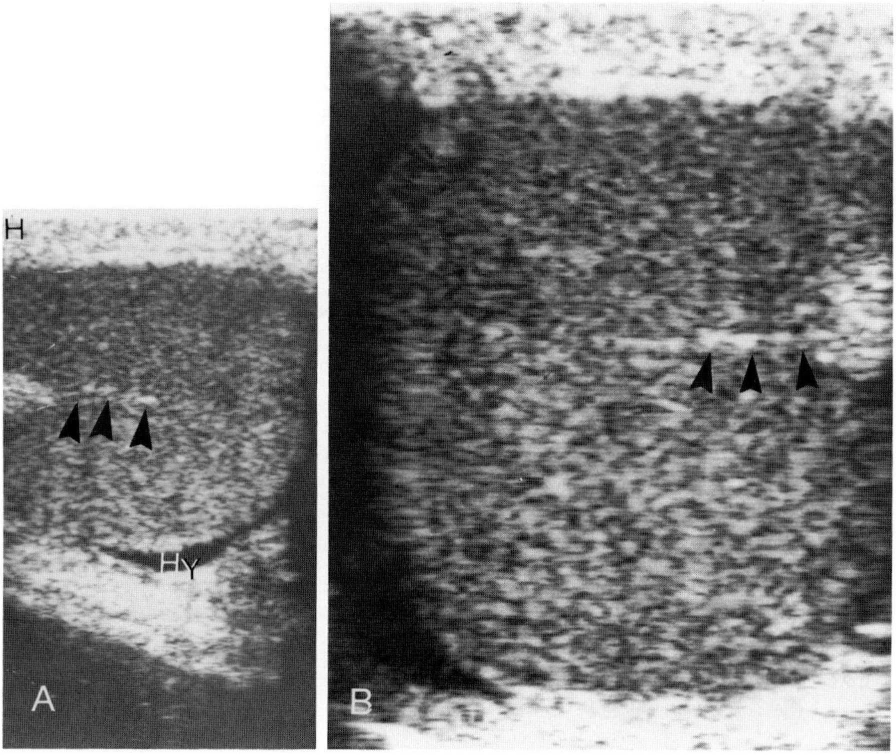

Figure 13.8. Real-time high-resolution ultrasound of the testis. Longitudinal (**A**) and transverse (**B**) images demonstrate a brightly echogenic thick band, the mediastinum testis (*arrowheads*). A small hydrocele (*Hy*) is present. *H,* toward patient's head.

testicular plexus of the sympathetic trunk), and the vas deferens. Duplex real-time scanning with Doppler ultrasound and color Doppler can be used to evaluate venous and arterial flow in these structures (Fig. 13.12) (19, 20).

CONGENITAL ANOMALIES

Undescended Testicle

Shortly before birth or early within the neonatal period, the testes begin their descent through the inguinal canal into the scrotum. On occasion, the process may fail to be initiated or becomes disrupted. Undescended testes are not uncommon in premature infants, being present in an estimated 20 to 33% of all preterm males (3, 21). The prevalence of this condition is close to 100% in neonates weighing less than 1 kg at birth (22). Approximately 3.4% of male children weighing greater than 2500 g will have undescended testes. By 3 to 4 months of age, the incidence declines to 0.7%. Cryptorchidism is bilateral in 10% of cases and, of those that go to surgery, anorchia is found in 3 to 5% (3, 11, 23, 24).

Most often, the testis comes to rest just above or within the external inguinal ring but may on occasion be femoral or intraabdominal. About 80% of undescended testes will be found at or below the level of the inguinal canal (3). An abdominal testicle is commonly small and nonpalpable. It is often abnormally developed. Intracanalicular testes, which lie within a hernial sac in the inguinal canal, are also frequently not palpable. This testis is commonly small and elongated. An emergent undescended testis lies outside the external inguinal ring, usually within a hernial sac. The testis may be malpositioned within the scrotum, generally situated in a more cephalad position, as a result of the late descent of the testicle into the scrotum. As a general rule, the testis that is partially or completely undescended is smaller than the contralateral testis (11).

The etiologies of cryptorchidism are multiple, including familial inheritance (prune belly

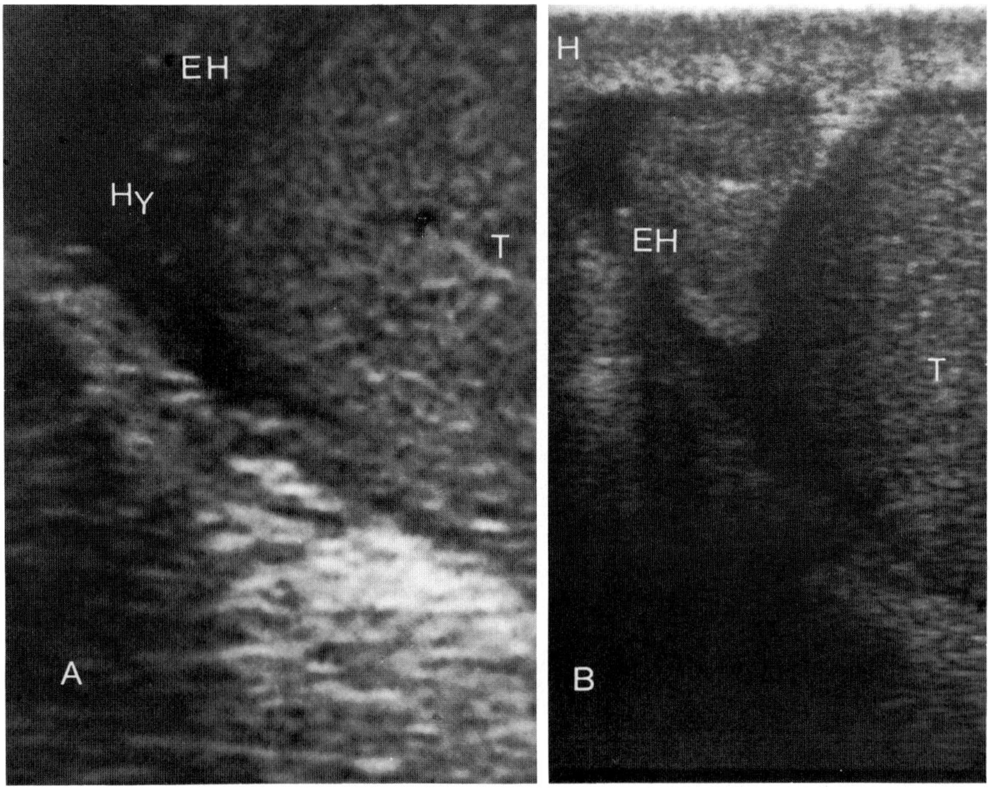

Figure 13.9. Normal epididymal head. The echogenicity of the epididymal head (*EH*) may be slightly greater than or equivalent to that of the testis (*T*). Its appearance on longitudinal images may be rounded (**A**) or triangular (**B**). *Hy,* small hydrocele; *H,* toward patient's head.

syndrome), mechanical obstruction, congenital abnormality of the testicle and abnormal hormonal effects (especially dihydrotestosterone) during embryogenesis (22). Mechanical obstruction results from fibrous encroachment upon the descending contents into the inguinal region with obstruction of the growing processus vaginalis. If a septum forms at the scrotal neck, the testis will come to reside within the superficial inguinal pouch. Cryptorchidism may be associated with other anomalies of the urogenital tract, including renal ectopia, renal agenesis, and the previously mentioned prune belly syndrome. A common association with congenital hernias has been noted. Sterility may result when either one or both testes are undescended, although this occurs more commonly in the latter instance. The abnormally placed testis is more prone to injury by accidental trauma. Testicular torsion may occur because the normal attachments of the spermatic cord are lacking (3, 11, 22).

Testicular malignancy occurs 4 to 5 times more frequently in males with an undescended testicle in the inguinal region than in males with normally situated testes. The incidence is even greater when the testis is located within the abdomen. Sarcomatous degeneration is the most ominous complication (Fig. 13.13) (3, 11, 23, 25, 26).

Infertility is also a complication of undescended testis. Infertility may ensue as a result of progressive pathologic abnormalities involving both the normal and undescended testis. These changes are progressive from the time the patient is a year old, and therefore surgery to correct this condition is usually performed at the age of 1 (22, 27, 28). If the undescended testis is brought into the scrotum by 6 years of age, sterility may still be avoided (3). Forty-four percent of patients who have had repair of bilateral undescended testes maintain fertility (3).

Many imaging techniques have been used to

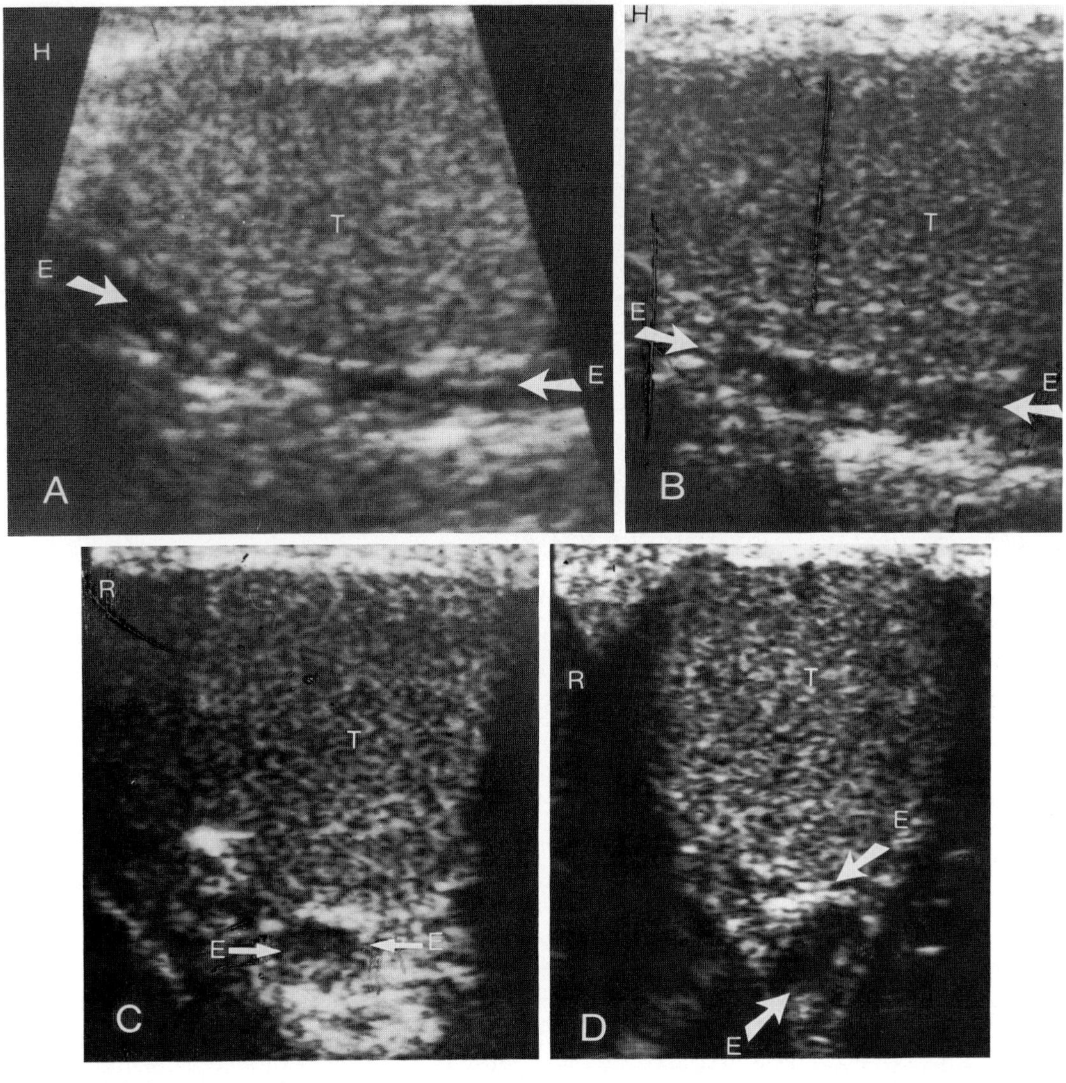

Figure 13.10. Normal epididymis. Real-time images demonstrate the appearance of the normal epididymis (*E*) on longitudinal (**A, B**) and transverse (**C, D**) images. The epididymal body may vary in size from 2 to 4 mm and is generally less echogenic than the testis (*T*). The epididymis is bounded by highly reflective margins, its fascial linings. *H,* toward patient's head; *R,* patient's right side.

define the location of the undescended testicle. Ultrasound has been particularly helpful when the suspected location is in the inguinal area (6, 22, 29–31). Comparison with the opposite normal side is helpful to look for asymmetry. In a location deep to the transversalis and internal oblique muscles, an asymmetric mass with acoustic characteristics equivalent to the normal testicle may be identified (Fig. 13.14). If the testis is atrophic, the acoustic characteristics may be atypical. It is more difficult and often impossible to locate aberrant testes in other locations (e.g., the abdomen) because they are small and difficult to distinguish from surrounding tissues. If an intraabdominal testis is comparable in size to the normal gland, malignant degeneration should be suspected.

Computed tomography (CT) (29, 32, 33) or magnetic resonance imaging (MRI) (21, 34) can be utilized for detection of the undescended testis and are preferred modalities for evaluating an intraabdominally located testis. The diag-

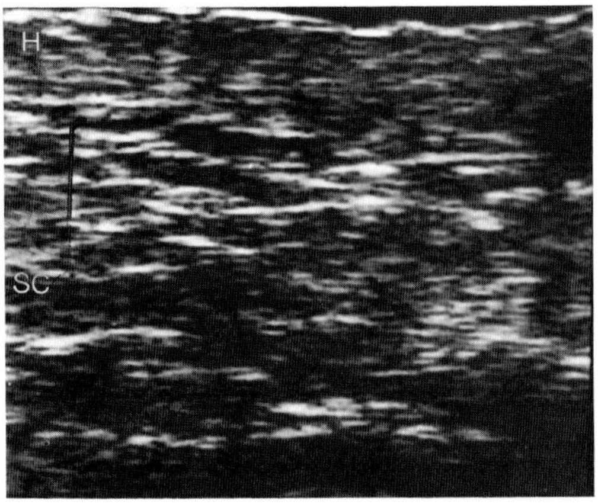

Figure 13.11. Normal spermatic cord. High-resolution real-time examination of the scrotum demonstrates multiple tubular structures representing the vascular structures of the spermatic cord (*SC*). Flow may be noted with some real-time equipment and with color Doppler. *H,* toward patient's head.

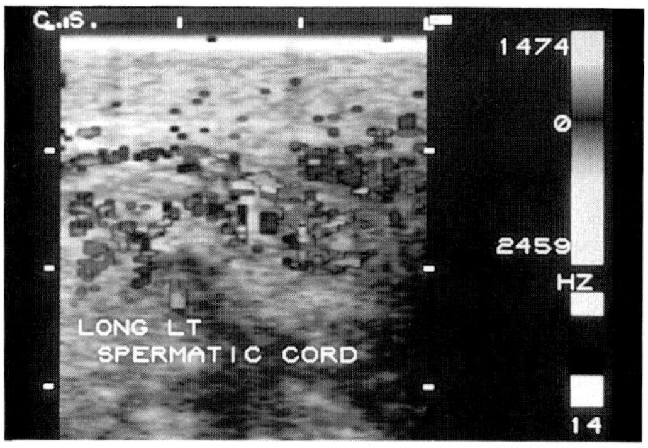

Figure 13.12. Color Doppler of normal spermatic cord. Flow toward and away from the transducer is seen in different segments of the tortuous testicular artery. *H,* toward patient's head. (See color plate 2.)

nosis is based on the recognition of an asymmetric, unilateral soft tissue density that is ovoid and is located along the course of testicular descent. The undescended testis is often smaller than the contralateral normal side, which may actually be hypertrophied. Fritzsche et al. (21) showed that both the transaxial and coronal planes could be used to detect the undescended testis. T2-weighted (long TE/TR) images were best in differentiating the undescended testis from surrounding fat when scans were obtained on a 1.5-tesla unit (21). Kier et al. (34) found that, although MR was of great value in the evaluation of young children with nonpalpable testes, it was not accurate enough to enable complete exclusion of an undescended testis. Failure to localize a testis with MR necessitates laparoscopy or surgical exploration (34).

In extremely difficult cases, venography may be needed to define the testis.

Atrophy

Congenital atrophy can be inferred in the newborn or prepubescent male with asymmetry of the testes. This entity is usually unilateral and can be diagnosed by computing testicular volume. It is easiest to use a simplified formula for calculating the volume of a prolated ellipse (35).

$$\frac{\text{length} \times \text{width} \times \text{thickness}}{2} = \text{volume in cc}$$

Volume may be more accurately calculated using a linear regression formula (36):

$$\text{Volume} = \text{length} \times \text{width} \times \text{depth} \times 0.65$$

In the prepubescent male, the average normal testicular volume is less than 1.5 cc (37). In the postpubescent period, the normal testicular volume is approximately 15 to 20 cc (37, 38), although variation in size in normal adults of different ethnic origins has been reported (39).

Acquired atrophy other than that occurring in the undescended testis may be associated with a variety of conditions. These include senility, infertility, prolonged hyperpyrexia, avitaminosis, hepatic cirrhosis, hypothyroidism, schizophrenia, estrogen therapy, and in diseases of the pituitary gland and hypothalamus (40). Acute atrophy has been reported as a complication following renal transplantation. This is a painful condition (6).

Polyorchidism

Polyorchidism may present as a scrotal mass palpated on physical examination. On occasion, it is diagnosed in the older child or adult, but frequently it may not be discovered until autopsy. The embryologic development of a duplicated or bifid testis has not been definitely established. Theories to explain this entity include (*a*) anomalous appropriation of cells from the degenerating mesonephros, which

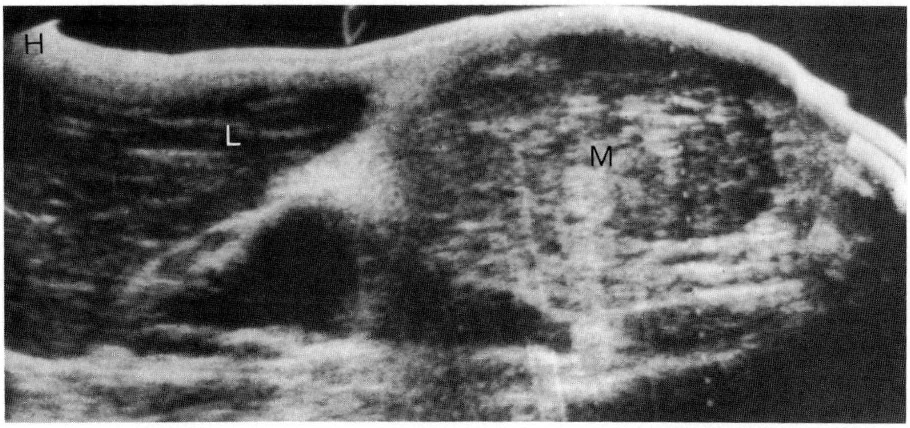

Figure 13.13. Malignant degeneration of abdominally located undescended testis. Longitudinal image demonstrates large complex mass (*M*) inferior to the liver margin (*L*) representing sarcomatous degeneration of an intraabdominal testis in a patient with prune belly syndrome. *H*, toward patient's head.

forms the vas deferens and epididymis; (*b*) duplication of the urogenital ridge (the precursor of the testis); (*c*) transverse as opposed to longitudinal division of the urogenital ridge; (*d*) incomplete degeneration of a portion of the mesonephros; and (*e*) development of peritoneal bands (41–44).

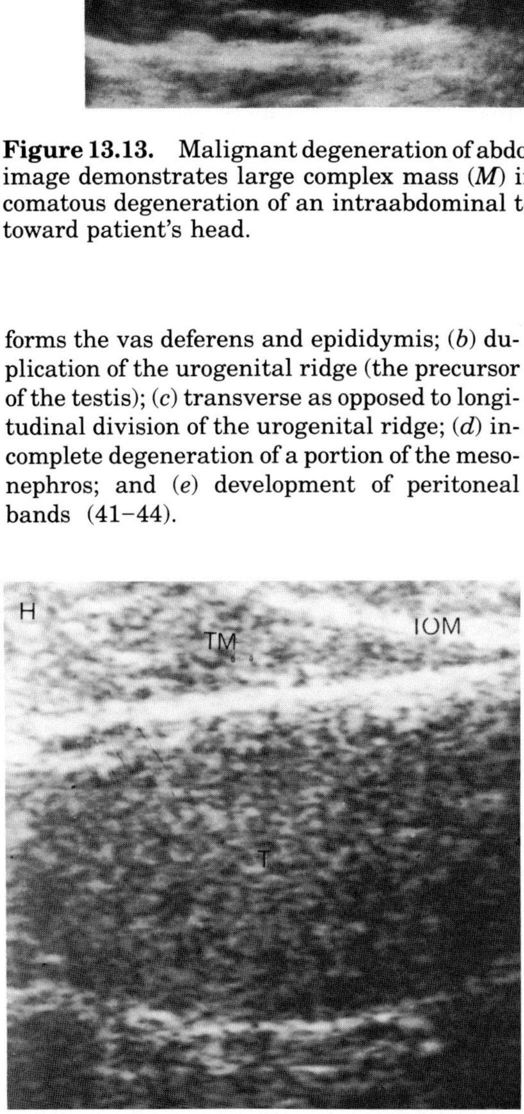

Figure 13.14. Undescended testis. Longitudinal real-time image of aberrant testis (*T*) located in the inguinal area. The transversalis muscle (*TM*) and internal oblique muscle (*IOM*) are visualized anterior to the testis. *H*, toward patient's head.

The size of the duplication of the testis and the number and position of the epididymis, vas deferens, and tunica vaginalis may depend on the stage of embryogenesis during which the anomalous development occurs. A bifid or duplicated testis with a single epididymis, vas deferens, and tunica albuginea surrounding both is more common than complete duplication of all structures. Ultrasound is the best modality to define this anomaly, demonstrating homogeneous echogenicity of the bifid testis (Fig. 13.15). Occasionally, the adjacent testis may demonstrate slightly different acoustic reflectivity than the adjacent testis (45).

Congenital Hydroceles

Hydroceles may be diagnosed in utero in male fetuses of at least 30 weeks' gestational age. Congenital hydroceles occur because of a communication between the funicular process and the peritoneum, allowing ascites present in the abdomen to descend into the scrotum (46). Abnormal lymphatic drainage may also explain their existence (47). Although hydroceles may normally be seen in a premature male, persistence into the neonatal period should arouse suspicion of an associated hernia or other pathology.

SCROTAL MASS

The differentiation of intratesticular from extratesticular pathology is essential. The vast majority of intratesticular lesions are malig-

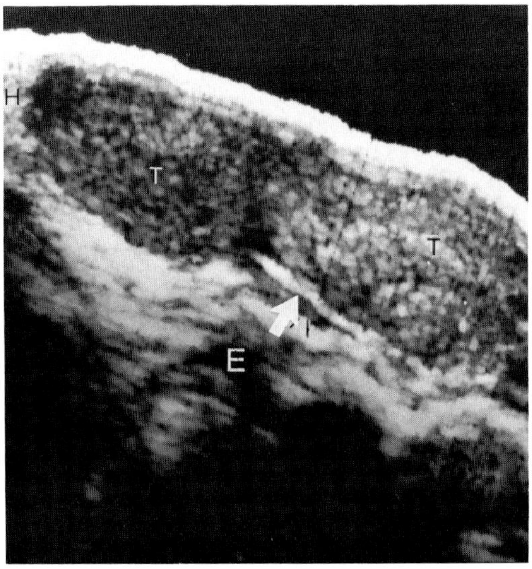

Figure 13.15. Bifid testis. A longitudinal image of the left side of the scrotum demonstrates two oval-shaped structures (*T*) with homogeneous echotexture. These represent a bifid testis. Note the presence of a single epididymis (*E*). *H,* toward patient's head.

nant, whereas extratesticular lesions are more likely to be due to inflammation or prior trauma or to represent benign tumors (3, 48). In this regard, ultrasound is most useful, with a diagnostic accuracy approaching 90 to 95% (3). As a generalization, testicular neoplasms present sonographically as focal alterations of the normal homogeneous echo texture. Although most tumors are hypoechoic, hyperechoic lesions may be seen if hemorrhage, fibrosis, or calcification is present (3, 10, 49). Unfortunately, some neoplasms are more diffuse in appearance and resemble processes such as abscess, infarction, or hemorrhage. Focal echogenic scars may represent areas of infarction, granuloma, or "burned-out" neoplasm. Calcification of the testis may be seen without a distinct mass and may signify an "inactive" or treated germ cell tumor (3, 50). Calcification in an active testicular tumor is unusual but has been seen (49).

Since there is extensive overlap in the ultrasonographic appearance of benign and malignant intratesticular pathology (e.g., malignant infiltration versus orchitis or missed torsion), the following criteria may be used to help separate these entities (51): (*a*) with tumor, there is often some residual normal testicular tissue present; (*b*) with tumor, the epididymis is generally spared; (*c*) with orchitis, the epididymis is frequently affected; (*d*) with chronic torsion, the epididymis may or may not be normal; (*e*) a diffusely homogeneous hyperechoic testis is almost certainly benign; (*f*) skin thickening suggests an inflammatory process.

Focal, clinically nonpalpable testicular neoplasms are often easily diagnosed by ultrasound (49, 52–55). These patients may present with gynecomastia or evidence of metastatic disease to the retroperitoneum or mediastinum. Lesions as small as 2 to 3 mm have been identified within the testicle on ultrasound (Fig. 13.16) (11, 49, 56).

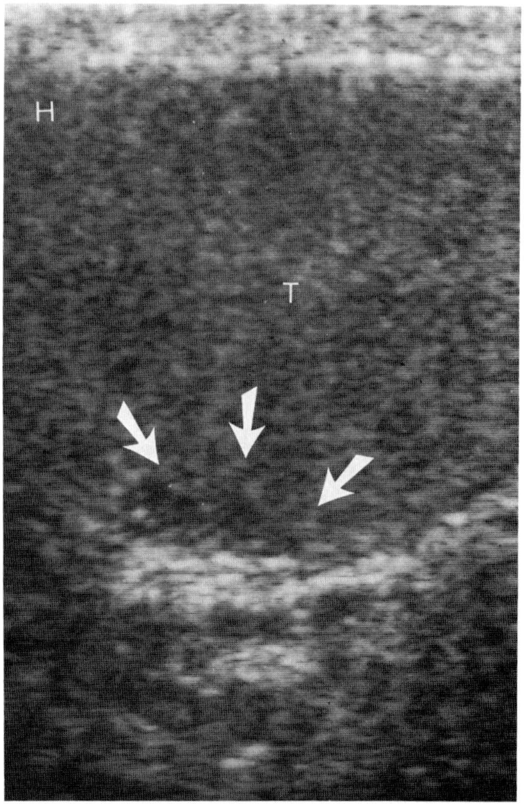

Figure 13.16. Nonpalpable seminoma. There is a 2 × 4 mm hypoechoic area in the posterior aspect of the testis (*T*) on this longitudinal image (*arrows*). The patient had retroperitoneal adenopathy and no known primary. Surgical resection revealed seminoma. *H,* toward patient's head.

Intratesticular Masses

Testicular neoplasms constitute approximately 1 to 2% of all male malignancies and 4 to 6% of all male genitourinary tumors. These neoplasms are among the most common malignancies in men aged 15 to 34 years and constitute the fifth most common cause of cancer death in this age group (3, 49, 57–59). Geographic predilections include an increased incidence in the United States and Denmark. Whites are affected 6 to 10 times more frequently than blacks. Tumor histology is age related. Endodermal sinus tumors and teratomas occur during the first decade, choriocarcinoma is seen commonly in the second and third decades, embryonal cell carcinoma in the third decade, and seminomas in the fourth decade (60). Most tumors are discovered on physical examination as a painless, nodular surface contour abnormality. Less commonly, testicular neoplasm may present as a testicular enlargement that may be painless or slightly painful (61). Ten percent present as an acute scrotum with sudden hemorrhage or necrosis, accounting for symptomatology. Most testicular malignancies are unilateral, but approximately 8% of testicular tumors subsequently recur in the contralateral testis. Approximately 4 to 14% of patients will present with symptoms secondary to metastatic disease. This is seen more commonly in patients with nonseminomatous germ cell tumors (3).

Of primary testicular neoplasms, 95% are of germ cell origin, with seminomas being the most common. The remainder of testicular malignancies are of Sertoli cell, Leydig cell, or mesenchymal origin (3, 52, 62, 63).

Although sonography alone cannot be used to make a specific diagnosis of malignant disease or to classify a neoplasm histologically, this modality is extremely useful in differentiating tumors from nonneoplastic scrotal pathologic conditions. It has been shown that the sensitivity and predictive value of a normal sonogram is as high as 100% (57). Sonography is also useful in the diagnosis of retroperitoneal adenopathy, with accuracy rates ranging from 77 to 82%, specificity 57 to 98%, and sensitivity 67 to 93% (64–67). Computed tomography (68–70) and MRI (71) are, however, currently the modalities of choice for staging disease. Sonography of the testes should be performed in patients who present with gynecomastia without explainable cause to exclude the presence of a nonpalpable neoplasm (56, 74). Similarly, sonography of the testes should be performed in young males who present with metastasis (i.e., retroperitoneal or mediastinal adenopathy) to exclude the presence of a clinically occult testicular malignancy (52, 54, 74). Ultrasound of the testes should be performed at regular intervals in patients with a history of primary testicular malignancy, as this may allow earlier detection of recurrence (3).

Magnetic resonance imaging of the testes for detection of tumor reveals neoplasms to be inhomogeneous and decreased in signal intensity on T2-weighted images relative to the normal parenchyma. Visualization of the tunica albuginea is a distinct advantage, allowing assessment of its margins to determine extragonadal extension of tumor (72, 73).

PRIMARY MALIGNANT TUMORS

Seminoma

Germ cell tumors represent 60% of all testicular malignancies. The most common germ cell tumor is the seminoma, which accounts for 40 to 50% of this class of tumors. Germ cell tumors, and in particular seminomas, are bilateral in 1 to 3% of cases and may be either synchronous or metachronous (75). Seminomas tend to occur in older men and, although they are less aggressive, 25% will be metastatic on initial presentation. They are usually confined within the tunica albuginea (3). Seminomas are the most common tumors seen in the cryptorchid testis. It is undetermined whether early orchiopexy is protective, providing a decreased risk of developing carcinoma, or whether surgery merely allows for earlier diagnosis and treatment (61). These tumors are radiosensitive and survival rates approach 95 to 100% for stage 1 disease (76).

Seminomas tend to produce a uniformly reduced reflectivity on ultrasound. This is compatible with the monotonous histology of the tumor. The echogenicity may vary depending on tumor size and the presence of calcification or cystic degeneration (Fig. 13.17) (3, 77).

On magnetic resonance images, these tumors appear mildly inhomogeneous with markedly decreased signal intensity on T2-weighted images (72).

Embryonal Cell Carcinoma

Embryonal cell carcinoma accounts for approximately 20 to 25% of germ cell tumors and

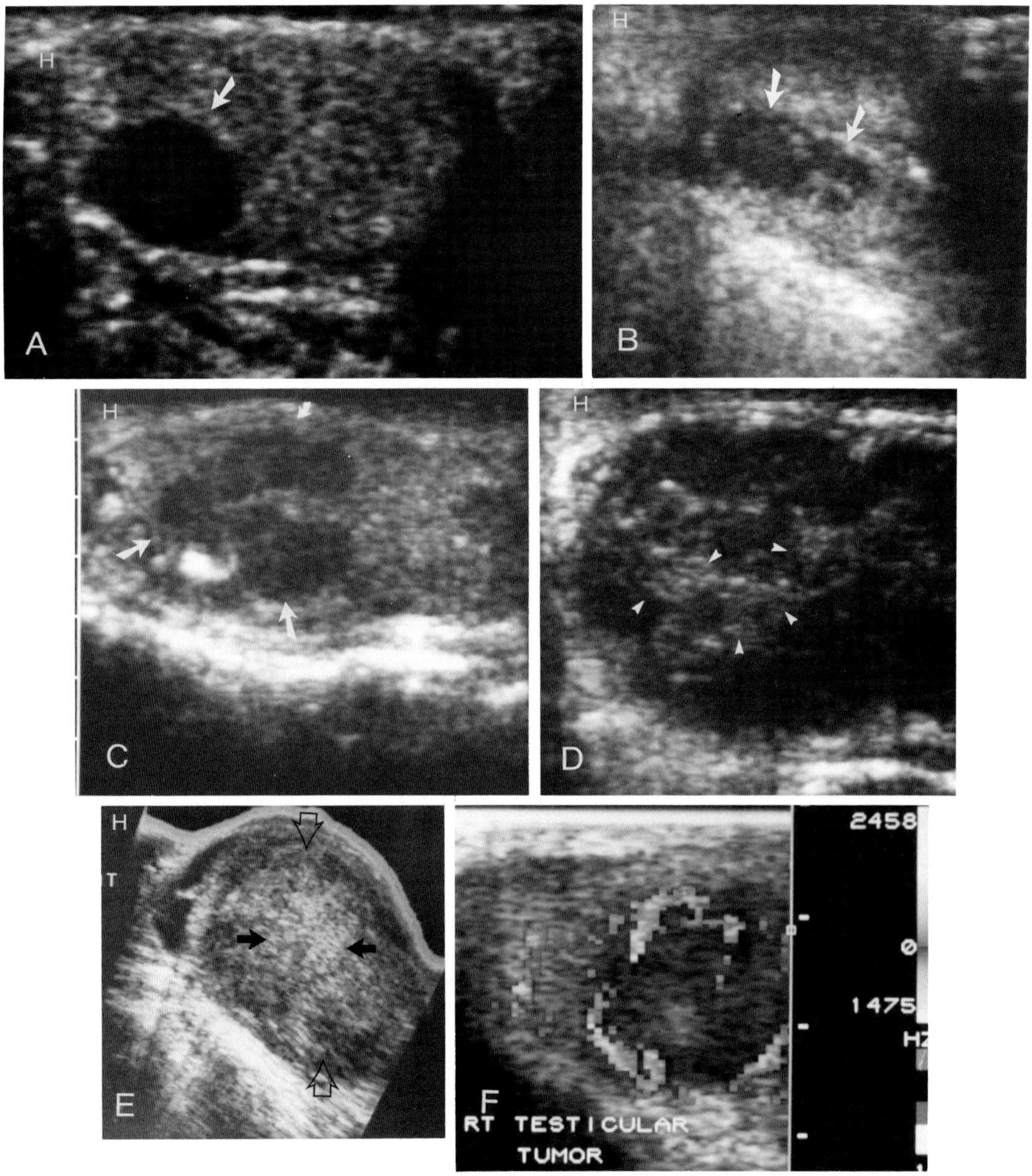

Figure 13.17. Seminoma. The majority of testicular malignancies are ultrasonically quite similar in appearance. Tumor echogenicity, however, is variable and is dependent on tumor size and the presence of calcification or cystic degeneration. **A,** An area of uniformly reduced reflectivity (*arrow*) within the testis represents a seminoma. **B** and **C,** Predominantly hypoechoic lobulated masses (*arrows*) in the testis contain hyperechoic regions, giving a slightly different appearance to these seminomas. **D,** Nearly total replacement of the testis with seminomatous tumor appears as poorly marginated hypoechoic infiltration with a small amount of normal-appearing testicular parenchyma centrally (*arrowheads*). **E,** A predominantly hyperechoic mass (*arrows*) with peripheral hypoechoic region (*open arrows*) also represents a seminoma. **F,** Color Doppler demonstrates displacement of intratesticular vessels by a predominantly hypoechoic mass (*M*). The mass is relatively hypovascular and at surgery, seminoma was found. *H,* toward patient's head. (See color plate 2.)

is the most aggressive germ cell neoplasm. Invasion of the tunica is commonly seen as well as the presence of hemorrhage and cystic degeneration. This tumor is much less sensitive to radiation therapy when compared with the seminoma. Embryonal cell carcinoma is equivalent to the "yolk sac" tumor seen in children less than 3 years of age. It is the most common infantile germ cell carcinoma which clinically presents with markedly elevated α-fetoprotein with or without human chorionic gonadotropin markers (3, 78).

On sonography, embryonal cell carcinoma presents as a hypoechoic mass that is usually more inhomogeneous in echogenicity and less well defined than the seminoma. The tunica albuginea may be invaded, resulting in distortion of the contour of the testicle. Cystic necrosis and areas of increased echogenicity resulting from focal hemorrhage may be seen (3).

Magnetic resonance imaging demonstrates greater fluctuation and inhomogeneity in signal intensity than that seen with seminoma. Disruption of the thin black line representing the tunica albuginea and invasion of the epididymis is not an uncommon finding (72).

Choriocarcinoma

Choriocarcinoma represents 1 to 3% of primary malignant testicular tumors. It is an aggressive tumor that most frequently presents as metastasis before the testicular mass is clinically apparent. The lesion itself may be very small. The echogenicity of these tumors is frequently mixed because of the presence of hemorrhage, necrosis, and calcification. Metastatic deposits of choriocarcinoma may be found without evidence of choriocarcinoma in the primary lesion (3). Azzopardi (79) studied this phenomenon in 17 patients who died of disseminated widespread choriocarcinoma and other nonseminomatous tumors and found a distinct fibrotic scar in the testicle, which represented the necrotic remnants of germ cell tumors, indicating a "burned out" primary testicular neoplasm. These "scars" consist of acellular, dense collagenous tissue, hematoxyphilic deposits composed of phospholipids, protein, and deoxyribonucleic acid and calcium phosphates. Sonographically, a highly echogenic focal lesion with or without shadowing is seen (Fig. 13.18). Although this is not specific, burned-out tumor may be strongly suggested in the appropriate clinical setting of metastatic disease. Ultrasound, however, cannot differentiate between active and inactive tumor (3).

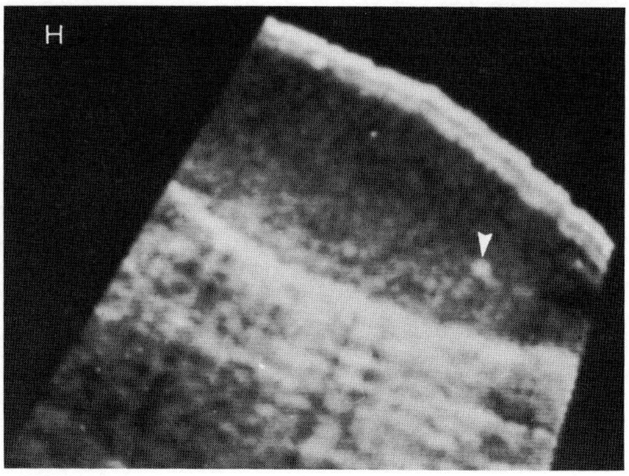

Figure 13.18. Nonpalpable regressed germ cell tumor. An echogenic focus (*arrowhead*) that does not cause shadowing represents an inactive germ cell tumor. In this case, there is no associated mass. *H,* toward patient's head.

Choriocarcinoma may be part of a mixed tumor including seminoma, embryonal cell carcinoma, or teratoma. Serum human chorionic gonadotropin levels are generally elevated (78).

Teratoma

Teratomas represent 5 to 10% of primary testicular neoplasms. By definition, they are composed of more than one germ cell layer and most are well-differentiated squamous cysts. Approximately one-third will show signs of metastatic disease within 5 years. Sonographically, these tumors are of mixed echogenicity, reflecting the individual components (bone, cartilage, smooth muscle, mucous gland, respiratory epithelium, and keratinaceous material) (Fig. 13.19) (3).

Mixed histologic tumors occur approximately 40% of the time. Teratocarcinoma, a mixture of teratoma and embryonal cell carcinoma, is the most common of this type and is the second most frequent germ cell tumor after the seminoma. These tumors are of mixed echogenicity, reflecting the components of cysts, hemorrhage, and necrosis. Metastasis occurs early (3).

METASTATIC DISEASE

Metastasis to the testes is more common than germ cell tumors in patients over 50 years of age. Most frequently, the primary neoplasm

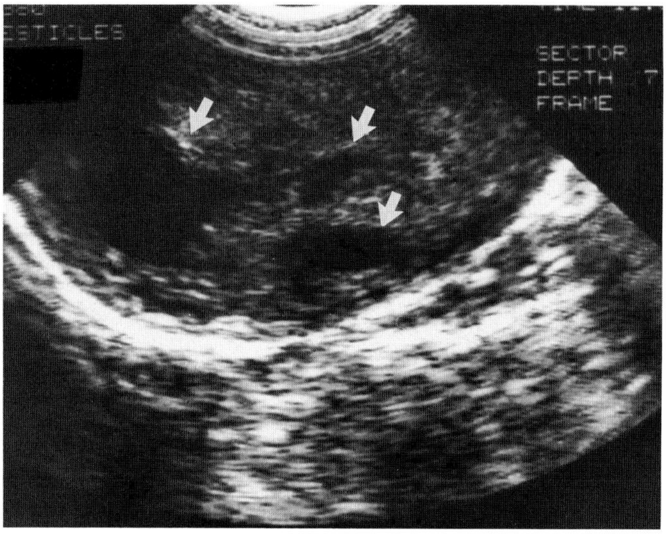

Figure 13.19. Teratoma. Complex, poorly marginated area of predominantly decreased echogenicity represents a teratoma (*arrows*). The appearance is nonspecific.

originates in the prostate or kidney, but metastatic melanoma, neuroblastoma, or tumor from the bronchi, pancreas, bladder, thyroid, and bowel have been observed (3, 80). Sonographically, these lesions may be hypoechoic, occasionally echogenic, and sometimes of mixed reflectivity (Fig. 13.20) (5).

LYMPHOPROLIFERATIVE DISEASE

The testes are a sanctuary for lymphoproliferative disease because the "gonadal barrier" inhibits concentration of chemotherapeutic agents, allowing for progression of disease (81). Malignant infiltration is more common in patients with acute leukemia than in patients with lymphoma. Clinically evident testicular involvement may be seen more frequently in patients with acute leukemia. Postmortem examinations reveal that overall, approximately one-third of males with lymphoproliferative disease demonstrate some degree of bilateral testicular involvement (82).

The frequency of testicular involvement on postmortem examination of patients with lymphoproliferative disease was greatest in patients having acute leukemia (64%) compared with patients with chronic leukemia (24%) and non-Hodgkin's lymphoma (18.6%). Hodgkin's disease involving the testicles is extremely rare (82).

As more effective therapeutic strategies have evolved, with successful eradication of bone marrow and CNS involvement, extramedullary relapse in other sites, especially the testis, is being recognized with greater frequency (81, 83).

Ultrasound has accurately demonstrated clinically occult involvement of the testis in patients with lymphoproliferative disease (7, 54). Two patterns of involvement have been recognized (Fig. 13.21). The most common is an "ill-defined" infiltration of the normal parenchyma that sonographically appears as an irregular, hypoechoic abnormality involving a part of or the entire testis. The second pattern consists of one or more focal, sharply marginated, intratesticular, anechoic or hypoechoic mass(es) surrounded by normal parenchyma. The latter may not be distinguishable from a primary malignancy involving the testis, except by history or bilateral involvement (7, 84–86).

BENIGN TESTICULAR LESIONS

Benign intratesticular lesions are far less common than malignant disease. Sonography is useful in differentiating the solid versus cystic nature of intratesticular masses. With regard to solid masses, however, sonography cannot reliably distinguish benign from malignant testicular processes. An echo-poor or complex abnormality involving the testis could represent abscess, orchitis, torsion, or benign or malignant neoplasm. Although a purely hyperechoic or echogenic testicular lesion is frequently benign, representing scar or calcification, a malignant lesion cannot be excluded (10, 48, 87, 88).

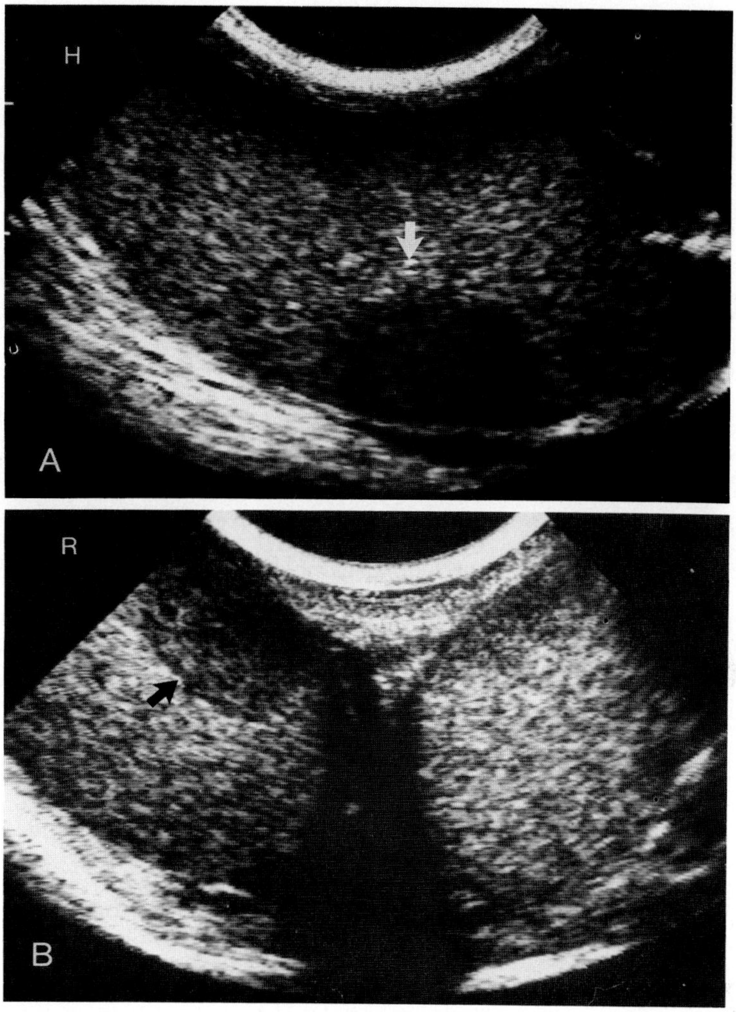

Figure 13.20. Metastatic melanoma. Longitudinal (**A**) and transverse (**B**) images of the right testis demonstrate hypoechoic regions, both anteriorly and posteriorly (*arrows*) that at surgical resection proved to be malignant melanoma. *H,* toward patient's head; *R,* patient's right side.

Testicular Cysts

Prior to the widespread use of high-resolution sonography, testicular cysts were considered rare. Recent studies, however, have demonstrated an occurrence rate of approximately 8 to 9.8% in patients referred for sonographic examination (89, 90). Ninety-two percent of intratesticular cysts are solitary. They usually range in size from approximately 2 mm to 1.8 cm and possess the characteristics of cysts: anechoic fluid collections with thin, sharply defined walls and good sound through transmission (Fig. 13.22) (91, 92). The primary differential consideration includes neoplastic cysts of which those in teratomas are the most common. Solid portions of the tumor help to differentiate these cystic lesions from benign cysts. Seminomas occasionally contain cystic structures, usually as a result of occlusion of the rete testis with subsequent cystic dilatation of the ducts or as a result of tumor necrosis. The rare epidermoid cyst may be confused with a simple cyst, particularly when it appears cystic with only a few low-level internal echoes. Some epidermoids, however, will appear as a hypoechoic solid mass with a thick capsule that is sometimes partially calcified. Frequently, these are located adjacent to the inner surface of the tunica albuginea (3, 57, 91).

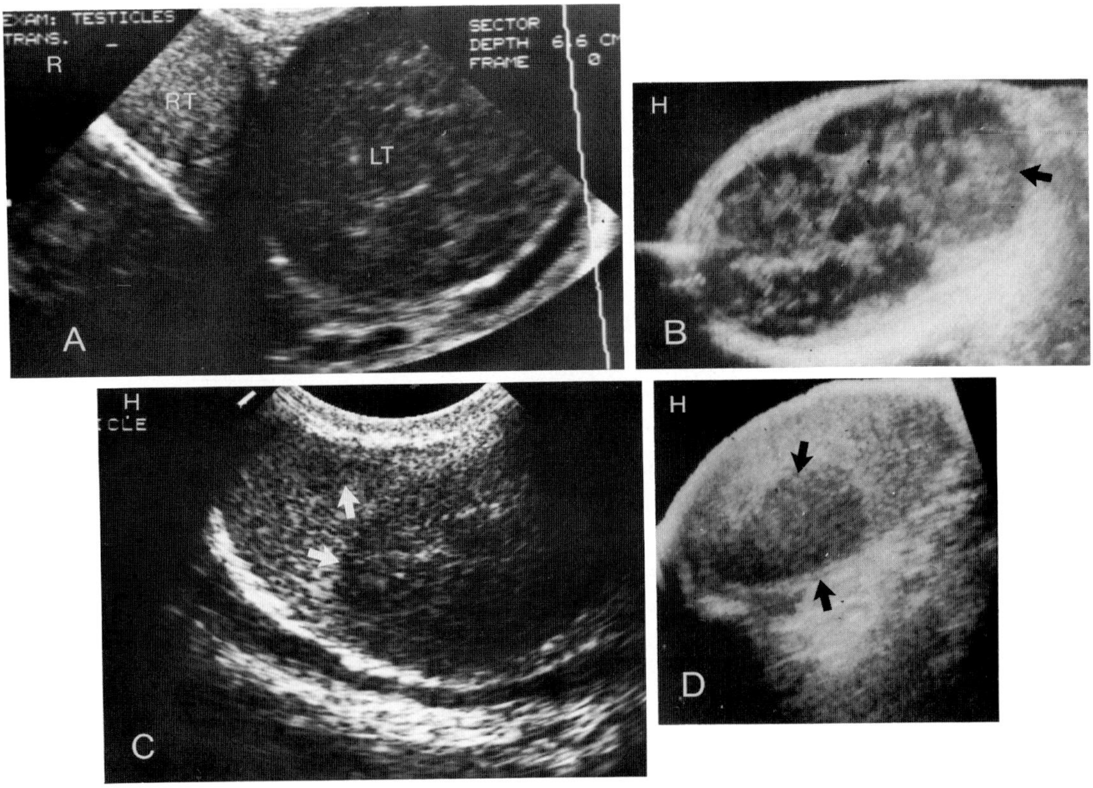

Figure 13.21. Lymphoproliferative disease. Two patterns of involvement may be seen on ultrasound in patients with lymphoma or leukemia with testicular involvement. **A,** Compare the enlarged left testis (*LT*) with the normal right testicle (*RT*) in this patient with lymphoma. The left testis is diffusely inhomogeneous in echo texture, signifying infiltration by tumor. **B,** Near total infiltration of the testis by hypoechoic tumor with a small residuum of normal parenchyma (*arrow*) is noted in this patient with lymphoma. **C,** There are at least two poorly demarcated hypoechoic regions (*arrows*) in the testis of this patient with leukemia. **D,** Leukemic involvement of the testis in another patient is more focal and better demarcated (*arrows*) compared with the infiltrative pattern. *H,* toward patient's head; *R,* patient's right side.

Two types of nonneoplastic cysts have been identified: intratesticular cysts and cysts of the tunica albuginea. Cysts of the tunica albuginea are palpable as small masses and are usually seen in middle-aged men. They are not actually within the testis but indent the parenchyma (91). Early reports suggested a traumatic or infectious etiology (93, 94), but recently it has been postulated that they originate in mesothelial rests as an embryonal remnant or from efferent ductules as they pass through the tunica albuginea (95, 96).

Intratesticular cysts are usually nonpalpable and are an incidental finding on sonography (3, 90). They may be found anywhere in the testes and, if peripheral in location, may be palpable. They are felt to arise from the rete testes since they histologically resemble this structure (97). Secondary lesions following trauma or inflammation and dysgenic predisposition are also potential causes (91). Cystic dysplasia of the testis develops from an embryogenic defect and is usually diagnosed in childhood (98).

Simple testicular cysts have characteristic appearances on magnetic resonance imaging. They are round, well-marginated, low-intensity masses on T1-weighted and proton density images. There is relatively increased signal intensity on T2-weighted images, in which the lesions become nearly isointense with normal testicular parenchyma (99).

Benign Testicular Neoplasms

The majority of benign testicular neoplasms originate from the Sertoli and Leydig cells, comprising the group known as gonadal stro-

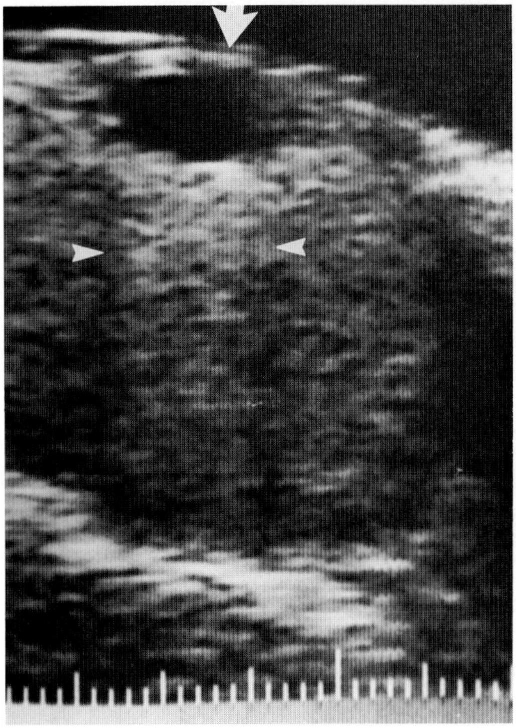

Figure 13.22. Testicular cyst. Peripheral, anechoic rounded lesion with thin, sharply defined walls (*arrow*) and good sound through transmission (*arrowheads*) represents an intratesticular cyst.

mal tumors. These tumors may be seen at any age. Ultrasonographically, they cannot be differentiated from malignant tumors and usually appear as a hypoechoic solid mass, occasionally with cystic components (3). The epidermoid (keratin) cyst was previously discussed.

Testiculiths

Testiculiths present sonographically as small, echogenic foci usually associated with distal shadowing. They are thought to represent venous phleboliths or spermatic granuloma. The differential diagnostic consideration is focal calcific scarring in an inactive ("burned-out") germ cell tumor. The latter can sometimes be delineated by the presence of an adjacent hypoechoic mass (5).

Microlithiasis

Testicular microlithiasis is a rare entity resulting from the deposition of calcific concretions in the seminiferous tubules. Although the exact etiology of this condition is unknown, microlithiasis has been found in patients with cryptorchidism, Kleinfelter's syndrome, and male pseudohermaphroditism. It has also been found in patients who have had similar calcifications in the lungs and central nervous system (100). The relationship of microlithiasis to infertility is uncertain, since the condition has been found in otherwise normal patients. The condition is usually asymptomatic and not treatable (101).

Sonographically, microlithiasis presents as multiple, punctate hyperechoic areas throughout both testes (Fig. 13.23) (101, 102). It is important to recognize this pattern and be aware that it may obscure other unrelated testicular pathology (101).

The differential diagnosis of microlithiasis includes other entities in which testicular calcification is found: tumors (before and after treatment), focal scars, spermatic granulomas, and adrenal rests (3). Sarcoid and torsion (101), which can present as diffuse testicular hyperechogenicity, should also be considered as differential possibilities.

Granulomatous Disease

Granulomatous disease of the testis presents as a solid mass, either unilateral or bilateral. Approximately 5% of patients with sarcoid will develop testicular or epididymal involvement. Sonographically, the lesion presents as a hyperechoic solid mass within or replacing the testis (5).

Testicular Abscess

Testicular abscess may be identified in the presence of epididymo-orchitis secondary to mumps, smallpox, tuberculosis, scarlet fever, influenza, typhoid, syphilis, cholecystitis, sinusitis, osteomyelitis, and appendicitis. Abscess secondary to epididymo-orchitis is often seen in the diabetic patient (3, 100, 103). The abscess may rupture into the tunica vaginalis, resulting in a pyocele. This is discussed in greater detail in the portion of this chapter on epididymitis and orchitis.

Sonographically, an abscess may present as a hypoechoic or mixed echogenic mass. Skin thickening and hydrocele may also be present. History is essential in differentiating this lesion from a neoplasm (104).

Infarct

Occasionally, a case of missed torsion will present as a focal, hypoechoic testicular mass or

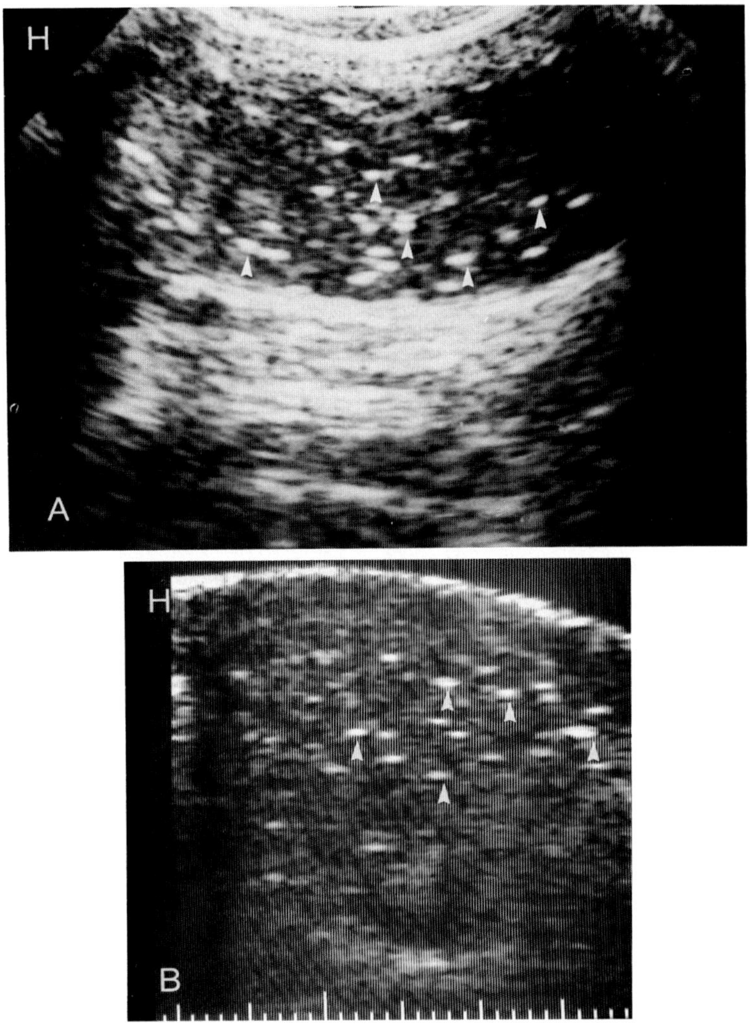

Figure 13.23. Testicular microlithiasis. Multiple punctate hyperechoic foci (*arrowheads*) scattered throughout the testicular parenchyma in two different patients. *H*, toward patient's head.

as a diffusely hypoechoic testis. There may be areas with increased echogenicity. Other etiologies for testicular infarction include trauma, leukemia, bacterial endocarditis, polyarteritis nodosa, and Henoch-Schönlein purpura (3, 105–107). History is important in differentiating this abnormality from testicular neoplasms because sonographically, hypoechoic infarcts are indistinguishable from malignancies. A diminution in size relative to the acute event favors the diagnosis of infarct (3, 105). Magnetic resonance imaging may be useful in selected cases, since fibrotic tissue is usually low in signal intensity on both T1- and T2-weighted images (71).

Schistosomiasis

Although uncommon in this country, bilharzial infection can involve the testis. Sonographically it has been reported to appear as echogenic testicular masses with scrotal edema (108).

Adrenal Rest

Ectopic adrenal rests are not uncommon in newborns, having been reported in approximately 50% of neonates. They are most commonly found in the kidney but may occur in the pelvis and scrotum, related to the common embryologic development. In most instances, these aberrant foci of tissue regress and disappear in the first few years of life (109, 110). These rests, however, may hypertrophy in patients with high levels of circulating adrenocorticoid hormones, as in congenital adrenal hyperplasia, Cushing's syndrome, or Addison's disease (111, 112). Clinically, they may present as a palpable mass located within the testis or spermatic cord (109, 111). Sonographically, adrenal rest tumors are seen as multiple hypoechoic nodules, most commonly located near the testicular hilus. If they become fibrotic, they may be hyperechoic and may cause acoustic shadowing. Malignant degeneration is very rare, but close clinical and sonographic follow-up is important to document stability or regression of tumor size during glucocorticoid therapy (112).

Magnetic resonance imaging of adrenal rest tumors demonstrates that these lesions are isointense with respect to normal parenchyma on T1-weighted images but are hypointense on T2-weighted images.

Extratesticular Processes

HYDROCELE

A hydrocele is the most common cause of testicular swelling and may be unilateral or bilateral (3, 48). A hydrocele of the testis results from the trapping of fluid between the visceral and parietal layers of the tunica vaginalis, whereas fluid trapped within the processus vaginalis along the spermatic cord is termed a hydrocele of the cord. The processus vaginalis is a connection between the peritoneal cavity and scrotum that normally closes off at about the time of birth. Fluid that is trapped around the testis at the time of closure is usually slowly reabsorbed during the first 18 months of life. On occasion, however, the processus vaginalis may remain patent during the first year of life. If the processus vaginalis fails to close, then a communicating hydrocele with a variable amount of fluid is established. Surgical ligation is often required, and if it is not performed the processus vaginalis eventually stretches in diameter. It will then accommodate an intraabdominal structure such as a loop of bowel, thereby forming an inguinal hernia (3). Hydroceles may be either congenital, primary (idiopathic), or secondary (reactive) to infarction, inflammation (epididymitis), neoplasm, or trauma (6, 113). Up to 50% of acquired hydroceles are secondary to trauma (40). Ten percent of testicular malignancies are associated with hydroceles that are generally smaller than their idiopathic counterparts (3, 51).

The diagnosis of a hydrocele is usually apparent on physical examination. It is, however, sometimes difficult to separate a hydrocele from a hernia, as both will transilluminate. Thickening of the tunica vaginalis in chronic epididymitis does not permit the transmission of light. Additionally, when a large amount of fluid is present, the scrotum becomes tense and palpation of the underlying testicle is impeded. Sonographically, simple hydroceles are anechoic fluid collections confined to the anterolateral portion of the scrotum, defined by the tunica vaginalis (Fig. 13.24). They provide an

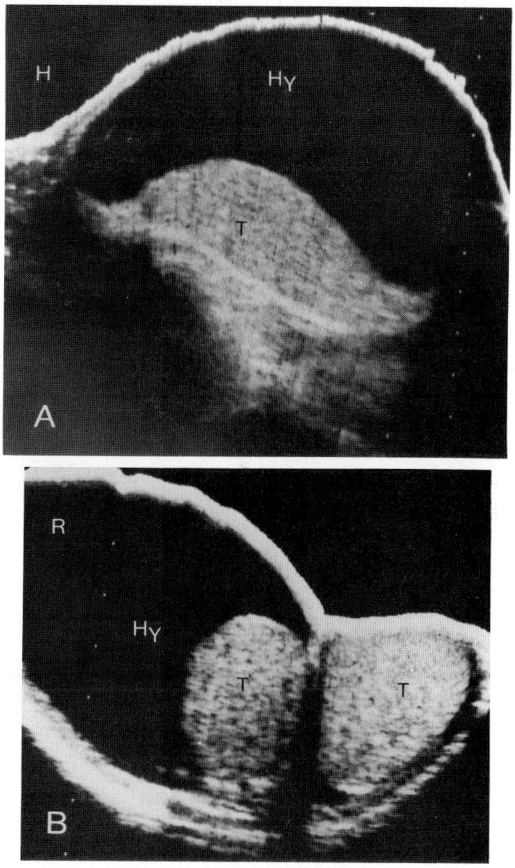

Figure 13.24. Large hydrocele. Simple hydroceles (*Hy*) are anechoic fluid collections confined to the anterolateral portion of the scrotum as seen on longitudinal (**A**) and transverse (**B**) images. Distortion of the testicle (*T*) may occur because of pressure effects from a large fluid collection, but the fluid also provides an optimal acoustic window for evaluation of the underlying testicle. *H*, toward patient's head; *R*, patient's right side.

optimal acoustic window for evaluation of the underlying testicle. Longstanding hydroceles and hydroceles complicated by pus (pyocele or pyogenic hydrocele) or hemorrhage (hematocele or hemorrhagic hydrocele) may contain homogeneous low-level echoes, debris, or septations (Figs. 13.25 and 13.26) (2, 3, 6, 11). Alternatively, homogeneous low-level internal echoes may indicate an increased cholesterol content within the fluid (Fig. 13.27). In some cases of pyocele, a fluid-fluid level may be seen as well as a comet-tail artifact, which indicates the presence of a gas collection (114). Air inside the scrotum secondary to the presence of a gas-forming organism is rare and is more commonly seen due to penetrating trauma, surgery, fistula, emphysema, or hernia (115). Calcifications have been reported within a hydrocele. Thickening of the scrotal wall is frequently present in complicated or chronic hydroceles (Fig. 13.28). The actual wall thickness can be overestimated if direct contact scanning is performed. This is known as the "bang effect" and can be avoided by using a block of gel mattress (11).

Magnetic resonance imaging demonstrates hydroceles to change in shape with patient position, conforming to the testicular contour. These collections appear low in signal intensity on T1-weighted images with increased signal intensity on T2-weighted images, characteristic of fluid (72, 73, 99).

EXTRATESTICULAR NEOPLASMS AND MISCELLANEOUS PROCESSES

Solid extratesticular neoplasms are uncommon. While most are benign, metastatic deposits and primary malignant lesions are encountered. Adenomatoid tumors of the epididymis are the most frequently encountered solid neoplasms, accounting for 30% of all extratesticular masses (3, 40). These tumors usually occur from the second to fourth decades of life and present clinically as a discrete mass. These are benign, slow-growing tumors of mesothelial origin that arise from the tunica vaginalis or the spermatic cord. The globus minor is a favored location. They range in size from several millimeters to 2 cm (113, 116). Adenomatoid tumors present sonographically as a well-marginated solid mass with echogenicity equivalent to or greater than that of the testis (Fig. 13.29) (6). Malignant mesotheliomas may occur but are much less common. Papillary cystadenomas have been found in patients from ages 16 to 68. They are usually unilateral, but

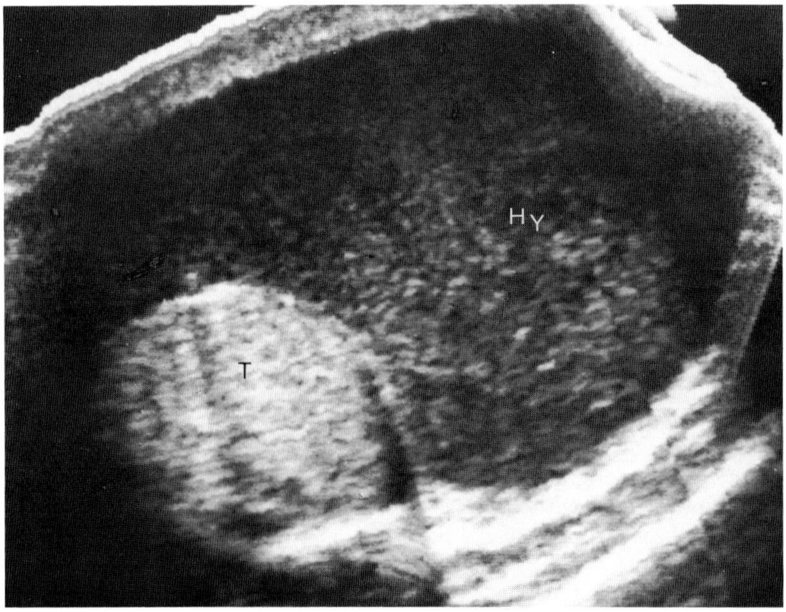

Figure 13.25. Complicated hydrocele. Homogeneous low-level echoes indicate a complicated hydrocele (*Hy*) such as a pyocele or hematocele. History is important to differentiate the two entities. The testis (*T*) is normal.

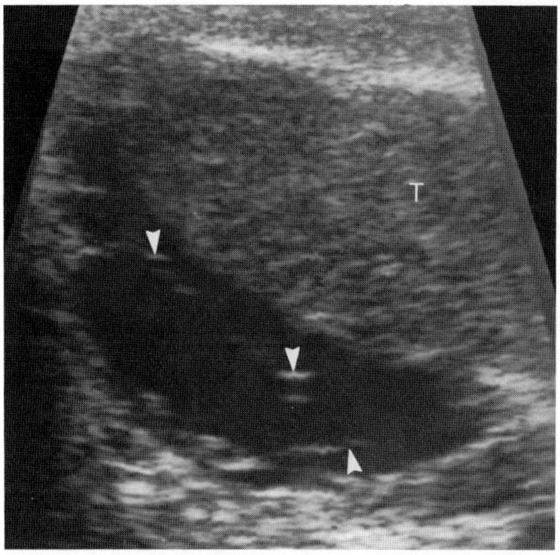

Figure 13.26. Hydrocele with adhesion. Multiple irregular linear acoustic reflections (*arrowheads*) are visualized within a fluid collection indicative of adhesions from a prior inflammatory process. *T,* testis.

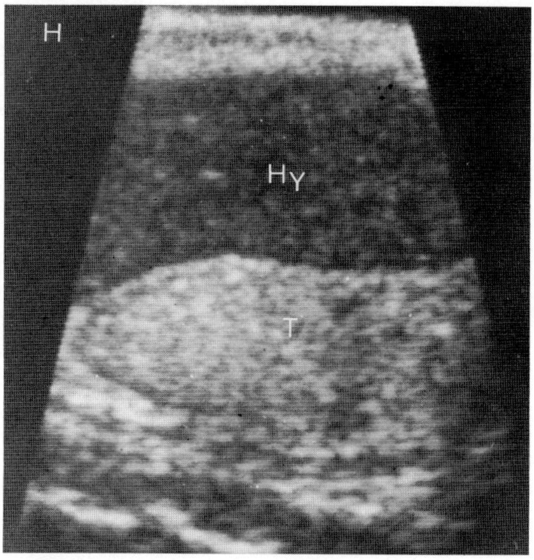

Figure 13.27. Cholesterol in hydrocele. A homogeneous low-level echogenic collection (*Hy*) located anterior to the testis (*T*) has the same sonographic appearance of a hematocele or pyocele. Aspiration of this collection revealed clear fluid with cholesterol deposits. *H,* toward patient's head.

when bilateral they may be associated with von Hippel-Lindau syndrome (117, 118). Other rare extratesticular neoplasms include fibromas, adrenal rests, and cholesteatomas (3).

Primary malignant neoplasms include fibrosarcoma (118), malignant histiocytoma, leiomyosarcoma (119), and lymphosarcoma. All are rare. Squamous cell carcinoma of the scrotum has been found in chimney sweeps and metal workers. Metastatic deposits have been identified in patients with malignant melanoma and gastric, renal, prostate, and colon carcinoma (120–125). Sonographically, these lesions present as a focal solid enlargement of the epididymis, separable from the testis (Fig. 13.30). Reactive hydroceles may be present.

Scrotal lipomas arise most commonly from

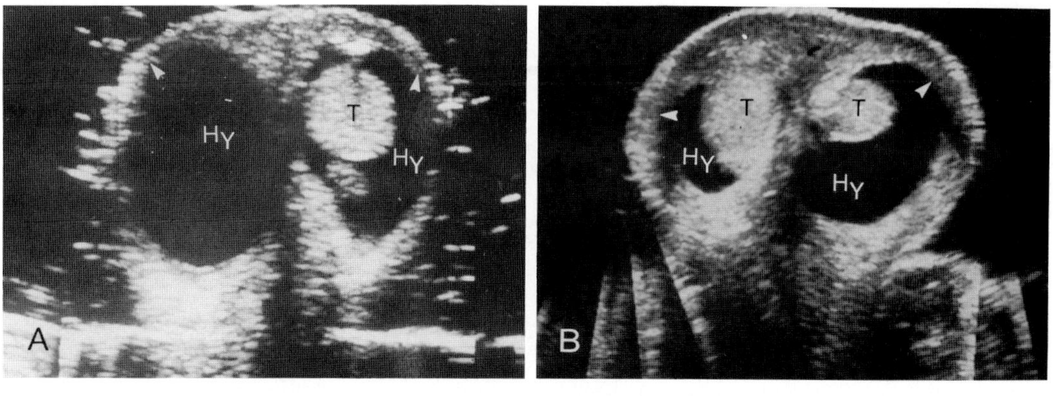

Figure 13.28. Subacute and chronic hydroceles with change in scrotal wall thickness. Compare bilateral hydroceles (*Hy*) and normal skin thickness (*arrowheads*) (**A**) with chronic hydroceles (**B**) with thickened skin (*arrowheads*). The testes are situated at different levels within the scrotal sac, accounting for the differences in appearance of the hemiscrotum in each case.

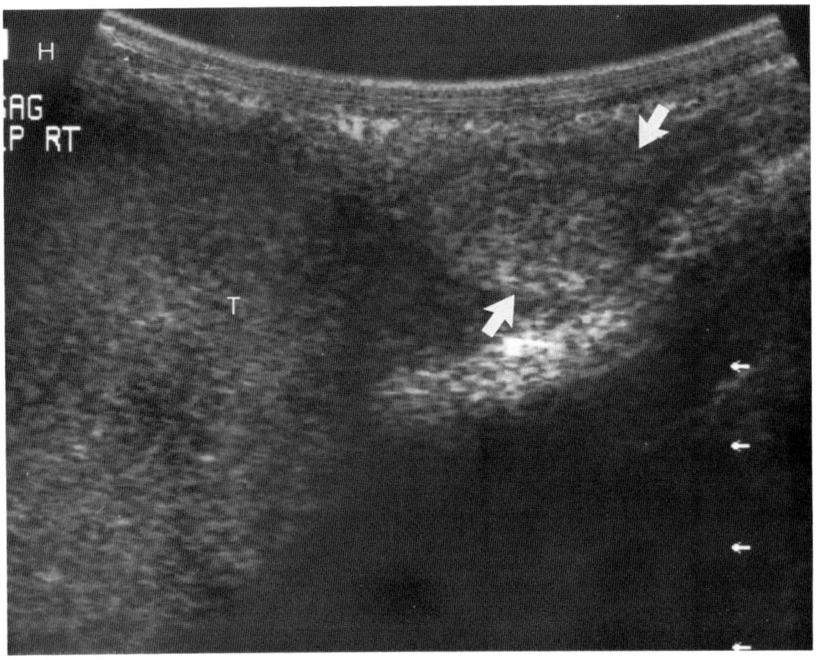

Figure 13.29. Adenomatoid tumor of the epididymis. A well-marginated solid mass (*arrows*) with echogenicity equivalent to the testis (*T*) is visualized inferior to and separate from the testis. This was found to be an adenomatoid tumor of the epididymis on surgical resection. *H,* toward patient's head.

the cord, occurring between the ages of 40 and 60 years. Rhabdomyosarcomas of the cord have been identified. The differential diagnosis of extratesticular neoplasms includes polyorchidism and focal chronic epididymitis. In polyorchidism, multiple testes may mimic an intrascrotal neoplasm. Sonographically, the appearance of this palpable mass should indicate the proper etiology (45).

Chronic epididymitis commonly presents as a focal nodular area within the epididymis, mimicking a neoplasm. It clinically presents as a painless mass that is difficult to delineate from the testis if fibrosis has occurred. Sonographically, the lesion is hyperechoic and separable from the testis (3).

SPERMATOCELE

Spermatoceles represent cysts composed of thick, creamy fluid containing nonviable spermatozoa, fat, cellular debris, and sediment of lymphocytes (126). These retention cysts are most often located in the epididymal head, arising in the region of the rete testis. They may be

Figure 13.30. Epididymal metastasis. Longitudinal ultrasound demonstrates a focal mass within the body of the epididymis (*arrowheads*). A secondary hydrocele (*Hy*) is present. The testis is normal. The patient had a primary lung carcinoma with metastases to the epididymis. *H,* toward patient's head.

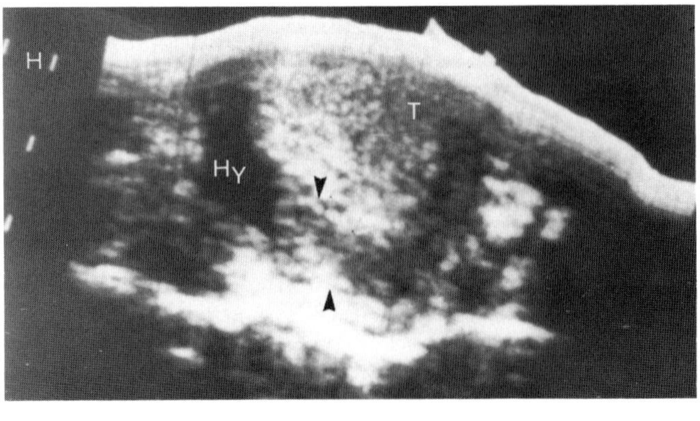

unilateral or bilateral, unilocular or multilocular, single or multiple. Septations may be present. A large spermatocele can be differentiated from a hydrocele because of location. A spermatocele will displace the testicle anteriorly, while a hydrocele will displace it posteriorly. On ultrasound, they have the characteristics of a simple cyst: no internal echoes, good sound through transmission, and sharp walls (Fig. 13.31) (3, 120).

EPIDIDYMAL CYST

Epididymal cysts contain clear, serous fluid, not sperm. They are less common than spermatoceles but may occur anywhere within the epididymis in a range of sizes (3, 120). Congenital epididymal cysts are more frequent in men with a history of antenatal diethylstilbestrol exposure (127). Cystic degeneration of the epididymis has been noted in male patients following vasectomy (120).

Epididymal cysts and spermatoceles have the same sonographic appearance and are not differentiable (Fig. 13.32). The cyst may be lobulated (Fig. 13.33), or multiple cysts may be present (Fig. 13.34). When cysts are large, compression of the adjacent testicular parenchyma may occur, giving the false impression of an intratesticular neoplasm (3, 11, 120).

Magnetic resonance imaging of spermatoceles frequently demonstrates a higher signal intensity than water on balanced images because of the proteinaceous content (72).

SPERM GRANULOMA

Sperm granuloma result from extravasation of sperm into the surrounding tissue. Granuloma formation results from necrosis. This may occur either within or external to the testis. In patients who have had a vasectomy, granuloma formation may result when rupture of dilated cystic tubules occur. Clinically, sperm granuloma present as painless masses. On ultrasound, they appear as solid, hypoechoic masses (3).

SARCOID

Sarcoidosis involving the genital tract is rare, being present in less than 1% of patients with the systemic disease. Clinically, it may present as acute or recurrent epididymitis or as painless enlargement on palpation. Sarcoid may affect the epididymis, although with lesser frequency than the testis (128, 129). On so-

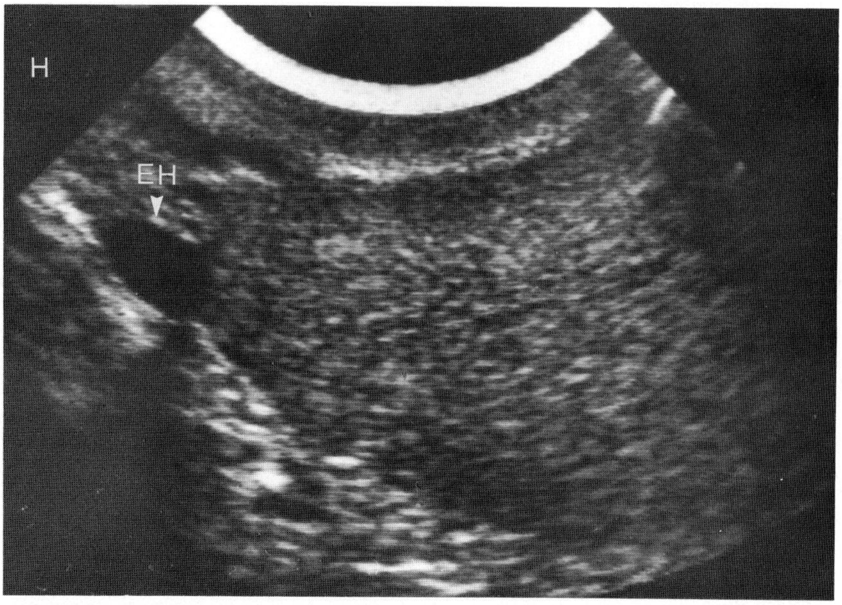

Figure 13.31. Spermatocele. A single anechoic fluid collection with good sound through transmission and sharp walls originating in the epididymal head (*EH*) represents a spermatocele (*arrowhead*). These have the same sonographic appearance as epididymal cysts. *H,* toward patient's head.

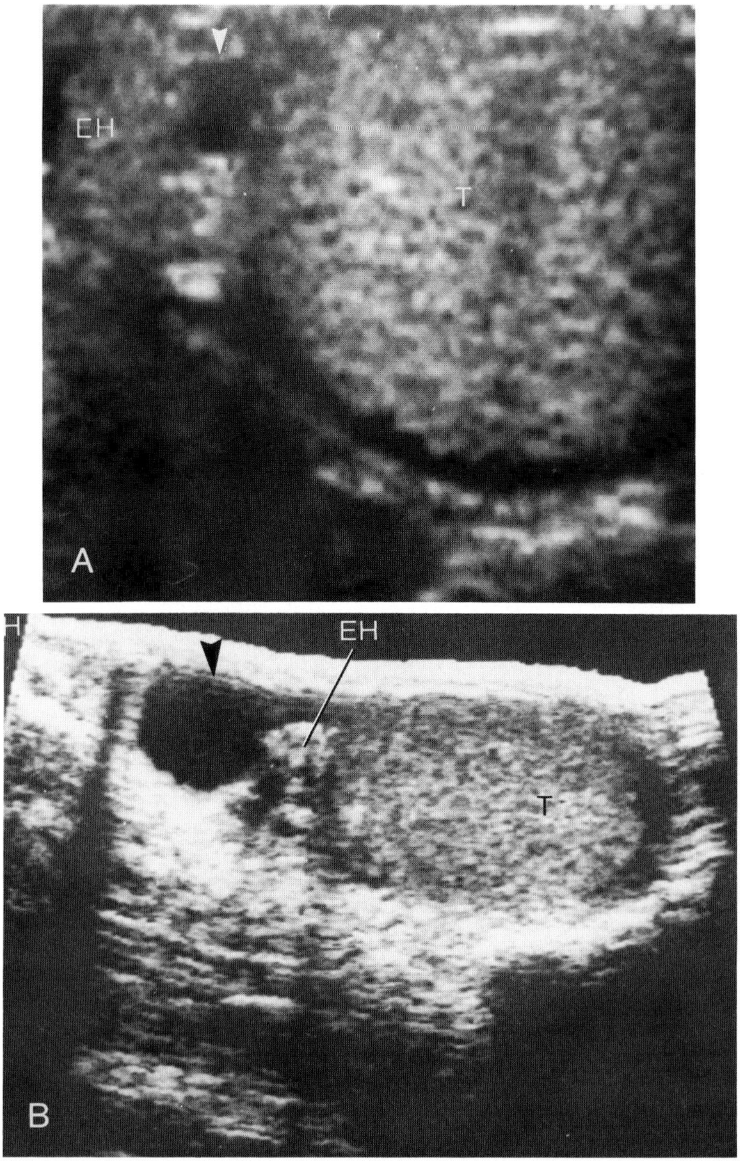

Figure 13.32. Epididymal head cyst. Two examples (**A, B**) of simple cysts: anechoic fluid collections with sound through transmission and smooth, well-defined walls (*arrowhead*). *EH*, epididymal head; *T*, testicle; *H*, toward patient's head.

nographic examination, sarcoid may appear as a solid, infiltrating testicular neoplasm. Epididymal sarcoid often appears as a solid, hypoechoic mass (Fig. 13.35) (120).

MECONIUM PERITONITIS

In children, healed meconium peritonitis has been imaged as brightly echogenic scrotal masses (Fig. 13.36) (130). Calcification is present in both the abdomen and scrotum and can be confirmed with plain films.

SCROTAL HERNIA

Although most hernias are clinically apparent, the diagnosis may on occasion be questioned. Sonography of the inguinal canal and scrotum serves to confirm or refute the diagnosis (131). The sonographic appearance of

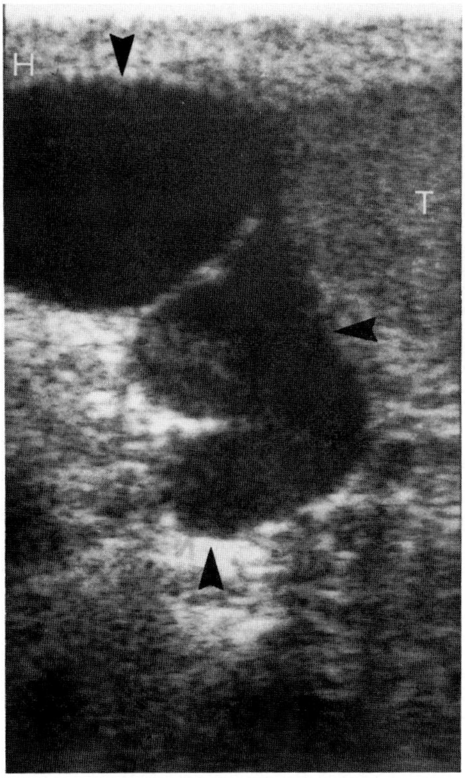

Figure 13.33. Lobulated epididymal cyst. The head of the epididymis has been replaced by a lobulated cystic mass (*arrowheads*). The testis (*T*) is normal. *H,* toward patient's head.

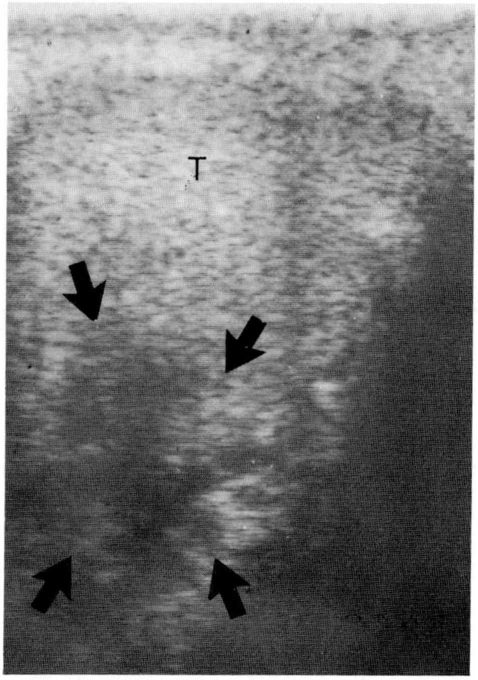

Figure 13.35. Epididymal sarcoid. A hypoechoic, irregularly marginated mass (*arrows*) that appears to infiltrate the posterior aspect of the testis (*T*) was identified in a patient with a palpable scrotal mass. Noncaseating granuloma involving the epididymis only was removed at surgery.

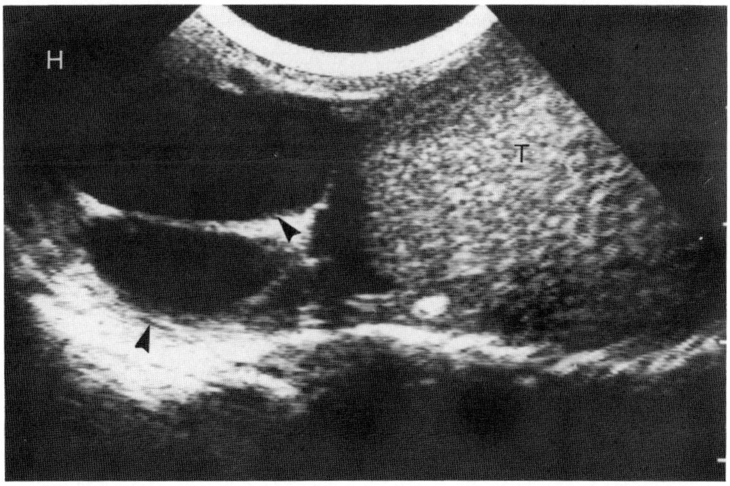

Figure 13.34. Multiple epididymal cysts. The region of the epididymal head has been replaced by multiple cystic structures (*arrowheads*). The testis (*T*) is normal on this sagittal image. *H,* toward patient's head.

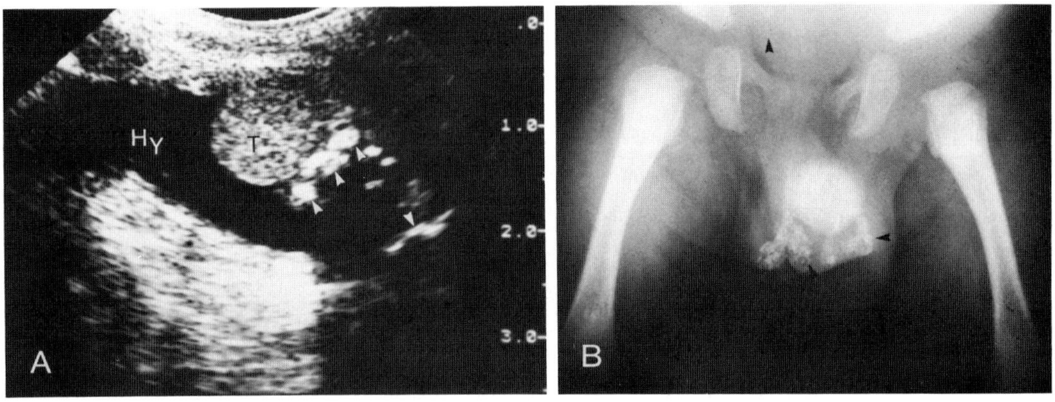

Figure 13.36. Meconium peritonitis. **A,** Real-time ultrasound demonstrates multiple echogenic masses (*arrowheads*) within the scrotum, some of which are contiguous with the testicle (*T*). A hydrocele is also identified (*Hy*). **B,** Radiographic examination of the pelvis confirms the presence of multiple calcifications in the scrotum (*arrowheads*) and abdomen (*arrow*).

fluid-filled structures with thick walls and the presence of peristalsis is diagnostic (Fig. 13.37). A scattered echogenic pattern (snow storm) may be seen due to the presence of gas in bowel, or an area of increased echogenicity may be seen because of the presence of fatty omentum within the hernia (77). A scrotal hernia may be accompanied by a hydrocele because of the associated patent processus vaginalis.

Sonography has been used to assess immediate and delayed complications in patients after inguinal herniorrhaphy (132). Local complications occur in approximately 8.7% of patients and include recurrence of hernia, scrotal swelling (secondary to hydrocele), hematoma, and ischemic orchitis (133–135). Scrotal hematoma may result from an inadequately ligated or unligated cremasteric artery (134). The hematoma, which dissects through the inguinal canal into the scrotum, is located anterolateral to the testis. The scrotal wall may be involved. Sonography may be beneficial in detecting the site of origin and the extent of the hematoma. The appearance of the hematoma is age related (137).

Infrequently, patients may present with epididymal enlargement, acute pain, and swelling following herniorrhaphy (136, 138). The etiology is unclear but may relate to hemorrhagic epididymitis, trauma, subclinical infection, or ischemia. Sonographically, the epididymis is enlarged with increased echogenicity (138). Enlargement and decreased echogenicity of the testis 4 to 6 hr following surgery signals ischemic orchitis (136, 138, 139). This is seen in approximately 0.3 to 0.5% of patients following inguinal hernia repair and is 10 times more common in patients with recurrent repairs (140). Doppler examination is sometimes useful, but radionuclide examination is the study of choice (141–146). If this abnormality goes unrecognized, testicular atrophy will result.

THE "ACUTE SCROTUM"

There are many etiologies of an acutely swollen and painful scrotum. The differential diagnosis includes epididymitis, orchitis, torsion of the testis, the appendix testis or appendix epididymis, Henoch-Schönlein purpura, trauma, scrotal fat, necrosis, hemorrhage or infarction in a testicular tumor, and idiopathic scrotal edema. Of these entities, epididymitis and torsion occur with the greatest frequency and often present the greatest diagnostic dilemma. It is imperative to make the distinction between these processes, as prompt surgical intervention is necessary to salvage the testis in the event of torsion. Epididymitis is treated medically. Both high-resolution real-time sonography and Doppler ultrasound, in conjunction with scintigraphy, can aid the clinicians in appropriate clinical management (137, 147).

Epididymitis

Epididymitis is the most common cause of an acute scrotum, constituting 75% of all intrascrotal inflammatory processes (148). Epididymitis is generally a clinical diagnosis; how-

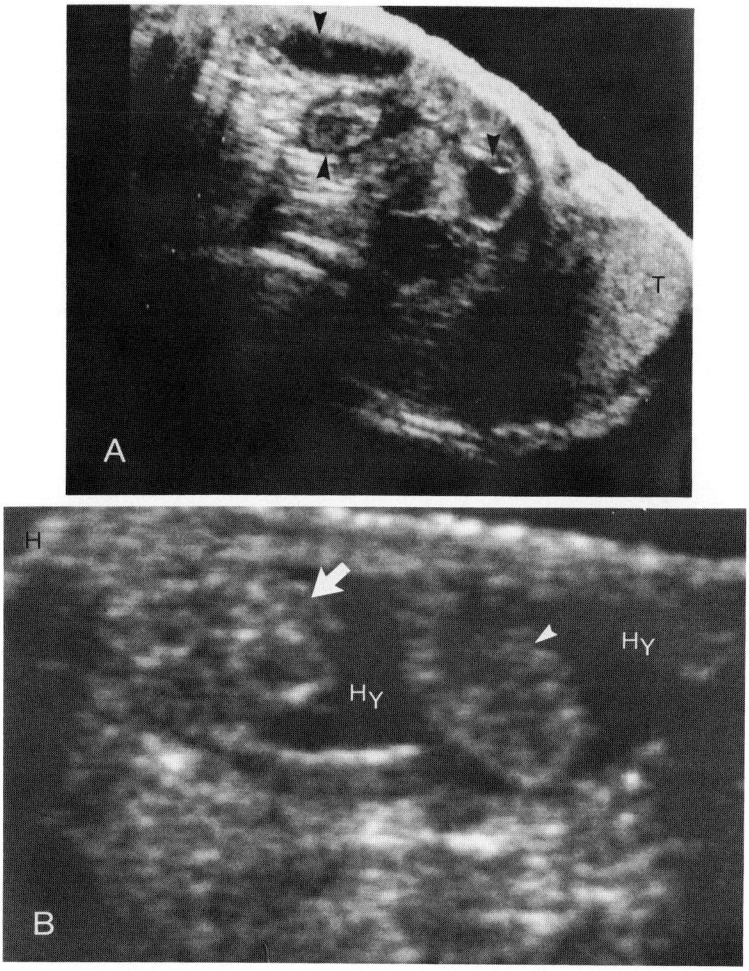

Figure 13.37. Hernia. Fluid-filled structures with thick walls (*arrowheads*) located within either the inguinal canal or the scrotal sac represent fluid-filled loops of bowel of a hernia. Solid material (*arrow*) may also be present within the lumen, indicative of feces. Peristalsis may be observed on real-time study. A scrotal hernia may be accompanied by a hydrocele (*Hy*) because of an associated patent processus vaginalis. *E,* epididymis; *H,* toward patient's head; *T,* testis.

ever, nuclear isotope studies and sonography are commonly used to confirm the diagnosis and assess for complication (141, 149, 150).

Although epididymitis is usually seen in adolescents and middle-aged men, it has been reported in infants and young children (151–154). Clinical distinction between epididymitis and spermatic cord torsion is often difficult, but in part it can be made on the basis of age. In patients younger than 20 years of age, epididymitis and torsion occur with a ratio of 3 to 2, whereas in patients older than age 20, the ratio approximates 9 to 1 (3). In addition to spermatic cord torsion, torsion of the epididymal or testicular appendages, orchitis, intrascrotal hematoma, and rarely tumor are considerations in the differential diagnosis (11, 155–160).

Clinical features of epididymitis include a swollen, erythematous, and tender scrotum. In most cases, one side is affected and the pain increases over 1 to 2 days. It is generally insidious in onset, helping to differentiate this entity from torsion. The patient may be febrile, and approximately 50% of patients will complain of dysuria. Sepsis, leukocytosis, and pyuria may be present (3, 10). The etiology is varied and in the younger age group it is typically infectious or idiopathic (120). Organisms that have been implicated include *Neisseria gonorrhoeae, Chlamydia trachomatis, Escherichia coli, Pseudomonas,* and *Aerobacter* (11, 120, 149). Cytomegalovirus has been reported in patients with acquired immunodeficiency syndrome (161). Less common causes include *Schistosoma haematobium* and granulomatous infections from *Mycobacterium tuberculosis,* histoplasmosis, blastomycosis, and coccidiomycosis (117, 151–154, 162–166). Granulomatous epididymitis is usually associated with pulmonary or renal infection. Symptoms are more chronic and present as painless swelling of the scrotum and palpable, hard, nontender epididymal masses (166). In older men, epididymitis is commonly related to prostatitis, urinary tract infection, trauma, and instrumentation (151). Retrograde reflux of urine through the vas deferens and congenital anomalies are other causative factors (167).

The imaging modalities available to diagnose this entity include nuclear isotope scanning, ultrasound, and magnetic resonance imaging.

The isotope scan may show early increased flow to the testis on the affected side in the angiographic phase. The activity may take the form of the epididymis being either linear or curvilinear, representing the inflamed epididymis. Central or medial displacement of the epididymis may be seen on static images. If the patient has an associated orchitis, unilateral increased flow through the spermatic cord vessels to the epididymis and testis will be seen. If the epididymitis is focal, a distinct area of increased isotope uptake is commonly seen, corresponding to the area of inflammation. Similarly, a focal area of increased activity in the location of the testis may represent focal orchitis (141–143, 168).

Sonography shows enlargement of the epididymis, particularly the head, with decreased echogenicity secondary to edema (Fig. 13.38) (4, 126). Longitudinal images may better demonstrate this than transverse images (11). Hyperechoic regions indicate early fibrosis, which can obstruct the seminiferous tubules (120, 141). The parietal layer of the tunica vaginalis is usually moderately thickened but indistinguishable from the remaining layers of the scrotal sac. Skin thickening may be seen on ultrasound. Acute hydroceles are not uncommon and are usually anechoic (Fig. 13.39)

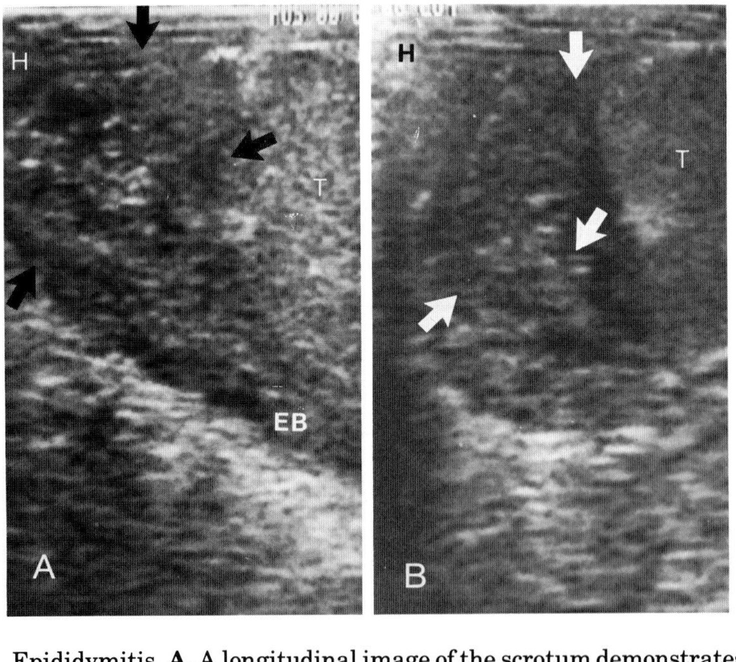

Figure 13.38. Epididymitis. **A,** A longitudinal image of the scrotum demonstrates enlargement of the epididymal head (*arrows*) with decreased echogenicity in a patient with epididymitis. The testis (*T*) is normal. *EB,* epididymal body. **B,** A similar case reveals enlargement of the epididymal head (*arrows*). *H,* toward patient's head.

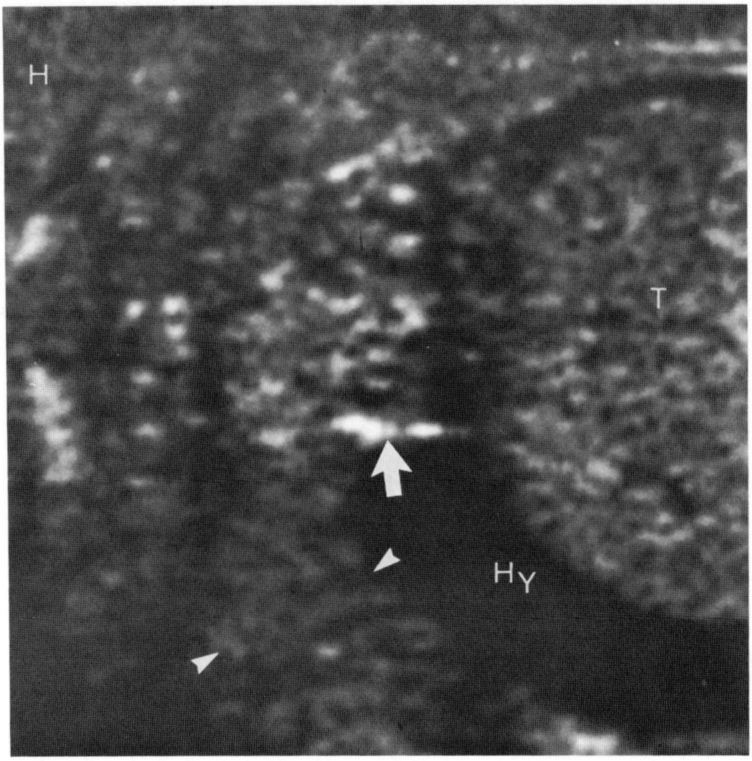

Figure 13.39. Epididymitis. Enlargement of the epididymal head (*arrow*), small reactive hydrocele (*Hy*), and skin thickening (*arrowheads*) are consistent with the clinical diagnosis of epididymitis. *H*, toward patient's head; *T*, testis.

(149). If internal echoes are present (i.e., pyocele) or if adhesions between the tunica vaginalis and epididymis are seen, a severe inflammatory process such as tuberculous epididymitis should be considered. Typically in tuberculous epididymitis, the epididymal head is enlarged if dissemination has occurred by a hematogenous route, and the vas deferens and epididymal tail are affected if spread has occurred in a retrograde fashion from the prostate or from reflux of infected urine (166). Isolated enlargement of the tail of the epididymis should also raise strong suspicion of a tuberculous etiology. Sonographically, the affected part may appear as a complex mass due to necrosis. Untreated, complicated epididymitis may lead to abscess formation (10, 11).

Twenty percent of patients with epididymitis will have an associated enlarged hypoechoic testicle, representing diffuse orchitis, or a focal area of decreased echogenicity, indicating focal orchitis (3). The abnormal focal area is usually located posteriorly in the testis in close relationship to the epididymis. Color Doppler may demonstrate a discrepancy in flow with an increase on the affected side compared with the normal side, corresponding to findings on isotope study (Figs. 13.40 and 13.41) (3).

Acute testicular ischemia is a severe complication of epididymitis, caused by compression of spermatic vessels by the enlarged epididymis and severe edema of the spermatic cord. Sonographically, the testis may demonstrate areas of markedly decreased echogenicity. A prompt epididymotomy can save the testis. Left untreated, ischemia may progress to infarction (Fig. 13.42) (169, 170). Distinction between testicular infarction secondary to epididymitis and orchitis associated with epididymitis may be difficult, as both entities can yield the same sonographic images (166). Color Doppler may be helpful, demonstrating a decrease or lack of blood flow in the infarcted testicule compared with the normal side (Fig. 13.43).

In most cases of untreated, uncomplicated epididymitis, the inflammatory process re-

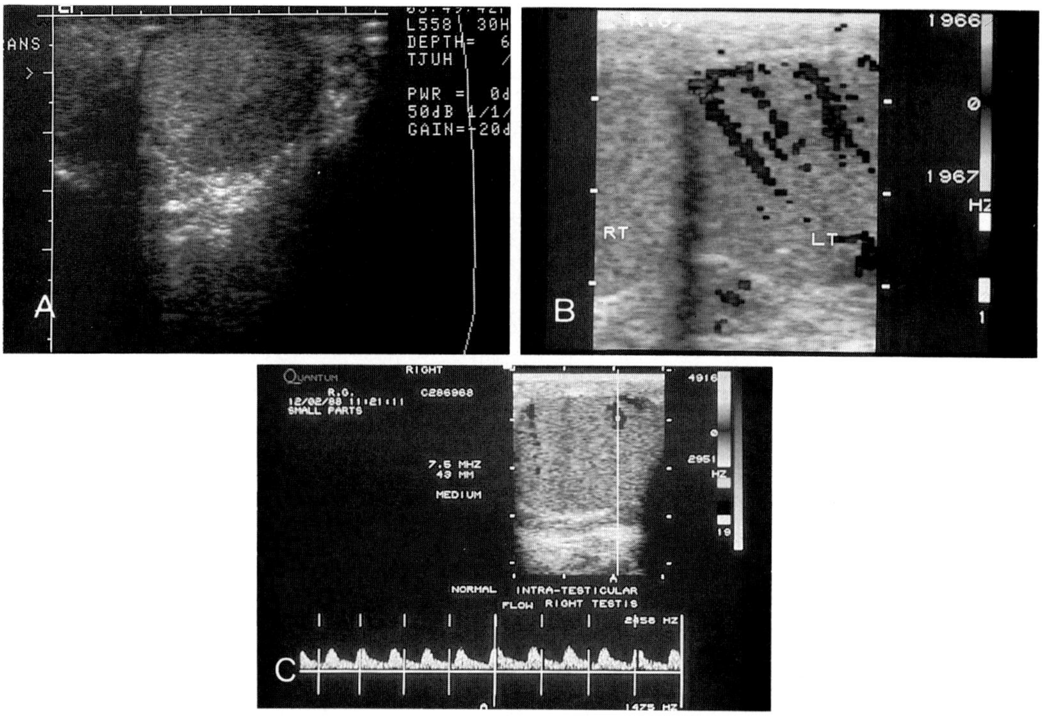

Figure 13.40. Epididymo-orchitis. **A,** Transverse sonogram of the left testis reveals a focal hypoechoic area (*arrowheads*) posteriorly in the testis. **B,** Color Doppler image of both testes in transverse view demonstrates an increased flow in the hyperemic left testis (*LT*) of this patient with epididymo-orchitis. Although no vessels are seen in the normal right (*RT*) testis in this view, normal flow is seen on an additional image (**C**) of the right testis. (See color plate 2.)

solves with concomitant decrease in size of the epididymis and return to normal echogenicity (117). In chronic epididymitis, the epididymis is frequently enlarged and may contain hyperechoic areas (Fig. 13.44). Sonography is useful to follow the course of these patients to rule out abscess development (2, 3, 10).

Magnetic resonance images are best obtained in the sagittal plane to demonstrate the long axis of the epididymis. With acute epididymitis, diffuse or focal epididymal enlargement is seen. The signal intensity may be normal, slightly greater than normal, or more heterogeneous on T2-weighted images com-

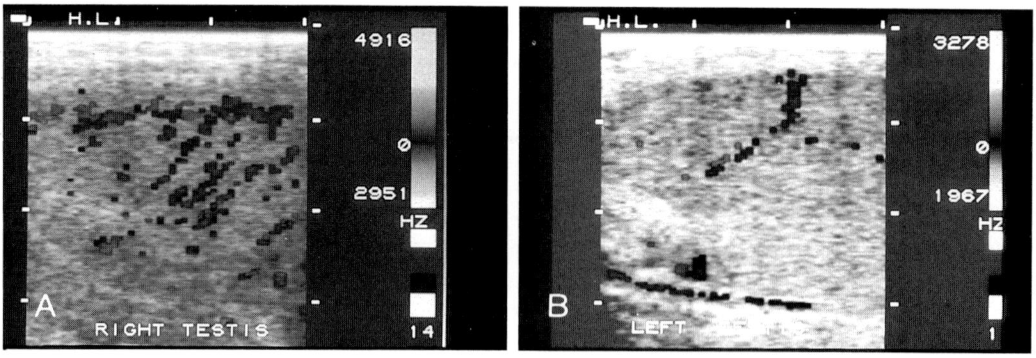

Figure 13.41. Orchitis. Color Doppler demonstrates a discrepancy in flow between the normal left testis (**A**) and the affected right side (**B**). Red and blue in the vessels denote flow toward and away from the transducer. (See color plate 3.)

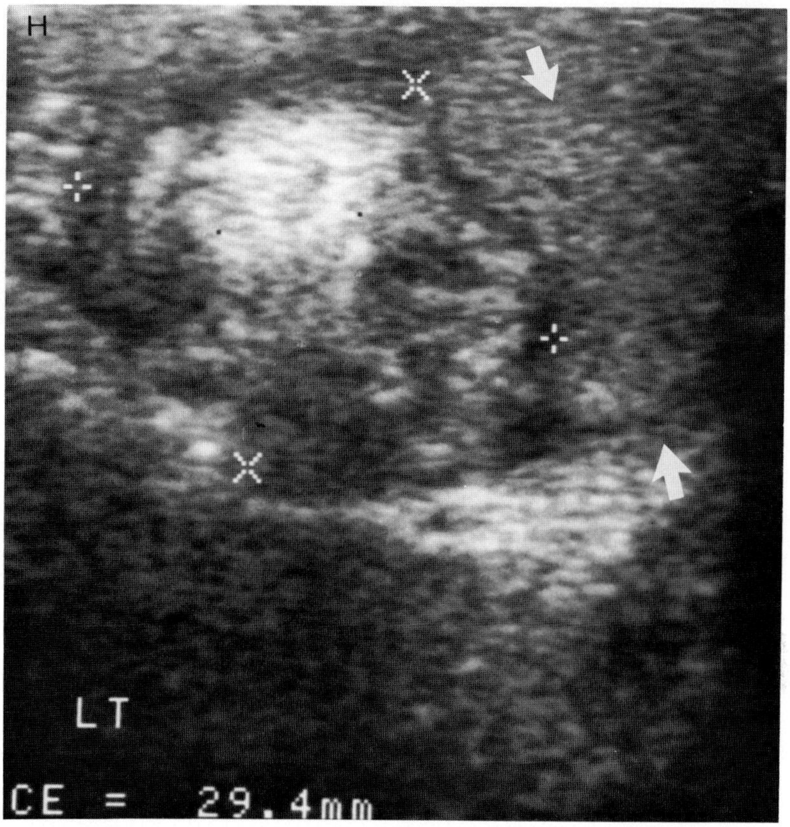

Figure 13.42. Testicular infarction secondary to epididymitis. An irregularly shaped region of heterogeneous echo texture, demarcated by measurement cursors, is visualized in the left testis of a patient with a clinical history of epididymitis. Areas of increased echogenicity are consistent with fibrosis. Following testicular infarction, a portion of the testicular parenchyma remains normal in echogenicity (*arrows*). *H,* toward patient's head.

pared with the normal side. Additionally, the signal intensity of the affected epididymis is slightly less than that of the testis on T2-weighted images rather than markedly less intense as seen with the normal side. Hypervascularity with increased flow in serpiginous tubular structures coursing through the spermatic cord has been demonstrated. As opposed to varicocele, serpiginous structures in the spermatic cord have low signal intensity corresponding to high flow. Complications of epididymitis including hydrocele, orchitis, and skin thickening are easily recognized with magnetic resonance imaging (72, 99).

Orchitis

Orchitis is an unusual finding without associated epididymitis. Symptomatology is similar to epididymitis with testalgia, scrotal swelling, erythema, leukocytosis, and fever as salient features. Frequently, urinary tract symptomatology is absent (10). The affected testis may be diffusely enlarged on palpation (11). Patients with mumps and coxsackievirus infections may also present with glandular enlargement. Differentiation of orchitis from epididymitis on radionuclide study alone is difficult. Flow to the testis may be mildly increased. Delayed images show increased uptake by the affected testis. The epididymis should be normal (141). On ultrasonography, the testis may appear normal in size or enlarged (51). The echogenicity may be diffusely decreased or heterogeneous in appearance when compared with the normal side (Figs. 13.45 and 13.46). Reactive hydroceles may be present (Fig. 13.47). Skin thickening is frequently seen (171).

Malakoplakia, a rare inflammatory process, has been reported to involve the testis. Sonographically, this entity mimics diffuse or-

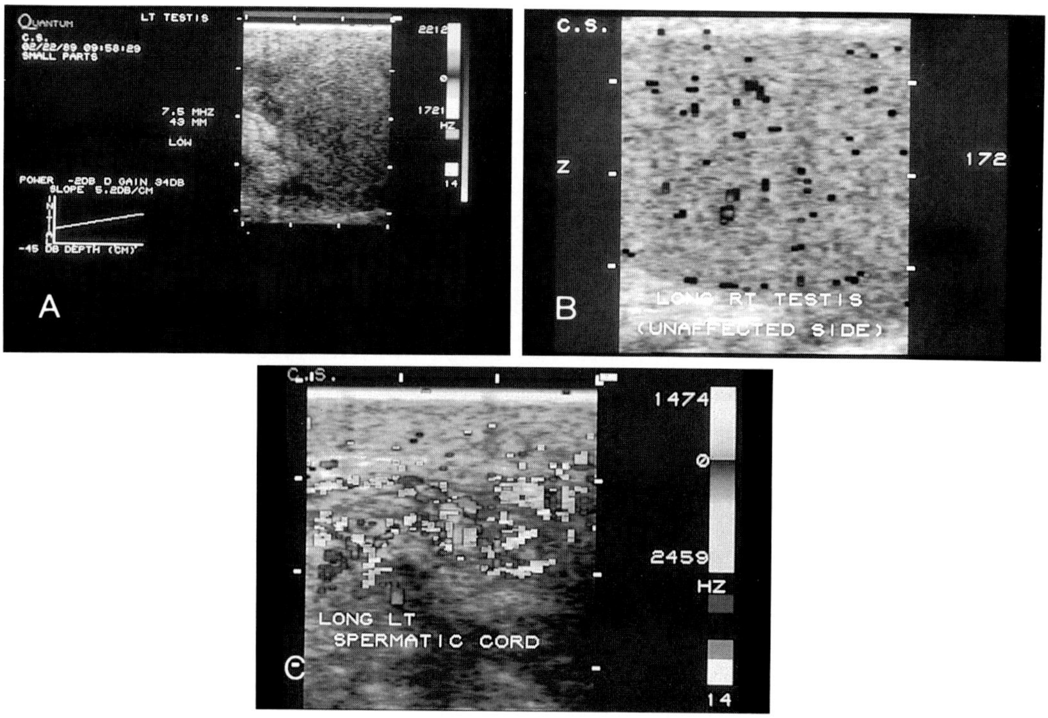

Figure 13.43. Testicular infarction. **A,** Color flow Doppler demonstrates a lack of blood flow in the infarcted left testis of the same patient as in Figure 13.42. **B,** Patient's normal right testis shows intratesticular flow. **C,** Flow is demonstrated in the patient's left spermatic cord vessels. (See color plate 3.)

chitis, appearing as a diffusely enlarged hypoechoic testicle (172).

Focal orchitis may occur without involvement of the epididymis, having the same sonographic appearance as an intratesticular neoplasm. In addition, epididymo-orchitis can be confused with intratesticular neoplasm with extension into the epididymis (11, 120). There are a few differentiating factors that would favor an inflammatory etiology. These include preservation of normal oval testicular shape, skin thickening, and clinical history (173). Approximately 10% of neoplasms present as an acute scrotum. Open biopsy may be required, particularly if clinical and sonographic improvement with time are not evident (11, 120).

Magnetic resonance imaging may be more sensitive than sonography in identifying intratesticular abnormalities, targeting patients who require closer clinical follow-up or surgical intervention. Focal orchitis may be best demonstrated on T2-weighted images as a focal area of decreased signal intensity superimposed on a testis with global decrease in signal intensity. The integrity of the tunica albuginea can be assessed as an intact or disrupted thin, black rim surrounding the testis. An abscess will have a signal intensity similar to water but is usually more inhomogeneous (72).

Torsion of the Spermatic Cord

Torsion of the spermatic cord is commonly termed testicular torsion. The condition occurs 3 times as frequently in males aged 11 to 20 years compared with older men, with a peak incidence of 13 years. The second highest frequency of incidence occurs in newborns. Clinically, the patient presents with a history of sudden onset of severe scrotal pain, usually during rest or sleep. Nausea and vomiting may occur. Symptomatology may be lacking in the newborn, in which the scrotum appears swollen and red (11, 174). The need to make an accurate early diagnosis is critical, since there is a 60 to 90% salvage rate for a testis in torsion operated on less than 24 hr after the onset of pain, compared with a salvage rate of less than 20% when surgery is delayed more than 24 hr (3, 136, 147). The differentiation between torsion and epididymitis may present a diagnostic di-

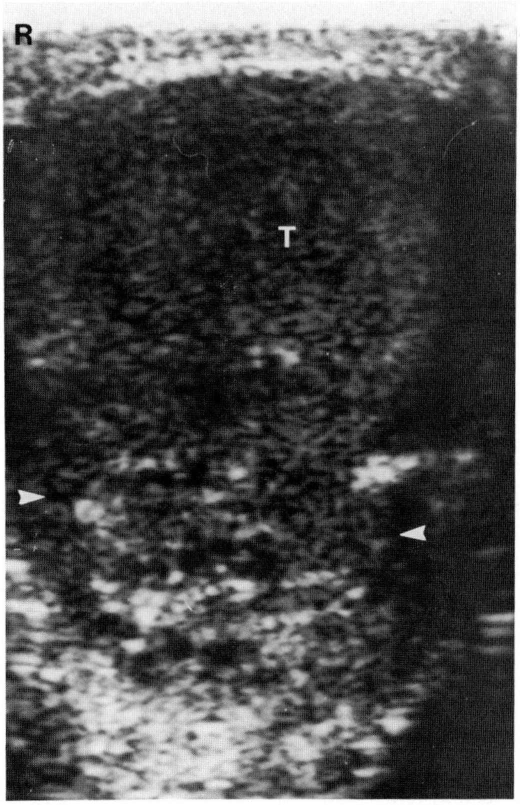

Figure 13.44. Chronic epididymitis. The epididymis is enlarged (*arrowheads*) and demonstrates heterogeneous echogenicity. The overall echogenicity is equivalent to or greater than that of the testicle (*T*) in this patient with chronic epididymitis. *R*, patient's right side.

lemma, as epididymitis on occasion has the same clinical presentation. Laboratory tests may be somewhat useful in that torsion, unlike epididymitis, rarely presents with pyuria of greater than 5 white blood cells per high-powered field (3).

Spermatic cord torsion results from abnormal embryological development in which the testis becomes suspended within the processus vaginalis rather than being applied to the posterior scrotal wall by the tunica vaginalis. The abnormality has been likened to a "bell and clapper." Intravaginal torsion is more common than extravaginal torsion, accounting for 20% of acute scrotal pathology in postpubertal males (3). In cases of intravaginal torsion, the tunica vaginalis completely invests the testis and epididymis, allowing for free rotation of the testis about the cord (147). Extravaginal torsion occurs almost exclusively in neonates (175). In this type of torsion, the testis and fascial layers rotate about the spermatic cord above the level of the tunica vaginalis before it attaches to the scrotal wall (147).

Radionuclide scintigraphy has been the gold standard for diagnosis of torsion of the spermatic cord. This examination can be divided into multiple phases demonstrating the physiologic effects of torsion over time. In the acute phase (within 7 hr), uptake is not increased on the affected side but a "nubbin" sign, indicating an abrupt cutoff of isotope activity, is noted at the level of the iliac artery. By comparison, the normal side may appear to have increased flow

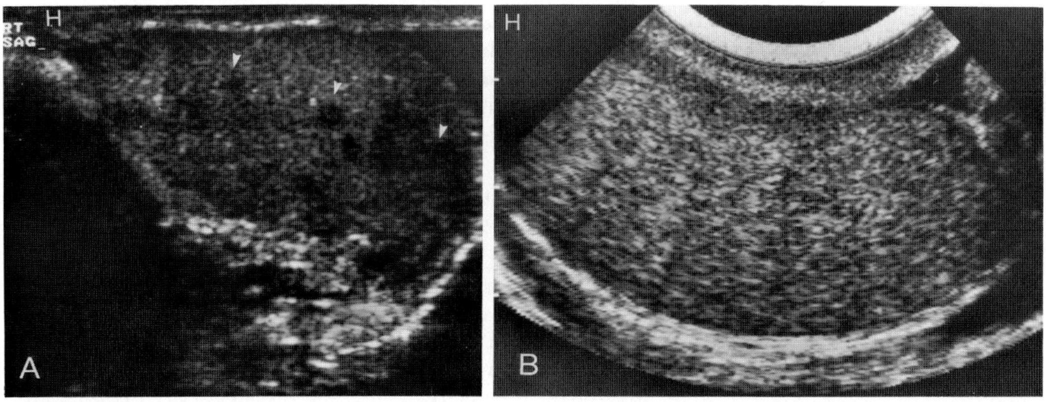

Figure 13.45. Longitudinal image of the right testicle (**A**) reveals multiple hypoechoic areas (*arrowheads*) that are no longer identified on follow-up examination (**B**) 2 months later. A normal testis was visualized. The patient had orchitis that was resolved with medical therapy. *H*, toward patient's head.

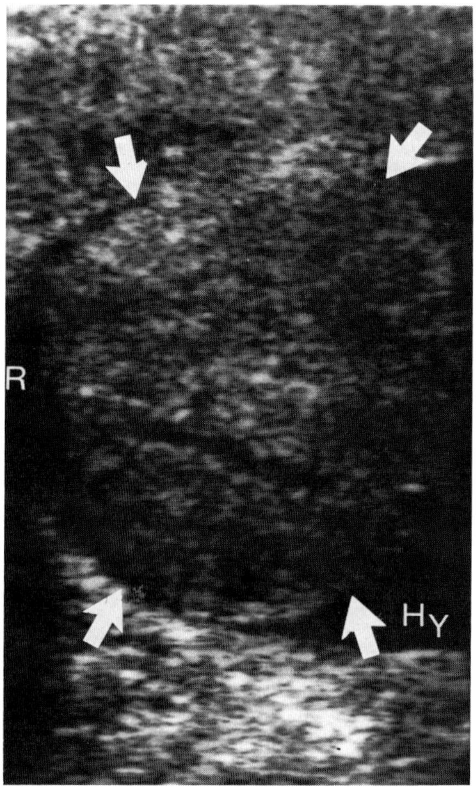

Figure 13.46. Chronic orchitis. The testis (*arrows*) demonstrates a heterogeneous echo texture. A small hydrocele (*Hy*) is present. The patient had longstanding orchitis. *R*, patient's right side.

because of lack of activity on the affected side. Delayed scans demonstrate a cold defect in the location of the testis (141–143, 168).

In the subacute phase (1 to 10 days after torsion), a nubbin sign with perfusion to the dartos fascia may be seen. The testicle will be represented by a cold defect. Arterial perfusion to the dartos fascia can produce the "halo" on static images (141–143, 168).

Late findings seen with missed torsion will show a nubbin sign with flow to the dartos fascia but not the testis and a halo sign on static images (141–143, 168).

Ultrasound B-scanning is usually not diagnostic because the appearance of testicular torsion on gray-scale sonography is variable (158, 176). The study is at best complementary to scintigraphy. However, B-scanning combined with Doppler becomes an accurate procedure for the diagnosis of torsion. In the immediate posttorsion period (1 to 7 hr), the testis is enlarged, inhomogeneous, and hypoechoic, although focal or diffuse hypoechoic areas have been reported. The epididymis is also enlarged and may have a varied sonographic appearance (Fig. 13.48). The twisted spermatic cord may be visualized as an enlarged hyperechoic tubular structure (vessel filled with clot), approximately 1 cm in diameter, situated superior to the testis. Scrotal skin thickening and reactive hydrocele are sometimes present. At 24 hr and beyond, anechoic areas may be seen within the testis secondary to hemorrhage and infarction (Fig. 13.49) (6, 11). A large echogenic or complex extratesticular mass caused by hemorrhage is sometimes seen (139). Late findings include an atrophic testicle with increased or decreased echogenicity (Fig. 13.50). Increased echogenicity is frequently due to fibrosis (Fig. 13.51). The epididymis may be enlarged. Doppler ultrasound (duplex and color flow) have been used to detect the presence (or absence) of intratesticular arterial pulsations (Figs. 13.52 and 13.53). Burks et al. (177) found that color Doppler was 86% sensitive, 100% specific, and 97% accurate in the diagnosis of testicular torsion and ischemia in the painful scrotum when the single criterion of presence or absence of intratesticular flow was used. Comparison with the opposite normal side is helpful to demonstrate diminished blood flow. It may be possible to detect lack of perfusion resulting from torsion; however, Doppler may be misleading, since in the posttorsion period, venous stasis and preserved arterial pulsation have been reported. Doppler can, however, help differentiate torsion from epididymitis. In the latter, increased perfusion is seen, whereas flow is diminished or absent with torsion (6). This is therefore an important distinction.

Experience with magnetic resonance imaging and testicular torsion is limited. It may be useful, as the entire course and caliber of the spermatic cord may be traced in a coronal plane and compared with the contralateral side. Edema of the cord appears as low signal intensity on T1-weighted and high signal intensity on T2-weighted images. The point of torsion may be identified. Associated intratesticular hemorrhages can be identified in acute and chronic phases because of change in signal characteristics (72).

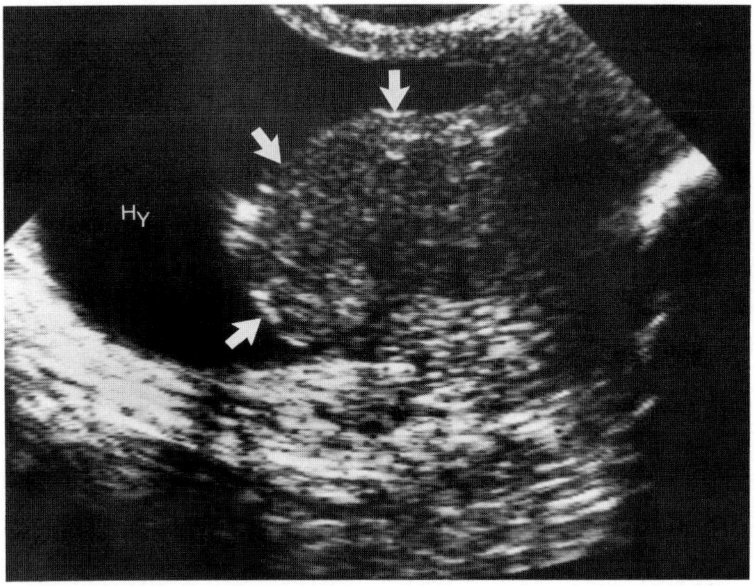

Figure 13.47. Chronic orchitis. The testicle (*arrows*) is heterogeneous in echo texture with areas of decreased and increased echogenicity. A moderately large, reactive hydrocele is present (*Hy*). The patient had chronic orchitis.

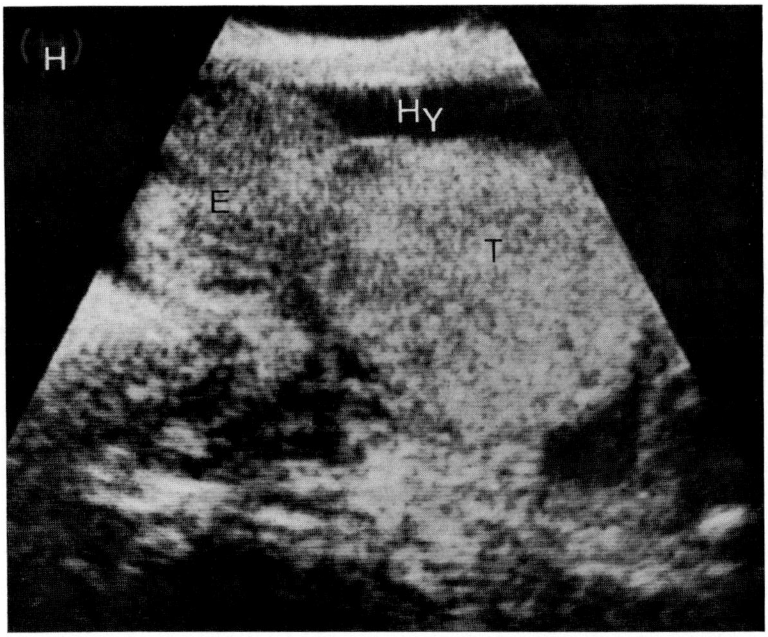

Figure 13.48. Acute torsion. Longitudinal image demonstrates an enlarged hypoechoic epididymis (*E*). The testis (*T*) has a heterogeneous echo texture. A small hydrocele is present (*Hy*). The patient underwent surgery for acute spermatic cord torsion. *H,* toward patient's head.

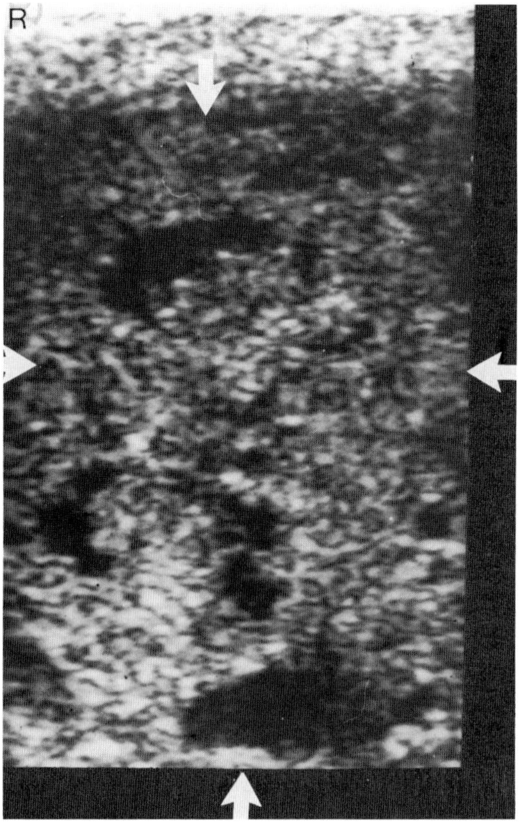

Figure 13.49. Subacute torsion. The testis (*arrows*) demonstrates multiple areas of decreased echogenicity due to hemorrhagic cystic changes. This may be seen 1 to 10 days following the acute event. *R*, patient's right side.

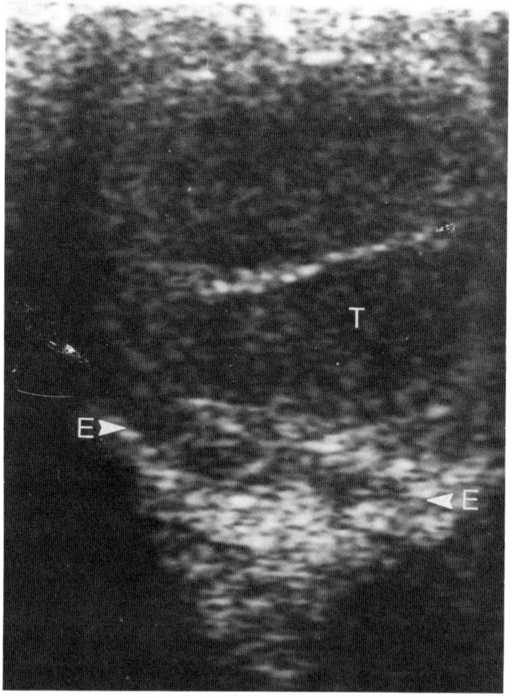

Figure 13.50. Missed torsion, atrophy. The testis (*T*) is diffusely hypoechoic and small measuring 2 × 2 × 2 cm. The epididymis (*E*) has a normal appearance.

INFERTILITY

Varicoceles

Varicoceles represent dilatation of the veins of the pampiniform or cremasteric plexus. They are present in 8 to 15% of the normal male adult population (178). Greater than 90% of unilateral varicoceles are found on the left side and are the result of the drainage pattern of the more tortuous left internal spermatic vein into the left renal vein before reaching the inferior vena cava. Several etiologies of varicoceles have been proposed, including obstruction of the internal spermatic vein or left renal vein, incompetent valves in the spermatic vein, and collateral bypass of competent valves with reflux into the pampiniform plexus (179–181). While a unilateral right-sided varicocele may be innocuous when detected, a search for a pelvic neoplasm or other abnormality obstructing venous return is warranted (e.g., left-sided vena cava) (11, 182). Bilateral varicoceles have been reported, with an incidence of 10 to 70% (1983).

Varicoceles that cause venous stasis lead to increased scrotal heat, which may cause decreased sperm motility. They are an important cause of infertility, being present in 21 to 39% of infertile men (184, 185). In 1952, Tulloch (186) reported successful impregnation following bilateral varicocelectomies in an azospermic patient. This event and subsequent clinical and laboratory studies provided evidence of significant detrimental effects on spermatogenesis by the presence of varicoceles regardless of their size (186, 187). Small, subclinical, and unilateral varicoceles have been shown to decrease sperm motility to the same degree as large or bilateral lesions (184, 187). Since small but clinically significant varicoceles may be missed on careful physical examination, physicians have used a variety of imaging modalities to make the diagnosis. These modalities have included angiography (188), ultrasound (189,

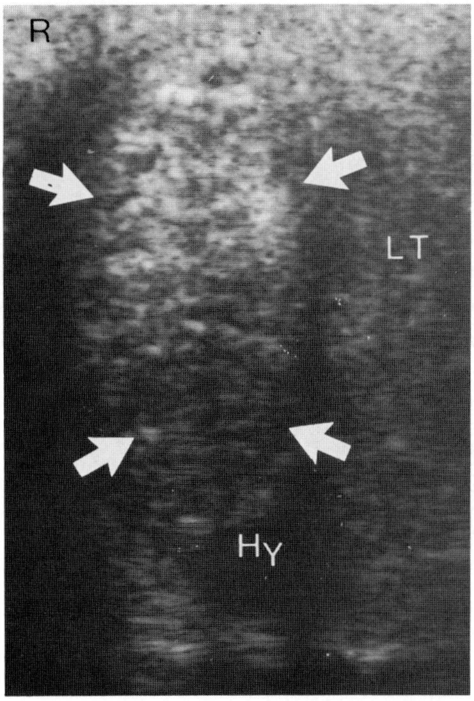

Figure 13.51. Missed torsion, testicular fibrosis. The right testis (*arrows*) is small (1.5 × 3 cm) and echogenic compared with the normal left testis (*LT*). Increased echogenicity is due to fibrosis. A small associated hydrocele (*Hy*) is present. *R*, patient's right side.

190) with Doppler (191, 192), thermography (193, 194), and radionuclide studies (141, 168, 194, 195).

Although venous angiography is the most objective method of diagnosis, it is also the most invasive. The procedure has been performed via the femoral or jugular veins demonstrating abnormal retrograde flow into the left renal and internal spermatic veins. Occasionally, retrograde filling of the dilated testicular veins and pampiniform plexus may be seen (188). While this technique is not usually employed for diagnosis, this procedure has been successfully used for various therapeutic procedures, including sclerotherapy (196), embolization (197), and occlusion with detachable balloons (198, 199).

Radioisotope imaging using ^{99m}Tc pertechnetate, human serum albumin, or a combination of ^{99m}Tc pertechnetate and stannous pyrophosphate–labeled red blood cells has been used for evaluating varicoceles. The isotope angiogram detects increased uptake in the varicocele in the late venous phase, which can persist and be seen on delayed static images (168, 194). This method is helpful in confirming the diagnosis of clinically obvious varicoceles.

Gonda et al. (187) have shown that sonography is superior to radionuclide scanning in the diagnosis of subclinical varicoceles. A source of difficulty in the radionuclide diagnosis of subclinical varicoceles was the presence of bilateral varicoceles. Small varicoceles also escaped detection because of lack of blood pooling in the majority of these cases (187).

Thermography has been employed in an attempt to determine increased scrotal heat caused by the venous stasis in varicoceles (193). Large varicoceles with constant reflux were detected with great accuracy. Hamm (185) reported an accuracy of 98.4% compared with 92.7% for sonography. However, lesions with only intermittent reflux or minimal stasis often failed to be diagnosed by thermography. Also, the test has been shown to be inadequate in patients with a single or atrophic testicle, a small valve, or bilateral varicoceles. The test is inadequate since the diagnosis relies on temperature differences on both sides of the scrotum (183, 185).

Ultrasound evaluation appears to have the most success of the noninvasive imaging modalities for defining subtle varicoceles (11). The Doppler stethoscope, which uses continuous-wave Doppler, was commonly used in the past to make the diagnosis. Venous reflux has been graded as follows: grade I, representing stasis; grade II, intermittent reflux; and grade III, continuous reflux (191). Spontaneous venous reflux of grades II and III was reported in 18% of fertile and 54% of infertile patients. The incidence of grade III varicoceles in infertile men was twice that of fertile men (192).

High-resolution real-time ultrasound is currently the method of choice to confirm the presence of clinically apparent varicoceles and to detect subclinical varicoceles (187). Examination is conducted in both supine and erect positions, and the Valsalva maneuver may be used to accentuate subtle dilatation of veins (Fig. 13.54). Normal veins in the spermatic cord appear as numerous linear, fluid-filled structures in the pampiniform plexus that are less than 1.5 mm in diameter. These can increase in diameter to 5 or 6 mm in patients with varicoceles (Figs. 13.55 and 13.56). Particulate flow can be visualized with high-resolution real-time imaging, and quantitative flow can be determined

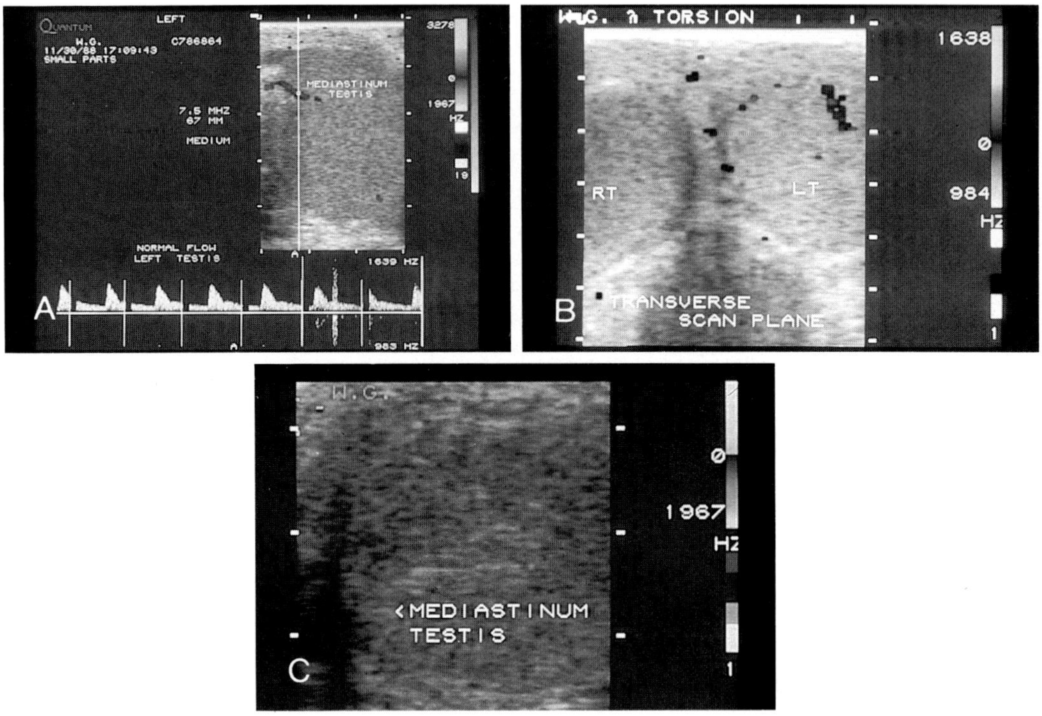

Figure 13.52. Acute spermatic cord torsion. Normal flow is visualized in the mediastinum (**A**) and elsewhere within the normal left testis on an additional transverse image (**B**). On the patient's right side following torsion, there is a lack of intratesticular flow and flow could not be demonstrated in the mediastinum (**C**). (See color plate 4.)

by duplex and color Doppler to confirm the presence of venous channels differentiating varicoceles from spermatoceles (Fig. 13.57) (3). Sonography is also helpful in differentiating a very large varicocele from a hydrocele, although the latter is located anterior to the testis and the former usually posterior. Differentiation from herniation of bowel into the scrotum can be made by observation of peristalsis or shadowing due to gas with real-time imaging (2, 11).

Magnetic resonance imaging has the ability to demonstrate the entire spermatic cord from the inguinal ring to the mediastinum testis, an advantage over ultrasound. Varicoceles appear as a widening of the spermatic canal and prominence of the intrascrotal spermatic cord. Dilated serpiginous structures representing veins frequently possess high signal intensity on T2-weighted images because of slow flow and phase shift artifact. This is seen on both balanced and T2-weighted images (72).

TRAUMA

Blunt trauma to the scrotum may result in testicular contusion, rupture, or peritesticular hematoma or hematocele (200, 201). Due to the mobility of the testis and scrotal elasticity, the testis frequently escapes injury in blunt trauma (31). However, rupture can occur if the scrotum is forcefully compressed against the symphysis pubis. Rupture occurs when the testis is struck with enough force to burst the tunica albuginea, such as with blunt injuries (e.g., in cases of kick injury to the scrotum or in baseball or straddle injuries. Seminiferous tubules extrude through the broken capsule and a hematocele usually forms (202).

Patients with testicular rupture present with a tender, indurated scrotal mass and ecchymosis. Transillumination is not possible and delineation of the testis or epididymis from the remaining scrotal contents on physical examination is difficult. Rapid surgical intervention

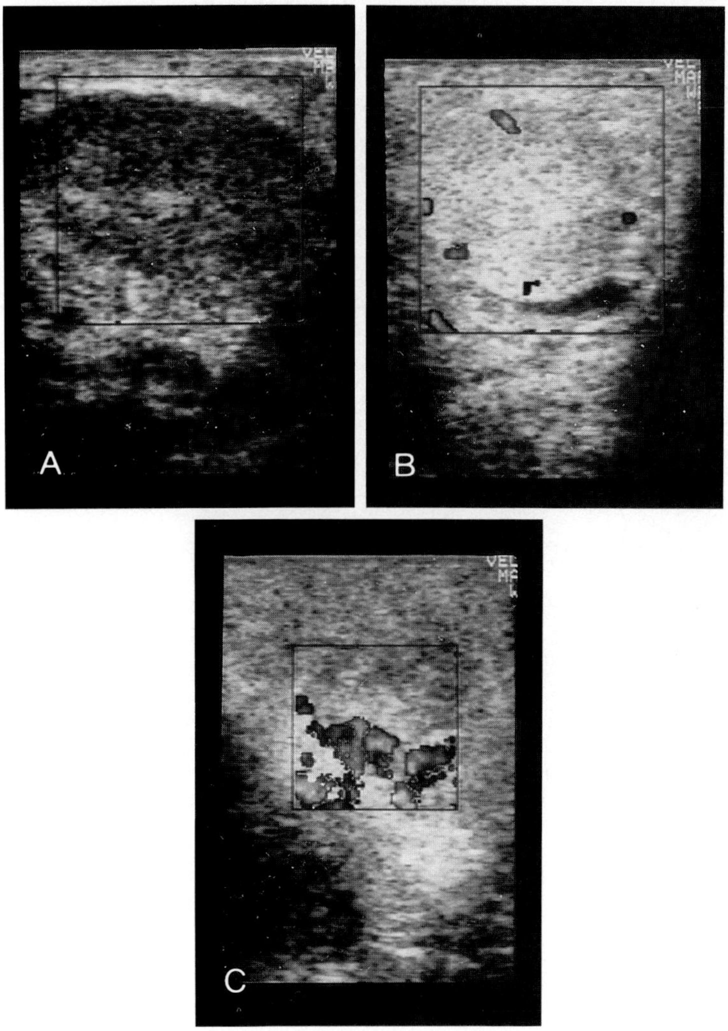

Figure 13.53. Chronic spermatic cord torsion. Color Doppler examination reveals a lack of intratesticular flow in a patient with spermatic cord torsion (**A**). Flow is present in the contralateral testis (**B**) as well as in the region of the epididymis on the abnormal side (**C**). These vessels likely represent hyperemic collateral vessels supplying the epididymis. (See color plate 5.)

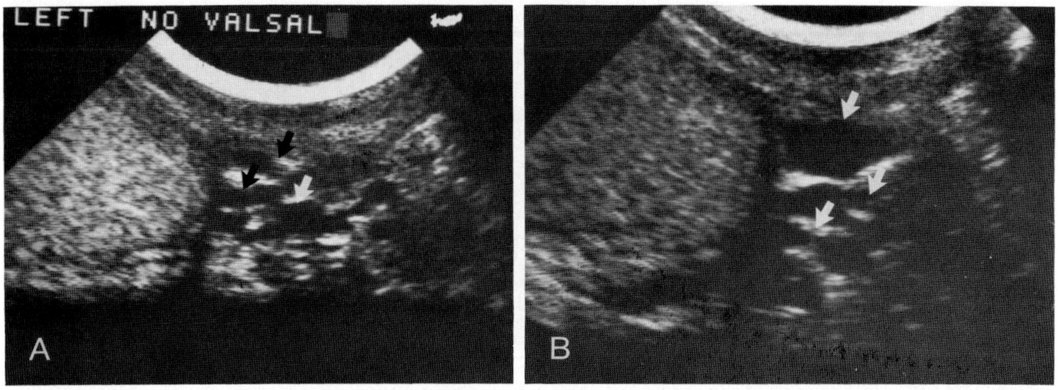

Figure 13.54. Valsalva maneuver to accentuate varicocele. **A,** Real-time image of the scrotum demonstrates slightly dilated serpiginous veins of the pampiniform plexus (*arrows*). **B,** Valsalva maneuver accentuates the degree of dilatation (*arrows*).

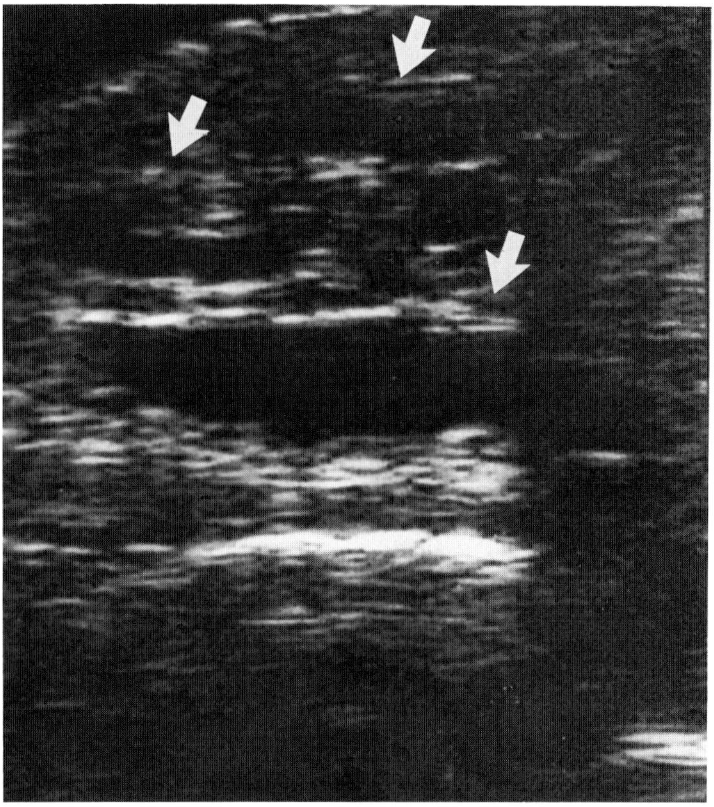

Figure 13.55. Subclinical varicocele. Longitudinal image of the spermatic cord demonstrates dilatation of the veins of the pampiniform plexus (*arrows*). They measure 2 to 5 mm.

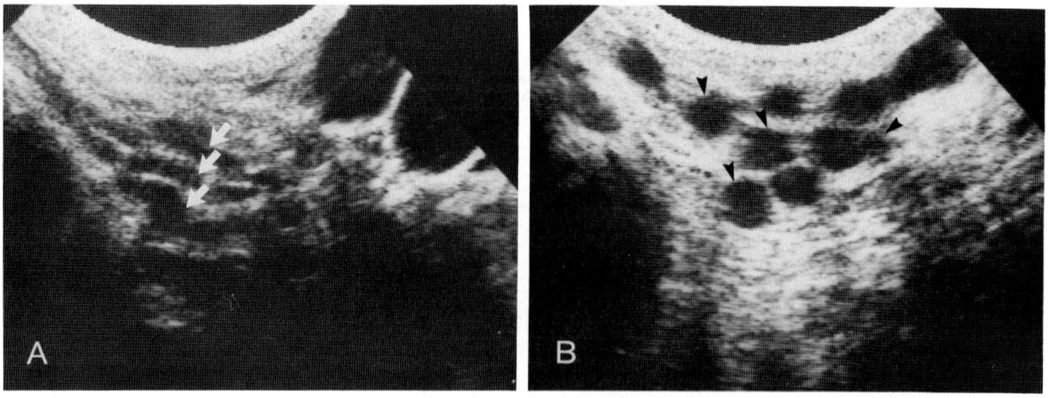

Figure 13.56. Varicocele. Dilated veins of the pampiniform plexus may appear as (**A**) serpiginous tubular structures (*arrows*) or (**B**) rounded anechoic structures (*arrowheads*), depending on the plane of scan. Particulate flow may be visualized with real-time imaging.

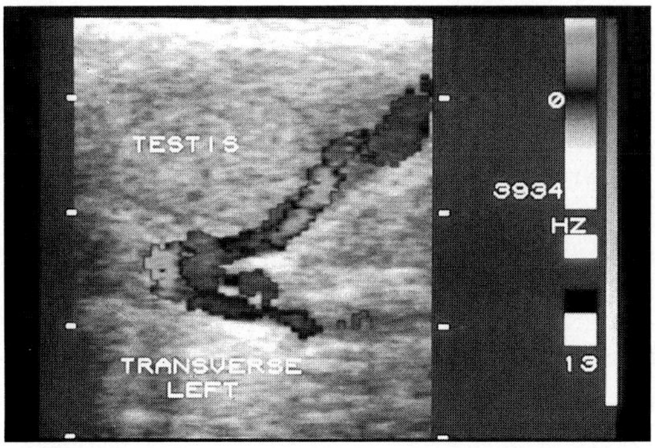

Figure 13.57. Varicocele. Color Doppler image of the left hemiscrotum reveals increased flow in a dilated tortuous vessel posterior to the testis. Flow toward and away from the transducer reflects the tortuosity of the vein within the plexus. (See color plate 5.)

is required to prevent the complication of hypoperfusion and necrosis (202). Salvageability of a ruptured testis depends directly on the time of intervention. Ninety percent of rupture testes can be saved if surgical intervention occurs within 72 hr of the injury. Beyond this time limit, salvageability drops to 55% (3). Identification of a normal testis is equally as important to obviate the need for surgery.

Testicular radionuclide studies are helpful in the diagnosis if a photopenic region corresponding to the hematoma, extruded tubules, or hypoperfused testis is demonstrated (202, 203).

Sonography is usually the most accurate imaging modality (204, 205). Scanning of the scrotum should be performed from the posterior aspect of the testicle as well as anteriorly. A large hematocele will displace the testis posteriorly. A false diagnosis of rupture may be made if the testicle is not imaged from a posterior approach, as it may not be visualized when the scrotum is scanned from the anterior position (6).

With rupture, there is loss of the echogenic linear structures of the tunica albuginea and mediastinum testis on ultrasound. Hematoma within the substance of the testis and contour irregularity may be present (Fig. 13.58). The fracture plane may be visualized (137, 205). Rupture may occur with or without an accompanying hematocele (3). A hematocele is a collection of blood between the two layers of the tunica vaginalis, which may be an isolated finding or may be seen in association with rupture or testicular hemorrhage. Sonographically, a hematocele appears as a hypoechoic fluid collection with multiple internal echoes (205). If the hematocele is longstanding, the tunica vaginalis becomes abnormally thick-

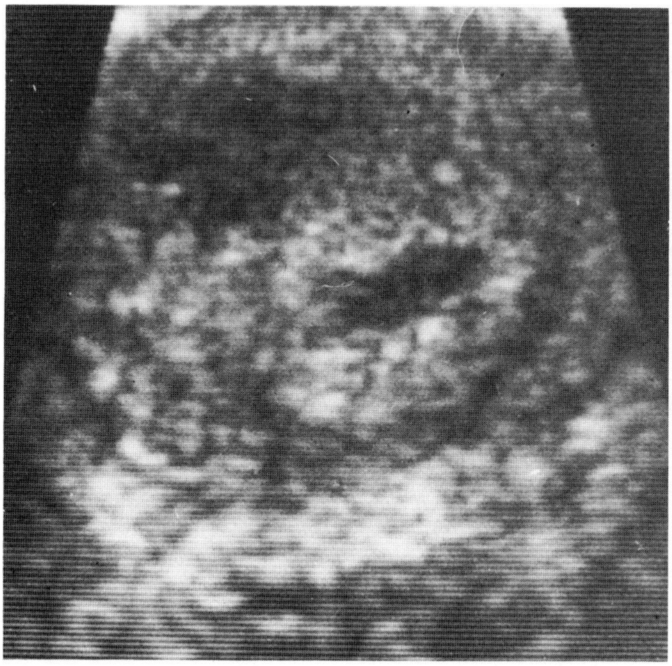

Figure 13.58. Testicular rupture. The parenchyma is markedly inhomogeneous in echogenicity in this patient with a ruptured testicle. The mediastinum testis is not visualized, nor is the plane of fracture.

ened with dense fibrous tissue and appears as a thick-walled fluid collection indistinguishable from abscess or chronic hydrocele. The tunica albuginea (or even the tunica vaginalis) may become partially calcified (Fig. 13.59) (6, 206).

Exploratory surgery is indicated when a hematocele is found following blunt scrotal trauma (206). A hematocele following minor trauma should signal the possibility of an occult testicular neoplasm. A delayed diagnosis or misdiagnosis increases the likelihood of disease progression and potentially worsens long-term prognosis.

Focal alterations in testicular echogenicity are seen with infarction or hemorrhage secondary to trauma. Depending on the age of infarction, the sonographic appearance will vary from hyperechoic to hypoechoic (3, 6). A diffuse, moderate decrease in echogenicity usually represents edema, fluid, and hyperemia. The scrotal wall may be thickened and an accompanying reactive hydrocele may be found. Epididymal enlargement may be present (11).

Significant trauma may lead to rupture of the bulbous urethra with involvement of the deep fascia of the penis. Urine can extravasate through the perforation into the scrotum, resulting in a fluid collection with the same acoustic properties as a hydrocele (3).

Extratesticular injuries may be diagnosed by ultrasound, which aids in the diagnosis of site and severity (149). A scrotal wall hematoma is an effusion of blood within the tissue of the scrotal wall (1, 40). The blood can collect beneath the tunica dartos, between the tunica vaginalis and the fibrous coat, or within the scrotal septum. Sonographically, the appearance will vary with age and location. Acutely, the scrotal wall will appear thickened. Hypoechoic areas due to liquefaction are seen 2 to 3 days after trauma (6). These may be followed with serial scans until resolution if the testis is intact.

Ultrasound can demonstrate a hematoma or tear of the epididymis. It may be difficult to rule out an associated testicular fracture, due to the close proximity of these two structures. This is especially true when the abnormal image is located at the upper or lower pole of the scrotal sac. Surgery may therefore be required (149).

A small hemorrhagic effusion within the spermatic cord can be seen after minimal trauma. Sonographically, this appears as a small hypoechoic area posterior and superior to the testis. This will disappear 1 to 2 weeks following the injury (149).

If scrotal trauma has been caused by a foreign body, sonography may be useful in localizing the offending object, which will appear as a bright acoustic reflector if it is metallic or of a

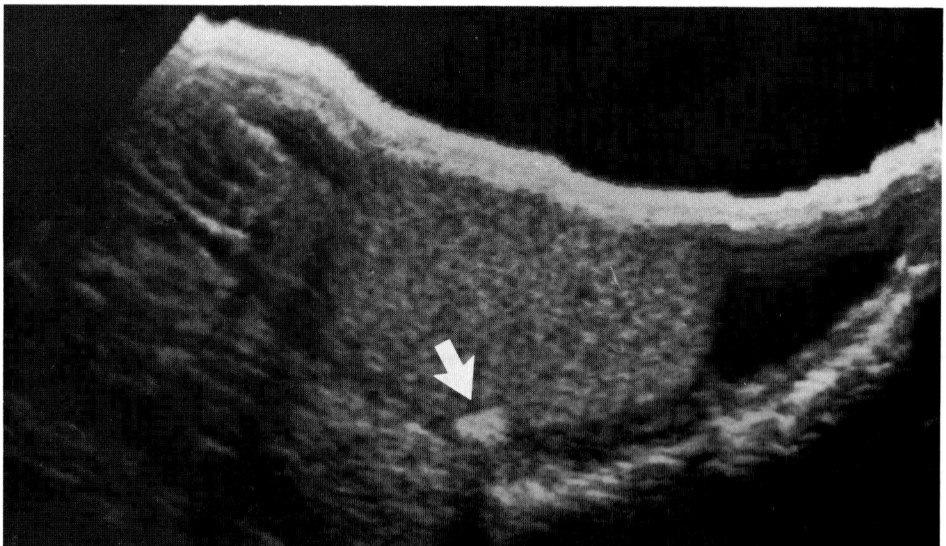

Figure 13.59. Tunical vaginalis calcification. A brightly echogenic area with shadowing (*arrow*) posterior to the testicle represents calcification within the tunica albuginea secondary to old trauma.

substance with high molecular density (Fig. 13.60) (11).

The value of magnetic resonance imaging in trauma rests in its ability to assess the integrity of the tunica albuginea. Disruption of this band of low signal intensity on T1-weighted images indicates the need for surgical intervention. The signal intensity of the traumatized testis is inhomogeneous, with areas of high and low to intermediate signal intensity representing hemorrhage in different stages of organization. An acute hematocele will demonstrate low signal intensity on balanced images and further decrease in signal intensity on T2-weighted images (72).

CONCLUSION

Ultrasound has become an invaluable tool in the diagnosis of scrotal diseases. It provides rapid, noninvasive imaging of the scrotal contents and does not require the use of ionizing radiation. For these reasons, the study may be repeated with impunity. With respect to other

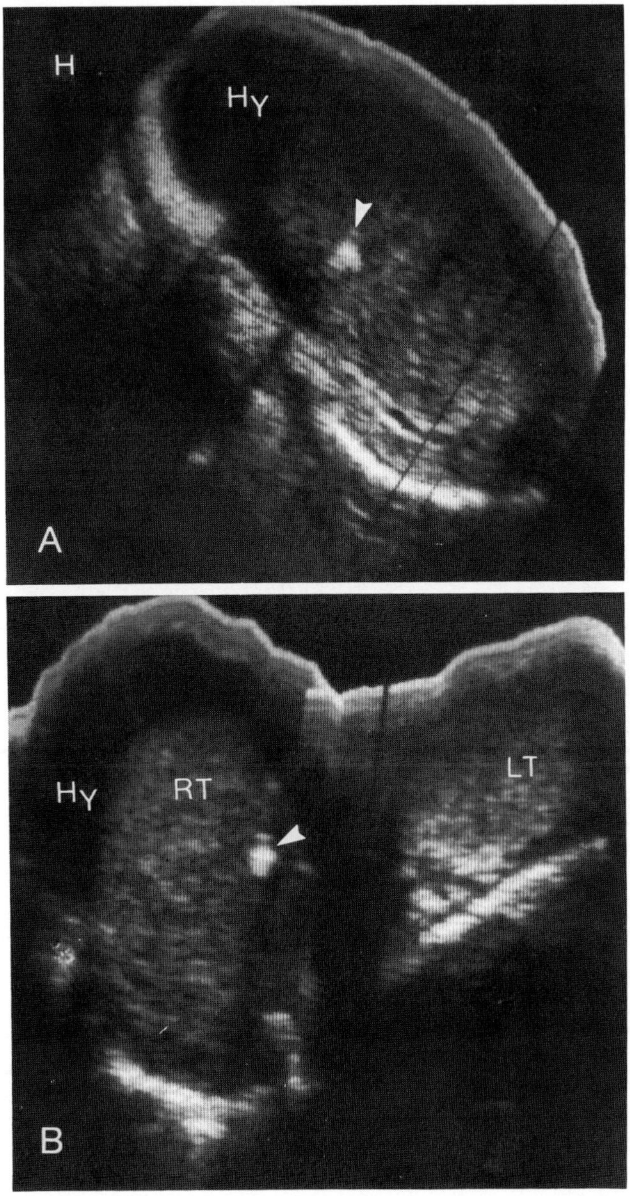

Figure 13.60. Foreign body and hematocele. An echogenic focus (*arrowhead*) imbedded within the right testis (*RT*) noted on both longitudinal (**A**) and transverse (**B**) images of the scrotum represents metallic pellets from a gunshot. An anechoic fluid collection (*Hy*) represents a hematocele. The left testis (*LT*) is normal. *H,* toward patient's head.

available imaging modalities, ultrasound is comparatively less expensive. If not used as a primary imaging modality, sonography plays an important complementary role in the diagnosis of multiple scrotal abnormalities. With the information gleaned from sonographic examination, unnecessary surgery may be avoided, and, if surgery is indicated, the surgeon is better able to determine which approach is best.

References

1. Bunce PL. Scrotal abnormalities. In: Glenn JF, ed. Urologic surgery. New York: Harper & Row, 1975:783–800.
2. Wald L, Rifkin, MD. Scrotal masses. In: Eisenberg RL, ed. Algorithmic approach to radiology. Philadelphia: JB Lippincott, 1988:401–411.
3. Krone KD, Caroll BA. Scrotal ultrasound. Radiol Clin North Am 1985;23:121–139.
4. Arger PH, Mulhern CB Jr, Coleman BG, et al. Prospective analysis of the value of ultrasound. Radiology 1981;141:763–766.
5. Caroll BA, Gross DM. High-frequency scrotal sonography. AJR 1983;40:511–515.
6. Hricak M, Filly RA. Sonography of the scrotum. Invest Radiol 1983;18:112–121.
7. Phillips G, Kumari-Subaiya S, Sawitsky A. Ultrasonic evaluation of the scrotum in lymphoproliferative disease. J Ultrasound Med 1987; 6:169–175.
8. Nachtsheim DA, Scheible FW, Gosink BB. Ultrasonography of testis tumors. J Urol 1983;129:978.
9. Richie JP, Birnholz J, Garnick MB. Ultrasonography as a diagnostic adjunct for the evaluation of masses in the scrotum. Surg Gynecol Obstet 1982;154:695–698.
10. Vick CW, Bird KI Jr, Rosenfield AT, et al. Ultrasound of the scrotal contents. Radiology 1982; 4:147–153.
11. Rifkin M. Scrotum and contents. In: Diagnostic imaging of the lower genitourinary tract. New York: Raven Press, 1985;241–324.
12. DiGiacinto TM, Patten P, Willscher M, Daly K. Sonography of the scrotum. Med Ultrasound 1982;6:95–101.
13. Becker JM, Ritchie WGM, Goldenberg NJ. Ultrasound of the scrotum and its contents. Semin Ultrasound 1982;3:348–355.
14. Orr DP, Skolnick ML. Sonographic examination of the abnormal scrotum. Clin Radiol 1980;31:107–113.
15. Fornage BD, Touche DH, Rifkin MD. Small parts real-time sonography: a new "water-path." J Ultrasound Med 1984;3:355–357.
16. Moore KL. The urogenital system. In: The developing human. Clinical oriented embryology. Philadelphia: WB Saunders, 1977:220–258.
17. Basmajan JV. Grant's method of anatomy. Baltimore: Williams & Wilkins, 1971:192–199.
18. Rifkin MD. The testes and epididymis. In: Goldberg BB, ed. Atlas of normal ultrasound measurements. New York: Year Book Medical Publishers, 1990.
19. Middleton WR, Thorne DA, Melson GL. Color Doppler ultrasound of the normal testes. AJR 1989;152:293–297.
20. Gooding GA. Sonography of thc spermatic cord. AJR 1988;151:721–724.
21. Fritzsche PJ, Hricak H, Kogan BA, et al. Undescended testis: value of MR imaging. Radiology 1987;164:169–173.
22. Friedland GW, Chang P. The role of imaging in the management of the impalpable undescended testis. AJR 1988;151:1107–1111.
23. Blandy JP. Urology. Oxford, England: Blackwell Scientific Publications, 1976.
24. Harrison JH, Gittes RF, Perlmutter AD, et al., eds. Campbell's urology. 4th ed. Philadelphia: WB Saunders, 1979:1549–1561.
25. Batata MA, Whitmore WF Jr, Hilaris BS, Tukita N, Grabstald H. Cancer of the undescended or maldescended testis. AJR 1976; 126:302–312.
26. Batata MA, Whitmore WF Jr, Chu FCH, et al. Cryptorchidism and testicular cancer. J Urol 1980;124:382–387.
27. Kogan SJ. Cryptorchidism and infertility: an overview. Dialog Pediatr Urol 1981;4:2–3.
28. Lipshultz LL. Cryptorchidism and infertility: theoretical observations on endocrine and immunological aspects. Dialog Pediatr Urol 1981; 4:7–8.
29. Wolverson MK, Houttuin E, Heiberg E, Sundaram M, Shields JB. Comparison of computed tomography with high-resolution real-time ultrasound in the localization of the impalpable undescended testis. Radiology 1983;146: 133–136.
30. Weiss RM, Carter AK, Rosenfield AT. High-resolution real-time sonography in the location of the undescended testis. J Urol 1986; 135:936–938.
31. Finkelstein MS, Rosenberg HK, Snyder HM, Duckett JW. Ultrasound evaluation of the scrotum in pediatrics. Urology 1986;27(1):1–9.
32. Lee JKT, Glazer HS. Computed tomography in the localization of the nonpalpable testis. Urol Clin North Am 1982;9:397–404.
33. Rajifer J, Tauber A, Linner N, Naftalin E, Worthen N. The use of computerized tomography scanning to localize the impalpable testis. J Urol 1983;129:972–974.
34. Kier R, McCarthy S, Rosenfield AT, Rosenfield NS, Rapaport S, Weiss R. Nonpalpable testes in young boys: evaluation with MR imaging. Radiology 1988;169:429–433.
35. Daniel WA, Feinstein RA, Howard-Peebles P, Baxley WD. Testicular volume in adolescents. J Pediatr 1982;101:1010–1012.
36. Dornberger V, Dornberger G, Eggstein M. Volumetric des hodens mittels real-time sonographic. Ultraschall 1986;7:300–303.
37. Kaplan SA. Clinical pediatrics and adolescent endocrinology. Philadelphia: WB Saunders, 1982.
38. Handelsman DS, Staraj S. Testicular size: the effects of aging, malnutrition, and illness. J Androl 1985;6:144–151.

39. Diamond JM. Variation in human testis size. Nature 1986;320:488–489.
40. Mostofi FK. Testes, scrotum and penis. In: Anderson WAD, Kissane JM, eds. Pathology St. Louis: CV Mosby, 1977;2:1013–1037.
41. Wescott JW, Dy Khuizen RE. Polyorchidism. J Urol 1967;98:497–500.
42. Nocks BN. Polyorchidism with normal spermatogenesis and equal-sized testes: a theory of embryological development. J Urol 1978;120: 638–640.
43. Jichlinski D, Ward-McQuaid N. Duplication of the testis and infertility. J Urol 1963;90: 583–587.
44. Wilson WA, Littler J. Polyorchidism: a report of two cases with torsion. Br J Surg 1953;41: 302–307.
45. Rifkin MD, Kurtz AB, Pasto ME, Goldberg BB. Polyorchidism diagnosed preoperatively by ultrasound. J Ultrasound Med 1983;2:93–94.
46. McKay DG, Fowler, Jr. R, Barnett JS. The pathogenesis and treatment of primary hydroceles in infancy and childhood. Austr NZ J Surg 1958;28:1–11.
47. Rinker JR, Allen L. A lymphatic defect in hydrocele. Am Surg 1951;17:681–686.
48. Sample WF. Renal, adrenal, retroperitoneal, and scrotal ultrasonography. In: Sarti D, Sample W, eds. Diagnostic ultrasound text and cases. Boston: GK Hall, 1980:268.
49. Grantham JG, Charboneau JW, Janes EM, Kirschling RJ, Kvols LK, Segura JW, Wold LE. Testicular neoplasms: 29 tumors studied by high-resolution US. Radiology 1985;157: 775–780.
50. Shawker TH, Nasser J, O'Leary T, Shapiro E, Krudy AB. Ultrasonographic detection of "burned-out" primary testicular germ cell tumors in clinically normal testes. J Ultrasound Med 1983;2:477–479.
51. Rifkin MD, Kurtz AB, Pasto ME, et al. The sonographic diagnosis of focal and diffuse infiltrative intrascrotal lesions. Urol Radiol 1984; 6:20–26.
52. Kirschling RJ, Kvols LK, Charboneau JW, Grantham JG, Zincke H. High-resolution ultrasonographic and pathologic abnormalities of germ cell tumors in patients with clinically normal testes. Mayo Clin Proc 1983;58:648–653.
53. Peterson CJ, Catalona WJ, Koehler RE. Ultrasonic localization of a non-palpable testis tumor. J Urol 1979;122:843–844.
54. Glazer HS, Lee JKT, Melson GL, McClennan BL. Sonographic detection of occult testicular neoplasms. AJR 1982;138:673–675.
55. Moudy PC, Makhija JS. Ultrasonic demonstration of a non-palpable testicular tumor. J Clin Ultrasound 1983;11:54–55.
56. Emory TH, Charboneau JW, Randall RV, Scheithauer BW, Grantham JG. Occult testicular interstitial-cell tumor in patients with gynecomastia: ultrasonic detection. Radiology 1984;151:474.
57. Schwerk WB, Schwerk WN, Rodeck G. Testicular tumors: prospective analysis of real-time US patterns and abdominal staging. Radiology 1987;164:369–374.
58. Millen P, Behrendt H, Hassfeld D. Tumoren des hodens des nebendhodens und der hodenhullen. In: Hohenfellner R, Zingg EJ, eds. In: Urologie. Stuttgart: Thieme, 1982;1.
59. Silverberg E. Cancer statistics, 1984. CA 1984; 34:7–23.
60. Morrison AS, Cole P, Maclure KM. Epidemiology of urologic cancers. In: Javadpour N, ed. Principles and management of urologic cancer. 2nd ed. Baltimore: Williams & Wilkins, 1983:12–31.
61. Martin DC. Germinal cell tumors of the testis after orchiopexy. J Urol 1979;121:422.
62. Ekman P. Current concepts in the management of testicular germ cell tumors in adults: a review. Int J Androl 1982;5:356–366.
63. Murphy GP. Testicular cancer. CA 1983;33: 100–104.
64. Behrendt H, Heckemann R, Meyer-Schickerat M, Hartung R. Ergebnisse aus sonographischen stagings bei hodentumoren. Verh Dtsch Ges Urol 1982;34:146–150.
65. Burney B, Klatte E. Ultrasound and computed tomography of the abdomen in the staging and management of testicular carcinoma. Radiology 1979;132:415–419.
66. Hutschenreiter G, Alken P, Schneider H. The value of sonography and lymphography in the detection of retroperitoneal metastases in testicular tumors. J Urol 1979;122:766–769.
67. Williams R, Feinberg S, Kneight L, Traley E. Abdominal staging of testicular tumors using ultrasonography and computed tomography. J Urol 1980;123:872–875.
68. Thoeni RF. Computed tomography of the pelvis. In: Moss A, Gamsu G, Genant H, eds. Computed tomography of the body. Philadelphia: WB Saunders, 1983:987–1053.
69. Husband JE, Macdonald JS, Peckham MJ. Computed tomography in testicular disease: a review. J R Soc Med 1981;74:441–447.
70. Pillari G, Rubenstein WA, Siess J. Seminoma: improved imaging and tumor characterization with computed tomography. J Urol 1980; 123:41–43.
71. McCarthy S, Fritzsche PJ. Male pelvis. In: Stark D, Bradley W, eds. Magnetic resonance imaging. St. Louis: CV Mosby, 1987:1233–1264.
72. Baker LL, Hajek PC, Burkhard TK, et al. MR imaging of the scrotum: pathologic conditions. Radiology 1987;163:93–98.
73. Seidenwurm D, Smathers RC, Lo RK, et al. Testes and scrotum: MR imaging at 1.5 T. Radiology 1987;164:393–398.
74. Scott RF, Bayliss AP, Calder JF, Garvie WH. Indications for ultrasound in the evaluation of the pathological scrotum. Br J Urol 1986; 58:178–182.
75. Aristizabal S, Davis JR, Miller RC, et al. Bilateral primary germ cell testicular tumors: report of four cases and review of the literature. Cancer 1978;42:591.
76. Caldwell WL, Kudemian MT, Frias Z, et al. The management of testicular seminomas, 1979. Cancer 1980;45 (suppl):1768–1774.

77. Desai KM, Haworth JM, Gingell JC. Scrotal ultrasound. J R Soc Med 1985;78:710–714.
78. Bosl GL, Lange PH, Nochomovitz LE, et al. Tumormakers in advanced nonseminomatous testicular cancer. Cancer 1981;47:572.
79. Azzopardi JG, Mostofi FK, Theiss EA. Lesions of the testes observed in certain patients with widespread choriocarcinoma and related tumors. Am J Pathol 1961;38:207.
80. Casola G, Scheible FW, Leopold GR. Neuroblastoma metastatic to the testis: ultrasonographic screening as an aid to clinical staging. Radiology 1984;151:475–476.
81. Stoffel TJ, Nesbitt ME, Levitt SH. Extramedullary involvement of the testes in childhood leukemia. Cancer 1975;35:1203–1211.
82. Giuler RL. Testicular involvement in leukemia and lymphoma. Cancer 1969:23:1290.
83. Saiontz HI, Gilchrist GS, Smithson WA, Burgert EO Jr, Cupps RT. Testicular relapse in childhood leukemia. Mayo Clin Proc 1978; 53:212.
84. Lupetin AR, King W, Rich P, Lederman RB. Ultrasound diagnosis of testicular leukemia. Radiology 1983;146:171–172.
85. Portalez D, Song MY, Marty MH, et al. Ultrasonographic patterns of testicular non-Hodgkins lymphoma: a report of five cases. Eur J Radiol 1982;2:222–225.
86. Rayor RA, Scheible FW, Brock WA, et al. High resolution ultrasonography in the diagnosis of testicular relapse in patients with acute lymphoblastic leukemia. J Urol 1982;128:602–603.
87. Leopold GR, Woo VL, Scheible FW, Nachtsheim D, Gosink BB. High-resolution ultrasonography of scrotal pathology. Radiology 1979; 131:719–722.
88. Sample WF, Gottesman JE, Skinner DG, Ehrlich RM. Gray scale ultrasound of the scrotum. Radiology 1978;127:225–228.
89. Gooding GAW, Leonhardt W, Stein R. Testicular cysts: US findings. Radiology 1987;163: 537–538.
90. Leung ML, Gooding GAW, Williams RD. High-resolution sonography of scrotal contents in asymptomatic subjects. AJR 1984;143:161–164.
91. Hamm B, Frobbe F, Loy V. Testicular cysts: differentiation with US and clinical findings. Radiology 1988;168:19–23.
92. Rifkin MD, Jacobs JA. Simple testicular cyst diagnosed preoperatively by ultrasound. J Urol 1983;129:982–983.
93. Frater K. Cysts of the tunica albuginea (cysts of the testis.) J Urol 1929;21:135–142.
94. Arcadia JA. Cysts of the tunica albuginea testis. J Urol 1952;68:631–635.
95. Mancilla JR, Matsuda GT. Cysts of the tunica albuginea: report of 4 cases and review of the literature. J Urol 1975;114:730–733.
96. Mennemeyer RP, Mason JT. Non-neoplastic cystic lesions of the tunica albuginea: an electron microscopic and clinical study of 2 cases. J Urol 1979;121:373–375.
97. Trainer TD. Histology of the normal testis. Am J Surg Pathol 1987;11:797–809.
98. Cho CS, Kosek J. Cystic dysplasia of the testis: sonographic and pathologic findings. Radiology 1985;156:777–778.
99. Rholl KS, Lee JK, Ling D, Heiken JP, Glazer HS. MR imaging of the scrotum with a high-resolution surface coil. Radiology 1987;163: 99–103.
100. Nistal M, Paniagua R, Diez-Pardo JA. Testicular microlithiasis in 2 children with bilateral cryptorchidism. J Urol 1979;121:535–537.
101. Jaramillo D, Perez-Atayde A, Teele RL. Sonography of testicular microlithiasis. Urol Radiol 1989;11:55–57.
102. Doherty FJ, Mullins TL, Sant BR, Drinkwater MA, Ucci A Jr. Testicular microlithiasis: a unique sonographic appearance. J Ultrasound Med 1987;6:389–392.
103. Hermansen MC, Chusid MJ, Sty JR. Bacterial epididymo-orchitis in children and adolescents. Clin Pediatr 1980;19:812–815.
104. Grutman H, Golimbu M, Subramanyam BR. Diagnostic ultrasound of scrotum. Urology 1986;27:72–75.
105. Blei L, Sihelnik S, Bloom D, et al. Ultrasonographic analysis of chronic intratesticular pathology. J Ultrasound Med 1983;2:17–23.
106. Stein BS, Kendall AR, Harke HT, et al. Scrotal imaging in the Henoch-Schönlein syndrome. J Urol 1980;124:568–569.
107. Vick CW, Bird KI Jr, Rosenfield AT, et al. Scrotal masses with a uniform hyperechoic pattern. Radiology 1983;184:209–211.
108. Abul-Khair MT, Arafa NM, Sobeth AM, et al. Sonography of bilharzial masses of the scrotum. J Clin Ultrasound 1980;8:239–240.
109. Schechter DC. Aberrant adrenal tissue. Ann Surg 1968;167:421.
110. Feldman AE, Rosenthal RS, Shaw JL. Aberrant adrenal tissue: an incidental finding during orchiopexy. J Urol 1975;113:706–708.
111. Burke EF, Gilbert E, Ushling DR. Adrenal rest tumors of the testes. J Urol 1973;109:649–652.
112. Seidenwurm D, Smathers RL, Kan P, Hoffman A. Intratesticular adrenal rests diagnosed by ultrasound. Radiology 1985;155:479–481.
113. McDonald DF, Donald F. Urology. In: Schwartz SI, ed. Principles of surgery. New York: McGraw-Hill, 1974;2:1552, 1579–1580.
114. DiDonna A, Rizzatto G. Pyocele of the scrotum: sonographic demonstration of fluid level and a gas-forming component. J Ultrasound Med 1986;5:99–100.
115. Burt TB, Knochel JQ, Lee TG. Gas as a contrast agent and diagnostic aid in abdominal sonography. J Ultrasound Med 1982;1:179.
116. Broth G, Bullock WK, Morrow J. Epididymal tumors: 1. Report of 15 new cases including review of literature. 2. Histochemical study of the so-called adenomatoid tumor. J Urol 1968; 100:530–536.
117. Price EB. Papillary cystadenoma of the epididymis: a clinicopathologic analysis of 20 cases. Arch Pathol 1971;91:456.
118. McCormack M. Bilateral fibrosarcoma of the epididymis. J Clin Pathol 1975;28:576–579.
119. Davides KC, King LM, Paat F. Primary

leiomyosarcoma of the epididymis. J Urol 1975; 114:642–644.
120. Rifkin MD, Kurtz AB, Goldberg BB. Epididymis examined by ultrasound. Radiology 1984;151:187–190.
121. Kovi J, Jackson AG, Jackson MA, Sampson CC. Solitary epididymal metastasis from carcinoma of prostate. Urology 1974;3:644–645.
122. Burger R, Guthrie TH. Metastatic colonic carcinoma to epididymis. Urology 1973;2:566–567.
123. Addonizio JC, Thelmo W. Epididymal metastasis from prostatic carcinoma. Urology 1981; 18:490–491.
124. Selli C, Woodward BH, Paulson DF. Late intrascrotal metastases from renal cell carcinoma. Urology 1982;20:423–425.
125. Algaba F, Santaularia JM, Villavicencio H. Metastatic tumor of the epididymis and spermatic cord. Eur Urol 1983;9:56–59.
126. Wakley CPG. Cysts of the epididymis: the so-called spermatocele. Br J Surg 1943;31:165–171.
127. Bibbo M, Gill WB, Azizi F, et al. Follow-up study of male and female offspring of DES-exposed mothers. Obstet Gynecol 1977;49:1–9.
128. Opal SM, Pittman DL, Hofeldt FO. Testicular sarcoidosis. Am J Med 1979;67:147–150.
129. Gerstenhaber BJ, Green R, Sachs FL. Epididymis sarcoidosis: a report of two cases and a review of the literature. Yale J Biol Med 1977; 50:669–675.
130. Friedman AP, Haller JO, Goodman JD. Sonography of scrotal masses in healed meconium peritonitis. Urol Radiol 1983;5:43–46.
131. Subramanyam BR, Balthazar EG, Raghavendra BN, et al. Sonographic diagnosis of scrotal hernia. AJR 1982;139:535–538.
132. Archer A, Choyke PL, O'Brien W, Maxted WC, Grant EG. Scrotal enlargement following inguinal herniorrhaphy: ultrasound evaluation. Urol Radiol 1988;9:249–252.
133. Rydell W, Hanover WH. Inguinal and femoral hernias. Arch Surg 1963;87:150–157.
134. Pollack R, Nyhus LM. Complications of groin hernia repair. Surg Clin North Am 1983;63: 1363–1371.
135. Cunningham J. Sonographic findings in clinically unsuspected acute and chronic scrotal hematocele. AJR 1983;140:749–752.
136. Hricak H, Hoddick WK. Scrotal ultrasound. In: Hricak H, ed. Genitourinary ultrasound. New York: Churchill-Livingstone, 1986:219–240.
137. Hricak H, Jeffrey RB. Sonography of acute scrotal abnormalities. Radiol Clin North Am 1983; 21:595–603.
138. Pintauro W, Klein F, Vick CW, Brocker B. The use of ultrasound for evaluating subacute unilateral scrotal swelling. J Urol 1985;133: 779–802.
139. Vick CW, Bird K, Rosenfield A, et al. Extratesticular hemorrhage associated with torsion of the spermatic cord: sonographic demonstration. Radiology 1986;158:401–404.
140. Wantz GE. Complication of inguinal hernia repair. Surg Clin North Am 1984;64:287–298.
141. Holder L, Melloul M, Chen DCP. Current status of radionuclide scrotal imaging. Semin Nucl Med 1981;11:232–249.
142. Chen DCP, Holder L, Melloul M. Radionuclide scrotal imaging: further experience with 210 patients. Part I: anatomy, pathophysiology, and methods. J Nucl Med 1983;24: 735–742.
143. Chen DCP, Holder L, Melloul M. Radionuclide scrotal imaging: further experience with 210 patients. Part II: results and discussion. J Nucl Med 1983;24:841–853.
144. Taylor KJW, Burns PN, Woodcock JP, Wells PNT. Blood flow in deep abdominal and pelvic vessels: ultrasonic pulsed Doppler analysis. Radiology 1985;154:487–493.
145. Wetzner SM, Kiser LC, Bezrek JS. Duplex ultrasound imaging: vascular application. Radiology 1984;150:507–514.
146. O'Leary OH. Vascular ultrasonography. Radiol Clin North Am 1985;23(1):35–36.
147. Sharer WC. Acute scrotal pathology. Surg Clin North Am 1982;62:955–970.
148. Symmers WSTC, ed. Systemic pathology. ed 2. London: Churchill Livingstone, 1979;4.
149. Martin B, Conte J. Ultrasonography of the acute scrotum. J Clin Ultrasound 1987;15: 37–44.
150. Chen DCP, Holder LE, Kaplan GN. Correlation of radionuclide imaging and diagnostic ultrasound in scrotal diseases. J Nucl Med 1986; 27:1774–1781.
151. Mittemeyer BT, Lennox KW, Borski AA. Epididymitis: a review of 610 cases. J Urol 1966; 95:390–392.
152. Gislason T, Noronha RFX, Gregory JG. Acute epididymitis in boys: a 5-year retrospective study. J Urol 1980;124:533–534.
153. Williams CB, Litvak AS, McRoberts JW. Epididymitis in infancy. J Urol 1979;121: 125–126.
154. Wolin LH. On the etiology of epididymitis. J Urol 1971;105:531–533.
155. Rifkin MD, Goldberg BB. The lower genitourinary tract and testes. In: Goldberg BB, ed. Abdominal ultrasonography. 2nd ed. New York: John Wiley & Sons, 1984:425–480.
156. Holland JM, Graham JB, Ignatoff JM. Conservative management of twisted testicular appendages. J Urol 1981;125:213–214.
157. Bigley HA, Hardin NJ, Chenault OW Jr. Epididymitis and testis tumor. JAMA 1977;238: 244–245.
158. Vordermark JS II, Favila MO. Testicular necrosis: a preventable complication of epididymitis. J Urol 1982;128:1322–1324.
159. Haynes BE, Bessen HA, Haynes VE. The diagnosis of testicular torsion. JAMA 1983;249: 2522–2527.
160. Kelalis PP, Stickler GB. The painful scrotum: torsion US epididymo-orchitis. Clin Pediatr 1976;15:220–221.
161. Randazzo RF, Hulette CM, Gottlieb MS, Rajfer J. Cytomegaloviral epididymitis in a patient with the acquired immune deficiency syndrome. J Urol 1986;136(5):1095–1097.
162. Berger RE, Alexander ER, Harnisch JP, et al. Etiology, manifestations and therapy of acute

epididymitis: prospective study of 50 cases. J Urol 1979;121:750–754.
163. Reeve HR, Weinerth JL, Peterson LJ. Tuberculosis of epididymis and testicle presenting as hydrocele. Urology 1974;4:329–331.
164. Eltayeb AA. Schistosomiasis of the epididymis. Br J Surg 1969;56:552–553.
165. Kazzaz BA, Salmo NAM. Epididymitis due to *Schistosoma hematobium* infection. Trop Geogr Med 1974;26:333–336.
166. Wechsler H, Westfall M, Lattimer JK. The earliest signs and symptoms in 127 male patients with genitourinary tuberculosis. J Urol 1960; 83:801–803.
167. Kissane JM, ed. Anderson's pathology. 8th ed. St. Louis: CV Mosby, 1985;1:796–811.
168. Holder LE, Matire JR, Holmes ER III, Wagner HN Jr. Testicular radionuclide angiography and static imaging: anatomy, scintigraphic interpretation, and clinical indications. Radiology 1977;125:739–752.
169. Bird K, Rosenfield AT. Testicular infarction secondary to acute inflammatory disease: demonstration by B scan ultrasound. Radiology 1984; 152:785–788.
170. Witherington R, Harper WM IV. The surgical management of acute bacterial epididymitis with emphasis on epididymotomy. J Urol 1982; 128:722–725.
171. Bird K, Rosenfield AT. B-scan ultrasonography of acute focal orchitis and its sequelae. AJR 1984;142:239.
172. Goodman A, Lipinski JK. Sonographic findings in malacoplakia of the testis with pathologic review. J Clin Ultrasound 1984;12:45–47.
173. Subramanyam BR, Horii SC, Hilton S. Diffuse testicular disease: sonographic features and significance. AJR 1985;145:121–124.
174. Williamson RCN. Death in the scrotum: testicular torsion. N Engl J Med 1977;296:338.
175. Smith SP, King LR. Torsion of the testis: techniques of assessment. Urol Clin North Am 1979;6(2):429–443.
176. Bird K, Rosenfield AT, Taylor KJW. Ultrasonography in testicular torsion. Radiology 1983;147:527–534.
177. Burks DD, Markey BJ, Burkhard TK, Balsara ZN, Haluszka MM, Canning DA. Suspected testicular torsion and ischemia: evaluation with color Doppler sonography. Radiology 1990; 175:815–822.
178. Clarke BG. Incidence of varicocele in normal men and among men of different ages. JAMA 1966;198:1121–1122.
179. Belker AM. The varicocele and male infertility. Urol Clin North Am 1981;8(1):41–51.
180. Etriby AAE, Ibrahim AAA, Mahmoud KZ, Elhaggar S. Subfertility and varicocle. I. venogram demonstration of anastomosis sites in subfertile men. Fertil Steril 1975;26:1013.
181. Sayfan J, Adam YG, Soffer Y. A natural "venous bypass" causing postoperative recurrence of a varicocele. J Androl 1981;2:108.
182. Rogers WF, Ralls PW, Boswell WD. Obstruction of the inferior vena cava by seminoma. J Urol 1980;124:613–614.
183. McClure RD, Hricak H. Scrotal ultrasound in the infertile man: detection of subclinical unilateral and bilateral varicoceles. J Urol 1986; 135:711–715.
184. Amelar RD, Dubin L. Male infertility: current diagnosis and treatment. Urology 1973;1: 1–31.
185. Hamm B, Fobbe F, Sorensen R, Felsenberg D. Varicoceles: combined sonography and thermography in diagnosis and post therapeutic evaluation. Radiology 1986;160:419–424.
186. Tulloch WS. A consideration of sterility factors in the light of subsequent pregnancies II: subfertility in the male. Edinburgh Medical Journal 1952;59:29.
187. Gonda RL, Karo JJ, Forte RA, O'Donell KT. Diagnosis of subclinical variococele in infertility. AJR 1987;184:71–75.
188. Ahlberg NE, Bartley O, Chidekel N, Fritjofsson A. Phlebography in varicocele scroti. Acta Radiol (Diagn) 1966;4:517–528.
189. Rifkin MD, Foy PM, Kurtz AB, Pasto ME, Goldberg BB. The role of diagnostic ultrasonography in varicocele evaluation. J Ultrasound Med 1983;2:271–275.
190. Wolverson MK, Houttuin E, Heiberg E, Sundaram M, Gregory J. High-resolution real-time sonography of scrotal varicocele. AJR 1983; 141:775–779.
191. Greenberg SH, Lipshultz LI, Morganroth J, Wein AJ. The use of Doppler stethoscope in the evaluation of varicoceles. J Urol 1977;117: 296–298.
192. Hirsh AV, Kellett MJ, Robertson G, Pryor JP. Doppler flow studies, venography and thermography in the evaluation of varicoceles of fertile and subfertile men. Br J Urol 1980;52: 560–565.
193. Gold RH, Ehrlich RM, Samuels B, Dowdy A, Young RT. Scrotal thermography. Radiology 1977;122:129–132.
194. Freund J, Handelsman DJ, Bautovich GJ, Conway AJ, Morris JG. Detection of varicocele by radionuclide blood-pool scanning. Radiology 1980;137:227–230.
195. Wheatley JK, Fajman WA, Witten FR. Clinical experience with the radioisotope varicocele scan as a screening method for the detection of subclinical varicoceles. J Urol 1982;128: 57–59.
196. Seyferth W, Jecht E, Zeitter E. Percutaneous sclerotherapy of varicocele. Radiology 1981; 139:335–340.
197. Formanek A, Rusnak B, Zollikofer C, Castaneda-Zuniga WR, Narayan P, Gonzalez R, Amplatz K. Embolization of infertility: a new approach. Radiology 1981;139:315–321.
198. White RI Jr, Kaufman SL, Barth KH, Kadir S, Smyth JW, Walsh PC. Occlusion of varicoceles with detachable balloons. Radiology 1981; 139:327–334.
199. Kaufman SL, Kadir S, Barth KH, Smyth JW, Walsh PC, White RI Jr. Mechanisms of recurrent varicocele after balloon occlusion of surgical ligation of the internal spermatic vein. Radiology 1983;147:435–440.

200. Ashkar LN, Schreck WR. Traumatic rupture of the testis and epididymis. J Urol 1968;99: 774–775.
201. Rao KG. Traumatic rupture of the testis. Urology 1982;20:624–625.
202. McConnell JD, Peters PC, Lewis SE. Testicular rupture in blunt scrotal trauma: review of 15 cases with recent application of testicular scanning. J Urol 1982;128:309–311.
203. Friedman SG, Rose JG, Winston MA. Ultrasound and nuclear medicine evaluation in acute testicular trauma. J Urol 1981;125:748–749.
204. Albert NE. Testicular ultrasound for trauma. J Urol 1980;124:558–559.
205. Lupetin AR, King W, Rich PJ, Lederman RB. The traumatized scrotum. Radiology 1983; 148:203–207.
206. Hricak H. Sonography of the scrotum. In: Margulis AR, Gooding GA, eds. Diagnostic radiology: San Francisco, University of California, 1982:371–377.

CHAPTER 14

Ultrasonography of Renal Transplants

LAURENCE NEEDLEMAN, M.D.

Renal transplantation is one of the great successes of modern medicine. Major advances in donor organ matching and preparation, surgical technique, and medical therapy to alter the immune response have made it the treatment of choice for end-stage renal disease.

Sonography has a central role in the postoperative and long-term follow-up of renal transplants. Ultrasound is the gold standard in some complications such as in initial evaluation of obstruction or fluid collections. Aspiration of peritransplant collections and transplant biopsies are performed under sonographic guidance in most instances. Many vascular complications that had previously required angiography or nuclear medicine scans for diagnosis can now be made with Doppler ultrasonography.

SURGICAL OVERVIEW

The transplant is implanted in the iliac fossa within the retroperitoneal space. It is preferable to put the kidney into the opposite side of the recipient (e.g., a donor right kidney is implanted into the recipient's left side) since this places the renal pelvis and ureter anteriorly and more accessible if subsequent surgery is necessary.

After the surgical incision the iliac vessels are dissected and the lymphatics are ligated to diminish lymph leak. The arterial anastomosis connects the renal artery to either the external or internal iliac artery. End-to-side anastomoses to the external iliac have less postoperative stenosis and fewer problems with disparity of the vessels (1). The hypogastric artery is usually avoided as a site since it is a frequent site of atherosclerotic plaque. Multiple arteries require other techniques. A very small upper polar artery may be sacrificed without significant problems. Lower-pole arteries are more important since they partially supply the ureter. If not reconstructed, significantly sized upper or lower polar arteries may cause segmental infarctions, possibly with a caliceal fistula (2). The venous anastomosis is more difficult. Adequate dissection is necessary to make a mobile vein that will not kink. The renal vein is anastomosed to the iliac vein.

The urinary tract is reestablished by ureteroneocystostomy. This technique has few complications and it protects the ureter from reflux. Other techniques may be used, depending on the length and condition of the ureter and of the recipient bladder. Rarely, ureteroureterostomy, pyeloureterostomy, or ileal conduits are necessary (2).

SONOGRAPHIC TECHNIQUES

The renal transplant is a superficial organ, and scanning with a 5-MHz transducer is often possible. Real-time scanning can define an optimal window in most cases even if bandages cover the surgical site. If the bandages need to be removed before the wound has healed, a sterile covering between the transducer and the skin can be applied to facilitate scanning.

Scanning Protocol

A series of scans through the entire transplant is performed by scanning across the transplant in long-axis as well as axial scans from above to below the organ. The longest length of the transplant is sought to define its long axis. Depending on the orientation of the transplant and the ultrasonic window this may be either a coronal or a sagittal scan. Axial scans are taken at right angles to the long axis. The longest length of the kidney defines the measurement of its length. The largest area in the axial plane defines the level at which the width and anteroposterior (AP) dimension of the kidney are taken. All three measurements are therefore at right angles to one another.

Renal volume is usually determined by the prolate ellipsoid method (length multiplied by width multiplied by AP dimension multiplied by 0.5233) (3).

The scan should evaluate the texture of the kidney, paying attention to the echogenicity and relative size and definition of the cortex, medulla, and central sinus. This requires careful attention to proper gain and power settings. Technical differences between scans (e.g., different machines doing different studies or different gain settings from study to study) as well as pathological processes may alter the kidney's appearance. Therefore, the relative echogenicity of the renal cortex and medulla are compared to the hepatic echogenicity based on scans of the liver taken with the same magnification, power, and gain settings as those used for the transplant. The central sinus should be evaluated for hydronephrosis, and the outer border of the kidney and the peritransplant region should also be evaluated.

If possible, the bladder should be full at the time of the ultrasonography. Sonograms of the bladder in transverse and sagittal planes are taken. The full bladder pushes bowel out of the pelvis and eases identification of fluid collections between the transplant and the bladder. If hydronephrosis is found, scans between the bladder and transplant are taken to identify a ureter. Postvoid scans are also performed to see if the dilatation is related to bladder distention (4).

Normal Findings

The normal renal transplant has a smooth, uninterrupted contour (Fig. 14.1). On axial scans the organ is elliptical and wider than it is thick. The cortex is slightly less echogenic or equal to the liver echogenicity. The cortex and medulla vary slightly in echogenicity, with fewer echoes in the medulla. In many, good corticomedullary distinction may be absent. The echogenicity of the transplant should be equal through the entire transplant as long as the ultrasound beam is not being attenuated or enhanced by overlying structures. The central echo complex should be well defined and be the most echogenic structure within the transplant. No peritransplant fluid should be present. Mild dilatation of the collecting system may be seen in otherwise normal transplants (Fig. 14.2) (4, 5).

Doppler Overview and Protocol

Doppler evaluation of the renal transplant may also be performed on transplant patients in whom vascular abnormalities are suspected. These include patients with malfunctioning transplants as well as those who develop hypertension or a bruit after transplant.

Medical Doppler ultrasound devices use the Doppler principle, by which moving objects reflect sound at a different frequency than that sent by the transducer (6). The difference between the transmitted frequency and the received frequency is the Doppler shift frequency. This shift may be positive or negative, depending on whether the motion of the object is toward or away from the transducer. The Doppler shifts are produced by moving red blood cells in blood vessels. At typical ultrasound frequencies and blood velocities the Doppler shifts are in the audible range and can be played over a speaker. Most modern systems also use spectrum analysis to display the Doppler signals

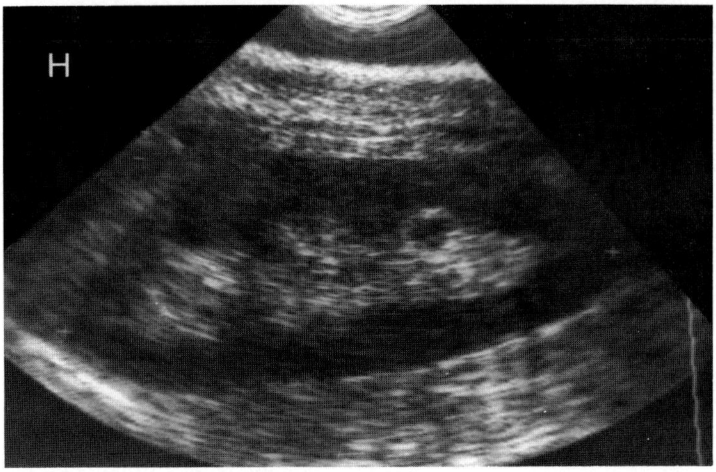

Figure 14.1. Longitudinal scan of a normal renal allograft. The renal sinus is normally echogenic. The renal cortex is minimally more echogenic than the medullary pyramids. *H,* toward the patient's head.

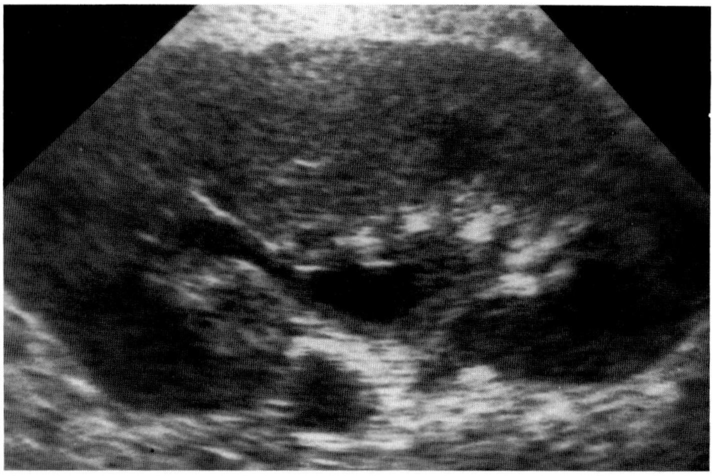

Figure 14.2. Normal renal transplant. There is mild dilatation of the intrarenal collecting system, which is a normal finding.

(Fig. 14.3). This allows a graphical representation of the Doppler shifts the machine is detecting. Forward or reverse flow is represented in the y axis while time is in the x axis. The amplitude of the signal is displayed by the gray scale of the spectrum. Doppler shift frequencies may be converted into velocities if the angle of the Doppler beam to the direction of blood flow is known or assumed. Most modern Doppler devices are duplex pulsed Doppler devices, which restrict the Doppler signals sampled to a small volume of tissue and allow the user to move this sample volume into a specific place within the ultrasound image. Color flow devices are also available that superimpose information about flowing blood on the gray scale image. Flow direction is encoded in different colors and the intensity or color shift indicates differences detected in the velocity of the blood.

Doppler signals are found by placing the sample volume in the region of the vessels and shifting its position until an appropriate signal is heard. It is not necessary to see a vessel sonographically to obtain a correct Doppler signal. An attempt should be made to place the sample volume along the entire length of the main renal artery from its anastomosis (Fig. 14.3) into the renal hilum (Fig. 14.4). The segmental renal vessels are insonated from the superior, middle, and inferior portions of the central sinus (Fig. 14.5); the interlobar arteries from between the renal pyramids (Fig. 14.6); and the upper, middle, and lower arcuate arteries from the corticomedullary junction (Fig. 14.7). Doppler signals from the main renal vein are also obtained (Fig. 14.8). Signals from these sites are adequate unless abnormalities are detected.

The normal renal arterial signal shows forward flow throughout the cardiac cycle. The pulsatility of the waveforms normally diminishes in the more distal renal circulation. This is identified by less difference in velocity between the systolic and diastolic components of the waveform. There is normally a small amount of disturbed flow in the main renal artery near the anastomosis (Fig. 14.3). Renal venous flow shows flow toward the heart. The waveform may be flat or show mild variation.

Color flow imaging may be helpful in identifying the vessels to place the sample volume in them more easily. In the vessels where color can be seen, the color should persist through the cardiac cycle. Color should vary based on the cardiac cycle. Different arteries or veins that are oriented in the same direction should have similar colors. Color in the veins should be relatively constant throughout the cardiac cycle.

PERITRANSPLANT FLUID COLLECTIONS

Fluid collections are frequent following transplantation. These are usually lymphoceles, urinomas, hematomas, seromas, or abscesses. The sonographic pattern of each collection and the time the collection presents after transplantation show that there is overlapping between the various forms. Aspiration and surgical exploration are the definitive means to define the type of fluid present.

In two studies that observed consecutive transplant recipients the incidences of perirenal fluid collections were 42% (7) and 41% (8). In both groups there were a large number of small collections in asymptomatic patients whose contents were not determined (in 10%

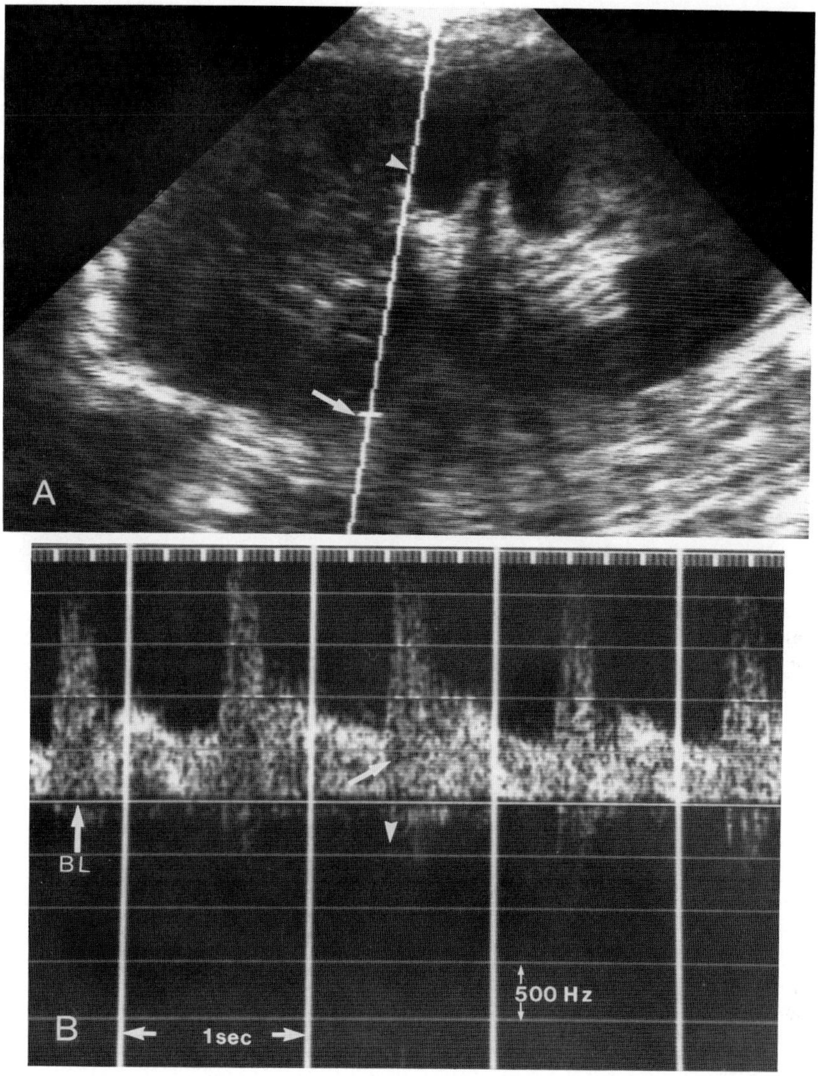

Figure 14.3. Doppler ultrasound of main renal artery. Longitudinal scan of the renal transplant (**A**) shows the line of sight for the Doppler ultrasound sample (*arrowhead*) and the site of the sample volume where the Doppler information is acquired (*arrow*). The main renal artery is sampled outside the confines of the transplant. **B,** Doppler spectral analysis of the main renal artery signal near the anastomosis. The baseline (*BL*) is identified, flow toward the Doppler transducer is above the baseline and flow away from the Doppler transducer is below the baseline. The arterial signal demonstrates flow in the forward direction throughout the cardiac cycle. Flow disturbances that are related to the anastomosis are identified by the lower-velocity signals in the Doppler signal (*arrow*) as well as some flow in the reverse direction (*arrowhead*). Each horizontal division represents 1 second. Each vertical division represents a Doppler shift of 500 Hz. These values may vary from scan to scan based on different machines or a particular machine's settings.

and 18% of transplants, respectively). In most cases these collections resolved or remained stable without compromise to the patient. Other studies suggest a smaller incidence of peritransplant collections. This wide variation reflects not only the different rate of complications among institutions but also the manner in which transplant patients are observed. If ultrasound is used aggressively, more collections (some incidental) will be found than if ultrasound is only called upon to scan patients with frank signs of collections.

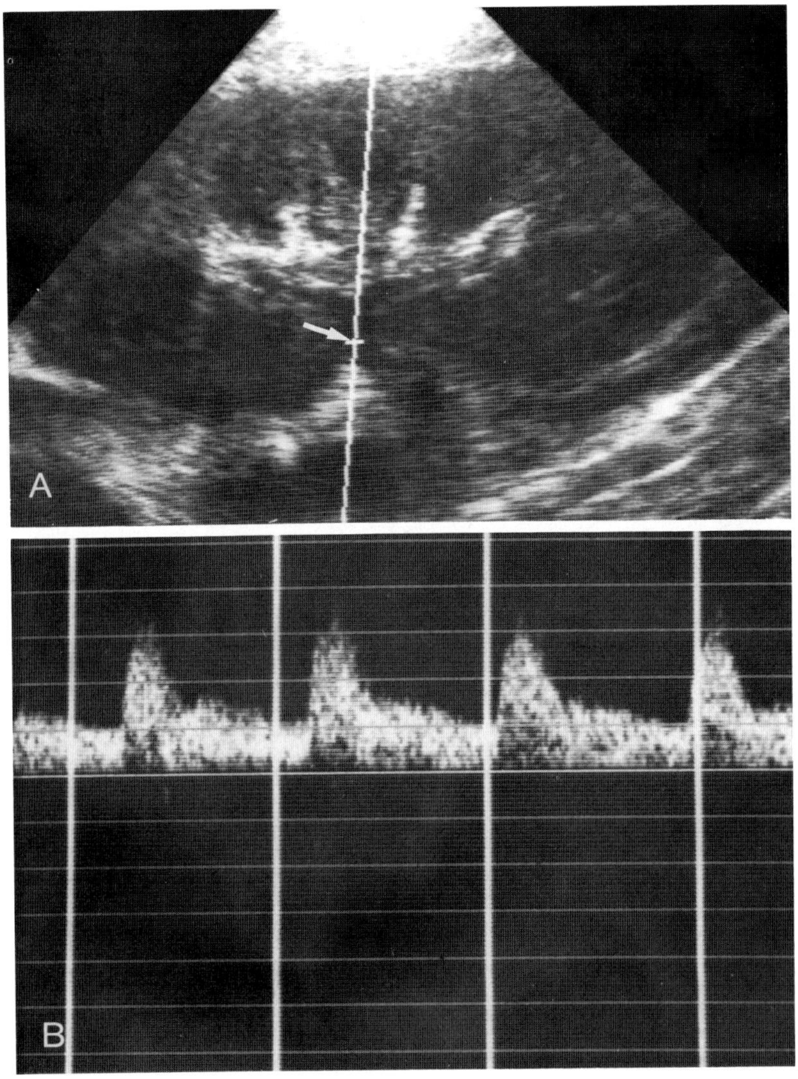

Figure 14.4. Doppler ultrasound of distal main renal artery. **A,** Longitudinal scan showing the sample volume to be in the main renal artery near the renal hilum (*arrow*). **B,** Doppler spectral analysis of the main renal artery shows flow in the forward direction throughout the cardiac cycle. The signal is more organized than the signal obtained in the main renal artery near the anastomosis.

In women the differential diagnosis of fluid collections must include ovarian cysts (9), and this entity should be considered and if possible excluded before aspiration is considered.

Lymphocele

A lymphocele is a collection of lymph that lies in the retroperitoneal space. The source of the lymph is unligated lymphatics rather than lymph production by the allograft (10). Lymphoceles are the most common peritransplant collection. They are seen in 10% to 20% of transplant recipients (7, 8). Small lymphoceles may be asymptomatic, although larger masses may cause transplant dysfunction by producing urinary obstruction or even pressure on hilar vessels. The lymphocele may press on the bladder, causing urinary frequency. Other signs and symptoms may include pain, ipsilateral leg edema, fever, pain and tenderness over the transplant, and persistent wound drainage (10–13). If the collection causes graft dysfunc-

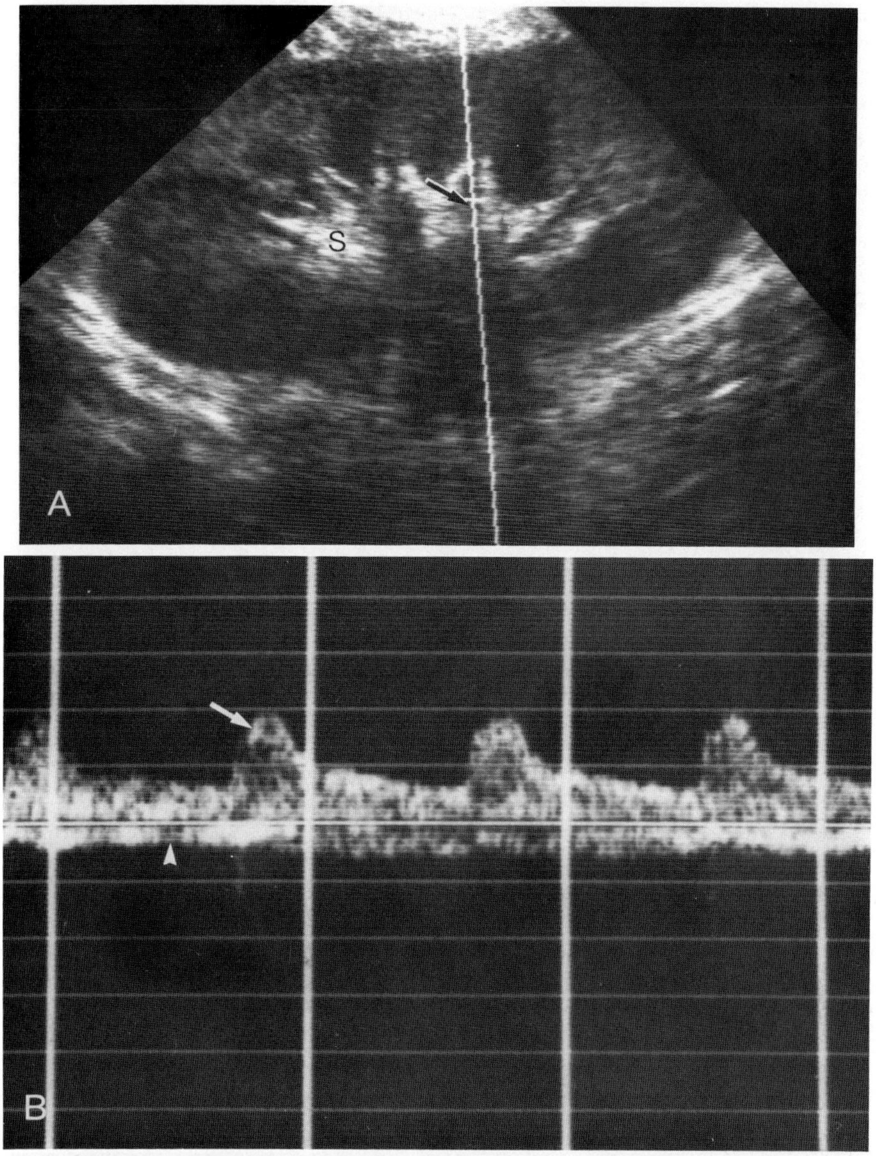

Figure 14.5. Doppler ultrasound of segmental vessels. **A,** Longitudinal scan of the renal transplant shows the sample volume (*arrow*) to lie within the vessels of the renal sinus (*S*). **B,** Doppler spectral analysis shows the arterial signal (*arrow*) flow throughout the cardiac cycle in the forward direction. The difference between systole and diastole is slightly less marked than in the main renal artery, indicating less pulsatility. A paired vein shows flow in the opposite direction below the baseline (*arrowhead*).

tion the collection may mimic rejection. Lymphoceles usually present within several months of the transplant (8, 14), although they have also been reported more than 1 year after the surgery (8, 11).

The sonographic appearance is of a fluid collection, typically related to the lower pole of the kidney (Fig. 14.9). The majority of the lymphoceles are medial to the kidney as well (5, 14). Linear septations have been described in many lymphoceles, 80% in one series (14), although they may also be purely cystic (9). Low-level internal echoes and fluid-fluid levels may rarely be seen in these collections. Layered

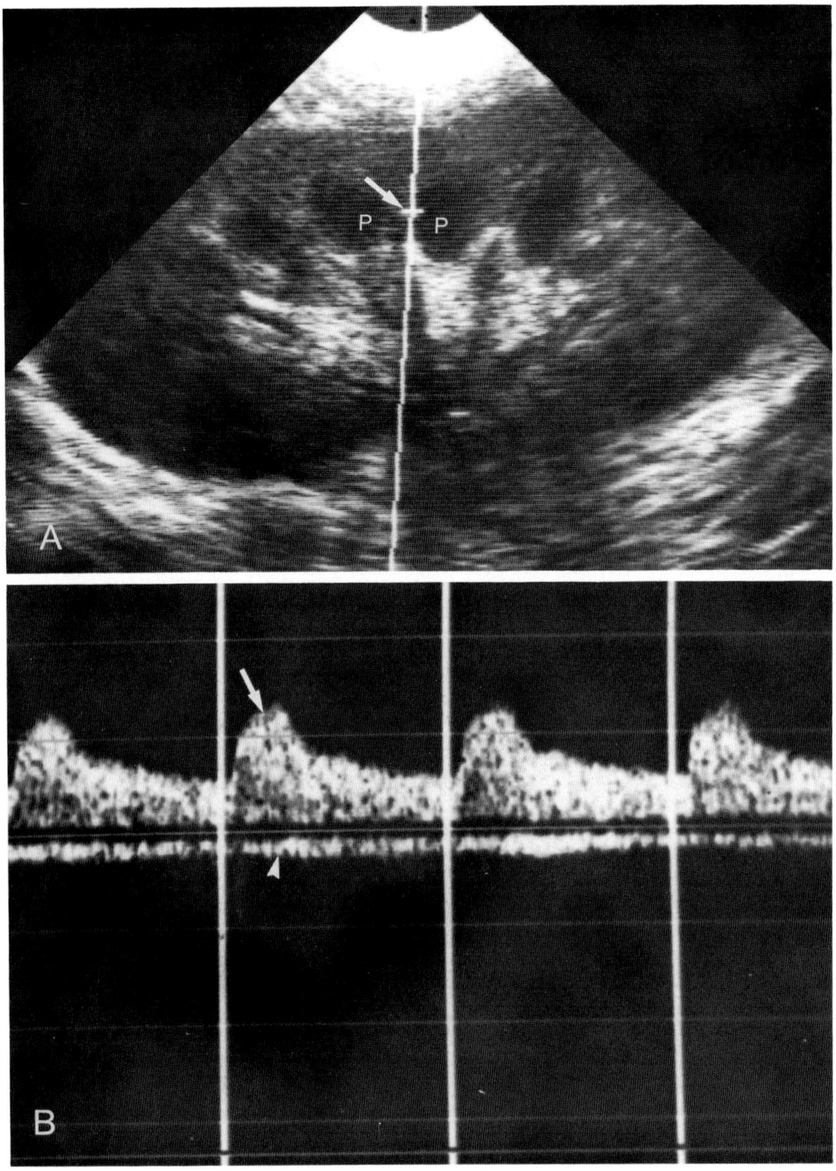

Figure 14.6. Doppler ultrasound of interlobar vessels. **A,** Longitudinal scan of the renal transplant shows the sample volume (*arrow*) to lie between two hypoechoic renal pyramids (*P*). **B,** Doppler spectral analysis reveals the interlobar artery signal (*arrow*) to have flow in the forward direction throughout the cardiac cycle. The paired vein (*arrowhead*) shows flow in the opposite direction.

debris or the development of echoes within previously anechoic fluid may suggest that the lymphocele has become infected (9, 13). Hydronephrosis may or may not be present, depending on the size and location of the collection.

Aspiration or repeated aspirations may treat the lymphocele (7, 8, 10). Problems with this therapy are that the fluid may reaccumulate or infection may be introduced (5, 7, 10, 11, 13). Definitive treatment consists of surgical marsupialization of the cyst into the peritoneal cavity (5, 10, 11).

Hematoma

Hematomas may develop after surgery in the early postoperative period (7, 12). They may also be due to allograft rupture or disruption of the vascular pedicle.

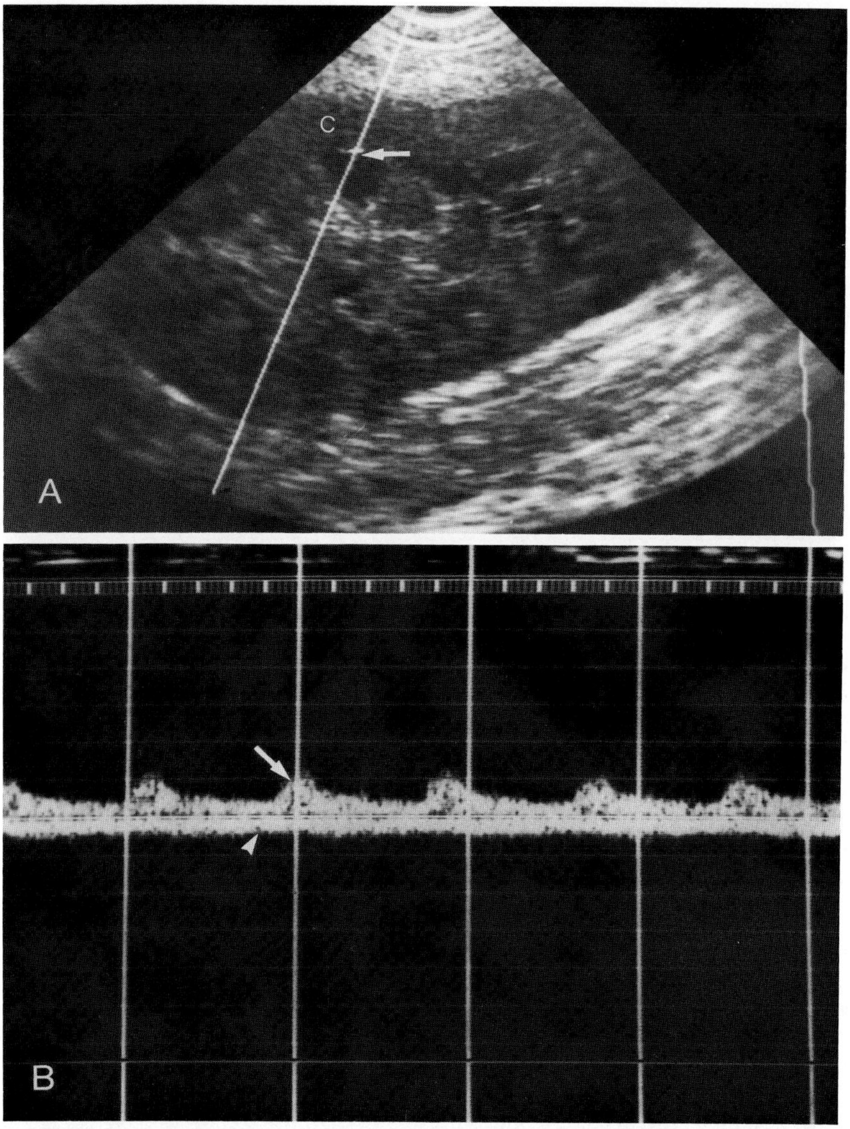

Figure 14.7. Doppler ultrasound of arcuate vessels. **A,** Longitudinal scan of the renal transplant reveals the sample volume (*arrow*) to lie at the corticomedullary junction (*arrow*). *C,* cortex. **B,** Doppler spectral analysis shows the arcuate arterial signal (*arrow*) to lie above the baseline and exhibit low pulsatility. The paired vein (*arrowhead*) shows flow in the opposite direction.

In acute hemorrhage, the onset of pain and a drop in hemoglobin with or without hypotension may be definitive. Some of these patients may be too ill to have imaging prior to surgery. In the less critically ill, symptoms may include pain over the transplant, decreased renal function, hematuria, or fever (9). On ultrasound the hematoma may have a variety of appearances based on its age (Fig. 14.10). Depending on the degree of liquefaction the hematoma may be anechoic or have internal echoes. An echogenic appearance of acute hematoma has also been reported (5, 15, 16). The echogenicity of the hematoma may make smaller collections difficult to separate from surrounding structures or from the kidney itself. A search for a mass effect on the kidney surface may aid the diagnosis. Septations may also be identified within hematomas. The sonographic appearance may be indistinguishable from a lymphocele or abscess.

Transplant rupture as a distinct cause of perirenal hematoma is felt to be due to acute

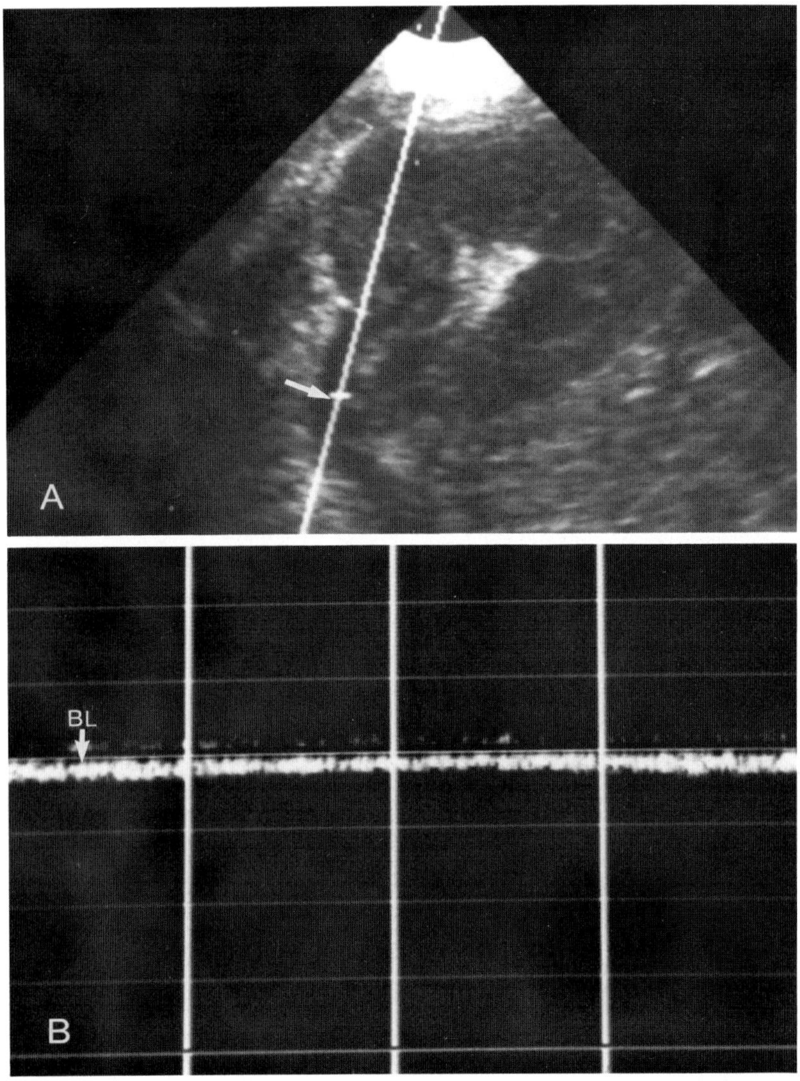

Figure 14.8. Doppler ultrasound of main renal vein. **A,** Transverse scan of the renal transplant shows the sample volume (*arrow*) to lie within the anterior vessel extending from the renal hilum. **B,** Doppler spectral analysis reveals flow below the baseline (*BL*), indicating flow away from the Doppler transducer. The flow is continuous, indicating its venous nature.

enlargement of the allograft. This may be associated with rejection, although the precise pathogenesis is still incompletely understood. Transplant rupture typically occurs within 3 weeks of surgery (15). The rupture typically occurs at the posterior convex surface of the kidney. A perirenal collection was observed in several case reports (15, 17), although the intrarenal component may not be appreciated. Small ruptures seen in association with rejection in children who received transplants were undetected in two cases reported by Slovis and his coworkers (16).

Abscess

Abscesses typically present within weeks of the surgery. The location of the collection is variable. Patients may present with fever and leukocytosis. Abscesses appear as a complex fluid collection, typically with low-level echoes. Septations are the exception in these masses (14). Because the transplant recipients are im-

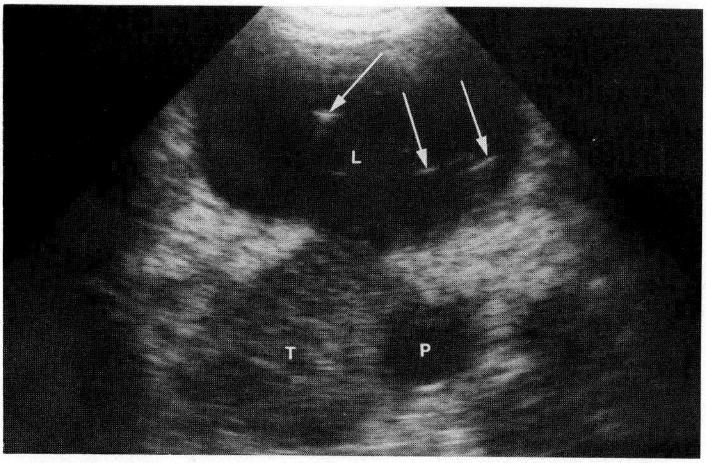

Figure 14.9. Lymphocele. There is a fluid collection anterior to the renal transplant (*L*) which contains several septations (*arrows*). An extrarenal pelvis (*P*) of the renal transplant (*T*) is identified.

munocompromised, the diagnosis of abscess should be made as rapidly as possible. Percutaneous aspiration with or without drainage should be freely used to confirm or exclude this diagnosis once it is entertained.

Seroma

A seroma is a sterile accumulation of serous fluid, which typically lies in the subcutaneous tissues. They rarely cause any significant complications, although they may be confused with wound abscesses.

Urinary Extravasation and Urinomas

Leakage of urine is usually seen in the first month after transplantation. In 15 patients with extravasation, Smolev et al. found 13 to have extravasated within 30 days of transplant, and seven within 7 days (18). The bladder and ureterovesical anastomosis accounted for the sites in two-thirds. The source is usually a necrotic ureter or pelvis. In most instances this is due to ischemia from a compromised blood supply. Rejection is also implicated in ureteral ischemia, although it is less common to produce leaks than postsurgical ischemia (19). Leakage from the kidney itself is quite rare and may be postischemic or occur at the site of biopsy. Caliceal-cutaneous fistula is a potentially devastating complication that can cause loss of the graft and sepsis. These fistulas are more commonly seen when there are multiple renal arteries.

The signs and symptoms of a urine leak are diminished urine output, pain, and swelling

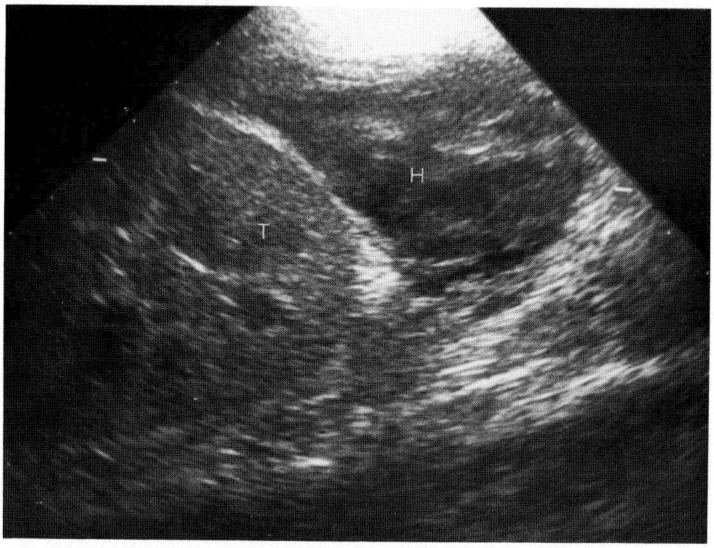

Figure 14.10. Hematoma. A longitudinal view of the lower pole of the renal transplant (*T*) reveals a complex collection (*H*) beneath the transplant.

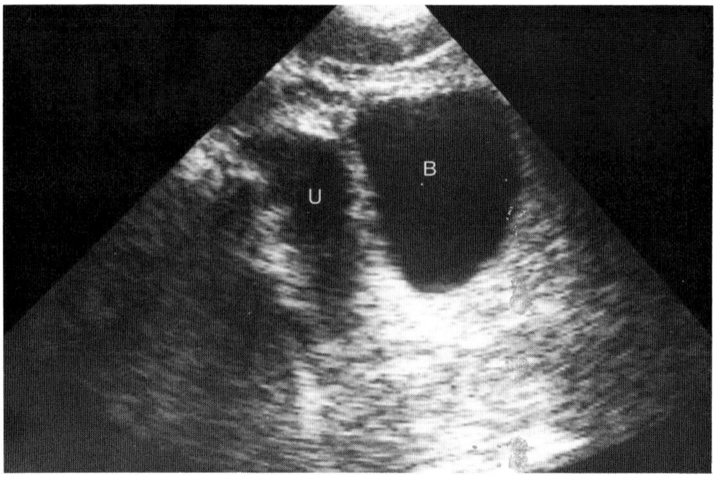

Figure 14.11. Urinoma. A fluid collection (*U*) is located behind the urine-filled bladder (*B*). The fluid is anechoic and without septations. On aspiration this collection was proven to be a urinoma.

over the graft. Creatinine may be elevated due to resorption of the urine.

Sonographically, the urine is usually in the form of a localized fluid collection (urinoma). This is frequently near the ureterovesical junction (Fig. 14.11) but may also be in a less typical extraperitoneal space (Fig. 14.12). Free intraperitoneal fluid representing urine ascites may also be seen in association with the collection. Urine ascites without a discrete urinoma is quite rare. Urinomas are usually simple collections, although fluid levels or septations have been seen (9, 14). Hydronephrosis may not be present since the urinoma may actually decompress the urinary system. The actual tract between the kidney and a cutaneous fistula has been seen sonographically (9). After injecting fluid into the bladder, another group observed bubbles in the bladder and an adjacent fluid collection, thus confirming the vesical leak (20).

The definitive diagnosis of extravasation is made by renal scan or aspiration of the fluid. A creatinine level in the fluid above the blood level is diagnostic of urinoma. A level equal to blood suggests seroma or lymphocele. Ultrasound is the method of choice to direct aspiration of the collection as well as direct antegrade urography, should it be necessary (21, 22).

URINARY OBSTRUCTION

Urinary obstruction (Fig. 14.13) may occur any time after transplantation, although it is more frequently a late complication. The site is most commonly in the distal ureter or ureterovesical junction. The causes are diverse and include postischemic fibrosis, kinks, blood

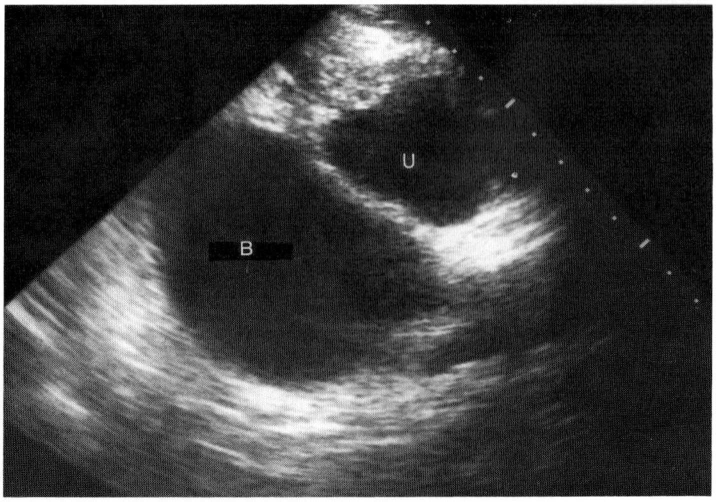

Figure 14.12. Urinoma. There is a simple fluid collection (*U*) anterior to the bladder (*B*) in the extraperitoneal space.

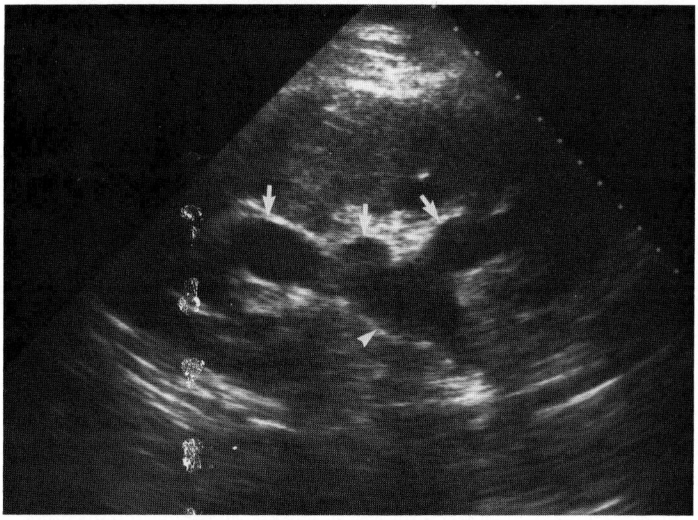

Figure 14.13. Hydronephrosis. Longitudinal view of the transplant reveals dilatation of the intrarenal collecting system (*arrows*) and the renal pelvis (*arrowhead*).

clots, and stones. The fibrosis that follows ischemia may be due to either poor initial ureteric blood supply or rejection and may involve a long segment. Rejection may alter ureteral dynamics and is another cause of dilatation (23). Extrinsic compression of the urinary system by fluid collections is one of the indications for their drainage. Occasionally mechanical obstruction is due to the altered anatomy from a full urinary bladder (21). Determining the site or cause of obstruction may be difficult sonographically since the entire ureter is not visualized. Usually ultrasound can reveal only the ureter near the graft and next to the bladder.

If dilatation of the collecting system is noted and the bladder is full, a postvoid study is necessary. Most times the degree of dilatation will decrease, confirming that there is no fixed obstruction (4). The presence of pelvocaliceal dilatation, even with an empty bladder, does not always indicate obstruction (4, 22). Slight separation of the renal pelvis is essentially a normal finding in the transplant (5). Even when there is marked distention of the pelvis with dilated calices, obstruction may not be present (4). In a study of 49 patients with pelvocaliceal dilatation who subsequently underwent antegrade pyelography, 86% were obstructed while 14% were not. In this study the criteria for a dilated collecting system were not stated, however.

GRAFT DYSFUNCTION

In the postoperative period approximately 10 to 30% of transplants are anuric (1). This depends on the donor matching, the condition of the kidney, maintenance of blood volume, and degree of immunosuppression. The differential diagnosis of anuria in the postoperative period includes obstruction, acute tubular necrosis (ATN), vascular occlusion, and acute rejection. When faced with this condition the clinician will irrigate the bladder catheter to rule out an obstructing clot, order an ultrasound scan to exclude hydronephrosis or fluid collection, and order a nuclear scan to rule out arterial occlusion. If Doppler ultrasound is available it may also be used to exclude an arterial occlusion.

Graft dysfunction may occur anytime. Acute tubular necrosis is rare outside of the immediate postoperative period. Most episodes of acute rejection occur in the first year following transplantation. Cyclosporine nephrotoxicity and chronic rejection may be seen anytime.

Rejection

Rejection is an immunological response by the host to the histocompatibility differences of the transplant. In hyperacute and accelerated rejection, there are preexisting antibodies that produce a rapid failure of the transplant. Hyperacute rejection is recognized at the time of surgery, while accelerated rejection takes hours to days to present. When it is recognized, the transplant is removed. In accelerated rejection two-thirds of transplants are lost acutely and only one-tenth will have a long-term survival.

Acute rejection is most common in the weeks to months following the surgery and it is rare after 1 year. Histologically two patterns are described: interstitial (or cellular) rejection and vascular (or humeral) rejection (24). Often there is a combination of the two, although interstitial rejection, which is milder, is more likely to be present without vascular rejection than the reverse. In interstitial or cellular rejection there is interstitial infiltration and cellular infiltration and damage in the intertubular capillaries. In vascular rejection the vascular endothelium is the site of antibody-induced damage. Glomerular capillaries, venules, and sometimes arterioles show microthrombi and platelet aggregation. There is necrosis of small arteries and arterioles. These vascular changes produce thrombosis and progressive ischemia of the transplant. Interstitial rejection is more likely to respond to therapy than vascular rejection.

The clinical presentation of rejection has been changed by the widespread use of cyclosporine. This immunosuppressive has attenuated the immunological response and the clinical signs of rejection. Acute rejection was formerly accompanied by renal failure, fever, tenderness and swelling over the transplant, hypertension, and weight gain. With cyclosporine the clinical signs may be minimal or absent, and the only clue to the diagnosis may be a rise in serum creatinine during routine surveillance. At our institution any patient who exhibits a 25% increase in creatinine level is considered at risk for acute rejection and given a pulse of steroids. An ultrasound scan and possibly a nuclear scan will be ordered. Further evaluation will be based on the patient's response to steroids and the results of the imaging studies. If the studies indicate a cause other than rejection for the elevated creatinine, that problem will be addressed. A biopsy will be considered if the diagnosis remains uncertain, particularly after the steroids have been allowed to work.

Chronic rejection is characterized by pathological changes in arteries, glomeruli, or both. Arterial narrowing, especially in interlobular or arcuate arteries, is characteristic.

SONOGRAPHY OF ACUTE REJECTION

Although a great deal of the sonographic literature of renal transplants addresses the ability to diagnose or exclude acute rejection, most clinicians either treat or perform biopsy based on the clinical suspicion of rejection, with the diagnosis confirmed clinically by an appropriate response to increased immunosuppression or pathologically by the findings at biopsy.

SONOGRAPHIC TEXTURE

The most common sonographic features associated with acute rejection are enlargement of the transplant (3, 25–30), increased cortical echogenicity (27, 31), increased size of renal pyramids (25, 27, 31, 32), decreased echogenicity of the renal pyramids (31, 32), decreased size and echogenicity of the renal sinus (25, 27, 28, 31, 32), and focal areas within the transplant exhibiting decreased echogenicity (25, 27, 30–32). Other features reported have included perirenal fluid collections (presumably from rupture) (27), distortion of the renal outline (31), cortical thickening (25, 28, 33), increased corticomedullary distinction (30, 31), and indistinct corticomedullary boundaries (25, 27).

Many of these signs have been correlated with histologic changes. The medullary enlargement and diminished echogenicity are associated with edema, congestion, and hemorrhage (Figs. 14.14 and 14.15) (25, 31). The increased cortical echogenicity is associated with cellular infiltration (Fig. 14.14) (25). Focal areas of decreased echogenicity are often hemorrhagic infarction (Fig. 14.16) (25, 31) and occasionally cortical necrosis (25). The decreased echogenicity and size of the central echo complex are due to rejection in this portion of the kidney as well. There is cellular infiltration, edema, microhemorrhages, and infarctions. Fat atrophy and replacement by fibrous tissue play a large role in changing the central sinus echogenicity and diminishing the distinction between the parenchyma and the central sinus echoes (34).

TRANSPLANT VOLUME

The rejecting transplant does enlarge (3, 27, 35, 36). The normal transplant also enlarges after implantation, so the amount of increase must be taken into account before suggesting rejection on this basis. Hricak et al. found normal hypertrophy to be 7 to 25% by the end of the second week after transplant and 14 to 32% by the end of the third week (27). The volume of the normal transplant rarely increases by more than 30% (3, 36). Cochlin et al. found volume changes of up to 30% in over half of 13 transplants (36). The kidney volume should not continue to increase beyond 6 months (37).

In one study, rejection was correctly detected in 83% by a volume increase of greater than 30% between ultrasound scans (3). In another,

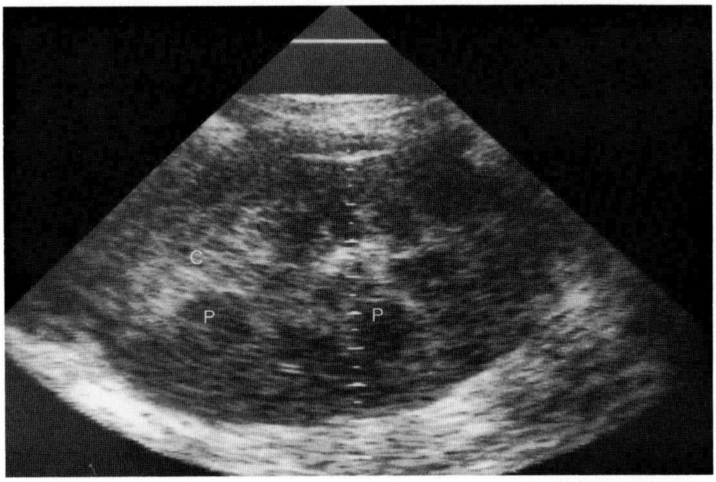

Figure 14.14. Acute rejection. The transplant is swollen, showing the transplant to be quite wide compared to its length. The pyramids (*P*) are more prominent than in normal transplants. The cortical echogenicity is increased and nonhomogeneous, and there is an area of very echogenic cortex in the superior aspect of the transplant (*C*). The central sinus is poorly defined.

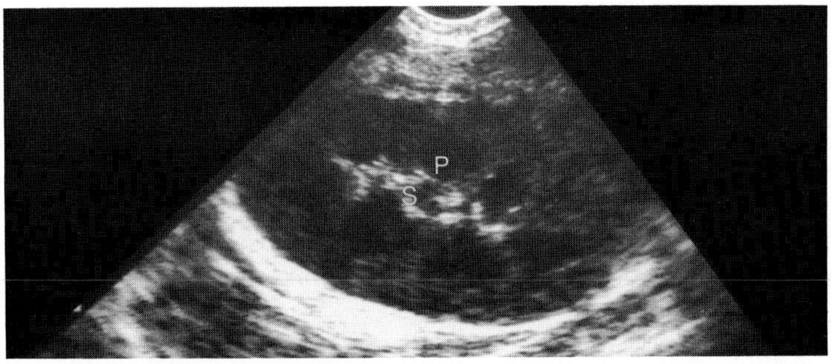

Figure 14.15. Acute rejection. The transplant is swollen. The pyramids (*P*) are larger and more prominent than normal. The cortical echogenicity is normal. The central sinus (*S*) is slightly less defined than normal.

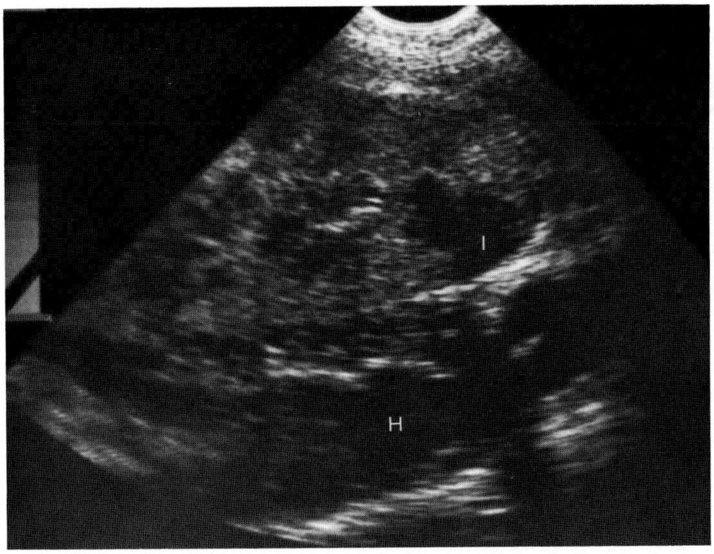

Figure 14.16. Renal infarction. There is a small anechoic area at the lower pole of the kidney (*I*). Its appearance did not change over studies in subsequent months. Incidentally noted is a hematoma (*H*) in the scan obtained during the immediate postoperative period.

a volume increase of greater than 20% over 5 days or 25% by the second week yielded an 84% sensitivity (27). Volume changes of greater than 30% can also be used in children, although the sensitivity and specificity are less than in adults.

DOPPLER OF ACUTE REJECTION

Even in the early stages of acute rejection, there is diminished blood flow and cortical ischemia. This is due to vasoconstriction as well as damage to the capillary network. There is also ischemia produced by the thrombosis in the arterial tree (38–40). The blood flow pattern changes in rejection, with a decrease in diastolic flow and a rapid rise and fall in the systolic portion as shown in both electromagnetic (40) and Doppler studies (41–43). The pattern is due to increased renovascular resistance (43). In severely elevated resistance, the diastolic flow may be absent or even reverse in diastole (Fig. 14.17).

A variety of indices have been devised to evaluate the relationship of the various components of the Doppler flow velocity waveforms in an attempt to quantitate the amount of pulsatility or resistance. A modified Pourcelot index, which some investigators term the resistance index (RI), is a simple measure of resistance. It is calculated by taking the peak systolic frequency (or velocity) minus the end-diastolic frequency (or velocity) and dividing it by the peak systolic frequency (or velocity).

$$\frac{\text{Systole} - \text{diastole}}{\text{systole}}$$

A slightly more complex index, sometimes re-

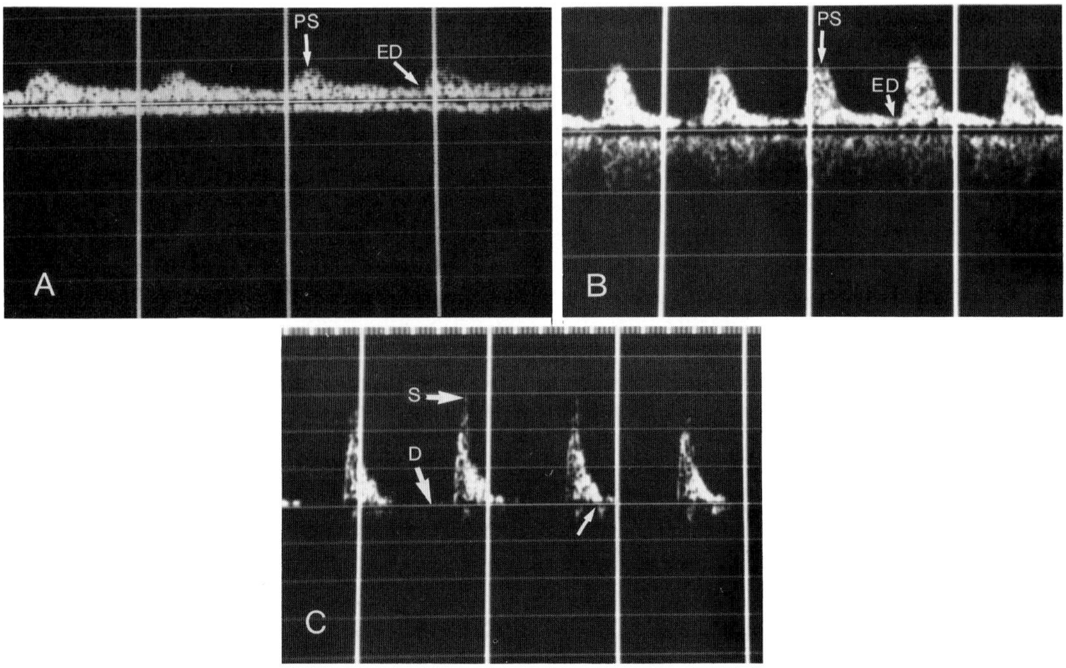

Figure 14.17. **A,** Normal and abnormal pulsatility in the arcuate artery (above the baseline) and arcuate vein (below the baseline) show the arterial signal to have low pulsatility. There is forward flow throughout the cardiac cycle and a small difference in the frequency at peak systole (*PS*) and end-diastole (*ED*). **B,** Increased pulsatility in the arcuate signal with marked difference in the frequencies during the systolic and diastolic components of the waveform. There is still flow in the forward direction throughout the cardiac cycle. A venous waveform is below the baseline. This waveform was taken from a patient with acute rejection. **C,** Doppler ultrasound of an extremely pulsatile arcuate artery. There is no flow during the bulk of the diastolic portion of the cardiac cycle (*D*). The systolic portion (*S*) shows a rapid upstroke and return to the baseline. There is a small component of flow reversal in the artery during the cardiac cycle (*arrow*). This waveform was obtained from a patient with acute rejection.

ferred to as the pulsatility index (PI), is the peak systolic frequency (or velocity) minus the end-diastolic frequency (or velocity) divided by the mean frequency (or velocity).

$$\frac{\text{Systole} - \text{diastole}}{\text{mean}}$$

Other indices of resistance also exist. The RI and PI increase with elevating resistance. Since the pulsatility varies in different vessels, normal values vary according to the indices as well as the vessel insonated.

There are significantly higher pulsatility indices in transplants with acute rejection compared to normals (44–47). Transplants with ATN may have elevated pulsatility indices as well. Some groups found significant differences between rejection and ATN (46), while others did not (45). There is significant overlap of the Doppler waveforms from the two groups. In several studies the most pulsatile Doppler waveforms were 100% specific for rejection, although at a reduced sensitivity of 11% (45), 13% (46), and 55% (47). This was by using a more restrictive RI of greater than 0.90 or a PI of 1.8. In several more recent studies the most pulsatile waveforms have been shown to be produced by diseases other than rejection. These include ATN (48, 49), renal vein obstruction or thrombosis (45, 49, 50), extrarenal compression of the graft (including excessive compression by the transducer) (49, 51), hypotension (49, 51), pyelonephritis (49), and cyclosporine toxicity (48). In one infant with an adult allograft, no diastolic flow was seen in the absence of any pathologic abnormalities, suggesting caution in interpreting indices in infants (48).

Several groups have reported a return to more normal waveforms in rejecting kidneys during treatment (52, 53). The value of serial Doppler examinations needs to be investigated further.

ACCURACY

In two recent studies comparing the sonographic diagnosis of rejection with pathology, the sensitivity of imaging was 72% overall and 85% if a volume increase above 30% was combined with a textural sign of rejection. The specificities were 33% (54) and 94% (3). The positive predictive values of these studies were high, which is to be expected since the prevalence of rejection is high in studies that use the biopsy as a standard. The negative predictive values were relatively low: 17% in one (54) and 79% in the other (3). The low negative predictive value means that a normal ultrasound cannot forestall a biopsy or treatment. In using both sonographic texture and Doppler, Townsend found the elevated resistance index to be better than the texture (55). A specificity of 100% was found with a sensitivity of 26%. If five sonographic criteria of rejection were present (swelling, medullary pyramid enlargement, pelvi-infundibular thickening, increased medullary conspicuity, and decreased renal sinus echogenicity), imaging had a sensitivity of 21% with 100% specificity. By combining Doppler and imaging, 33% of those with acute rejection were detected with 100% positive predictive value. This study consisted only of patients undergoing biopsy and so had a high prevalence of rejection and no cases of ATN. Presumably the specificity of their technique would decrease in a less restricted population.

Although sonographic findings are significantly different in the normal and rejecting transplant, there is sufficient overlapping between normal and abnormal texture and volume and sufficient lack of sensitivity and specificity of elevated Doppler pulsatility indices to hinder their use in clinical practice. No imaging study is consistently accurate enough to base a decision to treat or withhold treatment for rejection. Clinical impression, response to an antirejection treatment regimen, and biopsy continue to be the way rejection and suspected rejection are managed (56).

CHRONIC REJECTION

Chronic rejection may be seen as a normal-sized transplant with little distinction between the cortex, medulla, and central sinus (Fig. 14.18). A small nonhomogeneous kidney is also possible (31). Doppler does not appear to be helpful. Some investigators have shown no change in pulsatility (57, 58), while others have shown high resistance in some cases (44, 48, 55).

ACUTE TUBULAR NECROSIS

In several sonographic studies, in experimental studies of both animals and humans, the texture of the transplant has been sonographically normal (27, 30, 31, 59, 60). Elevated Doppler resistance has been found by several investigators (42, 45, 46, 48, 49). The etiology of the altered flow pattern is obscure. In comparing Doppler to radionuclide evalua-

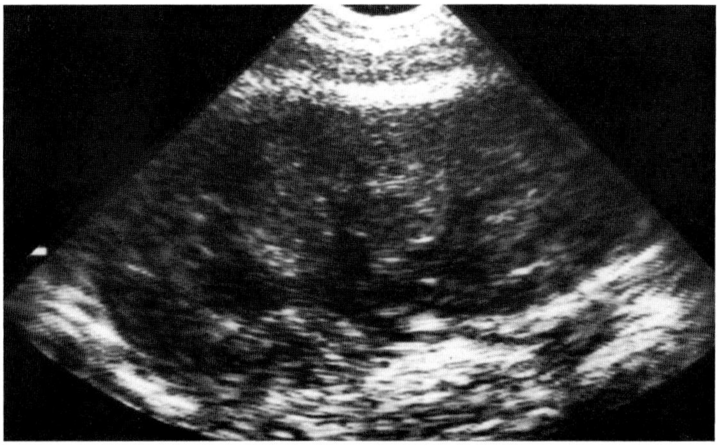

Figure 14.18. Chronic rejection. There is poor definition of the cortex, medullary, and central sinus. The overall size of the transplant is normal.

tion, the nuclear medicine study was superior to Doppler in distinguishing graft rejection from ATN in a study of 56 patients with 38 rejection episodes and 24 instances of ATN (45).

CYCLOSPORINE NEPHROTOXICITY

Cyclosporine toxicity is a cause of post-transplantation renal failure. Sonographic texture cannot be used to differentiate acute rejection from cyclosporine toxicity since many of these patients may also display an abnormal texture (61). Most groups have shown normal Doppler pulsatility in this entity (45, 46, 58), but diminution of diastolic flow has been shown in some cases (48, 62), making distinction of cyclosporine toxicity from other entities impossible in any particular case by duplex scanning alone.

VASCULAR COMPLICATIONS

Arterial Occlusion

Arterial occlusions may result from technical problems at the time of surgery or rejection. Complete occlusion is a catastrophic event, and the subsequent survival of the transplant depends on the rapid reestablishment of flow. Segmental infarction occurs when one of multiple renal arteries or branch vessels is occluded. If the vessels supply a small area there are no significant sequelae. If the devitalized portion is large, the loss of kidney may include the collecting system, producing a pyelocutaneous fistula. Loss of the lower polar artery is to be avoided since it may lead to ureteral or pelvic necrosis.

Infarction usually displays decreased echogenicity of the infarcted area (Fig. 14.16) (31, 63, 64). They extend to the capsule and may produce a mass effect. Rarely there may be a diffusely enlarged and hypoechoic kidney if there is massive infarction. Liquefaction necrosis may produce a sonolucent center, which could mimic other cystic lesions.

By Doppler, the diagnosis of complete occlusion is made by the absence of arterial signals from within the entire kidney after technical factors have been excluded. A high-resistance signal may be obtained in the vessel supplying the transplant. In segmental infarction there is local absence of signals in one part of the kidney with normal signals elsewhere in the transplant (Fig. 14.19). The identification of arterial thrombosis was one of the first reported uses of Doppler for transplants (65) and has been reported by several investigators (42, 57, 66). A diagnosis can usually be made with confidence (66), although confirmatory studies might still be performed because of the importance of the diagnosis.

Venous Occlusion

Venous thrombosis is rare and may be due to extrinsic compression, improper technique, or extension of deep venous thrombosis (67). The Doppler pulsatility of the arterial signal increases (68) and may show a long period of flow reversal during most or all of diastole (45, 49, 50). A venous signal will often be absent (50), although a nonocclusive clot may yield a weak venous signal.

Renal Artery Stenosis

The incidence of renal artery stenosis is 1 to 28% of patients, depending on the study. The higher value is seen in normotensive patients

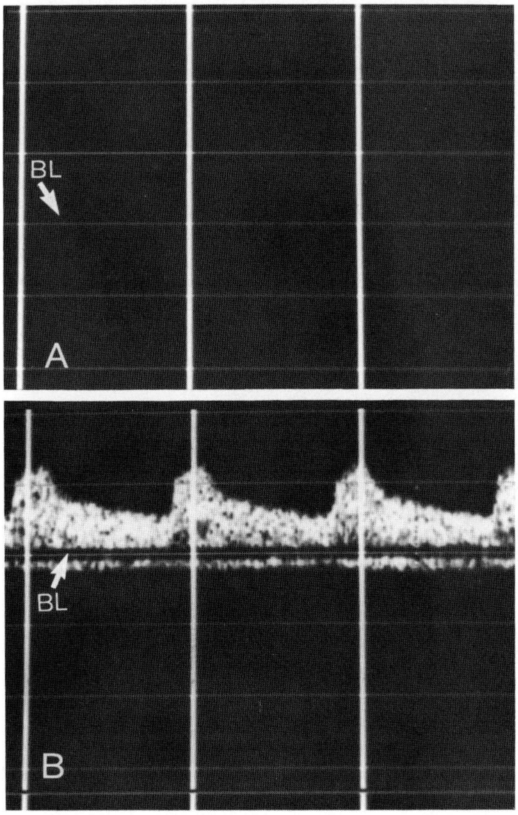

Figure 14.19. Doppler ultrasound of segmental infarction. **A,** Spectral analysis from the upper pole vessels revealed no arterial signal to be present. **B,** Normal arterial signals were obtained from all vessels in the lower pole. *BL,* baseline. The nonperfusion to the upper pole was confirmed by nuclear medicine and angiography. At surgery, a kink in an upper-pole artery was found as the cause of the occlusion to the upper-pole vessels. The patient underwent a heminephrectomy, and the remainder of his course was uneventful.

with routine posttransplantation angiography (67). Usually the diagnosis is suggested by clinical signs such as the new development of hypertension, worsening hypertension, or the appearance or change in a bruit over the transplant.

The diagnosis of renal artery stenosis depends on insonating the main renal artery throughout its course. The Doppler criteria of a significant stenosis are increased blood velocity through the stenosis (Fig. 14.20) and turbulence downstream from the stenosis. Downstream turbulence is detected by the presence of both forward and reverse flow and the shift of the blood velocity toward the baseline. Diminished pulsatility or diminished upstroke downstream from the stenosis might also be observed. A false-positive diagnosis may occur if there is increased velocity without turbulence or mild turbulence without detection of the jet. Mild turbulence may be produced by the anastomosis itself, and it should not be mistaken for a stenosis.

Taylor et al. used the criterion of a 7.5-kHz peak frequency (with a 3.0-MHz transducer) when associated with turbulence (66). This criterion was also used successfully by another group (69). A lower peak systolic frequency (greater than 3.0 kHz with a 5.0-MHz transducer) was used successfully in pediatric transplants (70). Several studies have shown Doppler to be reliable, with specificities varying between 86 and 100% (66, 69–72). In one study comparing 31 patients with angiography, duplex sonography detected 94% of patients with significant stenoses (69). In light of its high sensitivity and noninvasive character, Doppler is an excellent screening method for this entity.

Arteriovenous Fistulas

Arteriovenous fistulas (AVFs) in transplants are a well-recognized complication of renal biopsies. The vast majority are small and asymptomatic. Treatment is not necessary unless it produces hematuria or hypertension. The exact incidence following transplant biopsy is unknown, but 16% is quoted in native kidneys (73).

Duplex reveals marked turbulence due to the large pressure gradient and abnormal connection between vessels (Fig. 14.21) (66, 72). Increased velocities and diminished pulsatility in the arteries leading to the fistula may be noted (66, 73). The draining vein may show excessive pulsatility (73). On color Doppler imaging the artery feeding the AVF, and possibly its draining vein, may stand out by a difference in color than its neighbors, which have slower velocities. Extravascular color in the nearby parenchyma may also herald its presence (73).

CONCLUSION

Ultrasound has become a useful tool in the evaluation of the renal transplant. While the findings are not always diagnosis specific, the information obtained by the sonogram cer-

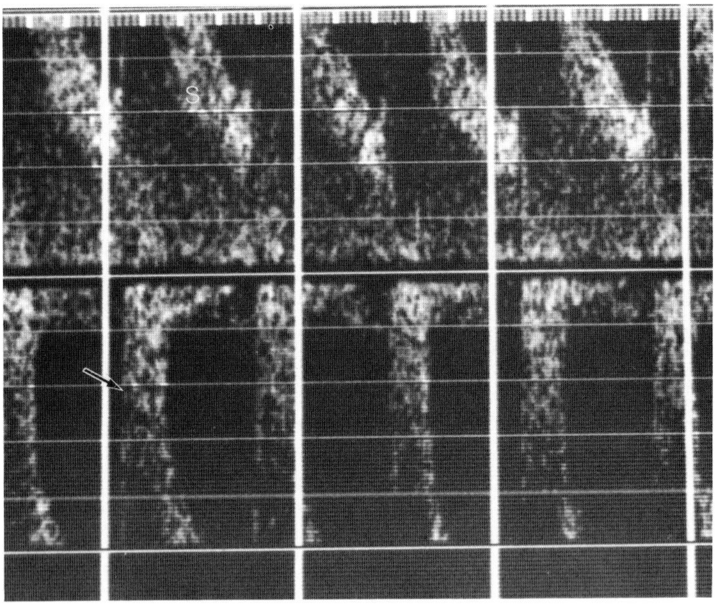

Figure 14.20. Doppler ultrasound of renal artery stenosis. Doppler spectral analysis from the main renal artery reveals extremely high-velocity flow related to the jet of blood produced by a stenotic segment of the renal artery. Although the blood is moving in the forward direction, it is moving so rapidly that the Doppler misinterprets this as flow in the reverse direction. This is known as aliasing. In this example, the most rapidly moving blood in the systolic portion of the waveform (*arrow*) is falsely placed by the spectrum analyzer below the baseline. Each gradation represents 1 kHz Doppler shift, and the actual frequency shift of the jet of blood is approximately 11 kHz. *S,* rapidly moving systolic portion of the jet, which is not aliased.

Figure 14.21. Arteriovenous fistula. Doppler spectral analysis reveals the extremely turbulent and high-velocity flow through this arteriovenous malformation. There is no organized signal, and flow is present both above and below the baseline. A large proportion of the flow is concentrating at the low velocities. The arteriovenous fistula was produced by renal biopsy. It was not visualized on ultrasound images.

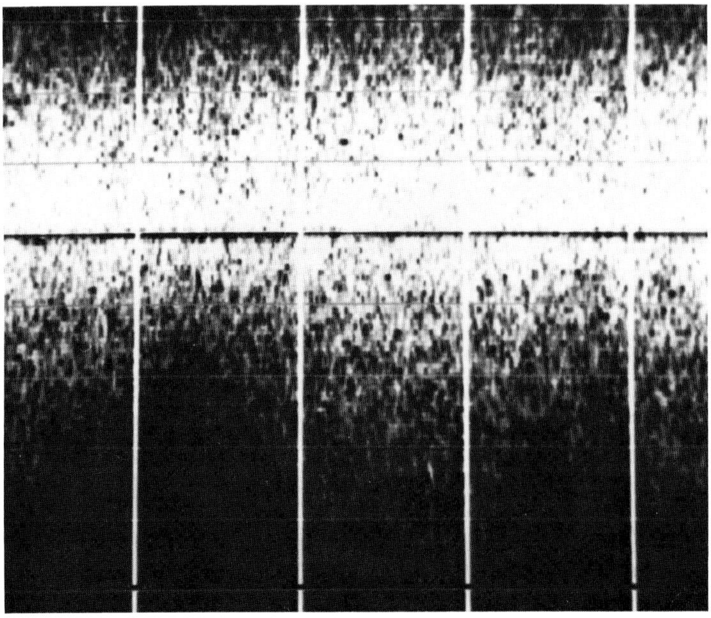

tainly is beneficial in the algorithm for the evaluation of renal transplantation.

References

1. Keown PA, Stiller CR. Kidney transplantation. Surg Clin North Am 1986;66:517–518.
2. Lee HM. Technical aspects of renal transplantation. In: Cerilli GJ, ed. Organ transplantation and replacement. Philadelphia: JB Lippincott, 1988:337.
3. Raiss GJ, Bree RL, Schwab RE, Schultz SR, Salem NG, Rosenberg BF. Further observations in the ultrasound evaluation of renal allograft rejection. J Ultrasound Med 1986;5:439–444.
4. Balchunas WR, Hill MC, Isikoff MB, Morillo G. The clinical significance of dilatation of the collecting system in the transplanted kidney. J Clin Ultrasound 1982;10:221–225.
5. Fleischer AC, James AE, MacDonnell RC, et al. Sonography of renal transplant patients. CRC Crit Rev Diagn Imaging 1982;18:197–242.
6. Burns PN. The physical principles of Doppler and spectral analysis. J Clin Ultrasound 1987; 15:567–590.
7. Yap R, Madrazo B, Oh HK, Dienst ST. Perirenal fluid collection after renal transplant. Am Surg 1981;47:287–290.
8. Morley P, Barnett E, Bell PRF, et al. Ultrasound in the diagnosis of fluid collections following renal transplantation. Clin Radiol 1975;26:199–207.
9. Coyne SS, Walsh JW, Tisnado J, et al. Surgically correctable renal transplant complications: an integrated clinical and radiologic approach. AJR 1981;136:1113–1119.
10. Benvenisty AI, Hardy MA. Selected complications of renal transplantation. In: Cerilli GJ, ed. Organ transplantation and replacement. Philadelphia: JB Lippincott, 1988:462.
11. Greenberg BM, Perloff LJ, Grossman RA, Naji A, Barker CF. Treatment of lymphocele in renal allograft recipients. Arch Surg 1985;120:501–504.
12. Kumar R, Wilson DD, Santa-Cruz FR. Postoperative urological complications of renal transplantation. RadioGraphics 1984;4:531.
13. Ridge JA, Manco-Johnson ML, Weil R III. Ultrasonographic diagnosis of infected lymphocele after kidney transplantation. Eur Urol 1987; 13:31–34.
14. Silver TM, Campbell D, Wicks JD, Lorber MI, Surace P, Turcotte J. Peritransplant fluid collections. Radiology 1981;138:145–151.
15. Rahatzad M, Henderson SC, Boren GS. Ultrasound appearance of spontaneous rupture of renal transplant. J Urol 1981;126:535.
16. Slovis TL, Babcock DS, Hricak H, et al. Renal transplant rejection: sonographic evaluation in children. Radiology 1984;153:659–665.
17. Ostrovsky PD, Carr L, Goodman JD, Moser FG. Ultrasound findings in renal transplant rupture. J Clin Ultrasound 1985;13:132–133.
18. Smolev JK, McLoughlin MG, Rolley R, Sterioff S, Williams GM. The surgical approach to urological complications in renal allotransplant recipients. J Urol 1977;117:10.
19. Salvatierra O Jr, Olcott C IV, Amend WJ Jr, Cochrum KC, Feduska NJ. Urological complications of renal transplantation can be prevented or controlled. J Urol 1977;117:421.
20. Rabinovici R, Rivkind A, Lebensart PD, Berlatzky Y. Ultrasonographic diagnosis of vesical leakage in a renal transplant recipient. Urol Radiol 1986;8:112–113.
21. Hunter DW. Evaluation and treatment of nonvascular problems of the transplanted kidney. Semin Interventional Radiol 1986;3:104–114.
22. Smith TP, Hunter DW, Letourneau JG, et al. Urinary obstruction in renal transplants: diagnosis by antegrade pyelography and results of percutaneous treatment. AJR 1988;151:507–510.
23. Hricak H, Mark AS, Alpers CE, Littleton RH. Sonographic evaluation of the rejecting ureter. Urol Radiol 1986;8:25–31.
24. Porter KA. Renal transplantation. In: Heptinstall R, ed. Pathology of the kidney. Boston: Little, Brown, 1983:1455–1547.
25. Hricak H, Toledo-Pereyra LH, Eyler WR, Madrazo BL, Zammit M. The role of ultrasound in the diagnosis of kidney allograft rejection. Radiology 1979;132:667–672.
26. Bartrum RJ Jr, Smith EH, D'Orsi CJ, Tilney NL, Dantono J. Evaluation of renal transplants with ultrasound. Radiology 1976;118:405–410.
27. Hricak H, Cruz C, Eyler WR, Madrazo BL, Romanski R. Acute post-transplantation renal failure: differential diagnosis by ultrasound. Radiology 1981;139:441–449.
28. Heckemann R, Rehwald U, Jakubowski HD, Donhuijsen K. Sonographic criteria for renal allograft rejection. Urol Radiol 1982;4:15–18.
29. Parvin SD, Rees Y, Veitch PS, Bell PRF. Objective measurement by ultrasound to distinguish cyclosporin A toxicity from rejection. Br J Surg 1986;73:1009–1011.
30. Singh A, Cohen WN. Renal allograft rejection: sonography and scintigraphy. AJR 1980;135:73–77.
31. Maklad NF, Wright CH, Rosenthal SJ. Gray scale ultrasonic appearances of renal transplant rejection. Radiology 1979;131:711–717.
32. Frick MP, Feinberg SB, Sibley R, Idstrom ME. Ultrasound in acute renal transplant rejection. Radiology 1981;138:657–660.
33. Hillman BJ, Birnholz JC, Busch GJ. Correlation of echographic and histologic findings in suspected renal allograft rejection. Radiology 1979;132:673–676.
34. Hricak H, Romanski RN, Eyler WR. The renal sinus during allograft rejection: sonographic and histopathologic findings. Radiology 1982;142: 693–699.
35. Lachance SL, Adamson D, Barry JM. Ultrasonically determined kidney transplant hypertrophy. J Urol 1988;139:497–498.
36. Cochlin DLL, Wake A, Salaman JR, Griffin PJA. Ultrasound changes in the transplant kidney. Clin Radiol 1988;39:373–376.
37. Absy M, Metreweli C, Matthews C, Khader AA. Changes in transplanted kidney volume measured by ultrasound. Br J Radiol 1987;60:525–529.
38. Rosen SM, Retik AB, Hollenberg NK, et al. Effect

of immunosuppressive therapy on the intrarenal distribution of blood flow in dog renal allograft rejection. Surg Forum 1966;17:233–234.
39. Hollenberg NK, Birtch A, Rashid A, et al. Relationships between intrarenal perfusion and function: serial hemodynamic studies in the transplanted human kidney. Medicine 1972;51: 95–106.
40. Henry WL, Kountz SL, Cohn R, et al. Changes in pulsatile blood flow in autograft and homograft kidneys during rejection. Transplantation 1969; 7:545–553.
41. Arima M, Ishibashi M, Michiyuki U, et al. Analysis of the arterial blood flow patterns of normal and allografted kidneys by the directional ultrasonic Doppler technique. J Urol 1979;122:587–591.
42. Berland LL, Lawson TL, Adams MB, et al. Evaluation of renal transplant with pulsed Doppler duplex sonography. J Ultrasound Med 1982;1: 215–222.
43. Norris CS, Barnes RW. Renal artery flow velocity analysis: a sensitive measure of experimental and clinical renovascular resistance. J Surg Res 1984;36:230–236.
44. Don S, Kopecky KK, Filo RS, et al. Duplex Doppler US of renal allografts: causes of elevated resistive index. Radiology 1989;171:709–712.
45. Allen KS, Jorkasky DK, Arger PH, et al. Renal allografts: prospective analysis of Doppler sonography. 1988;169:371–376.
46. Rifkin MD, Needleman L, Pasto ME. Evaluation of renal transplant rejection by duplex Doppler examination: value of the resistive index. AJR 1987;148:759–767.
47. Rigsby CM, Burns PN, Weltin GG, et al. Doppler signal quantification in renal allografts: comparison in normal and rejection transplants, with pathologic correlation. Radiology 1987;162: 39–42.
48. Genkins SM, Sanfilippo FP, Carroll BA. Duplex Doppler sonography of renal transplants: lack of sensitivity and specificity in establishing pathologic diagnosis. AJR 1989;152:535–539.
49. Warshauer DM, Taylor KJW, Bia MJ, et al. Unusual causes of increased vascular impedance in renal transplants: duplex Doppler evaluation. Radiology 1988;169:367–370.
50. Reuther G, Wanjura D, Bauer H. Acute renal vein thrombosis in renal allografts: detection with duplex Doppler US. Radiology 1989;170: 557–558.
51. Pozniak MA, Kelcz F, Stratta RJ, Oberley TD. Extraneous factors affecting resistive index. Invest Radiol 1988;23:899–904.
52. Murphy AM, Robertson RJ, Dubbins PA. Duplex ultrasound in the assessment of renal transplant complications. Clin Radiol 1987;38:229–234.
53. Rigsby CM, Taylor KJW, Weltin G, et al. Renal allografts in acute rejection: evaluation using duplex sonography. Radiology 1986;158:375–378.
54. Hoddick W, Filly RA, Blackman U, et al. Renal allograft rejection: US evaluation. Radiology 1986;161:469–473.
55. Townsend RR, Tomlanovich SJ, Goldstein RB, Filly RA. Combined Doppler and morphologic sonographic evaluation of renal transplant rejection. J Ultrasound Med 1990;9:199–206.
56. Imaging the transplanted kidney [Editorial]. Lancet 1986;1:781.
57. Arima M, Takahara S, Ihara H, et al. Predictability of renal allograft prognosis during rejection crisis by ultrasonic Doppler flow technique. Urology 1982;19:389–394.
58. Buckley AR, Cooperberg PL, Reeve CE, Magil AB. The distinction between acute renal transplant rejection and cyclosporine nephrotoxicity: value of duplex sonography. AJR 1987;149:521–525.
59. Hricak H, Toledo-Pereyra LH, Eyler WR, Madrazo BL, Sy GS. Evaluation of acute post-transplant renal failure by ultrasound. Radiology 1979;133:443–447.
60. Swobodnik WL, Spohn BE, Wechsler JG, et al. Real-time ultrasound evaluation of renal transplant failure during the early postoperative period. Ultrasound Med Biol 1986;12:97–105.
61. Linkowski GD, Warvariv V, Filly RA, Vincenti F. Sonography in the diagnosis of acute renal allograft rejection and cyclosporine nephrotoxicity. AJR 1987;148:291–295.
62. Ubhi CS, Irving HC, Norwood HM, Guillou PJ, Giles GR. Monitoring of renal allografts by Doppler ultrasound. Ann R Coll Surg Engl 1987; 69:229–232.
63. Becker JA, Butt K, Lipkowitz G. Segmental infarction of the renal allograft: ultrasound/MRI observations. Urol Radiol 1989;11:109–112.
64. Stuck KJ, Jafri SZ, Adler DD, Campbell DA, Dafoe DC, Silver TM. Ultrasound evaluation of uncommon renal transplant complications. Urol Radiol 1986;8:6–12.
65. Marchioro TL, Strandness DE, Krugmire RD. The ultrasonic detector for determining vascular patency in renal homografts. Transplantation 1969;8:296–298.
66. Taylor KJW, Morse SS, Rigsby CM, et al. Vascular complications in renal allografts: detection with duplex Doppler US. Radiology 1987;162: 31–38.
67. Tellis VA, Matas AJ, Veith FJ. Vascular complications of transplantation. In: Cerilli GJ, ed. Organ transplantation and replacement. Philadelphia: JB Lippincott, 1988:423.
68. Wood RFM, Nasmyth DG. Doppler ultrasound in the diagnosis of vascular occlusion in renal transplantation. Transplantation 1982;33:547.
69. Snider JF, Hunter DW, Moradian GP, Castaneda-Zuniga WR, Letourneau JG. Transplant renal artery stenosis: evaluation with duplex sonography. Radiology 1989;172:1027–1030.
70. Stringer DA, O'Halpin D, Daneman A, Liu P, Geary DF. Duplex Doppler sonography for renal artery stenosis in the post-transplant pediatric patient. Pediatr Radiol 1989;19:187–192.
71. Reinitz ER, Goldman MH, Sais J, et al. Evaluation of transplant renal artery blood flow by Doppler sound-spectrum analysis. Arch Surg 1983;118:415–419.
72. Ferretti G, Salomone A, Malfi B, Segoloni GP. Duplex scanning and the transplanted kidney. Lancet 1986;2:219.
73. Middleton WD, Kellman GM, Melson GL, Madrazo BL, Postbiopsy renal transplant arteriovenous fistulas: color Doppler US characteristics. Radiology 1989;171:253–257.

CHAPTER 15

Interventional Ultrasonography of the Genitourinary Tract

STEVEN M. COHEN, M.D.
MATTHEW D. RIFKIN, M.D.

Although nonsurgical percutaneous aspiration has been used for over a century, the technique was limited to large lesions. The development of fluoroscopy allowed more accurate needle placement, but with the development and use of diagnostic ultrasound in the 1970s smaller areas and normal structures not previously identifiable could be evaluated. This permitted accurate percutaneous needle placement into solid tissue for biopsy and fluid for aspiration. The advantages of ultrasonographic guidance include measurement of size, position, and depth from the skin surface of the lesion or collection. The absence of ionizing radiation and the availability of multiple scanning planes are also important advantages of ultrasound versus fluoroscopy. Both the tip of the aspiration or biopsy needle and the path of the needle can be monitored during puncture.

This chapter deals with the clinical applications and techniques of percutaneous needle placement and intervention in the genitourinary tract (including extracorporeal shock wave lithotripsy) using ultrasound.

EQUIPMENT

There has been considerable technologic advancement in the field of diagnostic and therapeutic interventional sonography since its introduction in the 1970s. Whereas the prototype equipment used A-mode aspiration transducers with a frequency of 2.25 MHz (1, 2), the advent of B-scan technology introduced improved and more easily adaptable transducers for use in interventional procedures.

Today, most ultrasound-guided interventional procedures are performed using real-time equipment. These enable the physician or operator to have constant, dynamic image updating of the position of various anatomic structures and physiologic motion associated with these structures. The units used today are more mobile than the scanners used in the past, permitting studies and interventional procedures to be performed outside the confines of the ultrasound facility.

Several basic types of transducers have been designed for real-time use in interventional techniques, including the following:

1. A linear array scanner with a central channel in which the needle can be inserted perpendicular to the scan plane. Once the needle has been placed in the designated mass or collection, the transducer can then be removed and the procedure completed (3) (Fig. 15.1).
2. Another type of liner array scanner with side attachment permits needle angulation.
3. A phased array scanner with a detachable needle guide.
4. A mechanical sector scanner with either a permanent or a detachable guidance system.
5. Endoluminal scanners for endorectal or endovaginal use (4) (Fig. 15.2).

A free-hand technique without a specific needle guide attachment may be used with just about any type of real-time transducer.

Biopsy guides vary depending on the type of transducer. For example, a clip-on device has been developed for use on the mechanical sector scanners. A benefit of the sector scanner is that the needle path (which is slightly oblique from the ultrasound beam) is visualized in its entirety more often than when using a linear array transducer. This permits immediate redirection of the needle if needed and accurate placement in the desired location (Fig. 15.3). If the biopsy needle becomes obscured during the procedure, manipulation of the needle (by moving it slightly back and forth or up and down)

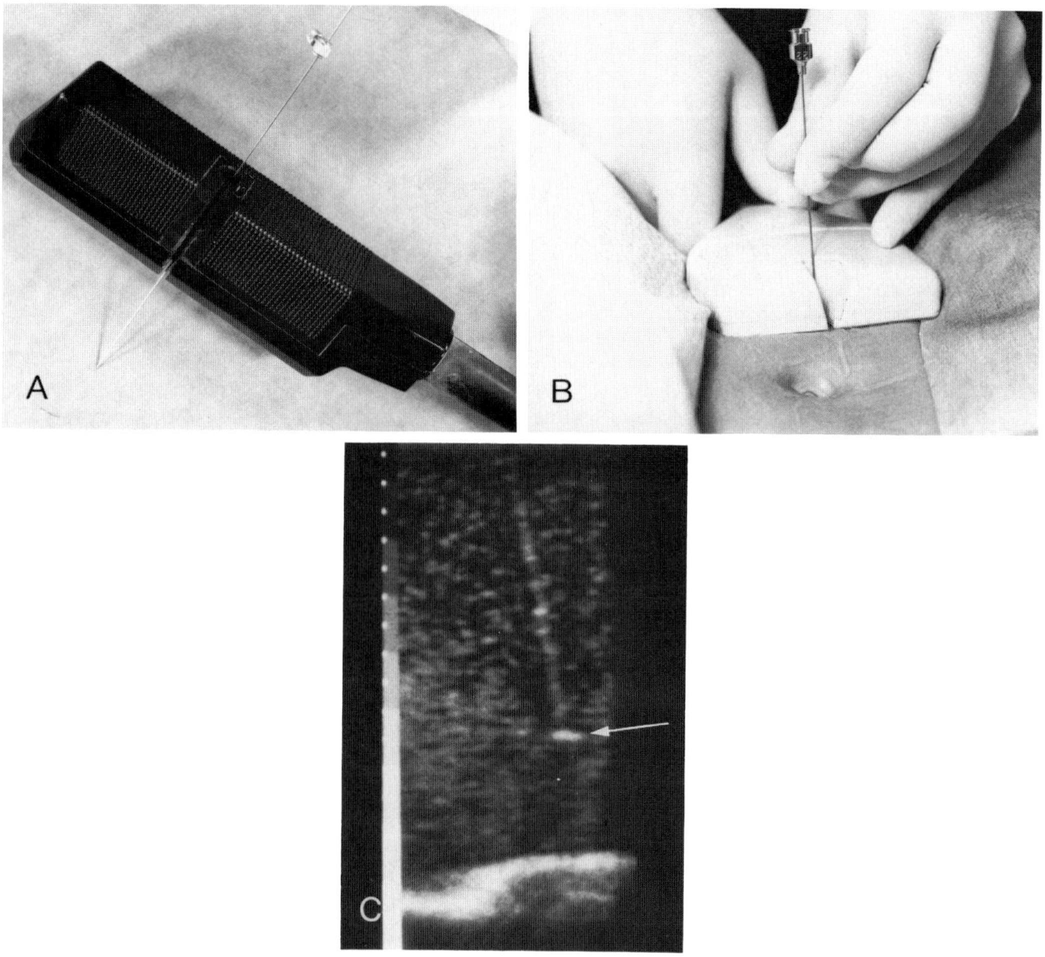

Figure 15.1. **A,** Linear transducer with central biopsy port. **B,** Use of a linear transducer with a centrally placed needle guide; the targeted lesion is placed at the center of the sonic field and a biopsy needle is advanced percutaneously toward it. **C,** Using real-time imaging, any slight deviation from a directly perpendicular path can be corrected for by angling the needle appropriately (*arrow* indicates needle tip).

will immediately help to reestablish its position. This is a time-saving advantage when compared with computed tomography, in which rescanning to confirm needle placement is necessary.

In addition to the actual hardware and imaging equipment, other items needed for most of the interventional procedures performed on the genitourinary tract may include the following (Fig. 15.4):

1. Antiseptic cleansing agent (i.e., Betadine),
2. Sterile gauze,
3. Various size venopuncture needles for skin and deeper anesthesia,
4. A variety of syringes,
5. Local anesthetic (i.e., xylocaine),
6. No. 11 scalpel blade,
7. Needle stop,
8. Sterile drapes,
9. Sterile gloves,
10. A ruler,
11. Extension tubing,
12. Various 18- to 23-gauge needles (i.e., Chiba and/or cutting needles, depending on the clinical situation and procedure to be performed).

Several varieties of thin, noncutting needles for cytologic evaluation and sampling are avail-

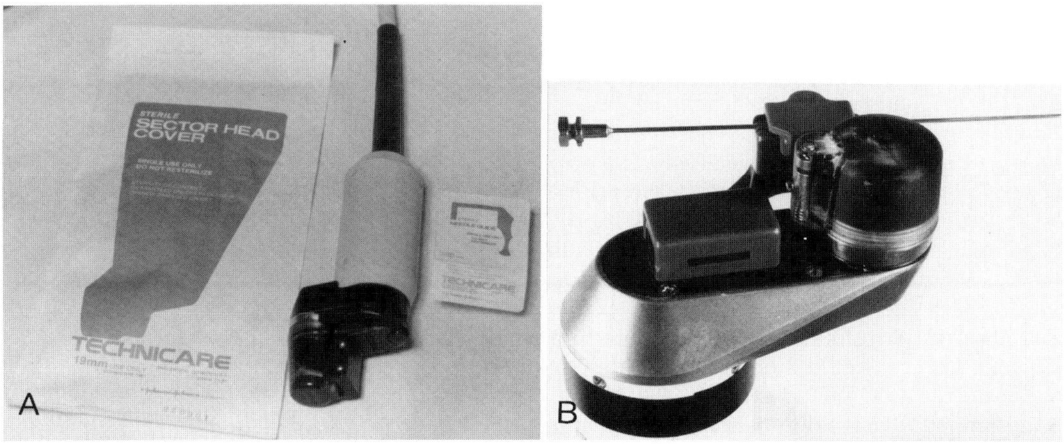

Figure 15.2. **A,** Mechanical sector transducer, with form-fitting sterile rubber cover and needle guide attachment. **B,** Close-up view of mechanical sector transducer with needle guide attachment engaged. Care should be taken to set the biopsy guide on the ultrasound machine to the proper side (left vs. right, superior vs. inferior).

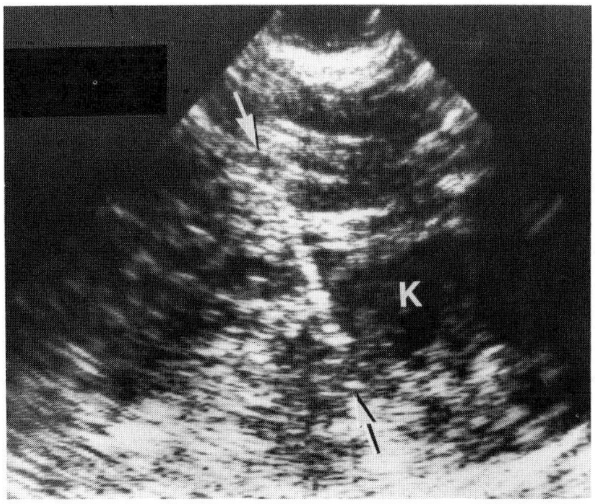

Figure 15.3. Real-time image of a biopsy needle (*arrows*) entering the lower pole of a native kidney (*K*).

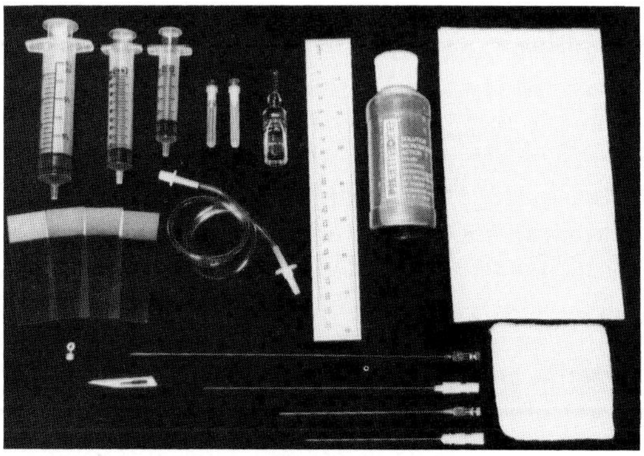

Figure 15.4. A typical aspiration or biopsy tray setup (see list in text).

able. While spinal needles can be used, a popular and frequently used needle is the "Chiba," which has a noncutting, short-angle beveled tip and is available in 18- to 23-gauge sizes and various lengths (5). Other needles have also been specifically designed for ultrasonically guided punctures. These have a corrugated Teflon coating that does not cause any increased tissue trauma but permits easier needle identification on ultrasound. A screw biopsy stylet may also be used to aid in needle tip localization (6).

Cutting needles are usually used to obtain larger tissue cores. These include, among others, the Westcott, Lee, Tru-cut or one of the Tru-cut type needles, which may have side-hole slots; the Madayag and Green needles with beveled tips; and the Franseen needle which has a Teflon tip with cutting teeth. A Rotex needle with a tapered screw tip is also available. These needles are obtained in various gauges and lengths, depending on the clinical situation and anatomic location to be biopsied (7, 8). If a core of tissue for histologic examination is needed, an automatic trigger device or a biopsy "gun" has been developed to facilitate sampling. This device simplifies core biopsies by all but eliminating disjoint movements, crush artifacts, and obscuration by blood; shortening procedure time; and decreasing patient discomfort (9).

The needle used is determined by the clinical situation (10). The anatomic site and character of the mass or collection must be considered. Additional considerations include the possible need for a guidewire if drainage is to be performed. For example, if a 0.038-inch guidewire is to be inserted, an 18-gauge needle is needed.

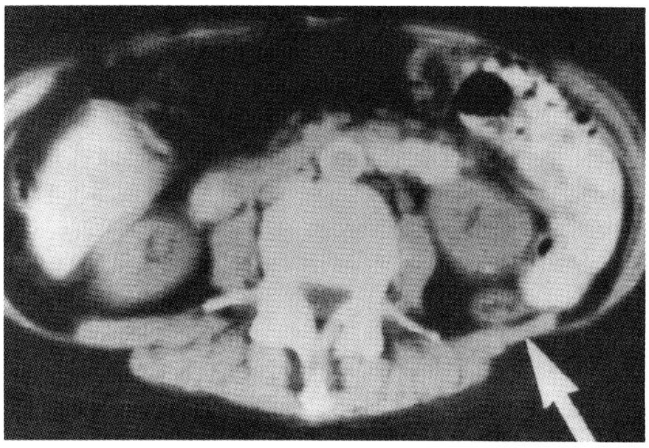

Figure 15.5. Computed tomographic scan through the level of the kidneys, depicting a retrorenal descending colon (*arrow*). Access to the left kidney is therefore compromised, as the commonly used posterolateral approach would transgress the colon.

GENERAL TECHNICAL CONSIDERATIONS

Ultrasonically guided aspirations and biopsies permit continual visualization of the entire needle during the actual procedure, and therefore the path and placement of the needle can be rapidly and dynamically determined. Areas to be avoided may also be identified. Correlation is usually obtained with previously obtained diagnostic images (including intravenous urography, pyelography, computed tomography, or ultrasound). If it is anticipated that fluoroscopy may be needed, a portable ultrasound unit can be used in a fluoroscopy or interventional radiological suite. An important consideration is the ability to actually visualize the region of interest on ultrasound if outside films are provided using other imaging modalities. If the structure is adequately identified using ultrasound, however, then this modality is the one of choice for guidance. Another important consideration is the presence or absence of significant overlying (intervening) structures. If a percutaneous nephrostomy, for instance, is considered, the remote possibility of retrorenal colon may be ascertained by correlating with other imaging modalities obtained before the start of the procedure (i.e., computed tomography) (Fig. 15.5). Real-time sonography performed at the time of the procedure should be able to delineate the possibility of this as well.

Informed consent, inquiry about the patient's allergic history, and an assessment of the patient's coagulation profile are imperative, as most major complications related to genitourinary interventional procedures are secondary to hemorrhage (11–15). A prothrombin time (PT), partial thromboplastin time (PTT), and platelet count are usually obtained. Additionally, if clinically warranted, a bleeding time may also be obtained. The shortest distance from the skin to the lesion that traverses the least dangerous course is then determined by imaging. Generally, the puncture of two or more spaces (that is, pleural, peritoneal, or retroperitoneal) or multiple organs should be avoided. Because the needle is visualized during the procedure, a perpendicular position from the skin to the lesion is not required. Therefore, angled needle placement can be used when necessary. The appropriate position for needle puncture may be marked and the patient is prepared in a sterile manner. The skin and deeper subcutaneous anesthesia is administered and then, if necessary, the skin is incised with a No. 11 scalpel blade to facilitate needle placement. This is particularly useful to help avoid deviation from the desired path when a very thin or flexible needle (such as the Chiba needle) is used, or if use of a large-bore needle or placement of a catheter for drainage is anticipated.

Prior to the biopsy or aspiration, the transducer is covered with a sterile rubber drape, and confirmation of the angle of needle entry into the lesion is then obtained. A stop may be placed on the needle to avoid inadvertent placement of the tip through the desired tissue. At this point, the decision can be made whether to use a clip-on biopsy guidance system or a freehand technique. If a guidance system is selected, the needle is placed in the orifice of the biopsy transducer and through the skin and is continually monitored as it is positioned into the lesion. As noted previously, if the needle becomes obscured, rapid back and forth motion of the needle tip or up and down motion of the needle obturator may be useful to regain visualization. When entering a cyst, a quick thrust of the needle directly into the cyst may be necessary to puncture the cyst wall.

For aspiration biopsy techniques, when the needle has reached the desired position, a 10-ml syringe is attached to the hub and strong suction is applied. At the same time, the needle is moved up and down several times within the mass and at slightly different angulations. Suction is then released and the needle is withdrawn (16, 17). The aspirated material can then be placed onto a glass slide for rapid cytological evaluation. It is generally helpful to have a member of the cytology team present at diagnostic aspiration to confirm the presence of appropriate cellular material. If a diagnosis can be made immediately, further aspirations may be avoided. Otherwise, several additional passes may be performed until the desired information is obtained or as the clinical situation permits.

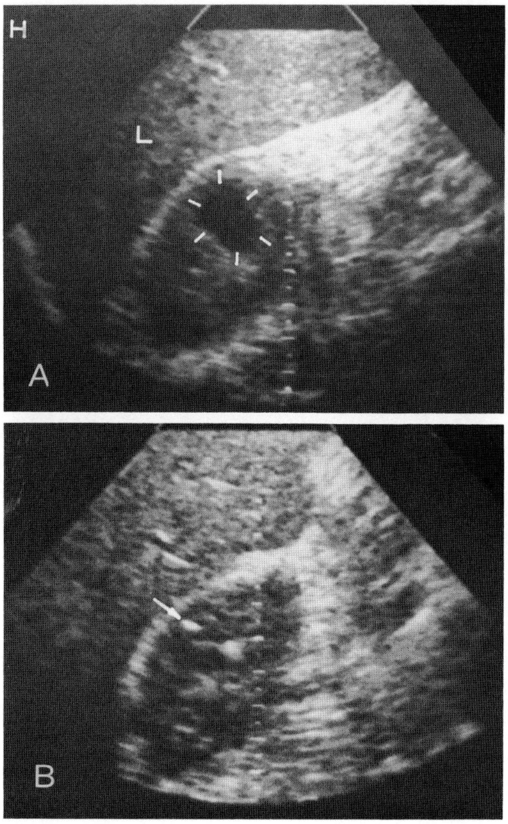

Figure 15.6. **A,** Hypoechoic mass (*lines*) in the right kidney; the strict criteria for the diagnosis of a cyst are not met, as there are low-level internal echoes. *H,* toward patient's head; *L,* liver. **B,** *Arrow* points to a catheter placed after aspiration revealed the presence of pus. Final diagnosis: infected cyst.

PROCEDURES

Guided Puncture and Aspiration of Renal Cysts

Percutaneous punctures of renal cysts were among the earliest nonsurgical techniques performed. As early as 1867, percutaneous drainage of renal cysts was described (18). At present, differentiating renal cysts from solid lesions is extremely accurate using sonography, and it is therefore no longer necessary to aspirate all renal cysts for diagnostic purposes if strict criteria for the presence of a cyst are met. These include (*a*) no internal echoes, (*b*) sharp walls, particularly the "far" wall, and (*c*) "good" sound through transmission. If a renal mass does not meet these criteria, then aspiration is usually indicated (19) (Fig. 15.6). Other indications include the presence of a cyst causing obstruction to the collecting system, an inconclusive correlative computed tomographic examination, unexplained hematuria with an apparent cyst or calcification within a cyst wall. Additionally, therapeutic intervention may be considered if there are local symptoms referable to the cyst. Occasionally, a renal cyst may cause pain, focal or global obstruction and hydronephrosis, or renin-dependent hypertension. When especially large, renal cysts may even cause biliary obstruction. These cysts can be drained percutaneously (17, 19–21).

The lesion to be aspirated is localized and the patient is positioned for the procedure. Usually, a posterolateral or posterior approach, inferior to the hemidiaphragm, is used to avoid bowel, other abdominal organs, the pleural space, and lung parenchyma. After the distance from the skin is marked and the angle of entry is identified, a small-gauge non-cutting needle is advanced into the region of the cyst. Note should be made that a somewhat less flexible needle than a 23-gauge Chiba should be used because there is less chance that the tip will change course during the insertion. Occasionally, it may be necessary to sharply thrust the needle into the cyst. Often, a "pop" is felt as the needle traverses the cyst wall. The stylet is then removed from the inserted needle. If there is increased pressure within the cyst relative to the atmosphere, the fluid will flow spontaneously. If the intracystic pressure is less than the surrounding atmospheric pressure, aspiration will then be required. A syringe is attached to extension tubing, which is then secured to the needle; the tubing is essential, as it allows for free movement of the needle during the patient's respiration and decreases the possibility of renal laceration that could occur if the hub of the needle were secured directly to a syringe, thus "fixing" the needle (22). The fluid is then removed for analysis.

Purely simple cysts are filled with clear, slightly yellowish serous fluid. Any turbidity or blood in the aspirate complicates the diagnosis, and further evaluation is indicated. Laboratory examination of cyst fluid can include determination of fat, LDH, and protein content. Benign cyst fluid is generally alkaline, with a pH of 7.5 to 8.5. It contains glucose and has less than 1000 mg of protein per deciliter. The LDH content of a simple cyst should be below that of serum. The fat content of the cyst has been one of the most frequently used of all laboratory criteria in cyst analysis (23). Renal cell carcinomas have been thought to have positive Sudan stains for fat, and inflammatory lesions should show no fat or at least only minimal amounts of fat. While this has been a source of some controversy in the literature, a negative fat preparation and the presence of clear fluid certainly suggests a benign etiology. Routine cytological evaluation should be obtained in all aspirated fluid (21, 24).

The sine qua non of malignancy is, of course, the identification of malignant cells. The reverse is not always true. While malignancy may be present with a negative cytological examination, it is rare. Additional confusion may arise when the lesion is of an inflammatory etiology and atypical cells are found on the initial cytology smears. If any doubt persists as to the character of these cysts, water-soluble iodinated contrast material can be instilled to evaluate the cyst wall (21, 24). This may help clarify the diagnosis: for example, a smooth cyst wall is compatible with a benign etiology, whereas an irregular cyst wall with filling defects and debris is indeterminate, suggesting possible malignancy.

A pseudocyst of the pancreas may present as a renal fossa cyst, and therefore obtaining amylase levels of the aspirate may help to exclude this possibility.

A simple aspiration procedure may render complete and permanent emptying. However, occasionally, the cyst may recur. If more definitive shrinkage is required, a variety of agents have been instilled into renal cysts to permanently decrease their size. These include quinacrine, talc, and Pantopaque. More recently, 95% ethanol has also been used. The cyst contents are aspirated in total and 25% of the initial cyst volume is replaced with 95% ethanol. The patient is then placed in the supine, prone, and both lateral decubitus positions for 5 min each. This allows contact of the ethanol with all the areas of the cyst wall. Then the alcohol is removed as well as the introducing catheter. The limited amount of time the alcohol is in contact with the cyst wall is enough to fix the epithelial lining cells, but not enough to penetrate the renal cyst capsule and damage normal renal parenchyma. It has been shown that the complications from this treatment have in general been no greater than those from simple cyst aspiration alone (25, 26).

A wide range of complications have been described in association with renal cyst puncture. The incidence of minor complications is approximately 10%. In institutions with very extensive experience, the major complication rate is approximately 0.75% and the overall mean incidence of major complications is approximately 1.4%, according to Lang (22). Major complications include perirenal hemorrhage, pneumothorax, arteriovenous malformation, and urinomas. These complications are more common when the needle is fixed directly to the aspiration syringe without any intervening extension tubing. In these particular cases, the kidney and cyst wall may be lacerated as they move with the patient's respiration. The use of nylon or Teflon sleeve trocars are associated with decreased incidence of hemorrhage. Pneumothorax and hemothorax are also important major complications. These are rare and directly related to the location of the cyst. Upper-pole cysts, particularly on the left, are associated with most of the cases of pneumothorax (22, 27).

No appreciable differences in the incidence of complications are associated with the number of puncture attempts. Additionally, the size of the needle does not appear to be important when comparison of the complication rates is made between the use of 18- and 22-gauge needles. Other rare complications include arteriovenous fistulas, infection, urinomas, and urine peritonitis. Rarely, renal rupture and inadvertent entry of the needle into the duodenum or colon have been reported. Minor complications include macrohematuria or microhematuria, occurring in 0.5 and 6% of the patients, respectively. Pain, fever, and extravasation of iodinated contrast material (if used) have also occurred. The incidence of pain and fever may be higher in patients in whom Pantopaque is instilled into the cyst (22, 27).

Renal Biopsy Localization

Renal biopsy is an extremely important tool for evaluating patients with renal disease. This may be characterized by hematuria, proteinuria, or chemical evidence of renal insufficiency, i.e., elevated BUN and creatinine. Although other radiological techniques, including radionuclide studies, have been used in the past to help localize the kidneys, ultrasound with continuous monitoring of the biopsy needle is an efficient, simple, and accurate modality for this purpose (27–29). The patient is placed in the prone position, and real-time sector transducers are generally used. These are excellent for placement over the flank because of their small size. Disposable clip-on biopsy guides are often used. An electronic range can delineate the proposed needle path into the lower pole of the kidney (30). A direct biopsy technique is most often used, although a tandem technique has been described (30, 31). All biopsy routes should avoid the renal medulla and cortomedullary junction. Additionally, the biopsy needle should enter the renal parenchyma perpendicular to the inferior renal cortex (Fig. 15.3).

When a core biopsy is required, a cutting VimSilverman or Tru-cut type biopsy needle is generally used. An automatic trigger device with a spring-loaded mechanism can also be used, which will lessen the risk of crush artifacts. The procedure time may be shortened, and the risk of complications will also decrease (9).

Ultrasound-guided renal biopsy is also an extremely important modality for use in children, with a higher success rate and fewer complications than are associated with blind biopsy (32).

Biopsy of Renal Masses

While ultrasound-guided biopsy using thin needles is an important tool in the diagnosis of many types of abdominal masses, the popularity of the procedure for renal masses is not widespread in this country. Elsewhere, several reports of ultrasonically guided fine-needle aspiration biopsy for renal masses have yielded fairly good results with a positive predictive value of malignant aspirate of 93% in one report (33). Some of the trepidation with regard to performing this procedure appears to be related to fear of hemorrhage, the very rare incidence of tumor seeding in the needle tract (34), and generalized trauma to a potentially localized tumor. There is somewhat less hesitation when metastatic disease is suspected or when the biopsy is done to confirm the diagnosis of renal cell carcinoma in a patient with already documented metastatic disease (35–37).

When the procedure is performed, localization with ultrasound aids in the proper location, depth, and angle of needle placement. Small-gauge (either 22- or 23-gauge) needles are generally used. These fine needles may be excessively flexible, and can be inserted through a larger 18- or 19-gauge localizing needle (38).

The needle is then inserted to the margin of the mass and the patient is instructed to cease respiration. With maximum continuous suction using a 10- or 20-ml disposable syringe, gentle up and down movements are then performed 5 or 6 times in rapid fashion within the mass. Suction is then released slowly and the needle is removed. Attempts should be made to avoid withdrawing large amounts of blood into the syringe, as this may obscure cytological diagnosis. The specimen is then emptied onto a slide and fixed in 95% ethanol. Additional material from the syringe may be emptied into fixative for cell block studies. Two to three aspirations may be needed to sample all areas of a lesion. Definitive cytological diagnosis can be made immediately (33, 38). Major complications are extremely rare, as has been alluded to previously (15, 33). Transient hematuria may occur. Significant bleeding is very rare with needle biopsy (33, 39).

At the completion of the biopsy, the patient can be rescanned at 10-min intervals to evaluate for evidence of possible complications such as perirenal bleeding. Other complications of percutaneous biopsy include macroscopic and microscopic hematuria, retroperitoneal hematoma, and arteriovenous fistula. Intraperitoneal hemorrhage has rarely been reported and is a serious complication (15, 40, 41).

There are a few caveats to observe when performing an aspiration cytology procedure. False-positive results are rare but do occur. Most problems occur when lesions are initially interpreted as well-differentiated adenocarcinoma. Therefore, Juul et al. recommend that cytological findings should be interpreted with caution (33). Additionally, a large mass may have areas of necrosis within it. Aspiration from this portion of the tumor may yield only insufficient or nondiagnostic material. Therefore, if necrosis is suspected and the tumor is large, biopsy from several portions of the tumor is suggested.

Antegrade Pyelography and Percutaneous Nephrostomy

Antegrade pyelography is a simple but extraordinarily useful procedure in terms of diagnostic and therapeutic yield. It can be performed rapidly using local anesthesia and is often used as a prelude to a variety of percutaneous interventional techniques (42, 43).

Percutaneous nephrostomy (PCN) has also evolved from merely a temporizing technique to an important longer-term therapeutic measure (44). PCN is more often used as a preliminary step for other uroradiologic techniques, such as ureteral dilatation, stone removal, therapy for urinomas, etc.

Both techniques can be performed with or without sonographic guidance, but the use of ultrasound often reduces the number of attempts, obviates the use of intravenous contrast material, determines the depth and angle of approach, and lessens complications (45–48). Fluoroscopy is a necessary adjunct tool whether the procedure is diagnostic or therapeutic (38).

Antegrade pyelography is indicated for determining morphologic and pathologic anatomy, performing urodynamic studies, gaining access for interventional procedures (42), and obtaining selective urine samples. The procedure is also invaluable for diagnosis and initial therapeutic intervention in nondilated obstructive uropathy (49–51). Antegrade pyelography is also performed in patients who are unable to undergo retrograde pyeloureterography because of contraindications to general anesthesia or previous ileal loop diversion.

Usually when performing antegrade pyelography, the patient is placed in the prone position and a direct, posterior percutaneous approach is used. Using sonographic guidance, a thin 22-gauge needle is advanced until it can be seen in the renal pelvis (if dilated) (Fig. 15.7). The needle guide is then snapped off the transducer and extension tubing is connected to the needle. Urine is collected for appropriate chemical and bacteriological studies. An opening pressure may be obtained if urodynamics are to be performed. Contrast material may be injected to opacify the collecting system, taking care not to overdistend the collecting system. This is to avoid the possibility of pyelovenous backflow, particularly in patients with infected urine (see below). *Over-aspiration* of urine should also be avoided, as the collecting system may collapse away from the needle. Both of these problems may be solved by withdrawing small amounts of urine and replacing it with equal amounts of contrast material (42).

Potential complications of antegrade pyelography include reaction to either the anesthetic agent or contrast material, local pain, pneumothorax, puncture of nearby organs, bleeding, urinoma, obstruction by clot formation, and infection. Urine extravasation may occur but is rare when the pelvis is punctured with a 22-gauge needle. The overall incidence of complications is generally under 1% (42).

Percutaneous nephrostomy may be performed in conjunction with antegrade pyelog-

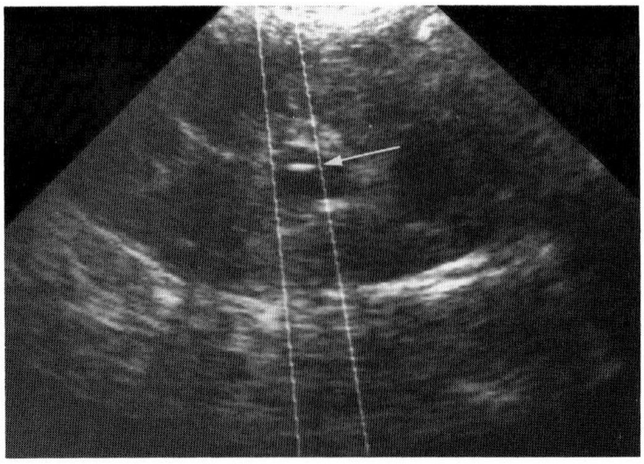

Figure 15.7. The tip of a 22-gauge needle (*arrow*) is seen within a mildly dilated renal pelvis after placement for antegrade pyelography.

raphy or as a separate procedure. Indications include relief of obstruction, therapy for pyonephrosis (Fig. 15.8), treatment of urinary tract leaks and fistulas, and as access for stent, guidewire, or catheter placement. A nephrostomy may also be used as an initial technique for subsequent ureteral dilatation, foreign body and calculus removal, YAG laser therapy, nephroscopy, and topical treatment (i.e., antibiotic irrigation in infection, stone dissolution, and chemotherapy) (43, 44, 52–56). The technique may also be applied successfully in children with upper urinary tract obstruction (57, 58).

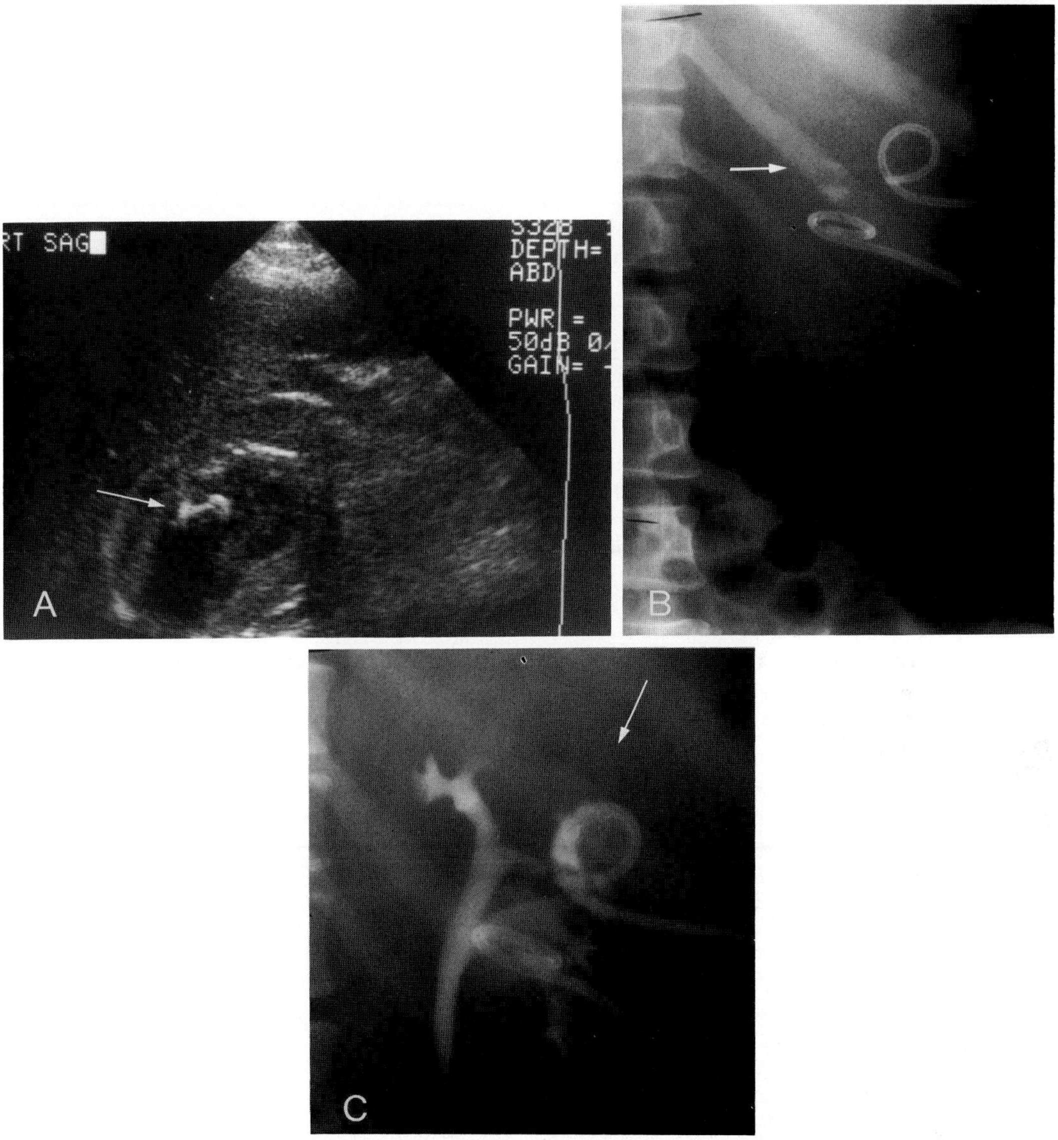

Figure 15.8. A, Segmental pyonephrosis secondary to obstruction by a relatively large right renal calculus (*arrow*). **B,** Scout film for antegrade pyelography performed after placement of two catheters. The upper catheter drains the superior interpolar calix and the lower catheter drains the inferior interpolar calix. Note the calculus in the interpolar portion of the kidney (*arrow*). **C,** Infundibular and upper catheter injection demonstrates an irregular, obstructed calix (*arrow*) and documents proper placement for drainage of the pyonephrosis.

There are no absolute contraindications to percutaneous nephrostomy, but coagulopathy does represent a relative contraindication. Technical difficulties may be encountered with extremely obese patients as well as in patients having undergone recent surgery or peritoneal dialysis. Antibiotics may be given prior to the procedure if urinary tract infection is present; often, a single dose of a penicillin derivative and aminoglycoside may be given 1 hr prior to the procedure (57). Premedication with short-acting sedatives may also be indicated.

A posterolateral approach is generally used, in contradistinction to the posterior approach used in antegrade pyelography. Besides avoiding hilar vessels, this path also generally courses through renal parenchyma, thus diminishing the frequency of urine extravasation and renal pelvis laceration. Before puncture, the kidneys should be visualized to include the dilated renal pelvis and at least one dilated calix (Fig. 15.9). This ensures an intraparenchymal path and avoids the vascular medulla and hilus. If there is no caliceal dilatation or if there is need to puncture a specific calix, opacification of the collecting system may be necessary prior to percutaneous nephrostomy (the so-called "second stick" technique). When the introducing needle is seen in the pelvis or calix, the stylet is withdrawn and extension tubing is connected to the needle. If urine is obtained, a small amount of contrast material may be instilled to opacify the collecting system. A guidewire may then be advanced until resistance is felt; at this point, fluoroscopy is used to complete the procedure (59, 60).

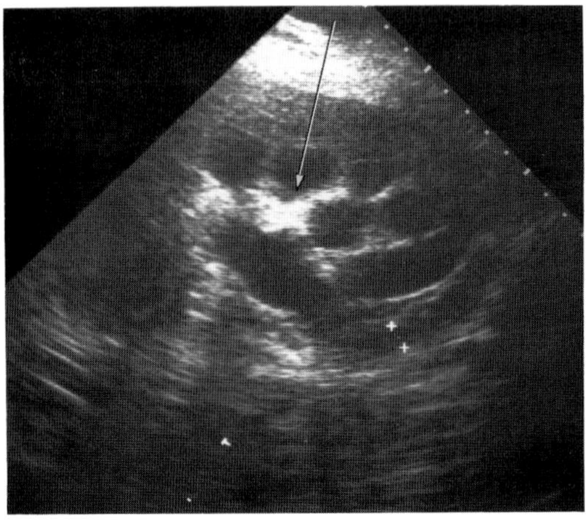

Figure 15.9. Determination of the proper plane and trajectory for percutaneous nephrostomy includes visualization of the dilated collecting system and desired calix to be entered (*arrow*). This ensures a transparenchymal route for catheter placement.

If no urine is initially obtained, the needle is withdrawn in a step-wise fashion with intermittent suction on the extension tubing.

Once the guidewire is in place, the needle is withdrawn and the tract may be dilated to the site of entry into the collecting system, usually to 8 or 9 French. A one-step procedure has been described that eliminates dilatation by using a puncture needle with an obturator and metal sheath, over which slides a soft polyethylene catheter (50). An 8.3 or 10.0 French pigtail nephrostomy catheter is then introduced into the pelvis over the guidewire. If percutaneous stone removal or ureteral stent placement is contemplated, a straight drainage catheter placed in the distal ureter is usually more useful than a simple pigtail catheter in the renal pelvis.

At the completion of the procedure, the catheter is then secured to the skin to prevent dislodgement. This may be accomplished using a commercially available disk system that secures itself around the catheter with a Teflon band and is then sutured to the skin (Molnar disk). Alternatively, a self-retaining pigtail catheter may be used which can also be fastened to the skin.

Generally, percutaneous nephrostomy is successful in 95 to 98% of cases (49, 53, 59). A somewhat lower success rate is seen when the urinary tract is not dilated or when staghorn calculi are present. Whereas mortality from surgical nephrostomy varies from 6 to 8% (often reaching nearly 12% in septicemic patients), death rates of only 0.2% were reported in a review of over 1200 percutaneous nephrostomies by Stables et al. in 1978 (53).

Complications include hemorrhage, particularly in patients with coagulopathies. Transient hematuria usually does occur and generally is not regarded as a complication. Care should be taken that the catheter is not obstructed by clot formation. If massive hematuria develops, then arterial injury may be postulated and the appropriate diagnostic and therapeutic measures should be promptly instituted.

It is also prudent to monitor the patient's hematocrit after percutaneous nephrostomy, as a sudden fall in hematocrit without definite evidence of gross hematuria may be due to retroperitoneal or perirenal hemorrhage.

Urinomas may also occur secondary to this procedure, but have been reported in only 1 to 2% of all patients. When they do occur, however, they usually require specific therapy. Pneumothorax and renopleural fistulas have also been reported.

Additionally, 1 to 2% of patients undergoing percutaneous nephrostomy may develop septicemia, particularly if pyonephrosis is present. This can be exacerbated by increasing the intrarenal pressure during percutaneous nephrostomy. Rarely, perinephric abscesses occur, usually in patients with previous underlying infection (57).

Percutaneous Drainage of Renal Abscesses and Perinephric Fluid Collections

Most intraabdominal abscesses can be treated by percutaneous drainage (61). Renal abscesses and related retroperitoneal collections are no exception; a recent study by Sacks et al. revealed that definitive therapeutic results occurred in 61% of their patients; absence of residual abscess at surgery was seen in the remaining 39% of patients (63).

Inflammatory disorders of the kidney and related retroperitoneal collections can be diagnosed using ultrasound and computed tomography (CT) (62). Included in this category of perinephric collections are urinomas and hematomas. Abscesses are generally hypoechoic and may be multiple; air can be seen if gas-forming organisms are present. Occasionally, abscesses may be hyperechoic and more difficult to diagnose using ultrasound. Urinomas are generally anechoic unless secondarily infected. The sonographic pattern of hematoma varies depending on its age. CT can be extremely useful to determine the anatomic extent of disease, more clearly delineate etiology, and determine whether or not hematomas are acute or chronic (63, 64).

Renal and perinephric abscess formation is relatively infrequent except in patients with predisposing factors, including diabetes, calculi, obstruction, and debilitation (63). Rapid diagnosis and intervention are therefore critical; even with the antibiotic arsenal we now employ, up to 50% of patients with renal abscess can die as a result of this disease (65).

One of the few contraindications to the procedure is a severe blood dyscrasia, except in a patient with disseminated intravascular coagulation secondary to sepsis caused by the abscess. Tumors may become infected and are usually drained only as a palliative procedure. It is necessary to remove calculi and relieve obstructions if these are predisposing causes for an infected collection (64, 66).

Diagnostic aspiration is performed before definitive drainage if a fluid collection is found in the GU tract. Ultrasound can be used in most cases, particularly if the lesion is well seen by this modality (64, 67). Before beginning the procedure, it is generally recommended to have an intravenous line in place; if infection is suspected, preprocedural antibiotics are appropriate. After the lesion is localized using a real-time transducer, a skin site is selected. Local anesthesia is given and a small skin incision is made.

The same basic principles used for abscess drainage elsewhere in the abdomen are used when draining renal abscesses and perinephric fluid collections. Care is taken not to traverse bowel, the intraperitoneal space, major vessels, or the pleura. Therefore, the posterior retroperitoneal approach is often used. Lesions that present in a more cephalad aspect of the perirenal space or renal fossa may require an angled approach to avoid the pleura. The initial puncture should be performed during suspended expiration to raise the level of the diaphragm.

The needle is inserted under sonographic guidance after local anesthesia has been given. For initial aspiration, generally a 20-gauge needle is used (Fig. 15.10). Occasionally, it may be necessary to use a larger-gauge needle if thick material is present within the collection. A larger-gauge needle or dilator is also needed to permit passage of a guidewire and subsequent drainage catheter (Fig. 15.11). The material obtained should be sent for microbiologic analysis. If clinically indicated, fungal cultures should also be obtained. If infection within a necrotic neoplasm is suspected, the material should be sent for cytological analysis. There has been a case report of lymphoma presenting as a pararenal collection (68).

Drainage techniques may be classified into two categories: the modified Seldinger type and the trochar technique (62).

The modified Seldinger technique has been previously described for antegrade pyelography and percutaneous nephrostomy. A thin guidewire is placed through the initial aspiration needle with subsequent tract dilatation

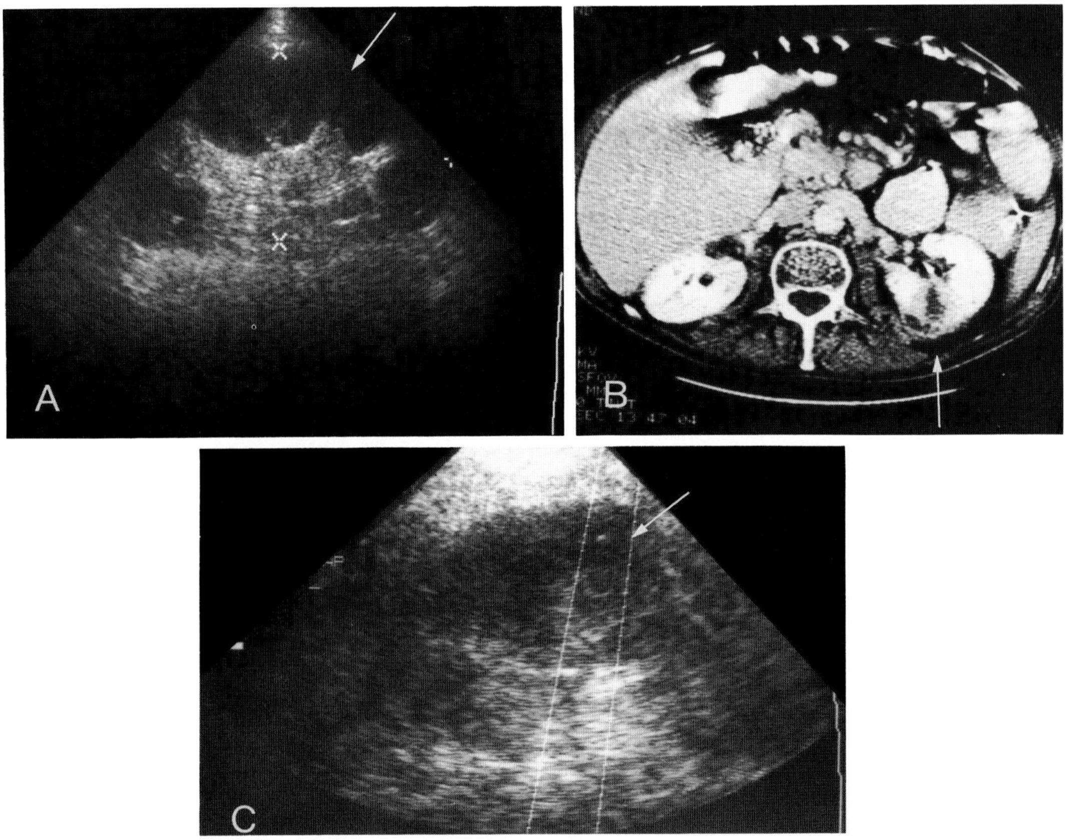

Figure 15.10. **A,** Coronal ultrasound of the left kidney in a 54-year-old man with flank pain, fever, and a history of diabetes. Note the mildly hypoechoic, focal bulge of the interpolar aspect of the left kidney (*arrow*). **B,** CT scan obtained following the ultrasound, demonstrating a focal, irregular area of decreased attenuation of the posterior interpolar portion of the left kidney (*arrow*). **C,** Using a posterior approach and ultrasound guidance a 20-gauge Chiba needle (*arrow*) was advanced into the abnormal region; pus and necrotic tissue were obtained. Diagnosis: lobar nephronia (focal pyelonephritis) with *Escherichia coli* infection.

Figure 15.11. Percutaneous drainage setup, including an 0.038-inch flexible J-tipped guidewire, stopcock, extension tubing, Molnar disk, aspiration needles, dilators and a pigtail catheter.

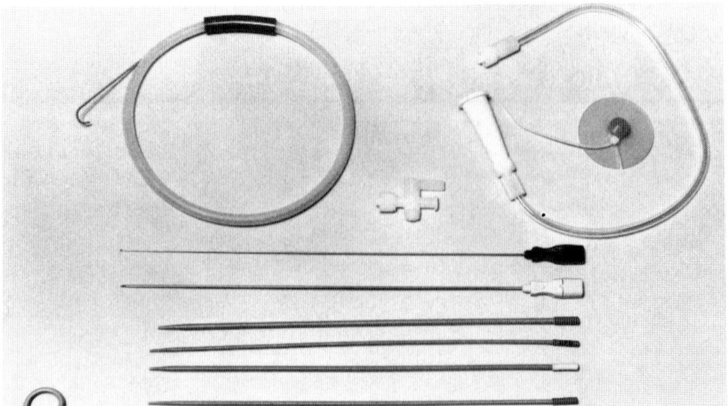

to accommodate a 0.038-inch guidewire. The catheter size is generally determined by the viscosity of the material collected (Figs. 15.12 and 15.13). A coaxial technique, using removable hub needles, may also be performed (69).

The trochar technique may also be used, thus eliminating the use of a guidewire. A larger skin incision is necessary, however, and this is usually performed at a second site adjacent to the aspiration needle using the tandem technique. With this method, the catheter with a cannula and internal stylet are pushed through the skin directly into the lesion. When the internal stylet is within the abscess cavity, the catheter is advanced over the cannula and it resumes its pigtail form. Then the cannula is removed and the catheter is fixed to the skin. This technique is generally used for larger and more superficial collections (70).

Regardless of the technique, once the catheter is in position a three-way stopcock can then be attached to the end of the catheter and a drainage bag attached to the stopcock. A closed method of drainage is used by connecting a large syringe to the stopcock and intermittently aspirating the material into the syringe. The syringe contents are then expressed in the closed drainage bag connected to another portion of the stopcock. The cavity should be emptied initially. Then, irrigation with small aliquots (approximately 10 to 15 ml) of saline will further débride the abscess cavity. The catheter is fixed to the patient's skin and left to gravity drainage or low suction. A subsequent imaging procedure, such as ultrasound, CT, or abscessogram is usually performed to determine whether the cavity has been drained adequately or if any residual loculations are present. If residual abscess cavities remain, additional aspirations and catheter placements may be needed. This concept is extremely important, as a major cause for failure of percutaneous abscess drainage is related to loculation or incomplete drainage of single or multiple cavities (60, 72).

Routine irrigation of the catheter may be performed, but in most cases irrigation is not necessary (60, 71). If clogging or poor drainage

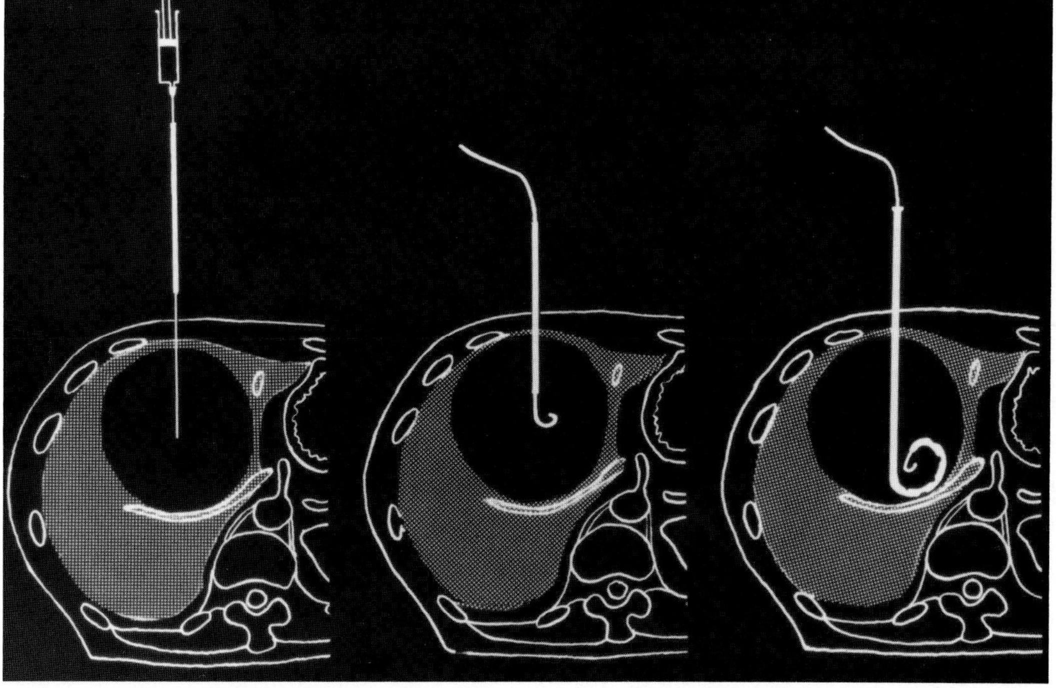

Figure 15.12. Diagrammatic representation of percutaneous drainage procedure. Diagnostic aspiration is performed using a small 20- to 22-gauge needle. The needle may be equipped with a Teflon dilator or a wire may be advanced through the needle into the collection. (Drawing courtesy of Wolfgang Dähnert, M.D.)

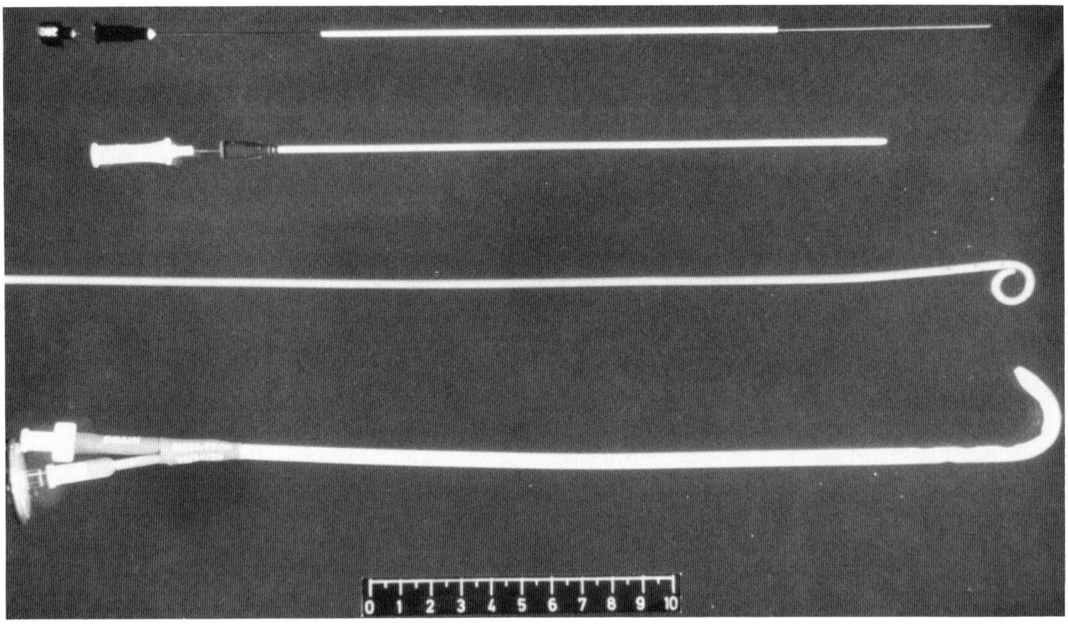

Figure 15.13. Several catheter types used for percutaneous drainage procedures. From top to bottom: single straight catheter/dilator; trocar type—APD; standard pigtail catheter with side holes; sump-type catheter.

occurs, the catheter may be irrigated with small aliquots of saline as necessary. Attempts should be made not to overirrigate, as this procedure may cause sepsis or bacteremia. The size of the abscess cavity may then be followed via fluoroscopic contrast injection and abscessogram. Monitoring of catheter drainage is imperative, and the catheter is generally removed when drainage has stopped, even if there is fluoroscopic evidence of a small residual abscess cavity. Although several weeks may pass before the catheter can be removed, the patient (if medically stable) need not remain hospitalized while the catheter is in place (73). If discharged from the hospital, the patient should be instructed to watch for evidence of reinfection such as recurrence of pain or fever. Immediate medical attention should be pursued if any of these symptoms occur (64).

As opposed to treatment by open surgical drainage, percutaneous abscess drainage results in decreased patient morbidity, obviates the use of general anesthesia, and is generally less costly (71).

The cure rates for percutaneous abscess drainage of genitourinary tract abscesses and fluid collections generally range from 60 to 80% (63, 64), depending on the type and location of the lesion, the expertise of the individual performing the procedure, and the patient's clinical situation, particularly the functional state of the patient's immune system. Even if complete cure is not obtainable, the percutaneous procedure may shorten and simplify the surgical procedure necessary to completely eradicate the abscess. Percutaneous procedures may be viewed as a temporizing measure in moribund patients, allowing clinical stabilization prior to surgical exploration.

Recurrence of collections may occur in 5 to 15% of cases (63, 71, 72). The major causes of recurrence include loculations, incomplete evacuation, and premature removal of the catheter. Also, the inability to successfully control a fistula or the presence of infected neoplasm have contributed to recurrence (64, 71, 72).

Not all processes in the anterior perinephric space are related to the kidney, and evaluation of the GI tract and pancreas is important if there is suspicion of a nonrenal source. Knowledge of the initial etiology of the collection will therefore also diminish the number of unsuccessful drainage procedures (Fig. 15.14). For example, it is imperative to diagnose the condition responsible for urinoma formation to determine proper treatment. If the collection has

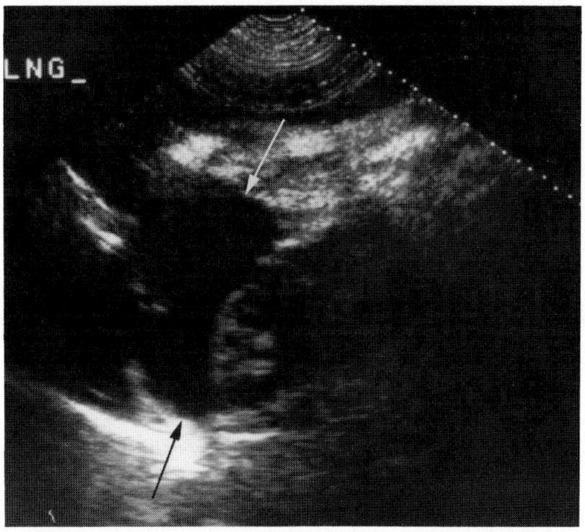

Figure 15.14. A left perirenal collection (*arrows*), initially thought to represent a urinoma or old hematoma. Diagnostic aspiration revealed a high amylase level; final diagnosis: pancreatic pseudocyst.

been caused by obstruction, then relief of the obstruction and reestablishment of normal urine flow should be accomplished. Any etiology for the obstruction needs to be corrected or simple drainage of the urinoma will effect only temporary relief (74).

Renal Transplants

Renal transplants are subject to many of the same pathological processes that may affect native kidneys. However, there is a special category of problems commonly associated with transplants and, additionally, a somewhat different approach to several of the problems that may be encountered (75, 76).

Allograft Biopsy

Renal transplants are generally placed in the iliac fossae in an extraperitoneal location. Renal transplants are not subject to the same type of extreme respiratory excursion as native kidneys. However, adherent anterior bowel or peritoneum is often present, particularly medially. As these patients are generally immunosuppressed, perforation of the adjacent bowel may be disastrous and care should be taken to avoid it. Either the upper or lower pole of the renal transplant may be biopsied, rather than the lower pole exclusively as in native kidneys (38). At times, overlying bowel can interfere with the upper pole approach, but a steeply oblique route can overcome this problem. Indications for biopsy generally include confirmation of rejection or suspected recurrent renal disease in the transplant (77). Techniques using a spring-loaded, automatic trigger device or "biopsy gun" have been described. Real-time sonography is performed to localize the allograft, to exclude hydronephrosis and perirenal collections, and to determine an appropriate needle path (Fig. 15.15). The path should maintain the needle within the cortex of the transplant. The skin entry site should be lateral to the skin incision to avoid peritoneum. The trigger device is loaded and a safety catch applied. The needle is then advanced through the biopsy guide, skin, and renal capsule to the level of the

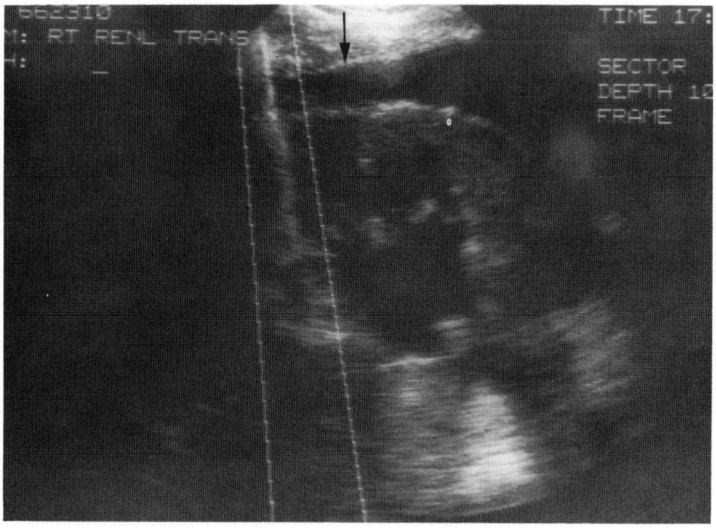

Figure 15.15. In this biopsy of a right lower quadrant renal transplant, the transducer is oriented sagittally and the biopsy guide is set so that the needle trajectory is from the superior aspect of the transducer head. Note the peritransplant lymphocele (*arrow*).

cortex of the transplant. The automatic trigger mechanism then pushes the needle cannula and obturator into the kidney in a precise, rapid manner (78).

In a series by Silver et al. in 1981, 51% of transplant recipients demonstrated abnormal peritransplant fluid collections, which were documented on ultrasonography (76). Additionally, significant urologic complications may occur in 12 to 13% of patients undergoing renal transplants (79). Untreated, some of these complications may have an associated mortality as high as 50%. Therefore, prompt diagnosis and treatment are critical. Ultrasound is an important tool in evaluating renal transplants, since it may be repeated as many times as necessary to assess both renal parenchyma and the peritransplant spaces. The integrity of the vasculature and intrarenal circulation can be evaluated using Doppler techniques.

The most common peritransplant collection is a lymphocele. In decreasing order of frequency, abscess, urinomas, and hematomas also occur. Common to all these lesions is their ability to be aspirated and drained percutaneously under sonographic guidance (75, 80) (Fig. 15.16).

Lymphoceles are a complication usually occurring several weeks following renal transplant surgery. Lymphoceles may also occur after any type of radical pelvic surgery. Histologically, a lymphocele is a lymph-filled space without a distinct epithelial lining (80–82). Any symptoms that occur with this entity are generally secondary to a space-occupying effect on the adjacent pelvic organs. They are usually unilocular and if there is any localized tenderness, erythema, or warmth, an associated inflammatory component is suspected (81). If there are no constitutional symptoms, many of these are never aspirated, since intervention may actually introduce infection in a previously sterile space. If symptoms force intervention, percutaneous aspiration and drainage is a viable alternative or supplement to eventual surgical marsupialization, or as a temporizing technique while rejection is treated. Sclerosis may be attempted with 10% povidone iodine, as recurrence is common after aspiration (75, 76, 78, 80, 82). In female transplant patients, care should be taken to differentiate lymphoceles from other cystic adnexal masses (83).

Owing to the generally immunosuppressed status of the renal transplant patient, an abscess is a potentially lethal complication. The presence of an abscess should be considered in any febrile transplant patient with a peritransplant fluid collection. In these patients, irreversible sepsis can develop extremely rapidly. Aspiration is performed in a manner similar to the one previously described, taking care to avoid overlying bowel and the peritoneum (75, 76).

Urinomas may also occur in the post–renal transplant patient. As in native kidneys, urinomas have several etiologies, including breach of the renal pelvis or caliceal leak. Somewhat more unique to transplants are the possibilities of ureteral necrosis or a disrupted ureterocystotomy. Most of these patients present with decreased urine output and rising BUN and creatinine levels. Pain and swelling may be seen over the renal transplant. Other uroradiographic examinations may be necessary to determine the exact origin of the leak. Urinary diversion or stenting may help alleviate the leak, and this may be performed using ultrasound as a guidance tool (75, 84). (Fig. 15.17).

Hematomas generally develop in the early postoperative period. These are less common than lymphoceles or abscesses. Evacuation and drainage may be required if renal function is compromised, and care should be taken that the hematoma is not secondary to ruptured graft. Another potential problem with hematoma is the possibility of secondary infection, particularly if an attempted drainage is incomplete. In fact, because of the extremely good culture medium afforded by blood, in addition to the variable viscosity of the hematoma, surgical drainage of peritransplant hematoma may be performed in lieu of percutaneous drainage (75, 76, 80).

The techniques of antegrade pyelography and percutaneous nephrostomy may also be used in patients with renal transplant hydronephrosis or extravasation (75, 84, 85). Several underlying etiologies are possible, including ureterovesical anastomatic stenosis, midureteral stenosis, and obstruction by extrinsic fluid collections. Extravasation may be the result of ureteral necrosis secondary to ischemia or rejection or caliceal perforation due to segmental infarct. Retrograde pyelograms may be difficult to perform in transplant patients and, if renal transplant function is compromised, intravenous urography may not yield diagnostic visualization. Diagnostic antegrade pyelography may need to be performed;

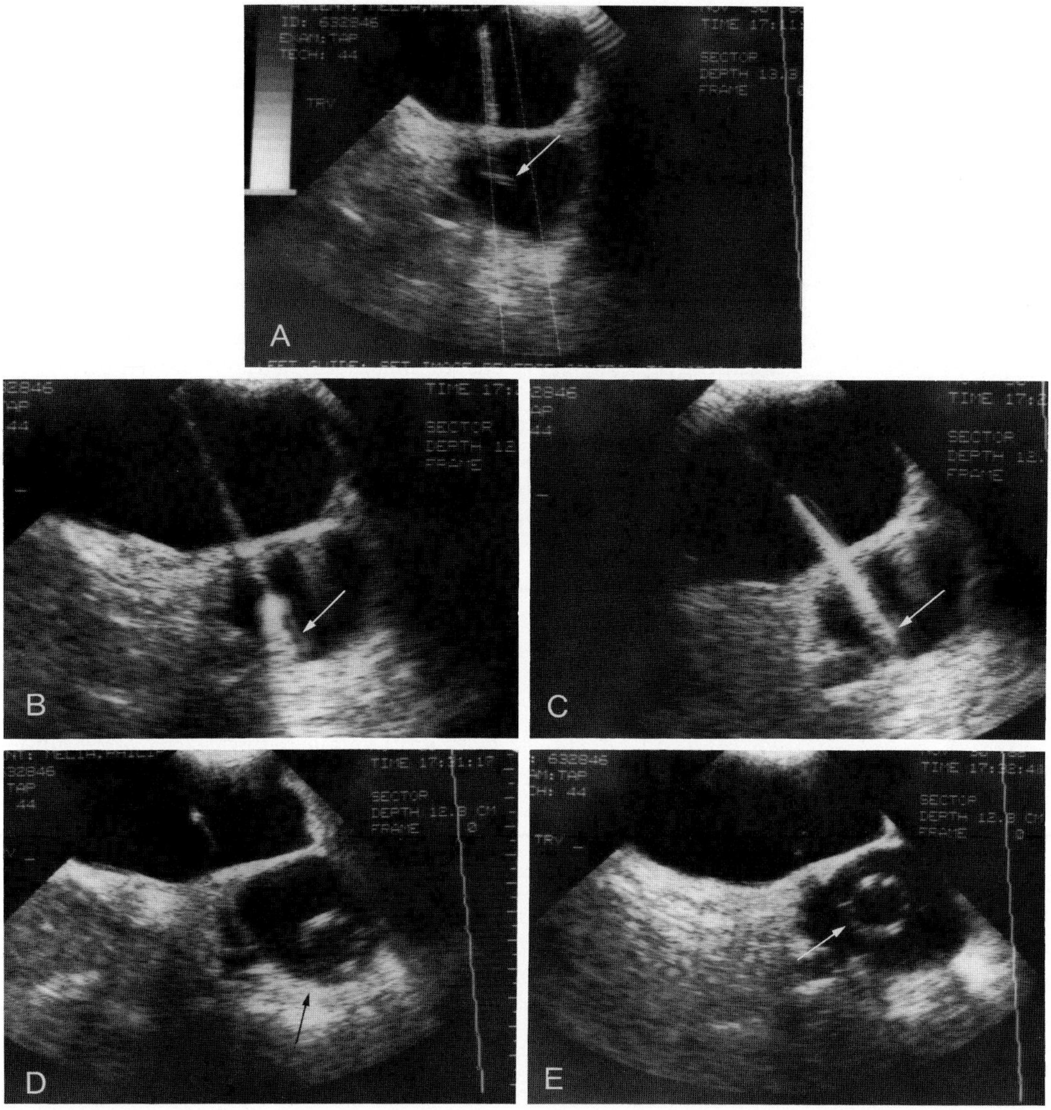

Figure 15.16. **A,** Percutaneous drainage of a loculated, infected lymphocele. Prior diagnostic aspiration had already been performed. Ultrasound was used exclusively in this particular procedure. An 18-gauge needle (*arrow*) has been advanced into the more dependent aspect of the collection. **B,** The needle has been removed after advancing an 0.038-inch guidewire (*arrow*) through it into the collection. **C,** A dilator (*arrow*) is seen within the collection; the ultimate drainage catheter used often requires dilatation of the tract for placement. **D,** A No. 8 French pigtail catheter with side holes has been advanced into the collection; the pigtail has reformed; the side holes will drain only the most dependent aspect of the collection (*arrow*). **E,** The catheter has been pulled back so that the side holes can also drain the more anterior aspect of the collection (*arrow*).

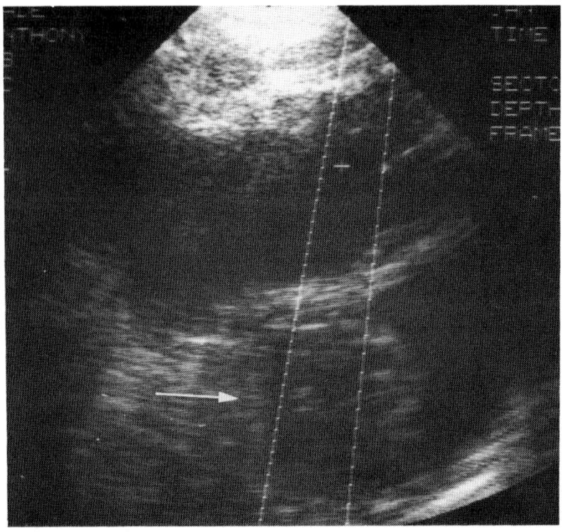

Figure 15.17. Sonographically guided aspiration of a prevesical collection in a young patient who experienced difficulty voiding after a right iliac fossa cadaveric renal transplant. Note the collapsed urinary bladder and Foley catheter (*arrow*) posteriorly. Laboratory analysis revealed a high creatinine in the fluid obtained, consistent with a urinoma. The collection was drained and a Foley catheter was left in the bladder; resolution occurred in 3 days.

subsequent percutaneous nephrostomy or stenting may also be necessary (75, 84, 85).

Adrenal Masses

Adrenal masses are of many varied etiologies, and the detection of an adrenal mass using either ultrasound or CT may be an incidental finding or may confirm clinical suspicion of metastatic disease. The demonstration of the lesion does not always confirm its etiology and biopsy is often required, particularly in patients with a known primary lesion. Fine-needle aspiration or core biopsy may be performed (86, 87). In general, CT is used for adrenal masses if they are not well seen on ultrasonography. However, if ultrasound can visualize the mass, its use as a guidance technique may be beneficial (86, 88).

The most common indication for adrenal mass biopsy is the exclusion of metastatic disease in patients with known primary lesions. With respect to clinical history, if pheochromocytoma is suspected, appropriate serological determinations (i.e., VMA determination) are obtained prior to biopsy (89). Abnormal bleeding is a relative contraindication to fine-needle aspiration biopsy.

A posterior approach is usually used when CT is used for guidance. The posterior approach with ultrasound may also be best, but in certain cases an anterior approach may be used for adrenal mass biopsy. Direct sonographic visualization is imperative to avoid major surrounding organs, vessels, and the pleural and peritoneal spaces. Using the anterior approach, the liver and peritoneum may be traversed, however. The technique used for biopsy is similar to that used in fine-needle aspiration of other abdominal masses, including confirmation of needle placement in the lesion, aspiration while performing a to-and-fro, up-and-down motion within the lesion, and gentle release of suction before removing the needle. Immediate cytology is obtained to confirm the presence of adrenal cells in the presence of an adrenal adenoma or malignant cells in metastatic disease. Samples should be taken from various portions of the lesion to reduce the possibility of sampling error. Material obtained should also be sent for cell block study (86, 87).

A pitfall unique to the location of the adrenal glands is the proximity of the pleural space. Often, an angled approach is necessary and a triangulated method described by van Sonnenberg (90) for CT can also be used in ultrasonography. However, angulation techniques are simpler with ultrasound than CT because of the ability to visualize the needle in its entirety during the biopsy. Insertion of the needle beneath the twelfth rib generally avoids violation of the posterior pleura at this level.

Bladder—Suprapubic Aspiration, Cystostomy, and Drainage of Perivesical Collections

Often, access to the urinary bladder is imperative for diagnostic purposes. A full bladder can often be percussed or palpated and therefore aspirated without using ultrasound (91). However, certain situations lend themselves to ultrasonographic guidance. This is useful most often in the neonatal and pediatric age groups in addition to older patients who have difficulty with bladder control. Patients in whom urethral catheterizations are contraindicated also merit sonographically guided suprapubic aspiration.

For uroradiologic procedures, a suprapubic route may be used for voiding cystourethrography when retrograde passage of a catheter cannot be accomplished secondary to urethral obstruction.

With the advent of ultrasound, suprapubic punctures allow more accurate needle placement and somewhat lower morbidity than that associated with nonvisually guided biopsies. The approach to the bladder is much like that used for renal cyst. A real-time transducer with a disposable needle guide is used to determine the needle path (17, 38).

Another advantage of suprapubic aspiration for cystourethrography is that the needle may be left in place and the study can be repeated if it is initially nondiagnostic. Other interventions and procedures may also be carried out in the genitourinary tract using the suprapubic route, including puncture and evaluation of ureteroceles and antegrade dilatation of urethral strictures (38, 92). This technique has also been advocated for puncture of Foley catheter balloons that have not been deflatable using any other means (93).

As has been described for renal transplants, several fluid collections may be seen alongside the urinary bladder. These also include lymphoceles, urinomas, abscesses, and hematomas. Bladder emptying should be performed prior to sonographically guided aspiration of these collections to avoid confusing the collection with the urinary bladder.

Percutaneous catheter drainage is generally the procedure of choice for the treatment of most pelvic abscesses (63, 71, 94). Although 85 to 90% of these abscesses can be drained safely by transabdominal percutaneous routes, safe access may be difficult to obtain in the pelvis due to surrounding bowel and adjacent organs. Therefore, a transvaginal method has also been described by Nosher et al. for catheter drainage of pelvic abscesses (94). The patient is placed in the lithotomy position with a vaginal speculum inserted in the introitus. After the cervix is identified, Betadine is used to cleanse the inside of the vagina. The cervix is then elevated to provide unobstructed access and visualization of the posterior fornix of the vagina. Simultaneously, real-time ultrasound is performed transabdominally with the patient's bladder distended. This is in contradistinction to the above-noted technique for transabdominal abscess drainage, in which bladder emptying is advocated. A one-step drainage catheter may be placed near the apex of the vagina, with the tip identified on ultrasound as an echogenic focus. The appropriate angulation of the needle is then confirmed and puncture of the center of the abscess collection via the posterior vaginal fornix is performed. The catheter is then advanced over the stylet, the stylet is removed, and fluid is aspirated and sent for appropriate bacteriologic study. The abscess can then be evacuated and gently lavaged with either Betadine or saline. The catheter is then sutured to the lateral vaginal wall with 1 or 2 sutures and left to drain by gravity. The transrectal approach can also be used, particularly in young nulliparous women and in men (95). One problem with the transrectal approach is the inability to secure the catheter, which may result in inadvertent expulsion of the catheter during defecation (94). Additionally, the transrectal route could introduce infection into a previously sterile collection.

Prostate

Over the past several years, great strides have been accomplished in imaging of the prostate and seminal vesicles (95). While the most cost-effective and simple means of diagnosis remains the digital rectal examination, new transducer technology has enabled exquisite imaging of this gland and identification of many nonpalpable lesions. In particular, endorectal scanning techniques have many indications, including evaluation of a palpable mass, screening for prostatic disease in patients with an otherwise normal examination, evaluation of inflammatory diseases of the seminal vesicles and prostate, evaluation of the urethra, and biopsy guidance. Additionally, endorectal ultrasonography has been used as a guide to prostatic abscess drainage (96).

There is some controversy as to whether ultrasound is necessary to guide a biopsy of an already palpable prostatic nodule. A recent study by Resnick (97) indicated that ultrasound-guided prostatic biopsy is not necessary as a routine procedure when a distinct nodule is palpable. However, if there is a distinctly abnormal examination but a negative digitally guided biopsy, then a repeat sonographically guided biopsy is necessary.

Additionally, subtle and nonpalpable lesions require biopsy by ultrasound guidance. Several approaches to ultrasound-guided biopsy of the prostate can be used, but the use of endorectal guidance is superior. Biopsies may be performed in either the lateral decubitus or the lithotomy position, and they are generally performed in an outpatient setting. The two major methods of biopsy are the transperineal and the transrectal techniques.

A small 18- to 20-gauge cutting needle will lessen patient discomfort and complications for prostatic biopsy, particularly when a biopsy needle specially fitted to a mechanical triggering device or "gun" is used. This ensures rapid and safe extraction of a tissue core and decreases the number of complications without loss of diagnostic accuracy. Fine-needle aspiration can also be used. Whereas the diagnostic accuracy of aspiration seems to be close to that of a large-core biopsy, cytology is more dependent on the pathologist or cytologist, and grading of the malignancy is also not as easy.

When using the transperineal approach, preliminary cleansing of the perineum is necessary. Shaving of the perineum is generally not needed. Although the biopsy can be performed while viewing the prostate in either the axial or sagittal plane, the use of a sagittally oriented plane allows visualization of the entire needle during the biopsy. One of the limitations of the axial orientation is that while the needle tip can be seen to enter the region of abnormality, the actual biopsy site is not delineated. Regardless of the orientation, the biopsy may be performed using a free-hand or transducer-guided technique. The use of a guide simplifies the procedure (Fig. 15.18).

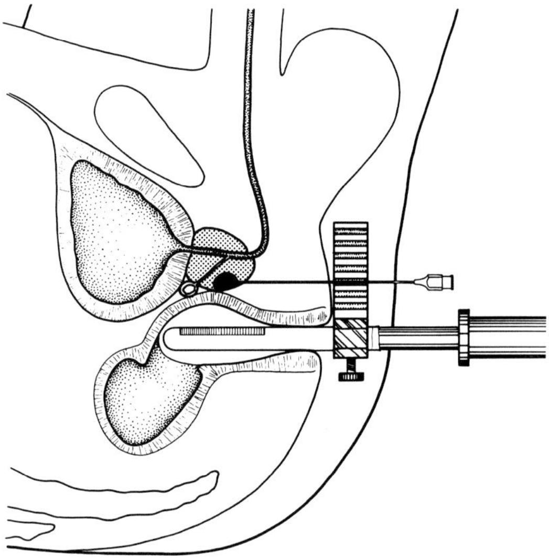

Figure 15.18. A transperineal biopsy using endorectal guidance. Note the guide attached to the ultrasound probe. The biopsy needle is placed through the guide and is fixed to the guide transducer complex. Under sonographic guidance, it is then placed into the abnormal area. (From Rifkin MD. Ultrasound of the prostate. New York: Raven Press, 1988.)

For the transperineal biopsy, the patient is placed in the lithotomy position. A preliminary scan is performed to ascertain the position of the lesion. The perineum is scrubbed with Betadine and local anesthesia (using 1% xylocaine) is administered with a 25-gauge needle. The ultrasound transducer (with a needle guide) is then placed into the rectum and the probe is positioned to reidentify the lesion in question. A 20- to 22-gauge needle may then be placed through the guide into the previously anesthesized subcutaneous tissues and anesthesia is then given to the deeper soft tissues to the prostatic capsule. The small biopsy needle can then be positioned into the lesion for aspiration biopsy or the needle can be withdrawn and a core biopsy needle then can be used (Fig. 15.19). With the advent of the mechanical trigger device, the biopsy can be performed quickly and with a minimal amount of local anesthesia.

The transrectal approach may also be used for ultrasound-guided biopsy. There are specially produced instruments that can be placed over the endorectal probe to guide the biopsy needle. These have been used predominantly in the sagittally oriented plane. No local antiseptic or anesthesia is required. However, a cleansing enema and pretreatment with antibiotics are essential to minimize the risk of sepsis. After the lesion is preliminarily demonstrated on sonography, an endorectal probe is then prepared with a biopsy guide. The patient is usually placed in the decubitus position, although the lithotomy position can be used. The probe is again placed in the rectum and angled until the line of needle insertion is visualized and is deemed appropriate to biopsy the suspected abnormality. The needle is then placed (using the guide) into the lesion and a core or aspiration biopsy is performed (Fig. 15.20).

Complications of prostatic biopsy include hematuria, hematospermia, periprostatic hematoma, urinary retention, and retroperitoneal hematoma. Sepsis and hematochezia can occur after transrectal biopsies. Vasovagal reaction has also been reported. With ultrasound guidance using thin needles, all are uncommon and usually clinically insignificant.

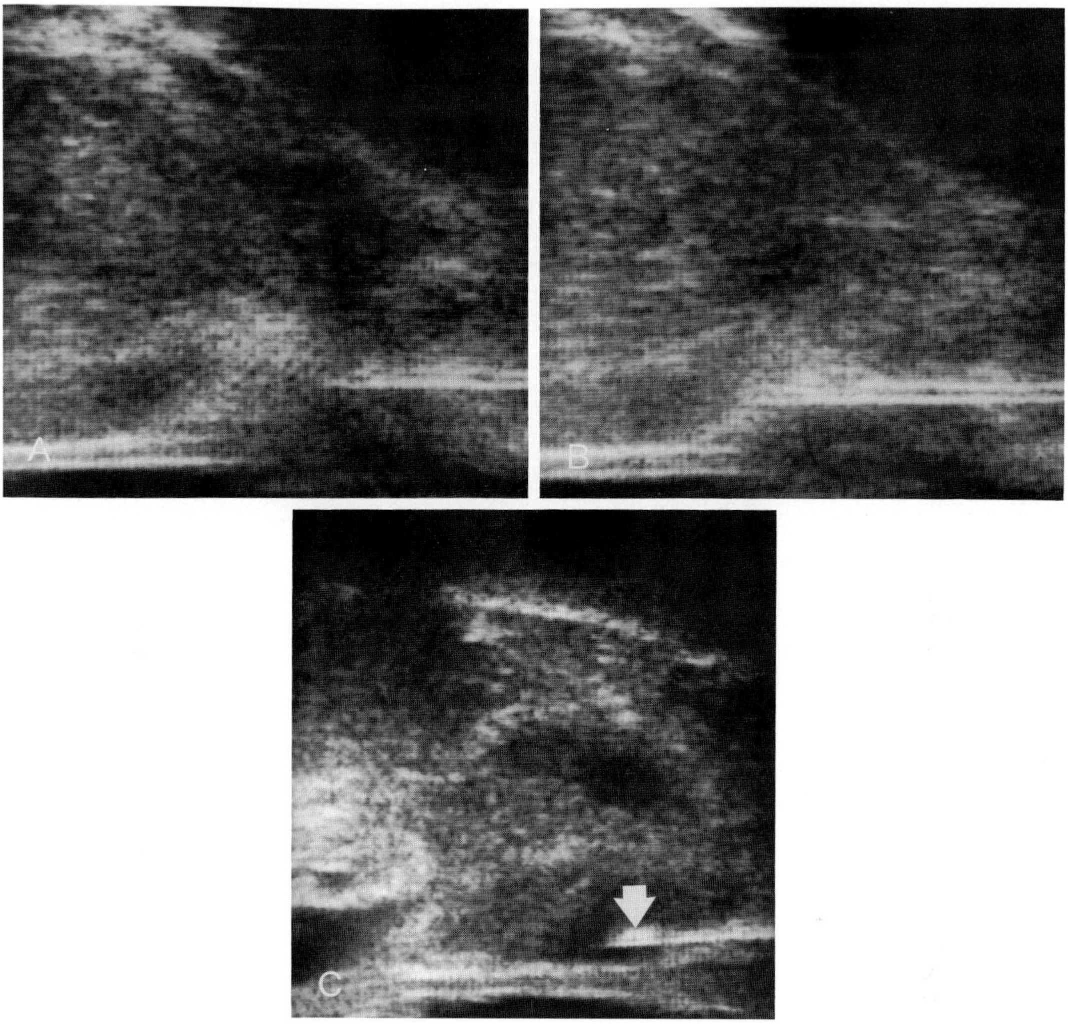

Figure 15.19. Transperineal biopsy of a hypoechoic prostate carcinoma. Sequential images depict the advancement of a biopsy needle placed through the perineum and guided into a posteriorly situated lesion. (From Rifkin MD. Ultrasound of the prostate. New York: Raven Press, 1988.)

Prostatic abscesses have also been the focus of ultrasonographic intervention in the prostate. These usually develop as processes secondary to prostatitis but can also originate from a hematogenous-borne infection. While most imaging techniques are nonspecific, CT and magnetic resonance imaging are useful adjunctive studies. Endorectal sonography can often delineate the area. The abnormal focus is usually somewhat hypoechoic and may be confused with a carcinomatous focus. Clinical symptoms referable to an abscess, such as fever leukocytosis, along with localized prostatic pain, help narrow the differential diagnosis. Endorectal ultrasound permits accurate aspiration to confirm the diagnosis and institute appropriate therapy (96).

Extracorporeal Shock Wave Lithotripsy

Extracorporeal shock wave lithotripsy (ESWL) has revolutionized the therapy of urinary tract calculi over the past several years (99–105). This technique is now considered by many to be the method of choice for treating most upper-tract calculi (99–102). Addition-

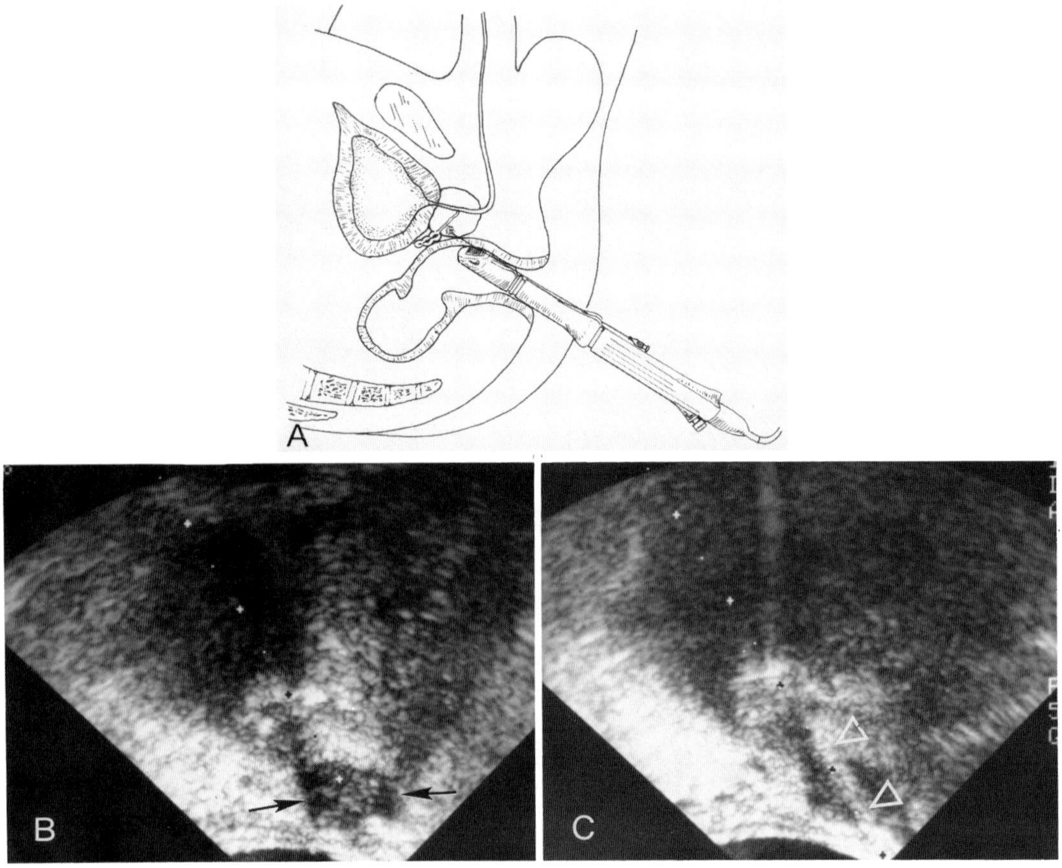

Figure 15.20. **A,** Diagnostic representation of a transrectal prostate biopsy. In this case, a longitudinally oriented sector scan is produced by the instrument shown. **B** and **C,** Transrectal prostate biopsy. Endorectal ultrasound with a longitudinally oriented sector scan demonstrates a hypoechoic lesion (*arrows*) in the apex of the prostate. The line of sight of the biopsy needle placement (electronic *dots* and *crosses*) is identified (**B**). The biopsy needle (*open arrowheads*) is then identified during the biopsy (**C**). (From Rifkin MD. Ultrasound of the prostate. New York: Raven Press, 1988.)

ally, calculi located in the ureter below the pelvic brim have also been treated successfully with ESWL (106).

ESWL has also been used to treat calculi in renal transplants (107). Although this is a relatively uncommon complication of renal transplant, kidney stones can be associated with significant morbidity, particularly because the patients are immunosuppressed and dependent on the solitary kidney.

While the technique is not universally accepted, Mayes et al. in a nonrandomized multicenter cohort study revealed that patients were more likely to be free of stones 3 months after treatment by nephrolithotomy than with lithotripsy. This was most evident in cases of staghorn calculi (108).

DEVELOPMENT AND TECHNIQUE

Initial clinical experimentation in ESWL began in February 1980. Protocol lithotripters were designed in Germany, and FDA approval for ESWL was received from the Food and Drug Administration late in 1984. Because of the obvious advantages of avoiding surgery, the popularity of lithotripsy spread rapidly (109).

The principal mechanism by which lithotripsy works entails the production of shock waves characterized by a positive-pressure pulse of short duration and rise time. This generates up to 1000 times atmospheric pressure within nanoseconds; the positive-pressure pulse is followed by a longer but lower-amplitude negative-pressure pulse (110).

Three basic designs are used by manufacturers to produce and focus shock waves: (*a*) underwater spark discharge, (*b*) piezoelectric crystals, and (*c*) an electromagnetic membrane. Shock waves may be focused using either a metal ellipsoidal reflector, several thousand piezoelectric crystals mounted on a spherical dish, or acoustic lenses, respectively. Spark-gap lithotripters can generate the highest acoustic energies per pulse (110); discussion in this chapter is limited to this technology.

The principles governing the success of spark-gap lithotripsy are based on the underwater generation of shock waves, which are focused onto either a fluoroscopically or sonographically localized renal calculus. If fluoroscopy is used, orthogonal fluoroscopic systems converge at the second focal point of a semi-ellipsoidal shock wave reflector. Diagnostic ultrasound localization can be used, however, as it provides two-dimensional real-time images in *any* plane without using ionizing radiation. The spatial coordinates of the stone are calculated using the main computer in the lithotripter control module based on the location of the tip of the ultrasound probe and its direction (Fig. 15.21). These are transmitted via a locating arm and a data input from distance measurements made using the ultrasound scanner. The coordinates are calculated several times to reduce the error of a single measurement. Once a set of coordinates has been validated, computer-assisted movement of the shock wave generator assembly is initiated, so that the second focus of the semi-ellipsoidal shell is at the stone coordinates (Fig. 15.22). The shock waves are generated by passing an 18- to 24-kV charge across an underwater electrode. This shock wave then passes through a bath of degassed water and then through the patient. Its energy is transmitted to objects of variable acoustic impedance, such as a calculus or air. Because of the ability to focus the energy, approximately 90% of the initial shock wave energy generated can reach a focal point localized to approximately a 2-cm sphere. The shock waves can be transmitted into the body either directly from a water bath or by a compressible water bag interfaced with the skin using ultrasound coupling gel. Underwater inflatable balloons help to displace water from the x-ray path to assist in locating the calculus if fluoroscopy is used. After the patient is localized and positioned, a series of shock waves triggered by the patient's electrocardiogram are generated. An impulse control system is built into the system which discharges the shock waves in cycles. Shock waves are then applied until the entire stone is fragmented into pieces no larger than 2 to 3 mm. Fluoroscopy or sonography is performed in an intermittent fashion to monitor the calculus disintegration and to recheck patient position. The fluoroscopic examination criteria for stone dis-

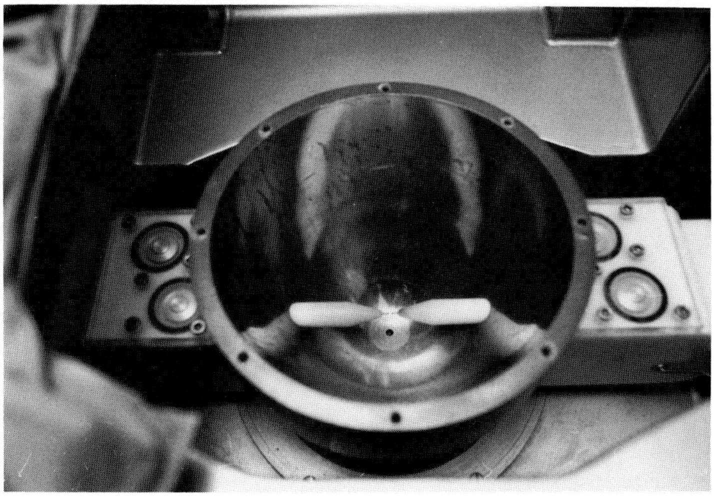

Figure 15.21. Spark gap lithotripter (in foreground), which can be used for biliary or urinary tract calculi. The transducer of the ultrasound unit is attached to an articulated arm, which in turn is connected to a computer console (background, left). The patient is scanned to determine the proper coordinates for placement of the ellipsoidal spark generator.

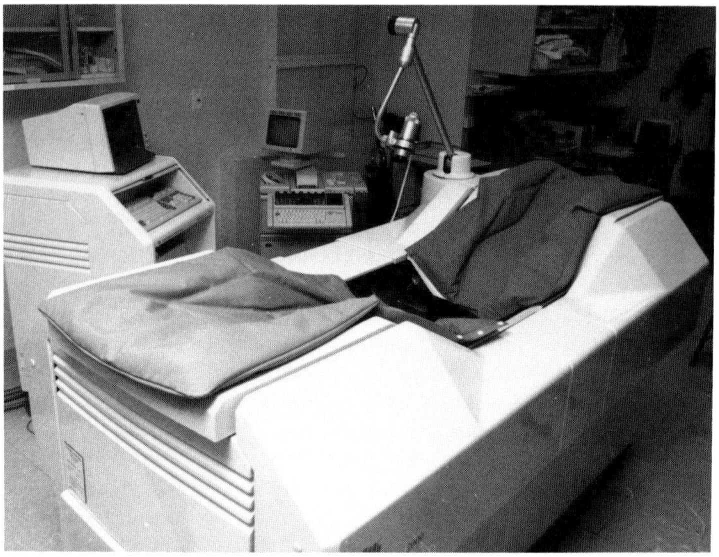

Figure 15.22. The stone coordinates are used to position the ellipsoid so that its second focus (area of maximum generated pressure) coincides with the region of the calculus.

solution is a change in stone density or migration of small pieces to form a cast of the collecting system (109). Typical renal calculi may require 800 to 2000 shock waves for fragmentation, with 1300 shock waves the average required. The procedure takes less than 1 hr and can be performed using general or epidural anesthesia. In some centers, only intravenous sedation with diazepam and mepridine is used.

Follow-up radiographs are usually obtained to follow the fragmented stone material as it passes down the ureter into the bladder. Although a significant portion of patients may need repeat ESWL therapy, the overall success rate reported from UCLA in 1988 was in the range of 80 to 85% (100).

It has also been documented that disintegration of ureteral stones is dependent on the amount of physical contact between the calculus and the ureteral wall. If the stone is wedged in a ureter that is edematous, disintegration may not occur, regardless of the number and strength of shock waves delivered (100). Therefore, successful stone fragmentation is dependent on the presence of a so-called expansion chamber, achieved by relocating the stone into the renal pelvis or into a ureteral segment amenable to ESWL treatment (100, 102). To facilitate ureteral stone relocation, the use of water-soluble, 2% lidocaine jelly mixed with normal saline or distilled water has been advocated (103). This material is injected by a No. 6 French ureteral catheter placed in a retrograde fashion. After the stone is repositioned in its desired location, a catheter is then attached to the patient's indwelling Foley catheter. If the stone is not able to be manipulated in a retrograde fashion, then repositioning may be achieved using a ureteroscope, again with ureteral lubrication as delineated above.

Whereas ESWL is considered the primary mode of therapy for most upper-tract calculi and some lower urinary tract calculi, this procedure alone is not as helpful if a patient has other distal pathology impeding fragment passage (e.g., ureteropelvic junction obstruction or ureteral stenosis). Additionally, patients with a very large number of stones or large stone burden may need several ESWL procedures, often complicated with bouts of ureteral obstruction. These patients might fare better with either percutaneous or nephroscopic removal (105, 108, 111, 112). In these cases, numerous other ancillary procedures are usually necessary to totally eradicate the stone burden, including ureteral stenting, percutaneous nephrostomy, and repeated ureteroscopy. In patients with large staghorn calculi, the combined approach is in fact advocated (111).

Approximately 1% of all renal calculi will not fragment with ESWL. Cystine stones are relatively impervious to these shock waves (109).

Passage of fragments and stone material is variable, with most patients showing radiographic evidence of retained stone material for 24 hr after therapy (109). The ultimate amount of residual stone material depends on the initial stone burden. A recent UCLA study described a 97% success rate in patients treated by a combined approach of stone repositioning and ESWL (100). This group felt that the presence of an adequate expansion chamber is the major variable in achieving success. In most patients, residual calculus fragments are passed without symptoms. If symptoms occur, oral analgesia is usually sufficient to alleviate pain. Transient asymptomatic renal obstruction can also be caused by the multiple stone fragments, but this alone is not cause for immediate intervention (99). Close follow-up is necessary, as there are reports of irreversible renal damage from asymptomatic obstructions (114). Adjunct procedures need to be performed if patients demonstrate evidence of obstruction or sepsis or if a particularly large volume of stone fragments are seen that do not pass spontaneously. If this so-called "Steinstrassen" occurs, removal is often achieved by retrograde ureteroscopy (109).

A potential shortcoming of ESWL is inadequate fragmentation, and thus the need for repeat study (99). This is usually not a problem unless obstruction or sepsis intervenes. The use of shock waves to disintegrate calculi causes some parenchymal changes in the affected kidney. Renal enlargement and a prolonged nephrographic phase, with delayed excretion of contrast medium (without evidence of obstruction) have been documented (99). Subcapsular hematomas may occasionally occur, but significant perinephric hemorrhage is rare (113–117) (Fig. 15.23). Magnetic resonance imaging has documented changes in 74% of treated kidneys, including subcapsular or perinephric fluid, focal or diffuse loss of the corticomedullary junction, and focal areas of signal intensity change (115). Most of these changes appear to be reversible and their clinical significance has been questioned. The potential for development of hypertension may be a late complication (117); other reported complications include posttreatment pain and sepsis (109). Nonurologic complications may include adjacent organ damage (e.g., pancreatitis) and arrhythmias (118). Interstitial emphysema has been noted on follow-up radiographs in ESWL patients secondary to epidural anesthesia (120).

Besides the use of ESWL in treating upper- and mid-ureteral calculi, reference has been made to treatment of calculi in the distal ureter using ESWL alone. In these patients, positioning to facilitate x-rays and shock waves to enter through the obturator foramen or greater sciatic notch is necessary (106). There has also been a report of treatment of unusual Koch pouch urinary calculi using ESWL (119).

"Difficult" calculi may be easier to position with the patient in the prone position (106, 107). The technique has also been advocated in selected renal transplant patients who develop calculi secondary to obstruction, secondary hyperparathyroidism, tubular acidosis, papillary necrosis, or recurrent infection. ESWL can usually be performed in conjunction with several of the other techniques delineated previously with regard to management of the renal transplant (107).

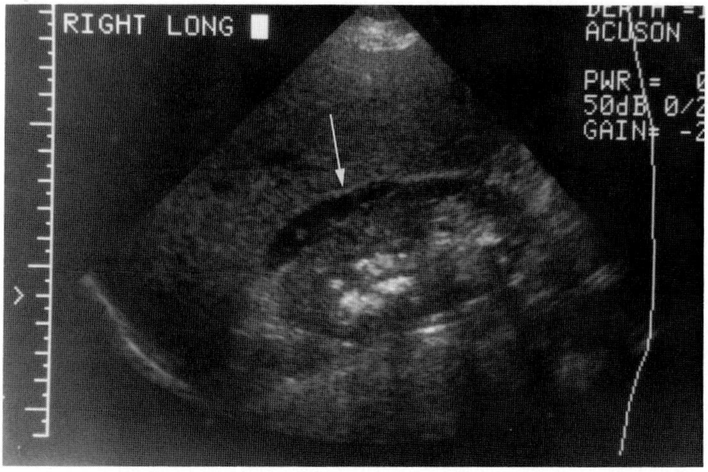

Figure 15.23. Right perirenal hematoma (*arrow*) that developed after ESWL therapy. Residual stone fragments are seen in the collecting system.

References

1. Goldberg BB, Pollack HM. Ultrasonic aspiration biopsy techniques. J Clin Ultrasound 1975; 4:141–151.
2. Goldberg BB, Pollack HM. Ultrasonic aspiration transducer. Radiology 1972;102:187–189.
3. Rizzatto G, Solbiati L, Croce F, Derchi LE. Aspiration biopsy of superficial lesions: ultrasonic guidance with a linear-array probe. Am J Radiol 1987;148:623–625.
4. Holm HH, Torp-Peterson S, Julla N, Carsen T. Instrumentation for sonographic interventional procedures. In: Clinics in Diagnostic Ultrasound. New York: Churchill Livingstone, 1987: 12–14.
5. Lamont AC, Fletcher EWL. Chiba needle in renal puncture guided by real-time ultrasound. Clin Radiol 1981;32:421–424.
6. Reading CC, Charboneau JW, Felmlee JP, James EM. US-guided percutaneous biopsy: use of a screw biopsy stylet to aid needle detection. Radiology 1987;163:280–281.
7. Haaga JR, LiPuma JP, Bryan PJ, Balsara VJ, Cohen AM. Clinical comparison of small- and large-caliber cutting needles for biopsy. Radiology 1983;146:665–667.
8. Qin D. Technical note a new needle for puncture biopsy. Am J Radiol 1986;147:543.
9. Parker SH, Hopper KD, Yakes WF, Gibson MD, Ownbey JL, Carter TE. Image-directed percutaneous biopsies with a biopsy gun. Radiology 1989;171:663–669.
10. Bernardino ME. Percutaneous biopsy. Am J Radiol 1984;142:41–45.
11. Nadel L, Baumgartner BR, Bernardino ME. Percutaneous renal biopsies: accuracy, safety, and indications. Urol Radiol 1986;8:67–71.
12. Livraghi T, Damascelli B, Lombardi C, Spagnoli I. Risk in fine-needle abdominal biopsy. J Clin Ultrasound 1983;11:77–81.
13. Phillips G, Schneider M. Ultrasonically guided percutaneous fine needle aspiration biopsy of solid masses. Cardiovasc Intervent Radiol 1981; 4:33–38.
14. Rezrek RH, Talner LB. Percutaneous nephrostomy. Radiol Clin North Am 1989;22:402.
15. Ralls PW, Barakos JA, Kaptein EM, et al. Renal biopsy–related hemorrhage: frequency and comparison of CT and sonography. J Comput Assist Tomogr 1987;11:1031–1034.
16. Hueftle MG, Haaga JR. Effect of suction on biopsy sample size. Am J Radiol 1986;147: 1014–1016.
17. Rifkin MD, Goldberg BB. Aspiration and biopsy techniques. In: Abdominal Ultrasonography. 2nd ed. New York: John Wiley & Sons, 1984: 481–514.
18. Thompson H. Enormous sac connected with the kidney, recognized as such during life and repeatedly emptied by tapping. Transactions of the Pathological Society 1867;13:128.
19. Pollack HM, Banner MP, Arger PH, Peters J, Mulhern CB Jr, Coleman BG. The accuracy of gray-scale renal ultrasonography in differentiating cystic neoplasms from benign cysts. Radiology 1982;143:741–745.
20. Stanisic TH, Babcock JR, Grayhack JT. Morbidity and mortality of renal exploration for cyst. Surg Gynecol Obstet 1977;145:733–736.
21. Sandler CM, Houston GK, Hall JT, Morrettin LB. Guided cyst puncture and aspiration. Radiol Clin North Am 1986;24:527–537.
22. Lang EK. Renal cyst puncture and aspiration: a survey of complications. American Journal of Roentgenology 1977;128:723–727.
23. Lang EK. Coexistence of cyst and tumor in the same kidney. Radiology 1971;101:7–16.
24. Lang EK, Johnson B, Chance HL, et al. Assessment of avascular renal mass lesions: the use of nephrotomography, arteriography, cyst puncture, double contrast study and histochemical and histopathologic examination of the aspirate. South Med J 1972;65:1–10.
25. Bean WJ, Rodan BA. Hepatic cysts: treatment with alcohol. Am J Radiol 1985;144:237–241.
26. Bean WJ. Renal cysts: treatment with alcohol. Radiology 1981;138:329–331.
27. Branitz BH, Schlossberg IR, Freed SZ. Complications of renal cyst puncture. Urology 1976; 7:578–580.
28. Goldberg BB, Pollack HM, Kellerman E. Ultrasonic localization for renal biopsy. Radiology 1975;115:167–170.
29. Branger B, Oules R, Balducchi JP, Fourcade J, Bourgeois JM. Ultrasonically continuously guided renal biopsy. Uremia Invest 1986;9: 297–303.
30. Hightower DR, Laing FC, Jeffrey RB. A tandem guide for renal biopsy. J Ultrasound Med 1985;4:441–443.
31. Birnholz JC, Kasinath BS, Corwin HL. An improved technique for ultrasound guided percutaneous renal biopsy. Kidney Int 1985;27: 80–82.
32. Chan JCM, Brewer WH, Still WJ. Renal biopsies under ultrasound guidance: 100 consecutive biopsies in children. J Urol 1983;129: 103–107.
33. Juul N, Torp-Pedersen S, Grønvall S, Holm HH, Koch F, Larsen S. Ultrasonically guided fine needle aspiration biopsy of renal masses. J Urol 1985;133:579–581.
34. Bush WH Jr, Burnett LL, Gibbons RP. Needle tract seeding of renal cell carcinoma. Am J Roentgenol 1977;129:725–727.
35. Wein AJ, Rinj EJ, Freiman DB, et al. Applications of thin needle aspiration biopsy in urology. J Urol 1979;121:626.
36. Nosher JL, Amonsa JK, Leiman S, Platker J. Fine needle aspiration biopsy of kidney and adrenal gland. J Urol 1982;128:895.
37. Kutcher R, Greenebaum E, Rosenblatt R, Moussouris HF. Prostatic carcinoma metastasis to the kidney: diagnosis by thin needle aspiration biopsy. Urol Radiol 1986;8:98–100.
38. Coleman BG, Pollack HM. Interventional genitourinary sonography. In: Interventional Ultrasound, Clinics in Diagnostic Ultrasound. New York: Churchill Livingstone, 1987:115–148.
39. Livragi T, Damascelli B, Lombardi C, Spagnoli I. Risk in fine needle aspiration biopsy. J Clin Ultrasound 1983;11:77.

40. Low RN, Jeffrey RB. Intraperitoneal hemorrhage after renal biopsy: a grave prognostic sign. Am J Radiol 1988;151:113–114.
41. Leonard JC, Nanney SM, Tytle T. Arteriovenous fistula secondary to renal biopsy. Clin Nucl Med 1986;11:284.
42. Phisler R, Papinicalau N, Yoder I. Diagnostic morphologic and urodynamic antegrade pyelography. Radiol Clin North Am 1986;24:561–571.
43. Fritzsche P. Antegrade pyelography: therapeutic applications. Radiol Clin North Am 1986; 24:573–586.
44. Kutcher R, Rosenblatt R. Sonographically guided percutaneous renal interventional procedures. JAMA 1984;251:3126–3129.
45. Burnett KR, Handler SJ, Conroy RM, Khonsari F, Nelson C. Percutaneous nephrostomy utilizing b-mode and real-time ultrasound guidance: the lateral approach and puncture facilitation with furosemide. J Clin Ultrasound 1982;10: 252–255.
46. Zegel HG, Pollack HM, Banner MP, et al. Percutaneous nephrostomy: comparison of sonographic and fluoroscopic guidance. Am J Radiol 1981;137:925–927.
47. Elyaderani ME, Kandzari SJ. Percutaneous antegrade pyelography and nephrostomy guided by ultrasound. WV Med J 1980;76:5–6.
48. Baron RL, Lee JKT, McClennan BL, Melson GL. Percutaneous nephrostomy using real-time sonographic guidance. Am J Radiol 1981;136: 1018–1019.
49. Maillet PJ, Pelle-Francoz D, Laville M, Gay F, Pinet A. Nondilated obstructive acute renal failure: diagnostic procedures and therapeutic management. Radiology 1986;160:659–662.
50. Schüller J, Schmeller NT, Kerstin H, Walther V. Ultrasound-guided percutaneous one-step nephrostomy. Br J Urol 1984;56:341–343.
51. Naidich JB, Rackson ME, Mossey RT, Stein HL. Nondilated obstructive uropathy: percutaneous nephrostomy performed to reverse renal failure. Radiology 1986;160:653–657.
52. Stables DP. Percutaneous nephrostomy: techniques, indications, and results. Urol Clin North Am 1982;9:15–29.
53. Stables DP, Ginsberg NJ, Johnson ML. Percutaneous nephrostomy: a series and review of the literature. Am J Roentgenol 1978;130: 75–82.
54. Perlmutt LM, Braun SD, Newman GE, Oke EJ, Dunnick NR. Percutaneous intervention in the solitary kidney. Cardiovasc Intervent Radiol 1987;10:223–225.
55. Picus D, Weyman PJ, Clayman RV, McClennan BL. Intercostal-space nephrostomy for percutaneous stone removal. Am J Radiol 1986; 147:393–397.
56. Ebisuno S, Fukatani T, Yoshida M, Kumeda K, Ohkawa T. Percutaneous dissolution of uric acid calculi with THAM irrigation. Urol Radiol 1987;9:146–148.
57. Stanley P, Diament MJ. Pediatric percutaneous nephrostomy experience with 50 patients. J Urol 1986;135:1223–1226.
58. Irving HC, Arthur RJ, Thomas DFM. Percutaneous nephrostomy in paediatrics. Clin Radiol 1987;38:245–248.
59. Rezrek RH, Talner LB. Percutaneous nephrostomy. Radiol Clin North Am 1984;22:393–405.
60. Winfield AC, Turner BI, Kirchner FK Jr, Braren HV. Practical experience with percutaneous nephrostomy: avoidance of common technical pitfalls. South Med J 1983;76:562–566.
61. vanSonnenberg E, Mueller PR, Ferrucci JT Jr. Percutaneous drainage of 250 abdominal abscesses and fluid collections. Radiology 1984; 151:337–341.
62. Gerzof SG. Percutaneous drainage of renal and perinephric abscess. Urol Radiol 1981;2: 171–179.
63. Sacks D, Banner MP, Meranze SG, Burke DR, Robinson M, McLean GK. Renal and related retroperitoneal abscesses: percutaneous drainage. Radiology 1988;167:447–451.
64. Cronan JJ, Amis ES Jr, Dorfman GS. Percutaneous drainage of renal abscesses. Am J Radiol 1984;142:351–354.
65. Finn DJ, Palestrant AM, DeWolf WC. Successful percutaneous management of renal abscess. J Urol 1982;127:425–426.
66. Tupper TB, Cronan JJ, Wald LM, Dorfman GS. Renal abscess: a complication of ethanol embolization. Radiology 1986;161:35–36.
67. Kuligowska E, Newman B, White SJ, Caldarone A. Interventional ultrasound in detection and treatment of renal inflammatory disease. Radiology 1983;147:521–526.
68. Lindgren PG, Magnusson A, Hagberg H, Paulsen K. Perirenal lymphoma. Acta Radiol Diagn 1986;27:433–435.
69. vanSonnenberg E, Wittich GR, Schiffman HR, et al. Percutaneous drainage access: a simplified coaxial technique. Radiology 1986;159: 266–268.
70. vanSonnenberg E, Mueller PR, Ferrucci JT Jr, Neff CC, Simeone JF, Wittenberg J. Sump catheter for percutaneous abscess and fluid drainage by Trocar and Seldinger technique. Am J Radiol 1982;139:613–614.
71. vanSonnenberg E, Ferrucci JT Jr, Mueller PR, Wittenberg J, Simeone JF. Percutaneous drainage of abscesses and fluid collections: technique, results and applications. Radiology 1982;142:1–10.
72. vanWaes PFGM, Feldberg MAM, Mali WPTM, et al. Management of loculated abscesses that are difficult to drain: a new approach. Radiology 1983;147:57–63.
73. Rifkin MD, Heffelfinger D, Kurtz AB, et al. Outpatient therapy of intrabdominal abscesses following early discharge from the hospital. Radiology 1985;155:333–334.
74. Lang EK, Glarioso L III. Management of urinomas by percutaneous drainage procedures. Radiol Clin North Am 1986;24:551–560.
75. Voegeli DR, Crummy AB, McDermott JC, Jensen SR, Montague TL. Percutaneous management of the urological complications of renal transplantation. Radiographics 1986;6: 1007–1022.
76. Silver TM, Campbell D, Wicks JD, Lorber MI,

Surace P, Turcotte J. Peritransplant fluid collections. Radiology 1981;138:145–151.
77. Spigos D, Capek V, Jonasson O. Percutaneous biopsy of renal transplants using ultrasonographic guidance. J Urol 1977;117: 699–700.
78. Ubhi CS, Irving HC, Guillou PJ, Giles GR. Short communication: a new technique for renal allograft biopsy. Br J Radiol 1987;60: 599–600.
79. Becker JA, Kutcher R. Urologic complications of renal transplantation. Semin Roentgenol 1978;13:341–351.
80. Yap R, Madrazo B, Oh HK, Dienst SG. Perirenal fluid collection after renal transplant. Am Surg 1981;47:287–290.
81. Spigos D, Capek V. Ultrasonically guided percutaneous aspiration of lymphoceles following renal transplantation: a diagnostic and therapeutic method. J Clin Ultrasound 1975;4: 45–46.
82. Basinger GT, Gittes RF. Lymphocyst: ultrasound diagnosis and urologic management. J Urol 1975;114:740–745.
83. Cohan RH, Saeed M, Sussman SK, et al. Percutaneous drainage of pelvic lymphatic fluid collections in the renal transplant patient. Invest Radiol 1987;22:864–867.
84. Smith TP, Hunter DW, Letorneu JG, et al. Urine leaks after renal transplantation: value of percutaneous pyelography and drainage for diagnosis and treatment. Am J Radiol 1988;-151:511–513.
85. Schmeller NT, Schüller J, Hofstetter A, Land W. Fine-needle antegrade pyelography of transplanted kidneys. Urol Radiol 1985;7:19–22.
86. Montali G, Solbiati L, Bossi MC, De Pra L, Di Donna A, Ravetto C. Sonographically guided fine-needle aspiration biopsy of adrenal masses. Am J Radiol 1984;143:1081–1084.
87. Bernardino ME. Management of the asymptomatic patient with a unilateral adrenal mass. Radiology 1988;166:121–123.
88. Reading CC, Charboneau JW, James EM, Hurt MR. Sonographically guided percutaneous biopsy of small (3 cm or less) masses. Am J Radiol 1988;151:189–192.
89. Casola G, Nicolet V, van Sonnenberg E, et al. Unsuspected pheochromocytoma: risk of blood-pressure alterations during percutaneous adrenal biopsy. Radiology 1986;159:733–735.
90. vanSonnenberg E, Wittenberg J, Ferrucci JT Jr, Mueller PR, Simeone JF. Triangulation method for percutaneous needle guidance: the angled approach to upper abdominal masses. Am J Radiol 1981;137:757–761.
91. Simon G, Berdon WE. Suprapubic bladder puncture for voiding cystourethrography. J Pediatr 1972;81:555–558.
92. Hare WSC, McOmish D, Nunn IN. Percutaneous transvesical antegrade passage of urethral strictures. Urol Radiol 1981;3:107–112.
93. Higgins WL, Mace AH. Puncture of a nondeflatable Foley balloon using ultrasound guidance. Radiology 1984;151:801.
94. Nosher JL, Winchman HK, Needell GS. Transvaginal pelvic abscess drainage with US guidance. Radiology 1987;165:872–873.
95. Rifkin MD. Biopsy techniques. In: Ultrasound of the Prostate. New York: Raven Press, 1988:113–139.
96. Weinberger M, Pitlik SD, Rabinovitz M, et al. Per-rectal ultrasonography for diagnosis of and guide to drainage of prostatic abscess. Lancet 1985;2:772.
97. Resnick MI. Transrectal ultrasound guided versus digitally directed prostatic biopsy: a comparative study. J Urol 1988;139:754–757.
98. Lee F, Littrup PJ, Kumasaka GH, Borlaza GS, McLeary RD. The use of transrectal ultrasound in the diagnosis, guided biopsy, staging and screening of prostate cancer. Radiographics 1987;7:627–644.
99. Grantham JR, Millner MR, Kaude JV, Finlayson B, Hunter PT II, Newman RC. Renal stone disease treated with extracorporeal shock wave lithotripsy: short-term observations in 100 patients. Radiology 1986;158:203–206.
100. Lupu AN, Fuchs GJ, Chaussy CG. Treatment of urethral calculi by extracorporeal shock-wave lithotripsy. Urology 1988;32:217–222.
101. Aronne LJ, Braham RL, Riehle R Jr, et al. Cost-effectiveness of extracorporeal shock-wave lithotripsy. Urology 1988;31:225–230.
102. Graff J, Pastor J, Funke PJ, et al. Extracorporeal shock wave lithotripsy for ureteral stones: a retrospective analysis of 417 cases. J Urol 1988;139:513–516.
103. Lupu AN, Chaussy CG, Fuchs GJ, Kaufman JJ. Use of 2% xylocaine jelly in retrograde displacement of ureteral stones [Abstract]. Presented at the Third World Congress on Endourology, New York, Sept. 20–22, 1985.
104. Wilbert DM, Reichenberger H, Noske E, et al. New generation shock wave lithotripsy. J Urol 1987;138:563–565.
105. Lingeman JE, Coury TA, Newman DM, et al. Comparison of results and morbidity of percutaneous nephrostolithotomy and extracorporeal shock wave lithotripsy. J Urol 1987;138: 485–490.
106. Becht E, Moll V, Neisius D, Ziegler M. Treatment of prevesical ureteral calculi by extracorporeal shock wave lithotripsy. J Urol 1988; 139:916–918.
107. Locke DR, Steinbock G, Salomon DR, et al. Combination extracorporeal shock wave lithotripsy and percutaneous extraction of calculi in a renal allograft. J Urol 1988; 139:575–577.
108. Mays N, Challah S, Patel S, et al. Clinical comparison of extracorporeal shock wave lithotripsy and percutaneous nephrolithotomy in treating renal calculi. Br Med J 1988;297: 253–258.
109. LeRoy AJ, Seymora JW. Extracorporeal shock wave lithotripsy. Radiol Clin North Am 1986;24:623–631.
110. Paumgartner G. Shock wave lithotripsy of gallstones. Am J Radiol 1989;153:235–242.
111. Cochran ST, Liu E, Barbaric ZL. Percutaneous nephrostomy in conjunction with ESWL in

treatment of nephrolithiasis. Am J Radiol 1988;151:103–106.

112. Cochran ST. Extracorporeal shock wave lithotripsy: clinical results. Urol Radiol 1988;10:46–47.
113. Rubin JL, Arger PH, Pollack HM, et al. Kidney changes after extracorporeal shock wave lithotripsy: CT evaluation. Radiology 1987; 162:21–24.
114. Hardy MR, McLeod DG. Silent renal obstruction with severe functional loss after extracorporeal shock wave lithotripsy: a report of 2 cases. J Urol 1987;137:91–92.
115. Baumgartner BR, Dickey KW, Ambrose SS, Walton KN, Nelson RC, Bernardino ME. Kidney changes after extracorporeal shock wave lithotripsy appearance on MR imaging. Radiology 1987;163:531–534.
116. Papanicolaou N, Stafford SA, Pfister RC, Althausen AF, Dretler SP. Significant renal hemorrhage following extracorporeal shock wave lithotripsy: imaging and clinical features. Radiology 1987;163:661–664.
117. Williams CM, Kaude JV, Newman RC, Peterson JC, Thomas WC. Extracorporeal shock-wave lithotripsy: long-term complications. Am J Radiol 1988;150:311–315.
118. Drach GW, Dretler SP, Fair W, et al. Report of the U.S. cooperative study of ESWL. J Urol 1986;135:1127–1133.
119. Boyd SD, Everett RW, Schiff WM, Fugelso PD. Treatment of unusual Koch pouch urinary calculi with extracorporeal shock wave lithotripsy. J Urol 1988;139:805–806.
120. Roberts MC, Pollack HM, Banner MP, Castro AD, VanArsdalen KN. Interstitial emphysema associated with epidural anesthesia for extracorporeal shock-wave lithotripsy. Am J Radiol 1987;148:301–304.

Index

Page numbers in italics denote figures; those followed by "t" denote tables.